SAUNDERS PHARMACEUTICAL WORD BOOK

1994

ELLEN DRAKE, CMT
RANDY DRAKE, BS

SAUNDERS PHARMACEUTICAL WORD BOOK

1994

W.B. SAUNDERS COMPANY
A Division of Harcourt Brace & Company
Philadelphia London Toronto Montreal Sydney Tokyo

W.B. SAUNDERS COMPANY
A Division of
Harcourt Brace & Company

The Curtis Center
Independence Square West
Philadelphia, Pennsylvania 19106

SAUNDERS PHARMACEUTICAL WORD BOOK 1994   ISBN 0-7216-5254-9

Copyright © 1994, 1992 by W.B. Saunders Company

All rights reserved. No part of this publication may be reproduced or transmitted in any form or by any means, electronic or mechanical, including photocopy, recording, or any information storage and retrieval system, without permission in writing from the publisher.
ISSN 1072-7779

Printed in the United States of America.

Last digit is the print number: 9   8   7   6   5   4   3   2   1

Authors' Dedication

To the Lord Jesus

"Now to Him who is able to do exceeding abundantly beyond all that we ask or think, according to the power that works within us, to Him be the glory in the church and in Christ Jesus to all generations forever and ever. Amen."

—EPHESIANS 3:20 21.

Preface

The *Saunders Pharmaceutical Word Book* has been improved in many ways for this second edition. First, all the drug names, whether trade, generic, or chemical, will be in bold print for greater ease of reading. Brand (trade) names will still appear with appropriate capitalization, with generic and chemical names shown in lower case—the way transcription style guides recommend they be typed. A total of 2554 new entries have been added to last year's book, and 2878 of last year's entries have been modified. There are 21,294 entries in this edition.

Saunders Pharmaceutical Word Book has been compiled primarily with the medical transcriptionist in mind, although it will certainly appeal to coders, quality assurance personnel, nurses, ward clerks, students of all allied health professions—anyone who has a need for a quick, easy-to-use drug reference that gives more information than just the spelling. Even physicians may find it useful to get quick information on medications their patients may be using for conditions outside their specialty. The "Notes on Using the Text" will explain the variety of information this book contains as well as how to find that information.

We think you will find this second edition more complete and more valuable than ever; however, no book is ever perfect. We plan to keep our database current by adding new entries as the information becomes available. Although we have diligently tried to be as accurate and comprehensive as possible, we will certainly welcome your comments regarding additions, inconsistencies, or inaccuracies. Please send them to us at W.B. Saunders Company, The Curtis Center, Independence Square West, Philadelphia, PA 19106. We welcome your suggestions.

ELLEN DRAKE, CMT
RANDY DRAKE, BS
Modesto, California

Acknowledgments

What wonderful families we have! We are grateful for them and to them for their continued support, understanding and prayers. They share in our success. We also appreciate our spiritual family and friends who are so important to us, especially Butch and Alice and Roland and Mardy.

Also, this book probably never would have been written were it not for the influence the American Association for Medical Transcription has had on us as well as the support and understanding of friends, peers, transcription students, and employers. I (Ellen) would like to acknowledge three special people: Brenda Hurley, CMT; Jenola Bradwell, ART, CMT; and Sally Pitman, MA, CMT. They have encouraged me, promoted me to others, and mentored me over many years, and I am grateful.

We would also like to thank Margaret Biblis, our editor at the W.B. Saunders Company, whose persistence and dogged determination got us into this in the first place. (She even tracked us down in the mission fields of Central America!) We appreciate her encouragement and, most of all, her patience.

Notes on Using the Text

The purpose of the *Saunders Pharmaceutical Word Book* is to provide the medical transcriptionist (as well as medical record administrators and technicians, coders, nurses, ward clerks, court reporters, legal secretaries, medical assistants, allied health students, and even physicians) a quick, easy-to-use reference that gives not only the correct spellings and capitalizations of drugs, but the designated uses of those drugs, the cross-referencing of brand names to generics, and the usual methods of administration (e.g., capsule, IV, cream). The indication of the preferred nonproprietary (generic) names and the agencies adopting these names (e.g., USAN, USP) should be particularly useful to those writing for publication. The reader will also find various trademarked or proprietary names (e.g., Spansule, Dosepak) that are not drugs but are closely associated with the packaging or administration of drugs.

There are four different ways to refer to drugs. One of these ways is not by the name of the drug itself but by the class to which it belongs—aminoglycosides for example. Inexperienced transcriptionists sometimes confuse these classes with the names of drugs. If you cannot find what you think is a drug name in this reference, it may be that you are looking for a class of drugs. Try your dictionary. Every drug, however, has three names. The first is the *chemical name*, which describes its chemical composition and how the molecules are arranged. It is often long and complex, sometimes containing numbers, Greek letters, italicized letters, and hyphens between elements. This name is rarely used in dictation except in research hospitals and sometimes in the laboratory section when the blood or urine is examined for traces of the drug. The second name for a drug is the *nonproprietary* or *generic name*. This is a name chosen by the manufacturer or discovering agency and submitted to a nomenclature committee (the United States Adopted Names Council, for example). The name is simpler than the chemical name but often reflects the chemical entity. It is arrived at by using guidelines provided by the nomenclature committee and must be unique. There is increasing emphasis on the adoption of the same nonproprietary name by various nomenclature committees worldwide. The third name for a drug is the *trade* or *brand name*. There may be several trade names for the same generic drug, each marketed by a different company. These are the ones that are highly advertised, and sometimes have unusual capitalization. An interesting article on the naming of drugs is "Pharmaceutical Nomenclature: The Lawless Language" in *Perspectives on the Medical Transcription Profession*.[1] *Understanding Pharmacology*[2] also discusses the naming of drugs.

Special effort has been made to include experimental and investigational drugs (342 entries), chemotherapy drugs and drug protocols, drugs that have been recently discontinued by the manufacturer or withdrawn from the market by the

Food and Drug Administration (FDA), and orphan drugs (603 entries). Orphan drugs are those products that have limited commercial appeal and are used for the treatment of relatively rare disease conditions. The government and FDA encourage the marketing of orphan drugs through subsidized research and the streamlining of the approval process. A few familiar drugs, such as Valium (diazepam), and some surprising ones (caffeine) are designated as orphan drugs for specific application in certain diseases.

We have included many foreign names of drugs for our Canadian friends, and also because we have so many visitors to the United States from other countries (and they get sick, too). The international and British spellings of generic drugs are cross-referenced to the American spellings, and vice versa. Occasionally there will be three different spellings—one American, one international, and another British—which are all cross-referenced to each other. Other special features that may be useful, especially for students, are commonly used prescribing abbreviations and the sound-alike list which are found in the appendices. Another appendix gives the investigational codes (assigned to drugs before they are named), cross-referenced to their subsequent generic names.

This information was compiled from a variety of sources including direct communication with over 500 drug companies. The orphan entries are taken directly from the latest list issued by the FDA. When sources differed, we ranked our sources as to reliability and went with what we thought was the most reliable one. We recognize that there may be several published ways in which to type a single drug, but we have chosen to use only one of those ways. In the instance of internal capitalization (e.g., pHisoHex), it should be recognized that in most instances it is acceptable to type such words with initial capitalization only (Phisohex).

Although we have made every attempt to include as much necessary information as possible, we have by no means tried to provide *prescribing information* as defined by the FDA. Not only have we left out dosages, but the given uses/actions for a particular drug are not all-inclusive. Physicians should consult the *Physicians' Desk Reference*, package insert, or some other acceptable source for prescribing information.

How the Book is Arranged

All entries are in alphabetical order by word. Hyphenated entries are alphabetized as if they were one word. All numbers, chemical prefixes (*N*-, *p*-, *l*-, *d*-, etc.) and punctuation (prime, ampersands, etc.) are ignored. For example, L-dopa would be alphabetized under "dopa," but levodopa under "levo."

In compliance with standards set by the AMA[3] and AAMT,[4] we have indicated brand names with initial capital letters unless an unusual combination of capitals and lower case has been designated by the manufacturer (e.g.,

Notes on Using the Text xiii

pHisoHex, ALternaGEL). Generic names are rendered in lower case. If the same name can be either generic or brand, both have been included.

The general format of a *generic* entry is:

    entry   council(s)   *designated use*   [other references]
    └─#1─┘   └───#2───┘   └─────#3─────┘   └──────#4──────┘

1. The name of the drug (in bold).
2. The various agencies that have approved the name, which may be any or all of the following (ranked according to appearance in the book):

USAN	United States Adopted Name Council
USP	United States Pharmacopeial Convention
NF	National Formulary
FDA	U.S. Food & Drug Administration
INN	International Nonproprietary Name (a project of the World Health Organization)
BAN	British Approved Name

3. The designated use, sometimes referred to as the drug's "therapeutic action." This is provided only for official FDA-approved names or other names for the same substance (e.g., the British name of an official U.S. generic). This entry is always in italic.
4. The entry in brackets is one of four cross-references:

see:	refers the reader to the "official" name(s).
now:	for an older generic name no longer used, refers reader to the current official name(s).
also:	a substance that has two or more different names, each officially recognized by one of the above groups, will cross-reference the other name(s).
q.v.	Latin for *quod vide*; *which see*. Used exclusively for abbreviations, it invites the reader to turn to the reference in parentheses.

   If there is more than one cross reference, alternate names will follow the order of the above agency list; i.e., U.S. names, then international names, then British names. The first cross reference will always be to the approved U.S. name, unless the entry itself is the U.S. name.

The general format for a *brand name* entry is:

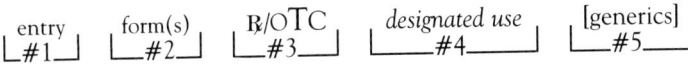

    entry   form(s)   R/OTC   *designated use*   [generics]
    └─#1─┘   └─#2─┘   └─#3─┘   └─────#4─────┘   └──#5──┘

1. The name of the drug (in bold), which almost always starts with a capital letter.
2. The form of administration; e.g., tablets, capsules, syrup. (Sometimes these are the very words that are slurred by the dictator causing confusion regarding the name.)

3. The ℞ or OTC status. A few drugs may be either ℞ or OTC depending on strength or various state laws.[5]
4. The designated use in italics as for generics. These are more complete or less complete as supplied by the individual drug companies.
5. The brackets that follow contain the generic names of the active ingredients to which the reader may refer for further information.

A Brief Note on the Transcription of Drugs

Many references are available describing several acceptable ways to transcribe drug information when dictated. For exhaustive discussions of these methods, the reader is referred to Fordney and Diehl's *Medical Transcription Guide: Do's and Don'ts*,[6] the American Association for Medical Transcription *Style Guide for Medical Transcription* by Tessier and Pitman, and the American Medical Association *Manual of Style*.

Although some institutions favor capitalizing every drug, others promote *not* capitalizing any drug, and yet others put drugs in all capital letters, the generally accepted style today for the transcription of medical reports for hospital and doctors' office charts (see the AMA *Manual of Style* for publications) is to capitalize the initial letter of brand name drugs and lower case generic name drugs. The institution may also designate that brand name drugs with unusual capitalization may be typed with initial capital letter only, or typed using the manufacturer's scheme.

In general, commas are omitted between the drug name, the dosage, and the instructions for purposes of simplification. Items in a series may be separated by either commas (if no internal commas are used) or semicolons. A simple series might be typed thus:

Procardia, nitroglycerin sublingual, and Tolinase

or

Procardia 10 mg three times a day, nitroglycerin 1/150 p.r.n., and Tolinase 100 mg twice a day.

or

Procardia 10 mg t.i.d., nitroglycerin 1/150 p.r.n., and Tolinase 100 mg b.i.d.

A more complex or lengthy list of medications, or a list with internal commas, may require the use of semicolons to separate the items in a series. For example,

Procardia 10 mg, one 3 times a day; nitroglycerin 1/150 p.r.n., to take one with onset of pain, a second in five minutes, and a third five minutes later, if no relief to go immediately to the ER; Tolinase 100 mg, one 2 times a day; and Coumadin 2.5 mg on Mondays, Wednesdays, and Fridays, and 5 mg on Tuesdays, Thursdays, and Saturdays . . .

Note that the "one" following Procardia 10 mg and Tolinase 100 mg is not necessary, but many doctors dictate something like this; when they do, it is acceptable to place a comma after the dosage.

An experienced transcriptionist can often predict whether or not the medications list is going to be short or long, simple or complex, and may habitually choose to use a semicolon to separate the items in a series rather than go back and change commas to semicolons when the need becomes apparent.

The typing of chemicals with superscripts or subscripts, italics, small capitals, and Greek letters often presents a problem to the medical transcriptionist. In general, Greek letters are written out (alpha-, beta-, gamma-, etc.). Italics and small capitals are written as standard letters followed by a hyphen (dl-alpha-tocopherol, L-dopa). Isotopes are written with a space and the isotope number following the name or abbreviation (iodine 131 or I 131, sodium iodide I 125).[7] Other combinations of letters and numbers are usually written without spaces or hyphens (OKT1, OKT3, T101, SC1), but this is a complex subject and is dealt with extensively in the AMA *Manual of Style*.

Endnotes

[1] Dirckx, John, M.D.: "Pharmaceutical Nomenclature: The Lawless Language," *Perspectives on the Medical Transcription Profession*, Vol. 1, No. 4. Modesto: Health Professions Institute, 1991, p. 9.

[2] Turley, Susan M., CMT: *Understanding Pharmacology*. Englewood Cliffs: Regents/Prentice Hall, 1991.

[3] American Medical Association: *Manual of Style*, 8th ed. Baltimore: Williams & Wilkins, 1989, §12.6.3, p. 212.

[4] Tessier, Claudia & Sally Pitman: *Style Guide for Medical Transcription*. Modesto: American Association for Medical Transcription, 1985, p. 14.

[5] Some states are moving toward the creation of a third class of drugs between ℞ and OTC. These medications, while not being readily available on the shelf, could be dispensed by a licensed pharmacist without a doctor's prescription.

[6] Fordney, Marilyn & Marcy Diehl: *Medical Transcription Guide: Do's and Don'ts*. Philadelphia: W.B. Saunders Co., 1990.

[7] American Medical Association: *Manual of Style*, op. cit., §12.13, pp. 235–238.

A (vitamin A) [q.v.]

A and D hand cream (discontinued 1989) OTC *moisturizer; emollient* [vitamins A & D]

A and D Medicated ointment OTC *topical diaper rash treatment* [zinc oxide; vitamins A & D]

A and D ointment OTC *moisturizer; emollient* [fish liver oil (vitamins A & D); cholecalciferol; lanolin]

A-200 Pyrinate gel (discontinued 1992) OTC *pediculicide* [pyrethrins; piperonyl butoxide technical; petroleum distillate]

A-200 shampoo OTC *pediculicide* [pyrethrins; piperonyl butoxide]

AA-HC Otic ear drops ℞ *topical corticosteroidal anti-inflammatory; antibacterial/antifungal* [hydrocortisone; acetic acid]

abamectin USAN, INN *antiparasitic*

Abbokinase IV or intracoronary artery infusion ℞ *thrombolytic* [urokinase]

Abbokinase Open-Cath liquid for catheter clearance ℞ *thrombolytic* [urokinase]

Abbo-Pac (trademarked form) *unit dose package*

Abbott HIVAB HIV-1 EIA test kit OTC *in vitro diagnostic aid for HIV-1 antibody in serum or plasma*

Abbott HIVAG-1 test kit OTC *in vitro diagnostic aid for HIV-1 antigen in serum or plasma*

Abbott HTLV I EIA test kit OTC *in vitro diagnostic aid for HTLV I antibody in serum or plasma*

Abbott HTLV III Confirmatory EIA test kit OTC *in vitro diagnostic aid for HTLV III antibody*

Abbott TestPack Plus hCG-Urine test kit ℞ *in vitro diagnostic aid for urine pregnancy test*

Abbott TestPack Strep A test kit ℞ *in vitro diagnostic aid for streptococci*

ABC (Adriamycin, BCNU, cyclophosphamide) *chemotherapy protocol*

ABC to Z tablets OTC *vitamin/mineral/iron supplement* [multiple vitamins & minerals; ferrous fumarate; folic acid; biotin]

ABCM (Adriamycin, bleomycin, cyclophosphamide, mitomycin) *chemotherapy protocol*

ABD (Adriamycin, bleomycin, DTIC) *chemotherapy protocol*

ABDIC (Adriamycin, bleomycin, DIC, [CCNU, prednisone]) *chemotherapy protocol*

ABDV (Adriamycin, bleomycin, DTIC, vinblastine) *chemotherapy protocol*

ABE (antitoxin botulism equine) [see: botulism equine antitoxin, trivalent]

abecarnil INN

Abitrexate IV or IM injection ℞ *antineoplastic for leukemia; systemic antipsoriatic; antirheumatic* [methotrexate sodium]

ABLC [see: TLC ABLC]

ablukast USAN, INN *antiasthmatic; leukotriene antagonist*

ablukast sodium USAN *antiasthmatic; leukotriene antagonist*

ABP (Adriamycin, bleomycin, prednisone) *chemotherapy protocol*

ABPP ℞ *investigational immunomodulator for AIDS* [bropirimine]

absorbable cellulose cotton [see: cellulose, oxidized]

absorbable dusting powder [see: dusting powder, absorbable]

absorbable gelatin film [see: gelatin film, absorbable]

absorbable gelatin powder [see: gelatin powder, absorbable]

absorbable gelatin sponge [see: gelatin sponge, absorbable]

absorbable surgical suture [see: suture, absorbable surgical]
Absorbase OTC *ointment base*
absorbent gauze [see: gauze, absorbent]
Absorbine Antifungal cream, powder OTC *topical antifungal* [tolnaftate]
Absorbine Arthritic Pain lotion OTC *counterirritant* [methyl salicylate; camphor; menthol; methyl nicotinate]
Absorbine Jock Itch powder OTC *topical antifungal* [tolnaftate]
Absorbine Jr. Antifungal spray liquid OTC *topical antifungal* [tolnaftate]
Absorbine Jr. Extra Strength liquid OTC *counterirritant* [menthol]
Absorbine Jr. liniment OTC *counterirritant; topical antiseptic* [menthol; acetone; chloroxylenol]
abunidazole INN
ABV (actinomycin D, bleomycin, vincristine) *chemotherapy protocol*
ABV (Adriamycin, bleomycin, vinblastine) *chemotherapy protocol*
ABVD (Adriamycin, bleomycin, vinblastine, dacarbazine) *chemotherapy protocol*
AC (Adriamycin, CCNU) *chemotherapy protocol*
AC; A-C (Adriamycin, cyclophosphamide) *chemotherapy protocol*
acacia NF *suspending agent; emollient; demulcent*
Acacia senegal [see: acacia]
acadesine USAN, INN, BAN *platelet aggregation inhibitor*
A-Caine Rectal ointment OTC *topical anesthetic; vasoconstrictor; astringent* [diperodon HCl; pyrilamine maleate; phenylephrine HCl; bismuth subcarbonate; zinc oxide]
acamprosate 6473 INN
acamylophenine [see: camylofin]
acaprazine INN
acarbose USAN, INN, BAN *α-glucosidase inhibitor*

Accu-Pak (trademarked form) *unit dose blister pack*
Accupep HPF OTC *oral nutritional supplement for GI problems*
Accupril film-coated tablets ℞ *antihypertensive; angiotensin-converting enzyme inhibitor* [quinapril HCl]
Accurbron liquid ℞ *antiasthmatic* [theophylline]
Accusens T multi-sample kit OTC *in vitro diagnostic aid for taste dysfunction*
Accutane capsules ℞ *internal keratolytic for acne* [isotretinoin]
ACD solution (acid citrate dextrose; anticoagulant citrate dextrose) [see: anticoagulant citrate dextrose solution]
ACe (Adriamycin, cyclophosphamide) *chemotherapy protocol*
ACE (Adriamycin, cyclophosphamide, etoposide) *chemotherapy protocol*
acebrochol INN
aceburic acid INN
acebutolol USAN, INN, BAN *antiadrenergic (β-receptor)*
acebutolol HCl *antihypertensive; antiarrhythmic; antiadrenergic (β-receptor)*
acecainide INN *antiarrhythmic* [also: acecainide HCl]
acecainide HCl USAN *antiarrhythmic* [also: acecainide]
acecarbromal INN *CNS depressant; sedative; hypnotic*
aceclidine USAN, INN *cholinergic*
aceclofenac INN
acedapsone USAN, INN, BAN *antimalarial; antibacterial; leprostatic*
acediasulfone sodium INN
acedoben INN
acefluranol INN, BAN
acefurtiamine INN
acefylline clofibrol INN
acefylline piperazine INN [also: acepifylline]
aceglatone INN

aceglutamide INN *antiulcerative* [also: aceglutamide aluminum]

aceglutamide aluminum USAN *antiulcerative* [also: aceglutamide]

Acel-Imune IM injection ℞ *immunization against diphtheria, tetanus and pertussis (DTP)* [diphtheria & tetanus toxoids & pertussis vaccine, adsorbed]

acemannan USAN, INN *antiviral; immunomodulator*

acemetacin INN, BAN

acemethadone [see: methadyl acetate]

acenocoumarin [see: acenocoumarol]

acenocoumarol NF, INN [also: nicoumalone]

Aceon ℞ *investigational antihypertensive; ACE inhibitor*

aceperone INN

Acephen suppositories OTC *analgesic; antipyretic* [acetaminophen]

acephenazine dimaleate [see: acetophenazine maleate]

acepifylline BAN [also: acefylline piperazine]

acepromazine INN, BAN *veterinary sedative* [also: acepromazine maleate]

acepromazine maleate USAN *veterinary sedative* [also: acepromazine]

aceprometazine INN

acequinoline INN

ACES soft capsules OTC *vitamin supplement* [vitamins A, C & E; selenium methionine]

acesulfame INN, BAN

Aceta tablets, elixir OTC *analgesic; antipyretic* [acetaminophen]

Aceta with Codeine tablets ℞ *narcotic analgesic* [codeine phosphate; acetaminophen]

Aceta-Gesic tablets OTC *antihistamine; analgesic* [phenyltoloxamine citrate; acetaminophen]

p-**acetamidobenzoic acid** [see: acedoben]

6-acetamidohexanoic acid [see: acexamic acid]

4-acetamidophenyl acetate [see: diacetamate]

acetaminocaproic acid [see: acexamic acid]

acetaminophen USP *analgesic; antipyretic* [also: paracetamol]

acetaminophenol [see: acetaminophen]

acetaminosalol INN

acetanilid (or acetanilide) NF

acetannin [see: acetyltannic acid]

acetarsol INN, BAN [also: acetarsone]

acetarsone NF [also: acetarsol]

acetarsone salt of arecoline [see: drocarbil]

Acetasol ear drops ℞ *antibacterial/antifungal* [acetic acid]

Acetasol HC ear drops ℞ *topical corticosteroidal anti-inflammatory; antibacterial/antifungal* [hydrocortisone; acetic acid]

acetazolamide USP, INN, BAN *carbonic anhydrase inhibitor; anticonvulsant*

acetazolamide sodium USP *carbonic anhydrase inhibitor*

acetcarbromal [see: acetylcarbromal; acecarbromal]

acet-dia-mer-sulfonamide (sulfacetamide, sulfadiazine & sulfamerazine) [q.v.]

acetergamine INN

Acetest Reagent tablets OTC *in vitro diagnostic aid for ketones in the urine or blood*

acetiamine INN

acetic acid NF *acidifying agent*

acetic acid, aluminum salt [see: aluminum acetate]

acetic acid, calcium salt [see: calcium acetate]

acetic acid, diluted NF *bladder irrigant*

acetic acid, ethyl ester [see: ethyl acetate]

acetic acid, glacial USP *acidifying agent*

acetic acid, potassium salt [see: potassium acetate]
acetic acid, sodium salt trihydrate [see: sodium acetate]
acetic acid, zinc salt dihydrate [see: zinc acetate]
acetic acid 5-nitrofurfurylidenehydrazide [see: nihydrazone]
aceticyl [see: aspirin]
acetilum acidulatum [see: aspirin]
acetiromate INN
acetohexamide USAN, USP, INN, BAN *sulfonylurea-type antidiabetic*
acetohydroxamic acid (AHA) USAN, USP, INN *urease enzyme inhibitor*
acetol [see: aspirin]
acetomeroctol
acetone NF *solvent; antiseptic*
acetophen [see: aspirin]
acetophenazine INN *antipsychotic* [also: acetophenazine maleate]
acetophenazine maleate USAN, USP *antipsychotic* [also: acetophenazine]
p-acetophenetidide *(withdrawn from market)* [see: phenacetin]
acetophenetidin *(withdrawn from market)* [now: phenacetin]
acetorphine INN, BAN
acetosal [see: aspirin]
acetosalic acid [see: aspirin]
acetosalin [see: aspirin]
acetosulfone sodium USAN *antibacterial; leprostatic* [also: sulfadiasulfone sodium]
acetoxyphenylmercury [see: phenylmercuric acetate]
acetoxythymoxamine [see: moxisylyte]
acetphenarsine [see: acetarsone]
acetphenetidin *(withdrawn from market)* [now: phenacetin]
acetphenolisatin [see: oxyphenisatin acetate]
acetrizoate sodium USP [also: sodium acetrizoate]
acetrizoic acid USP

acetryptine INN
acetsalicylamide [see: salacetamide]
acet-theocin sodium [see: theophylline sodium acetate]
acetyl adalin [see: acetylcarbromal]
acetyl sulfisoxazole [see: sulfisoxazole acetyl]
p-acetylaminobenzaldehyde thiosemicarbazone [see: thioacetazone; thiacetazone]
acetylaminobenzene [see: acetanilid]
N-acetyl-p-aminophenol (APAP; NAPA) [see: acetaminophen]
acetylaniline [see: acetanilid]
acetylated polyvinyl alcohol *viscosity-increasing agent*
acetyl-bromo-diethylacetylcarbamide [see: acetylcarbromal; acecarbromal]
acetylcarbromal [see: acecarbromal]
acetylcholine chloride USP, INN, BAN *cardiac depressant; cholinergic; miotic; peripheral vasodilator*
acetylcysteine (N-acetylcysteine) USAN, USP, INN, BAN *mucolytic inhaler; investigational immunomodulator for AIDS;* (*orphan: severe acetaminophen overdose*)
acetyldigitoxin (α-acetyldigitoxin) NF, INN
acetyldihydrocodeinone [see: thebacon]
acetylin [see: aspirin]
acetylleucine INN
acetylmethadol INN *narcotic analgesic* [also: methadyl acetate]
l-acetyl-α-methadol (LAAM) [see: levomethadyl acetate]
acetyloleandomycin [see: troleandomycin]
2-acetyloxybenzoic acid [see: aspirin]
acetylphenylisatin [see: oxyphenisatin acetate]
N-acetylprocainamide (NAPA) (*orphan: aid in implantable cardioverter defibrillator therapy*)

acetylpropylorvinol [see: acetorphine]
acetylresorcinol [see: resorcinol monoacetate]
acetylsal [see: aspirin]
***N*-acetylsalicylamide** [see: salacetamide]
acetylsalicylate aluminum [see: aspirin aluminum]
acetylsalicylic acid (ASA) [now: aspirin]
acetylsalicylic acid, phenacetin & caffeine [see: APC]
***N*¹-acetylsulfanilamide** [see: sulfacetamide]
acetyltannic acid USP
acetyltannin [see: acetyltannic acid]
acevaltrate INN
acexamic acid INN
ACFUCY (actinomycin D, fluorouracil, cyclophosphamide) *chemotherapy protocol*
Aches-N-Pain tablets OTC *nonsteroidal anti-inflammatory drug (NSAID); antiarthritic; analgesic* [ibuprofen]
Achromycin IV or IM injection (discontinued 1992) ℞ *broad-spectrum antibiotic* [tetracycline HCl]
Achromycin ophthalmic suspension, ophthalmic ointment ℞ *broad-spectrum antibiotic* [tetracycline HCl]
Achromycin topical ointment OTC *broad-spectrum antibacterial* [tetracycline HCl]
Achromycin V oral suspension, capsules ℞ *broad-spectrum antibiotic* [tetracycline HCl]
aciclovir INN *antiviral* [also: acyclovir]
acid acriflavine [see: acriflavine HCl]
acid citrate dextrose (ACD) [see: anticoagulant citrate dextrose solution]
acid histamine phosphate [see: histamine phosphate]
Acid Mantle OTC *cream base*
acid trypaflavine [see: acriflavine HCl]

acidogen [see: glutamic acid HCl]
acidol HCl [see: betaine HCl]
acidophilus [see: *Lactobacillus acidophilus*]
acidulated phosphate fluoride (sodium fluoride & hydrofluoric acid) *dental caries prophylactic*
Acidulin Pulvules (capsules) (discontinued 1992) OTC *gastric acidifier* [glutamic acid HCl]
acidum acetylsalicylicum [see: aspirin]
acifran USAN, INN *antihyperlipoproteinemic*
aciglumin [see: glutamic acid HCl]
Aci-Jel vaginal jelly OTC *acidity modifier* [acetic acid; oxyquinolone sulfate]
acinitrazole BAN *veterinary antibacterial* [also: nithiamide; aminitrozole]
acipimox INN, BAN
acitemate INN
acitretin USAN, INN, BAN *antipsoriatic*
acivicin USAN, INN *antineoplastic*
aclacinomycin A [now: aclarubicin]
aclantate INN
aclarubicin USAN, INN, BAN *antineoplastic*
aclatonium napadisilate INN, BAN
Aclophen long-acting tablets ℞ *decongestant; antihistamine; analgesic* [phenylephrine HCl; chlorpheniramine maleate; acetaminophen]
Aclovate ointment, cream ℞ *topical corticosteroidal anti-inflammatory* [alclometasone dipropionate]
ACM (Adriamycin, cyclophosphamide, methotrexate) *chemotherapy protocol*
A.C.N. tablets OTC *vitamin supplement* [vitamins A, B₃ & C]
Acne-10 lotion OTC *topical keratolytic for acne* [benzoyl peroxide]
Acne-Aid cleansing bar OTC *medicated cleanser for acne* [surfactant blend]

Acne-Aid cream OTC *keratolytic for acne* [benzoyl peroxide]
AcneCleanse pads OTC *acne*
Acnederm lotion (discontinued 1993) OTC *topical acne treatment* [sulfur; zinc sulfate; zinc oxide; isopropyl alcohol]
Acno Cleanser liquid OTC *topical acne cleanser* [isopropyl alcohol]
Acno lotion OTC *topical acne treatment* [sulfur; salicylic acid]
Acnomel cream OTC *topical acne treatment* [sulfur; resorcinol; alcohol; titanium dioxide]
Acnophill ointment (discontinued 1992) OTC *topical acne treatment* [sulfur; zinc oxide]
Acnotex lotion OTC *topical acne treatment* [sulfur; salicylic acid; methylbenzethonium chloride; isopropyl alcohol; acetone]
acodazole INN *antineoplastic* [also: acodazole HCl]
acodazole HCl USAN *antineoplastic* [also: acodazole]
aconiazide INN *(orphan: tuberculosis)*
aconitine USP
ACOP (Adriamycin, cyclophosphamide, Oncovin, prednisone) *chemotherapy protocol*
ACOPP; A-COPP (Adriamycin, cyclophosphamide, Oncovin, procarbazine, prednisone) *chemotherapy protocol*
acortan [see: corticotropin]
acoxatrine INN
9-acridinamine monohydrochloride [see: aminacrine HCl]
acridinyl anisidide [see: amsacrine]
acridinylamine methanesulfon anisidide (AMSA) [see: amsacrine]
acridorex INN
acriflavine NF
acriflavine HCl NF [also: acriflavinium chloride]
acriflavinium chloride INN [also: acriflavine HCl]
acrihellin INN

acrisorcin USAN, USP, INN *antifungal*
acrivastine USAN, INN, BAN *antihistamine*
acrocinonide INN
acronine USAN *antineoplastic*
acrosoxacin BAN *antibacterial* [also: rosoxacin]
ACT oral rinse OTC *topical dental caries preventative* [sodium fluoride]
actagardin INN
Actagen tablets, syrup OTC *decongestant; antihistamine* [pseudoephedrine HCl; triprolidine HCl]
Actagen-C Cough syrup ℞ *decongestant; antihistamine; antitussive* [pseudoephedrine HCl; triprolidine HCl; codeine phosphate; alcohol]
Actamin; Actamin Extra tablets OTC *analgesic; antipyretic* [acetaminophen]
Actamin Super tablets OTC *analgesic; antipyretic* [acetaminophen; caffeine]
actaplanin USAN, INN, BAN *veterinary growth stimulant*
ACTH (adrenocorticotropic hormone) [see: corticotropin]
ACTH powder for IM or subcu injection ℞ *steroid* [corticotropin]
ACTH-40; ACTH-80 subcu or IM injection ℞ *steroid* [corticotropin repository]
Acthar powder for IM or subcu injection ℞ *steroid* [corticotropin]
Acthrel ℞ *(orphan: adrenocorticotropic hormone-dependent Cushing syndrome)* [ovine corticotropin-releasing hormone]
Acticort 100 lotion ℞ *topical corticosteroid* [hydrocortisone]
Actidil tablets (discontinued 1993) OTC *antihistamine* [triprolidine HCl]
Actidose with Sorbitol liquid OTC *adsorbent poisoning antidote; reduces intestinal transit time* [activated charcoal; sorbitol]

Actidose-Aqua liquid OTC *adsorbent poisoning antidote* [activated charcoal]

Actifed 12-Hour sustained-release capsules (discontinued 1993) OTC *decongestant; antihistamine* [pseudoephedrine HCl; triprolidine HCl]

Actifed capsules, tablets, syrup OTC *decongestant; antihistamine* [pseudoephedrine HCl; triprolidine HCl]

Actifed Plus caplets, tablets OTC *decongestant; antihistamine; analgesic* [pseudoephedrine HCl; triprolidine HCl; acetaminophen]

Actifed Sinus caplets (daytime/nighttime) OTC *decongestant; antihistamine; analgesic* [pseudoephedrine HCl; diphenhydramine HCl; acetaminophen]

Actifed with Codeine Cough syrup ℞ *decongestant; antihistamine; antitussive* [pseudoephedrine HCl; triprolidine HCl; codeine phosphate; alcohol]

Actigall capsules ℞ *gallstone dissolving agent; (orphan: primary biliary cirrhosis)* [ursodiol]

Actimmune subcutaneous injection ℞ *biologic response modifier; (orphan: chronic granulomatous disease)* [interferon gamma-1b]

Actinex cream ℞ *antineoplastic for actinic keratoses* [masoprocol]

actinium *element (Ac)*

actinomycin BAN *antineoplastic* [also: dactinomycin; actinomycin D]

actinomycin C BAN *antineoplastic* [also: cactinomycin]

actinomycin D BAN *antineoplastic* [also: dactinomycin; actinomycin]

actinoquinol INN *ultraviolet screen* [also: actinoquinol sodium]

actinoquinol sodium USAN *ultraviolet screen* [also: actinoquinol]

actinospectocin [see: spectinomycin]

Actisite periodontal fiber ℞ *investigational oral antibiotic* [tetracycline]

actisomide USAN, INN *antiarrhythmic*

Activase IV infusion ℞ *tissue plasminogen activator for acute MI and pulmonary embolism* [alteplase]

activated attapulgite [see: attapulgite, activated]

activated carbon

activated charcoal [see: charcoal, activated]

activated 7-dehydrocholesterol [see: cholecalciferol]

activated ergosterol [see: ergocalciferol]

activated prothrombin complex BAN

actodigin USAN, INN *cardiotonic*

ACU-dyne Douche solution OTC *antiseptic/germicidal; vaginal cleansing and deodorizing* [povidone-iodine]

ACU-dyne ointment, perineal wash concentrate, prep solution, skin cleanser, prep swabs, swabsticks OTC *broad-spectrum antimicrobial* [povidone-iodine]

Acular eye drops ℞ *ocular nonsteroidal anti-inflammatory* [ketorolac tromethamine]

Acupaque ℞ *investigational broad-spectrum contrast agent for x-ray and CT scans* [iodixanol]

Acutrim 16 Hour; Acutrim Late Day precision-release tablets OTC *diet aid* [phenylpropanolamine HCl]

Acutrim; Acutrim II tablets OTC *diet aid* [phenylpropanolamine HCl]

acycloguanosine [see: acyclovir]

acyclovir USAN, USP, BAN *antiviral* [also: aciclovir]

acyclovir redox [see: redox-acyclovir]

acyclovir sodium USAN *antiviral*

acylpyrin [see: aspirin]

adafenoxate INN

Adagen IM injection ℞ *enzyme replacement; (orphan: severe combined immunodeficiency disease)* [pegademase bovine]

Adalat capsules ℞ *antianginal* [nifedipine]
adamantanamine [see: amantadine]
adamantanamine HCl [see: amantadine HCl]
adamexine INN
adapalene USAN, INN *antiacne*
Adapettes for Sensitive Eyes solution OTC *contact lens rewetting solution*
Adapin capsules (discontinued 1991) ℞ *anxiolytic; antidepressant* [doxepin HCl]
adaprolol maleate USAN *ophthalmic antihypertensive (β-blocker)*
Adapt solution OTC *contact lens rewetting solution*
Adavite tablets OTC *vitamin supplement* [multiple vitamins; folic acid; biotin]
Adavite-M tablets OTC *vitamin/mineral/iron supplement* [multiple vitamins & minerals; iron; folic acid; biotin]
ADBC (Adriamycin, DTIC, bleomycin, CCNU) *chemotherapy protocol*
ADC with Fluoride drops ℞ *pediatric vitamin supplement and dental caries preventative* [vitamins A, D & C; fluoride]
Adcon-L gel ℞ *investigational agent to inhibit excess scar formation following back surgery*
ADD-Vantage (trademarked form) *intravenous drug delivery system*
ADE (ara-C, daunorubicin, etoposide) *chemotherapy protocol*
ADE cream, ointment OTC *topical antioxidant* [vitamins A, D & E]
Adeflor chewable tablets, drops (discontinued 1992) ℞ *pediatric vitamin supplement and dental caries preventative* [multiple vitamins; fluoride]
Adeflor M tablets ℞ *pediatric vitamin deficiency and dental caries prevention* [multiple vitamins; fluoride; calcium; iron]

ADEKs chewable tablets OTC *vitamin/mineral supplement* [multiple vitamins & minerals; folic acid; biotin]
ademetionine INN
Adenic injection ℞ *nutrient* [adenosine phosphate]
adenine USP *amino acid*
adenine arabinoside (ara-A) [see: vidarabine]
Adenocard IV injection ℞ *antiarrhythmic* [adenosine]
Adenoscan ℞ *cardiac diagnostic aid*
adenosine USAN, BAN *antiarrhythmic; (orphan: brain tumors)*
adenosine monophosphate (AMP) [see: adenosine phosphate]
adenosine phosphate USAN, INN, BAN *nutrient*
5'-adenylic acid [see: adenosine phosphate]
adepsine oil [see: mineral oil]
Adequate M Improved tablets ℞ *vitamin/mineral/iron supplement* [multiple vitamins & minerals; iron; folic acid]
adhesive bandage [see: bandage, adhesive]
adhesive tape [see: tape, adhesive]
adibendan INN
adicillin INN, BAN
adimolol INN
adinazolam USAN, INN, BAN *antidepressant; sedative*
adinazolam mesylate USAN *antidepressant*
Adipex-P capsules (discontinued 1991) ℞ *anorexiant* [phentermine HCl]
Adipex-P tablets ℞ *anorexiant* [phentermine HCl]
adiphenine INN *smooth muscle relaxant* [also: adiphenine HCl]
adiphenine HCl USAN *smooth muscle relaxant* [also: adiphenine]
adipiodone INN [also: iodipamide]
Adipost slow-release capsules ℞ *anorexiant* [phendimetrazine tartrate]

aditeren INN
aditoprim INN
Adlone injection ℞ *glucocorticoids* [methylprednisolone acetate]
adnephrine [see: epinephrine]
ADOAP (Adriamycin, Oncovin, ara-C, prednisone) *chemotherapy protocol*
Adolph's Salt Substitute; Adolph's Seasoned Salt Substitute OTC *salt substitute* [potassium chloride]
ADOP (Adriamycin, Oncovin, prednisone) *chemotherapy protocol*
adozelesin USAN, INN *antineoplastic*
Adphen tablets (withdrawn from market 1991) ℞ *anorexiant* [phendimetrazine tartrate]
ADR (Adriamycin) [see: doxorubicin HCl]
adrafinil INN
adrenal [see: epinephrine]
Adrenalin Chloride eye drops ℞ *antiglaucoma agent* [epinephrine HCl]
Adrenalin Chloride nose drops OTC *nasal decongestant* [epinephrine HCl]
Adrenalin Chloride solution for inhalation OTC *bronchodilator for bronchial asthma* [epinephrine HCl]
Adrenalin Chloride subcu, IV, IM or intracardiac injection ℞ *bronchodilator for bronchial asthma, bronchospasm and COPD; vasopressor used in shock* [epinephrine HCl]
adrenaline BAN *vasoconstrictor; bronchodilator; topical antiglaucoma agent; vasopressor for shock* [also: epinephrine]
adrenaline bitartrate [see: epinephrine bitartrate]
adrenaline HCl [see: epinephrine HCl]
adrenalone USAN, INN *ophthalmic adrenergic*
adrenamine [see: epinephrine]
adrenine [see: epinephrine]
adrenochromazone [see: carbazochrome salicylate]

adrenochrome [see: carbazochrome salicylate]
adrenochrome monosemicarbazone sodium salicylate [see: carbazochrome salicylate]
adrenocorticotrophin [see: corticotropin]
adrenocorticotropic hormone (ACTH) [see: corticotropin]
adrenone [see: adrenalone]
Adria + BCNU (Adriamycin, BCNU) *chemotherapy protocol*
Adriamycin PFS; Adriamycin RDF (ADR) IV injection ℞ *antineoplastic antibiotic* [doxorubicin HCl]
Adria-Oncoline Chemo-Pin ℞ *chemical-dispensing pin*
Adria-L-PAM (Adriamycin, L-phenylalanine mustard) *chemotherapy protocol* L-phenylalanine mustard)
Adrin tablets (discontinued 1993) ℞ *peripheral vasodilator* [nylidrin HCl]
Adrucil IV injection ℞ *antineoplastic; (orphan: adjuvant to colorectal and esophageal cancer)* [fluorouracil]
ADS (azodisal sodium) [now: olsalazine sodium]
adsorbed diphtheria toxoid [see: diphtheria toxoid, adsorbed]
Adsorbocarpine eye drops ℞ *antiglaucoma agent; direct-acting miotic* [pilocarpine HCl]
Adsorbonac Ophthalmic eye drops OTC *corneal edema reducing adjunct; diagnostic aid* [hypertonic saline solution]
Adsorbotear eye drops OTC *ocular moisturizer/lubricant*
Advance home test kit OTC *in vitro diagnostic aid for urine pregnancy test*
Advance liquid (discontinued 1993) OTC *total or supplementary infant feeding*
Advil, Children's oral suspension ℞ *nonsteroidal anti-inflammatory drug (NSAID); antiarthritic; analgesic* [ibuprofen]

Advil Cold & Sinus caplets OTC *decongestant; analgesic* [pseudoephedrine HCl; ibuprofen]

Advil tablets, caplets OTC *nonsteroidal anti-inflammatory drug (NSAID); antiarthritic; analgesic* [ibuprofen]

A-E-R pads OTC *astringent* [hamamelis water]

Aeroaid spray OTC *antiseptic; antibacterial; antifungal* [thimerosal; alcohol]

AeroBid; AeroBid-M oral inhalation aerosol ℞ *corticosteroid for bronchial asthma* [flunisolide]

AeroCaine; AeroTherm aerosol solution OTC *topical local anesthetic; antiseptic* [benzocaine; benzethonium chloride]

AeroChamber (trademarked form) *aerosol holding chamber*

Aerodine aerosol OTC *broad-spectrum antimicrobial* [povidone-iodine]

Aerolate oral solution ℞ *bronchodilator* [theophylline]

Aerolate Sr.; Aerolate Jr.; Aerolate III timed-action capsules ℞ *bronchodilator* [theophylline]

Aerolone solution for nebulization (discontinued 1991) ℞ *bronchodilator for bronchial asthma and bronchospasm* [isoproterenol HCl]

Aeropent inhalant *(orphan: Pneumocystis carinii penumonia)* [pentamidine isethionate]

Aeroseb-Dex aerosol spray ℞ *topical corticosteroid* [dexamethasone]

Aeroseb-HC aerosol spray ℞ *topical corticosteroid; antiseborrheic* [hydrocortisone]

aerosol OT [see: docusate sodium]

aerosolized pooled immune globulin [see: globulin, aerosolized pooled immune]

Aerosporin powder for IV, IM or intrathecal injection ℞ *bactericidal antibiotic* [polymyxin B sulfate]

aeroTherm; aeroCaine aerosol solution OTC *topical local anesthetic* [benzocaine; benzethonium chloride]

Aerotrol (trademarked form) *inhalation aerosol*

AeroZoin spray OTC *skin protectant* [benzoin; isopropyl alcohol]

AErrane ℞ *anesthetic*

aethylis chloridum [see: ethyl chloride]

afloqualone INN

AFM (Adriamycin, fluorouracil, methotrexate) *chemotherapy protocol*

Afrin Children's Nose Drops OTC *nasal decongestant* [oxymetazoline HCl]

Afrin nasal spray, nose drops OTC *nasal decongestant* [oxymetazoline HCl]

Afrin extended-release tablets OTC *nasal decongestant* [pseudoephedrine sulfate]

Afrin Saline Mist solution OTC *nasal moisturizer* [sodium chloride (saline)]

Afrinol (name changed to Afrin in 1993)

Aftate for Athlete's Foot gel, powder, spray powder, spray liquid OTC *topical antifungal* [tolnaftate]

Aftate for Jock Itch gel, powder, spray powder OTC *topical antifungal* [tolnaftate]

afurolol INN

A/G Pro tablets OTC *dietary supplement* [protein hydrolysate; multiple vitamins, minerals & amino acids]

AG-337 ℞ *investigational antineoplastic*

aganodine INN

agar NF *suspending agent*

agar-agar [see: agar]

aggregated albumin [see: albumin, aggregated]

aggregated radio-iodinated I 131 serum albumin [see: albumin, aggregated iodinated I 131 serum]

agofollin [see: estradiol]

Agoral emulsion OTC *laxative* [mineral oil; phenolphthalein]

Agoral Plain emulsion OTC *emollient laxative* [mineral oil]

agurin [see: theobromine sodium acetate]

AHA (acetohydroxamic acid) [q.v.]

AH-chew chewable tablets ℞ *decongestant; antihistamine; anticholinergic* [phenylephrine HCl; chlorpheniramine maleate; methscopolamine nitrate]

AHF (antihemophilic factor) [q.v.]

AHG (antihemophilic globulin) [see: antihemophilic factor]

A-Hydrocort IV or IM injection ℞ *glucocorticoids* [hydrocortisone sodium succinate]

AIDS vaccine *investigational vaccine for AIDS*

air, compressed [see: air, medical]

air, medical USP *medicinal gas*

Akarpine eye drops ℞ *antiglaucoma agent; direct-acting miotic* [pilocarpine HCl]

AK-Biocholine tablets OTC *vitamin supplement* [choline bitartrate; citrus bioflavonoids]

AK-Chlor eye drops, ophthalmic ointment ℞ *ophthalmic antibiotic* [chloramphenicol]

AK-Cide eye drop suspension, ophthalmic ointment ℞ *topical ophthalmic corticosteroidal anti-inflammatory; bacteriostatic* [sulfacetamide sodium; prednisolone acetate]

AK-Con eye drops ℞ *topical ocular vasoconstrictor* [naphazoline HCl]

AK-Con-A eye drops ℞ *topical ocular decongestant/antihistamine* [naphazoline HCl; pheniramine maleate]

AK-Dex eye drops, ophthalmic ointment ℞ *ophthalmic topical corticosteroidal anti-inflammatory* [dexamethasone sodium phosphate]

AK-Dilate 2.5%; AK-Dilate 10% eye drops ℞ *ocular decongestant/vasoconstrictor; mydriatic* [phenylephrine HCl]

AK-Fluor 10%; AK-Fluor 25% IV injection ℞ *corneal disclosing agent* [fluorescein]

AK-Homatropine 5% eye drops ℞ *mydriatic; cycloplegic* [homatropine hydrobromide]

Akineton IV or IM injection ℞ *anticholinergic; antiparkinsonian agent* [biperiden lactate]

Akineton tablets ℞ *anticholinergic; antiparkinsonian agent* [biperiden HCl]

aklomide USAN, INN, BAN *coccidiostat for poultry*

AK-Mycin ophthalmic ointment ℞ *ophthalmic antibiotic* [erythromycin]

AK-NaCl 5% ophthalmic ointment OTC *corneal edema-reducing agent; diagnostic aid* [hypertonic saline solution]

AK-Nefrin eye drops OTC *topical ocular decongestant* [phenylephrine HCl]

Akne-mycin ointment, topical solution ℞ *topical antibiotic for acne vulgaris* [erythromycin]

AK-Neo-Cort eye drop suspension (discontinued 1992) ℞ *topical ophthalmic corticosteroidal anti-inflammatory; antibiotic* [hydrocortisone acetate; neomycin sulfate]

AK-Neo-Dex eye drops ℞ *topical ophthalmic corticosteroidal anti-inflammatory; antibiotic* [dexamethasone sodium phosphate; neomycin sulfate]

Akoline C.B. capsules, caplets OTC *dietary lipotropic with vitamin supplementation* [choline; inositol; methionine; multiple B vitamins; vitamin C; lemon bioflavonoids]

Akoline CB with Zinc caplets OTC *dietary lipotropic with vitamin and zinc supplementation* [choline; inositol; methionine; multiple B vitamins; vitamin C; bioflavonoid; zinc amino acid chelate]

AK-Pentolate eye drops ℞ *mydriatic; cycloplegic* [cyclopentolate HCl]

AK-Poly-Bac ophthalmic ointment ℞ *ophthalmic antibiotic* [polymyxin B sulfate; bacitracin zinc]

AK-Pred 0.125%; AK-Pred 1% eye drops ℞ *ophthalmic topical corticosteroidal anti-inflammatory* [prednisolone sodium phosphate]

AK-Rinse ophthalmic solution OTC *extraocular irrigating solution* [balanced saline solution]

AK-Spore H.C. ear drops, otic suspension ℞ *topical corticosteroidal anti-inflammatory; antibiotic* [polymyxin B sulfate; neomycin sulfate; hydrocortisone]

AK-Spore H.C. ointment ℞ *antibiotic; anti-inflammatory* [polymyxin B sulfate; bacitracin zinc; neomycin sulfate; hydrocortisone]

AK-Spore H.C. Ophthalmic eye drop suspension ℞ *topical corticosteroidal anti-inflammatory; antibiotic* [polymyxin B sulfate; neomycin sulfate; hydrocortisone]

AK-Spore ophthalmic ointment ℞ *ophthalmic antibiotic* [polymyxin B sulfate; neomycin sulfate; bacitracin]

AK-Spore ophthalmic solution ℞ *ophthalmic antibiotic* [polymyxin B sulfate; neomycin sulfate; gramicidin]

AK-Sulf eye drops, ophthalmic ointment ℞ *ophthalmic bacteriostatic* [sulfacetamide sodium]

AK-Sulf Forte eye drops (discontinued 1991) ℞ *ophthalmic bacteriostatic* [sulfacetamide sodium]

AK-Taine eye drops ℞ *topical ocular anesthetic* [proparacaine HCl]

AK-Tracin ophthalmic ointment ℞ *ophthalmic antibiotic* [bacitracin]

AK-Trol eye drop suspension, ophthalmic ointment ℞ *topical ophthalmic corticosteroidal anti-inflammatory; antibiotic* [dexamethasone; neomycin sulfate; polymyxin B sulfate]

AK-Vaso-A ophthalmic solution (discontinued 1991) ℞ *ocular decongestant* [naphazoline HCl; antazoline phosphate]

AK-Vernacon eye drops (discontinued 1991) ℞ *topical ocular decongestant/antihistamine* [phenylephrine HCl; pheniramine maleate]

Akwa Tears eye drops, ophthalmic ointment OTC *ocular moisturizer/lubricant*

Akwa Tears ophthalmic solution OTC *contact lens cushioning; artificial tears* [polyvinyl alcohol]

AK-Zol tablets ℞ *antiglaucoma; anticonvulsant; diuretic* [acetazolamide]

AL-721 *investigational antiviral for AIDS*

alacepril INN

Ala-Cort cream, lotion ℞ *topical corticosteroid* [hydrocortisone]

Aladrine Anti-Asthmatic tablets (discontinued 1991) OTC *decongestant; sedative* [ephedrine sulfate; amobarbital]

alafosfalin INN, BAN

Alamag suspension OTC *antacid* [aluminum hydroxide; magnesium hydroxide]

alamecin USAN *antibacterial*

alanine (L-alanine) USAN, USP, INN *nonessential amino acid; symbols: Ala, A*

alanine nitrogen mustard [see: melphalan]

alanosine INN

alaproclate USAN, INN *antidepressant*

Ala-Quin cream ℞ *topical corticosteroid; antifungal; antibacterial* [hydrocortisone; clioquinol]

Ala-Scalp lotion ℞ *topical corticosteroid* [hydrocortisone]

Alasulf vaginal cream ℞ *bacteriostatic; antiseptic; vulnerary* [sulfanilamide; aminacrine HCl; allantoin]

Ala-Tet capsules (discontinued 1992) ℞ *broad-spectrum antibiotic* [tetracycline HCl]

Alatone tablets ℞ *potassium-sparing diuretic* [spironolactone]

alazanine triclofenate INN

Alazide tablets ℞ *diuretic* [spironolactone; hydrochlorothiazide]

Alazine tablets ℞ *antihypertensive; vasodilator* [hydralazine HCl]

Albalon Liquifilm Ophthalmic eye drops ℞ *topical ocular vasoconstrictor* [naphazoline HCl]

Albalon-A Liquifilm eye drops ℞ *topical ocular decongestant/antihistamine* [naphazoline HCl; antazoline phosphate]

Albamycin capsules ℞ *bacteriostatic antibiotic* [novobiocin sodium]

Albay subcu or IM injection ℞ *venom sensitivity testing; allergenic hyposensitization therapy* [extract of honeybee, yellow jacket, yellow hornet, white-faced hornet, wasp & mixed vespid]

albendazole USAN, INN, BAN *anthelmintic*

albendazole oxide INN, BAN

Albright solution (sodium citrate and citric acid) *urine alkalizer; compounding agent*

albucid [see: sulfacetamide]

albumin, aggregated USAN *lung imaging aid*

albumin, aggregated iodinated I 131 serum USAN, USP *radioactive agent*

albumin, chromated Cr 51 serum USAN *radioactive agent*

albumin, human USP *blood volume supporter*

albumin, iodinated I 125 USP *blood volume test*

albumin, iodinated I 125 serum USAN, USP *blood volume test* [also: iodinated (^{125}I) human serum albumin]

albumin, iodinated I 131 USP *blood volume test*

albumin, iodinated I 131 serum USAN, USP *blood volume test* [also: iodinated (^{131}I) human serum albumin]

albumin, normal human serum [now: albumin, human]

Albuminar IV infusion ℞ *blood volume support* [human albumin]

Albuminar-5; Albuminar-25 IV infusion ℞ *blood volume expander; shock; burns; hypoproteinemia* [human albumin]

Albunex ℞ *investigational ultrasound heart imaging agent*

Albustix reagent strips OTC *in vitro diagnostic aid for protein in the urine*

Albutein 5%; Albutein 25% IV infusion ℞ *antihemophilic* [human albumin]

albuterol USAN, USP *bronchodilator* [also: salbutamol]

albuterol sulfate USAN, USP *bronchodilator*

albutoin USAN, INN *anticonvulsant*

Alcaine Drop-Tainers (eye drops) ℞ *topical ophthalmic anesthetic* [proparacaine HCl]

Alcare foam OTC *topical antiseptic* [ethyl alcohol]

alclofenac USAN, INN, BAN *anti-inflammatory*

alclometasone INN, BAN *topical corticosteroidal anti-inflammatory* [also: alclometasone dipropionate]

alclometasone dipropionate USAN, USP *topical corticosteroidal anti-inflammatory* [also: alclometasone]

alcloxa USAN, INN *astringent; keratolytic*

alcohol USP *topical anti-infective/antiseptic; astringent; solvent*

alcohol, dehydrated USP *antidote*

alcohol, diluted NF *solvent*

alcohol, rubbing USP, INN *rubefacient*

5% Alcohol and 5% Dextrose in Water; 10% Alcohol and 5% Dextrose in Water IV infusion ℞ *for caloric replacement and rehydration* [dextrose; alcohol]

Alconefrin 12; Alconefrin 25; Alconefrin 50 nasal spray, nose drops OTC *nasal decongestant* [phenylephrine HCl]

alcuronium chloride USAN, INN, BAN *skeletal muscle relaxant*
Aldactazide tablets ℞ *diuretic* [spironolactone; hydrochlorothiazide]
Aldactone tablets ℞ *potassium-sparing diuretic* [spironolactone]
alderlin [see: pronethalol]
aldesleukin USAN, INN, BAN *antineoplastic; biological response modifier; immunostimulant; (orphan: immunodeficiency diseases)*
aldesulfone sodium INN *antibacterial; leprostatic* [also: sulfoxone sodium]
aldioxa USAN, INN *astringent; keratolytic*
Aldoclor-150; Aldoclor-250 film-coated tablets ℞ *antihypertensive* [chlorothiazide; methyldopa]
aldocorten [see: aldosterone]
Aldomet Ester HCl IV injection ℞ *antihypertensive* [methyldopate HCl]
Aldomet tablets, oral suspension ℞ *antihypertensive* [methyldopa]
Aldoril 15; Aldoril 25; Aldoril D30; Aldoril D50 film-coated tablets ℞ *antihypertensive* [hydrochlorothiazide; methyldopa]
aldosterone BAN, INN
Alec *(orphan: neonatal respiratory distress syndrome)* [dipalmitoylphosphatidylcholine; phosphatidylglycerol]
alendronate sodium USAN *bone resorption suppressant*
alendronic acid INN
alentemol INN *antipsychotic; dopamine agonist* [also: alentemol HCl]
alentemol HCl USAN *antipsychotic; dopamine agonist* [also: alentemol]
alepride INN
Aler C 500 capsules OTC *vitamin supplement* [vitamin C]
Aler-Key capsules OTC *dietary supplement* [multiple vitamins; bioflavonoids; bovine adrenal concentrate]
Alersule Forte sustained-release capsules (discontinued 1992) ℞ *decongestant; antihistamine; anticholinergic* [phenylephrine HCl; chlorpheniramine maleate; methscopolamine nitrate]
Alersule sustained-release capsules ℞ *decongestant; antihistamine* [phenylephrine HCl; chlorpheniramine maleate]
aletamine HCl USAN, INN *antidepressant* [also: alfetamine]
alexidine USAN, INN *antibacterial*
alexitol sodium INN, BAN
alfacalcidol INN, BAN
alfadex INN
alfadolone INN [also: alphadolone]
alfaprostol USAN, INN, BAN *veterinary prostaglandin*
alfaxalone INN [also: alphaxalone]
Alfenta IV or IM injection ℞ *narcotic analgesic; anesthetic* [alfentanil HCl]
alfentanil INN, BAN *narcotic analgesic* [also: alfentanil HCl]
alfentanil HCl USAN *narcotic analgesic* [also: alfentanil]
Alferon LDO (low dose oral) ℞ *investigational AIDS drug* [interferon alfa-n3]
Alferon N intralesional injection ℞ *antineoplastic for condylomata acuminata* [interferon alfa-n3]
alfetamine INN *antidepressant* [also: aletamine HCl]
alfetamine HCl [see: aletamine HCl]
alfuzosin INN, BAN *antihypertensive (α-blocker)* [also: alfuzosin HCl]
alfuzosin HCl USAN *antihypertensive (α-blocker)* [also: alfuzosin]
algeldrate USAN, INN *antacid*
Algenic Alka Improved chewable tablets OTC *antacid* [aluminum hydroxide; sodium bicarbonate; magnesium trisilicate]
Algenic Alka liquid OTC *antacid* [aluminum hydroxide; magnesium carbonate; EDTA]
algestone INN *anti-inflammatory* [also: algestone acetonide]
algestone acetonide USAN, BAN *anti-inflammatory* [also: algestone]

algestone acetophenide USAN *progestin*

Algicon chewable tablets (discontinued 1992) OTC *antacid* [aluminum hydroxide; magnesium carbonate]

algin [see: sodium alginate]

alginic acid NF, BAN *tablet binder and emulsifying agent*

alginic acid, sodium salt [see: sodium alginate]

alglucerase *(orphan: Gaucher's disease)*

alibendol INN

aliconazole INN

alidine dihydrochloride [see: anileridine]

alidine phosphate [see: anileridine]

alifedrine INN

aliflurane USAN, INN *inhalation anesthetic*

alimadol INN

alimemazine INN *antipruritic* [also: trimeprazine tartrate]

alimemazine tartrate [see: trimeprazine tartrate]

Alimentum liquid OTC *hypoallergenic infant food* [soy protein formula]

alinidine INN, BAN

alipamide USAN, INN, BAN *diuretic; antihypertensive*

alisactide [see: alsactide]

alisobumal [see: butalbital]

alitame USAN *sweetener*

alizapride INN

Alkaban-AQ IV injection ℞ *antineoplastic* [vinblastine sulfate]

Alka-Mints chewable tablets OTC *antacid* [calcium carbonate]

Alka-Seltzer Advanced Formula effervescent tablets OTC *antacid; analgesic* [sodium bicarbonate; calcium carbonate; acetaminophen; citric acid; potassium bicarbonate]

Alka-Seltzer effervescent tablets OTC *antacid* [sodium bicarbonate; citric acid; potassium bicarbonate]

Alka-Seltzer Plus Cold Medicine; Alka-Seltzer Plus Sinus Allergy tablets OTC *decongestant; antihistamine; analgesic* [phenylpropanolamine bitartrate; brompheniramine maleate; aspirin]

Alka-Seltzer Plus Night-Time Cold tablets OTC *decongestant; antihistamine; analgesic* [phenylpropanolamine bitartrate; diphenhydramine citrate; aspirin]

Alka-Seltzer Plus tablets OTC *decongestant; antihistamine; analgesic* [phenylpropanolamine bitartrate; chlorpheniramine maleate; aspirin]

Alka-Seltzer with Aspirin effervescent tablets OTC *antacid; analgesic* [sodium bicarbonate; citric acid; aspirin]

alkavervir (veratrum viride alkaloids)

Alkeran tablets ℞ *antineoplastic for multiple myeloma and ovarian carcinoma* [melphalan]

Alkets chewable tablets OTC *antacid* [calcium carbonate; magnesium carbonate; magnesium oxide]

alkyl aryl sulfonate *surfactant/wetting agent*

alkylbenzyldimethylammonium chloride [see: benzalkonium chloride]

alkyldimethylbenzylammonium chloride [see: benzalkonium chloride]

allantoin USAN, BAN *topical vulnerary; keratolytic*

Allbee C-800 film-coated tablets OTC *vitamin supplement* [multiple B vitamins; vitamins C & E]

Allbee C-800 plus Iron film-coated tablets OTC *vitamin/iron supplement* [multiple B vitamins; vitamins C & E; ferrous fumarate; folic acid]

Allbee with C caplets OTC *vitamin supplement* [multiple B vitamins; vitamin C]

Allbee-T film-coated tablets OTC *dietary supplement* [multiple B vitamins; vitamin C; lactose; desiccated liver]

allegron [see: nortriptyline]

Allent sustained-release capsules ℞ *antihistamine; decongestant* [brompheniramine maleate; pseudoephedrine HCl]

Aller-Chlor tablets, syrup OTC *antihistamine* [chlorpheniramine maleate]

Allercon tablets OTC *decongestant; antihistamine* [pseudoephedrine HCl; triprolidine HCl]

Allercreme Skin lotion OTC *moisturizer; emollient*

Allercreme Ultra Emollient cream OTC *moisturizer; emollient*

Allerest, Children's tablets OTC *pediatric decongestant and antihistamine* [phenylpropanolamine HCl; chlorpheniramine maleate]

Allerest, No-Drowsiness tablets OTC *decongestant; analgesic* [pseudoephedrine HCl; acetaminophen]

Allerest 12 Hour nasal spray OTC *nasal decongestant* [oxymetazoline HCl]

Allerest 12 Hour sustained-release caplets OTC *decongestant; antihistamine* [phenylpropanolamine HCl; chlorpheniramine maleate]

Allerest eye drops OTC *topical ocular vasoconstrictor* [naphazoline HCl]

Allerest Headache; Allerest Sinus Pain Formula tablets OTC *decongestant; antihistamine; analgesic* [pseudoephedrine HCl; chlorpheniramine maleate; acetaminophen]

Allerest tablets OTC *decongestant; antihistamine* [pseudoephedrine; chlorpheniramine maleate]

Allerfrin OTC syrup OTC *decongestant; antihistamine* [pseudoephedrine HCl; triprolidine HCl]

Allerfrin tablets OTC *decongestant; antihistamine* [pseudoephedrine HCl; triprolidine HCl]

Allerfrin with Codeine syrup ℞ *decongestant; antihistamine; antitussive* [pseudoephedrine HCl; triprolidine HCl; codeine phosphate; alcohol]

Allergan Enzymatic tablets OTC *contact lens enzymatic cleaner*

Allergan Hydrocare Cleaning and Disinfecting solution OTC *contact lens disinfectant*

Allergan Hydrocare solution OTC *contact lens rinsing and storage solution* [preserved saline solution]

Allergan Sorbi-Care Saline solution (discontinued 1992) OTC *contact lens rinsing and storage solution* [preserved saline solution]

Allergen Ear Drops ℞ *topical local anesthetic; analgesic* [benzocaine; antipyrine]

Allergy Cold tablets OTC *decongestant; antihistamine* [pseudoephedrine HCl; triprolidine HCl]

Allergy Relief Medicine tablets OTC *decongestant; antihistamine* [phenylpropanolamine HCl; chlorpheniramine maleate]

Allergy tablets OTC *antihistamine* [chlorpheniramine maleate]

AlleRid capsules OTC *decongestant* [pseudoephedrine HCl]

AllerMax caplets OTC *antihistamine; motion sickness* [diphenhydramine HCl]

Allermed capsules OTC *nasal decongestant* [pseudoephedrine HCl]

Allerphed syrup OTC *decongestant; antihistamine* [pseudoephedrine HCl; triprolidine HCl]

Allersone ointment (discontinued 1992) ℞ *topical corticosteroid; anesthetic; astringent* [hydrocortisone; diperodon HCl; zinc oxide]

Allersule Forte sustained-release capsules (discontinued 1992) ℞ *decongestant; antihistamine; anticholinergic* [phenylephrine HCl; chlorpheniramine maleate; methscopolamine nitrate]

alletorphine BAN, INN

All-Nite Cold Formula liquid OTC *decongestant; antihistamine; antitussive; analgesic* [pseudoephedrine

HCl; doxylamine succinate; dextromethorphan hydrobromide; acetaminophen; alcohol]
allobarbital USAN, INN *hypnotic*
allobarbitone [see: allobarbital]
alloclamide INN
allocupreide sodium INN
allomethadione INN [also: aloxidone]
allopurinol USAN, USP, INN, BAN *xanthine oxidase inhibitor for gout; (orphan: kidney transplants)*
allopurinol riboside *(orphan: leishmaniasis; Chagas disease)*
allopurinol sodium *(orphan: ex vivo preservation of kidneys for transplantation)*
Allpyral subcu or IM injection ℞ *venom sensitivity testing; allergenic hyposensitization therapy* [extracts available: pollens, molds, epidermals, house dust, other inhalants & stinging insects]
all-*trans*-retinoic acid [see: tretinoin]
allyl isothiocyanate USAN
allylbarbituric acid [now: butalbital]
allylestrenol INN [also: allyloestrenol]
allyl-isobutylbarbituric acid [see: butalbital]
allylisopropylmalonylurea [see: aprobarbital]
4-allyl-2-methoxyphenol [see: eugenol]
***N*-allylnoretorphine** [see: alletorphine]
***N*-allylnoroxymorphone HCl** [see: naloxone HCl]
allyloestrenol BAN [also: allylestrenol]
allylprodine INN, BAN
5-allyl-5-*sec*-butylbarbituric acid [see: talbutal]
allylthiourea INN
allypropymal [see: aprobarbital]
Almacone chewable tablets, liquid OTC *antacid; antiflatulent* [aluminum hydroxide; magnesium hydroxide; simethicone]

Almacone II oral suspension OTC *antacid; antiflatulent* [aluminum hydroxide; magnesium hydroxide; simethicone]
almadrate sulfate USAN, INN *antacid*
almagate USAN, INN *antacid*
almagodrate INN
Alma-Mag, Improved liquid OTC *antacid; antiflatulent* [aluminum hydroxide; magnesium hydroxide; simethicone]
Alma-Mag #4 Improved chewable tablets OTC *antacid; antiflatulent* [aluminum hydroxide; magnesium hydroxide; simethicone]
Alma-Mag oral suspension OTC *antacid* [aluminum hydroxide; magnesium hydroxide]
almasilate INN, BAN
Almebex Plus B$_{12}$ liquid OTC *vitamin supplement* [multiple B vitamins]
almecillin INN
almestrone INN
alminoprofen INN
almitrine INN, BAN
almond oil NF *emollient and perfume; oleaginous vehicle*
Almora tablets OTC *magnesium supplement* [magnesium gluconate]
almoxatone INN
Alodopa-15; Alodopa-25 tablets ℞ *antihypertensive* [hydrochlorothiazide; methyldopa]
aloe USP
Aloe Grande lotion OTC *moisturizer; emollient; skin protectant* [vitamins A & E; aloe]
Aloe Vesta Perineal solution OTC *emollient/protectant*
alofilcon A USAN *hydrophilic contact lens material*
ALOMAD (Adriamycin, Leukeran, Oncovin, methotrexate, actinomycin D, dacarbazine) *chemotherapy protocol*

Alomide eye drops ℞ *(orphan: vernal keratoconjunctivitis)* [lodoxamide tromethamine]
alonacic INN
alonimid USAN, INN *sedative; hypnotic*
Alophen Pills No. 973 tablets OTC *laxative* [phenolphthalein]
alosetron HCl USAN *antiemetic*
aloxidone BAN [also: allomethadione]
aloxiprin INN, BAN
aloxistatin INN
alozafone INN
alpertine USAN, INN *antipsychotic*
alpha amylase (α-amylase) USAN *anti-inflammatory*
alpha interferon-2A [see: interferon alfa-2A]
alpha interferon-2B [see: interferon alfa-2B]
alpha interferon-N1 [see: interferon alfa-N1]
alpha interferon-N3 [see: interferon alfa-N3]
Alpha Keri Moisturizing Soap bar OTC *therapeutic skin cleanser*
Alpha Keri Spray; Alpha Keri Therapeutic Bath Oil OTC *bath emollient*
d-**alpha tocopherol** [see: vitamin E]
dl-**alpha tocopherol** [see: vitamin E]
d-**alpha tocopheryl acetate** [see: vitamin E]
dl-**alpha tocopheryl acetate** [see: vitamin E]
d-**alpha tocopheryl acid succinate** [see: vitamin E]
dl-**alpha tocopheryl acid succinate** [see: vitamin E]
Alpha Zeta tablets OTC *vitamin/mineral/iron supplement* [multiple vitamins & minerals; ferrous fumarate; folic acid; biotin]
alpha$_1$ antitrypsin, recombinant *(orphan: alpha$_1$-antitrypsin deficiency)*
alpha$_1$ PI (alpha$_1$-proteinase inhibitor) [q.v.]

alpha$_1$-proteinase inhibitor (alpha$_1$ PI) *(orphan: congenital alpha$_1$ PI deficiency)*
l-**alpha-acetyl-methadol (LAAM)** *(orphan: heroin addiction)*
alphacemethadone [see: alphacetylmethadol]
alphacetylmethadol BAN, INN
alpha-chymotrypsin [see: chymotrypsin]
Alphaderm cream (discontinued 1992) ℞ *topical corticosteroid* [hydrocortisone]
alphadolone BAN [also: alfadolone]
alpha-estradiol [see: estradiol]
alpha-estradiol benzoate [see: estradiol benzoate]
alpha-D-galactosidase *digestive enzyme*
alpha-galactosidase A *(orphan: Fabry's disease)*
1-alpha-hydroxy vitamin D2 *investigational osteoporosis treatment*
alpha-hypophamine [see: oxytocin]
alphameprodine INN, BAN
alphamethadol INN, BAN
alpha-methyldopa [now: methyldopa]
Alphamin IM ℞ *antianemic; vitamin supplement* [hydroxocobalamin]
Alphamul emulsion OTC *laxative* [castor oil]
AlphaNine powder for IV suspension ℞ *hemostatic; (orphan: hemophilia B)* [coagulation factor IX (human)]
alpha-phenoxyethyl penicillin, potassium [see: phenethicillin potassium]
alphaprodine INN, BAN [also: alphaprodine HCl]
alphaprodine HCl USP [also: alphaprodine]
AlphaRedisol IM (discontinued 1991) ℞ *antianemic; vitamin supplement* [hydroxocobalamin]
alphasone acetophenide [now: algestone acetonide]

Alphatrex cream, ointment, lotion ℞ *topical corticosteroid* [betamethasone dipropionate]
alphaxalone BAN [also: alfaxalone]
Alphosyl cream (discontinued 1992) OTC *topical antipsoriatic; antiseborrheic; vulnerary* [coal tar extract; allantoin]
Alphosyl lotion OTC *topical antipsoriatic; antiseborrheic; vulnerary* [coal tar extract; allantoin]
alpidem USAN, INN, BAN *anxiolytic*
alpiropride INN
alprazolam USAN, USP, INN, BAN *anxiolytic; sedative; treatment of panic disorders and agoraphobia*
alprenolol INN, BAN *antiadrenergic (β-receptor)* [also: alprenolol HCl]
alprenolol HCl USAN *antiadrenergic (β-receptor)* [also: alprenolol]
alprenoxime HCl USAN *antiglaucoma agent*
alprostadil USAN, USP, INN, BAN *vasodilator; platelet aggregation inhibitor*
Alramucil effervescent powder OTC *bulk laxative* [psyllium hydrophilic mucilloid]
Alramucil Instant Mix unit dose packets OTC *bulk laxative* [psyllium hydrophilic mucilloid]
Alredase ℞ *investigational aldose reductase inhibitor for diabetic neuropathy* [tolrestat]
alrestatin INN *aldose reductase enzyme inhibitor* [also: alrestatin sodium]
alrestatin sodium USAN *aldose reductase enzyme inhibitor* [also: alrestatin]
alsactide INN
alseroxylon *antihypertensive; rauwolfia derivative*
Altace capsules ℞ *antihypertensive; angiotensin-converting enzyme inhibitor* [ramipril]
altanserin tartrate USAN, INN *serotonin antagonist*
altapizone INN

alteconazole INN
alteplase USAN, INN, BAN *tissue plasminogen activator (tPA)*
ALternaGEL liquid OTC *antacid* [aluminum hydroxide gel]
althiazide USAN *antihypertensive* [also: altizide]
altizide INN *antihypertensive* [also: althiazide]
altoqualine INN
Altracin (orphan: *pseudomembranous enterocolitis*) [bacitracin]
altrenogest USAN, INN, BAN *veterinary progestin*
altretamine USAN, INN *antineoplastic;* (orphan: *ovarian adenocarcinoma*)
Alu-Cap capsules OTC *antacid* [dried aluminum hydroxide gel]
Aludrox oral suspension OTC *antacid; antiflatulent* [aluminum hydroxide; magnesium hydroxide; simethicone]
alukalin [see: kaolin]
alum, ammonium USP *topical astringent*
alum, potassium USP *topical astringent*
Alum Boro effervescent tablets, powder OTC
Alumadrine tablets ℞ *decongestant; antihistamine; analgesic* [phenylpropanolamine HCl; chlorpheniramine maleate; acetaminophen]
Alumid Plus liquid (discontinued 1991) OTC *antacid; antiflatulent* [aluminum hydroxide; magnesium hydroxide; simethicone]
Alumid suspension (discontinued 1991) OTC *antacid* [aluminum hydroxide; magnesium hydroxide]
alumina & magnesia USP *antacid*
aluminosilicic acid, magnesium salt hydrate [see: silodrate]
aluminum *element (Al)*
aluminum, micronized *astringent*
aluminum acetate USP *astringent*
aluminum acetate solution *astringent wet dressing; Burow solution*

aluminum aminoacetate [see: dihydroxyaluminum aminoacetate]
aluminum ammonium sulfate dodecahydrate [see: alum, ammonium]
aluminum bismuth oxide [see: bismuth aluminate]
aluminum carbonate, basic USAN, USP *antacid*
aluminum chlorhydroxide [now: aluminum chlorohydrate]
aluminum chlorhydroxide alcohol soluble complex [now: aluminum chlorohydrex]
aluminum chloride USP *topical astringent for hyperhidrosis*
aluminum chloride, basic [see: aluminum sesquichlorohydrate]
aluminum chloride hexahydrate [see: aluminum chloride]
aluminum chloride hydroxide hydrate [see: aluminum chlorohydrate]
aluminum chlorohydrate USAN *anhidrotic*
aluminum chlorohydrex USAN *topical astringent*
aluminum chlorohydrol propylene glycol complex [now: aluminum chlorohydrex]
aluminum clofibrate INN, BAN
aluminum dihydroxyaminoacetate [see: dihydroxyaluminum aminoacetate]
aluminum glycinate, basic [see: dihydroxyaluminum aminoacetate]
aluminum hydroxide gel USP *antacid*
aluminum hydroxide gel, dried USP *antacid*
aluminum hydroxide glycine [see: dihydroxyaluminum aminoacetate]
aluminum hydroxide hydrate [see: algeldrate]
aluminum hydroxychloride [now: aluminum chlorohydrate]
aluminum magnesium carbonate hydroxide dihydrate [see: almagate]
aluminum magnesium hydroxide carbonate hydrate [see: hydrotalcite]
aluminum magnesium hydroxide oxide sulfate [see: almadrate sulfate]
aluminum magnesium hydroxide oxide sulfate hydrate [see: almadrate sulfate]
aluminum magnesium hydroxide sulfate [see: magaldrate]
aluminum magnesium hydroxide sulfate hydrate [see: magaldrate]
aluminum monostearate NF
aluminum oxide
Aluminum Paste ointment OTC *occlusive skin protectant* [metallic aluminum]
aluminum phosphate gel USP *(disapproved for use as an antacid in 1989)*
aluminum potassium sulfate dodecahydrate [see: alum, potassium]
aluminum sesquichlorohydrate USAN *anhidrotic*
aluminum sodium carbonate hydroxide [see: dihydroxyaluminum sodium carbonate]
aluminum subacetate USP *astringent*
aluminum sulfate USP
aluminum zirconium tetrachlorohydrex gly USAN *anhidrotic*
aluminum zirconium trichlorohydrex gly USAN *anhidrotic*
Alupent inhalation aerosol powder, solution for inhalation, tablets, syrup ℞ *bronchodilator* [metaproterenol sulfate]
Alurate elixir ℞ *sedative; hypnotic* [aprobarbital]
alusulf INN
Alu-Tab tablets OTC *antacid* [dried aluminum hydroxide gel]
alverine INN, BAN *anticholinergic* [also: alverine citrate]
alverine citrate USAN, NF *anticholinergic* [also: alverine]

Al-Vite tablets (discontinued 1993) ℞ *vitamin supplement* [multiple vitamins]
amabevan [see: carbarsone]
amacetam HCl [now: pramiracetam HCl]
amacetam sulfate [now: pramiracetam sulfate]
Amacodone tablets ℞ *narcotic analgesic* [hydrocodone bitartrate; acetaminophen]
amadinone INN *progestin* [also: amadinone acetate]
amadinone acetate USAN *progestin* [also: amadinone]
amafolone INN, BAN
amanozine INN
amantadine INN, BAN *antiviral* [also: amantadine HCl]
amantadine HCl USAN, USP *antiviral; antiparkinsonian* [also: amantadine]
amantanium bromide INN
amantocillin INN
Amaphen capsules ℞ *analgesic; antipyretic; sedative* [acetaminophen; caffeine; butalbital]
Amaphen with Codeine #3 capsules ℞ *narcotic analgesic; sedative* [codeine phosphate; acetaminophen; caffeine; butalbital]
amaranth (FD&C Red No. 2) USP
amarsan [see: acetarsone]
Amatine ℞ *investigational hypotension treatment* [midodrine]
ambamustine INN
ambasilide INN
ambazone INN, BAN
ambenonium chloride USP, INN, BAN *anticholinesterase muscle stimulant*
ambenoxan INN, BAN
Ambenyl Cough syrup ℞ *antihistamine; antitussive* [bromodiphenhydramine HCl; codeine phosphate; alcohol]
Ambenyl-D liquid OTC *decongestant; antitussive; expectorant* [pseudoephedrine HCl; dextromethorphan hydrobromide; guaifenesin; alcohol]
Ambi 10 bar OTC *antiseptic skin cleanser* [triclosan]
Ambi 10 cream OTC *topical keratolytic for acne* [benzoyl peroxide]
Ambi Skin Tone cream OTC *hyperpigmentation bleaching agent; sunscreen* [hydroquinone; padimate O]
ambicromil INN, BAN *prophylactic antiallergic* [also: probicromil calcium]
ambicromil calcium [see: probicromil calcium]
Ambien film-coated tablets ℞ *imidazopyridine-type sedative/hypnotic* [zolpidem]
AmBisome ℞ *investigational antifungal* [liposomal formulation of amphotericin B]
ambomycin USAN, INN *antineoplastic*
ambroxol INN
ambruticin USAN, INN *antifungal*
ambucaine INN
ambucetamide INN, BAN
ambuphylline USAN *diuretic; smooth muscle relaxant* [also: bufylline]
ambuside USAN, INN, BAN *diuretic*
ambuterol [see: mabuterol]
ambutonium bromide BAN
ambutoxate [see: ambucaine]
amcinafal USAN, INN *anti-inflammatory*
amcinafide USAN, INN *anti-inflammatory*
amcinonide USAN, USP, INN, BAN *topical corticosteroid*
Amcon 250 tablets (discontinued 1991) OTC *contact lens rinsing and storage solution* [sodium chloride for normal saline solution]
Amcort IM injection ℞ *glucocorticoid* [triamcinolone diacetate]
amdinocillin USAN, USP *antibacterial* [also: mecillinam]
amdinocillin pivoxil USAN *antibacterial* [also: pivmecillinam]

ameban [see: carbarsone]
amebarsone [see: carbarsone]
amebucort INN
amechol [see: methacholine chloride]
amedalin INN *antidepressant* [also: amedalin HCl]
amedalin HCl USAN *antidepressant* [also: amedalin]
ameltolide USAN, INN *anticonvulsant*
Amen tablets ℞ *progestin; secondary amenorrhea; functional uterine bleeding* [medroxyprogesterone acetate]
amenozine [see: amanozine]
Americaine Anesthetic aerosol spray OTC *topical local anesthetic* [benzocaine]
Americaine Anesthetic Lubricant gel ℞ *anesthetic lubricant for upper GI procedures* [benzocaine; benzalkonium chloride]
Americaine ointment, anorectal ointment OTC *topical anesthetic; antiseptic* [benzocaine; benzethonium chloride]
Americaine Otic ear drops ℞ *topical local anesthetic; antibacterial/antifungal* [benzocaine; benzethonium chloride]
americium *element (Am)*
Amesec capsules OTC *antiasthmatic; bronchodilator; decongestant* [aminophylline; ephedrine HCl]
amesergide USAN *serotonin antagonist*
ametantrone INN *antineoplastic* [also: ametantrone acetate]
ametantrone acetate USAN *antineoplastic* [also: ametantrone]
ametazole BAN [also: betazole HCl; betazole]
A-Methapred powder for injection ℞ *glucocorticoids* [methylprednisolone sodium succinate]
amethocaine BAN *topical anesthetic* [also: tetracaine]
amethocaine HCl BAN *local anesthetic* [also: tetracaine HCl]
amethopterin [now: methotrexate]

amezepine INN
amezinium metilsulfate INN
amfebutamone INN *antidepressant* [also: bupropion HCl; bupropion]
amfebutamone HCl [see: bupropion HCl]
amfecloral INN, BAN *anorexic* [also: amphecloral]
amfenac INN, BAN *anti-inflammatory* [also: amfenac sodium]
amfenac sodium USAN *anti-inflammatory* [also: amfenac]
amfepentorex INN
amfepramone INN *anorexiant* [also: diethylpropion HCl; diethylpropion]
amfepramone HCl *anorexiant* [see: diethylpropion HCl]
amfetamine INN CNS *stimulant* [also: amphetamine sulfate; amphetamine]
amfetaminil INN
amfilcon A USAN *hydrophilic contact lens material*
amflutizole USAN, INN *gout suppressant*
amfodyne [see: imidecyl iodine]
amfomycin INN *antibacterial* [also: amphomycin]
amfonelic acid USAN, INN, BAN CNS *stimulant*
Amgenal syrup ℞ *antihistamine; antitussive* [bromodiphenhydramine HCl; codeine phosphate; alcohol]
amibiarson [see: carbarsone]
Amicar IV infusion, tablets, syrup ℞ *systemic hemostatic; control excessive bleeding* [aminocaproic acid]
amicarbalide INN, BAN
amicibone INN
amicloral USAN *veterinary food additive*
amicycline USAN, INN *antibacterial*
amidantel INN, BAN
amidapsone USAN, INN *antiviral for poultry*
Amidate IV ℞ *general anesthetic* [etomidate]

amidefrine mesilate INN *adrenergic* [also: amidephrine mesylate; amidephrine]

amidephrine BAN *adrenergic* [also: amidephrine mesylate; amidefrine mesilate]

amidephrine mesylate USAN *adrenergic* [also: amidefrine mesilate; amidephrine]

amidofebrin [see: aminopyrine]

amidol [see: dimepheptanol]

amidone HCl [see: methadone HCl]

amidopyrazoline [see: aminopyrine]

amidopyrine [now: aminopyrine]

amidotrizoate sodium [see: diatrizoate sodium]

amidotrizoic acid [see: diatrizoic acid]

amiflamine INN

amifloverine INN

amifloxacin USAN, INN, BAN *antibacterial*

amifloxacin mesylate USAN *antibacterial*

amifostine USAN, INN, BAN *topical radioprotectant; (orphan: chemoprotective agent for cisplatin and cyclophosphamide)* [USAN previously used: ethiofos]

Amigesic film-coated tablets, capsules ℞ *analgesic; antipyretic; anti-inflammatory; antirheumatic* [salsalate]

amikacin USP, INN, BAN *antibacterial*

amikacin sulfate USAN, USP *aminoglycoside bactericidal antibiotic*

amikhelline INN

Amikin IV or IM injection, pediatric injection ℞ *aminoglycoside-type antibiotic* [amikacin sulfate]

amilomer INN

amiloride INN, BAN *potassium-sparing diuretic* [also: amiloride HCl]

amiloride HCl USAN, USP *potassium-sparing diuretic; (orphan: cystic fibrosis)* [also: amiloride]

Amina-21 capsules OTC *dietary supplement* [multiple amino acids]

aminacrine BAN *topical anti-infective* [also: aminacrine HCl; aminoacridine]

aminacrine HCl USAN *topical anti-infective/antiseptic* [also: aminoacridine; aminacrine]

Amin-Aid Instant Drink powder OTC *oral nutritional supplement for renal failure*

aminarsone [see: carbarsone]

amindocate INN

amine resin [see: polyamine-methylene resin]

amineptine INN

Aminess 5.2% IV infusion ℞ *nutritional therapy for renal failure* [multiple essential amino acids]

aminicotin [see: niacinamide]

aminitrozole INN *veterinary antibacterial* [also: nithiamide; acinitrazole]

Amino LIV powder OTC *dietary supplement* [multiple amino acids]

Amino VIL powder OTC *dietary supplement* [multiple amino acids]

aminoacetic acid [now: glycine]

aminoacridine INN *topical anti-infective* [also: aminacrine HCl; aminacrine]

aminoacridine HCl [see: aminacrine HCl]

9-aminoacridine monohydrochloride [see: aminacrine HCl]

***p*-aminobenzene-arsonic acid** [see: arsanilic acid]

***p*-aminobenzenesulfonamide** [see: sulfanilamide]

***p*-aminobenzene-sulfonylacetylimide** [see: sulfacetamide]

aminobenzoate potassium USP *analgesic*

aminobenzoate sodium USP *analgesic*

aminobenzoic acid USP *ultraviolet screen*

***p*-aminobenzoic acid** [see: aminobenzoic acid]

aminobenzylpenicillin [see: ampicillin]

aminocaproic acid USAN, USP, INN, BAN *systemic hemostatic*

aminocardol [see: aminophylline]

Amino-Cerv pH 5.5 Creme ℞ *anti-inflammatory; pH restorant* [urea; sodium propionate; methionine; cystine; inositol]

aminodeoxykanamycin [see: bekanamycin]

2-aminoethanethiol [see: cysteamine; mercaptamine]

2-aminoethanethiol HCl [see: cysteamine HCl]

2-aminoethanol [see: monoethanolamine]

aminoethyl nitrate INN

amino-ethyl-propanol [see: ambuphylline]

aminoform [see: methenamine]

aminoglutethimide USP, INN, BAN *adrenocortical suppressant; antineoplastic*

6-aminohexanoic acid [see: aminocaproic acid]

aminohippurate sodium USP *renal function test*

aminohippuric acid USP

***p*-aminohippuric acid** [see: aminohippuric acid]

aminohydroxypropylidene diphosphonate (APD) [see: pamidronate disodium]

aminoisobutanol [see: ambuphylline]

aminoisometradine [see: methionine]

aminometradine INN, BAN

Amino-Min-D capsules OTC *dietary supplement* [multiple minerals; vitamin D; betaine HCl; glutamic acid HCl]

aminonat [see: protein hydrolysate]

Amino-Opti-C sustained-release tablets OTC *dietary supplement* [vitamin C; lemon & rose hips bioflavonoids; rutin; hesperidin]

aminopentamide sulfate [see: dimevamide]

aminophenazone INN [also: aminopyrine]

aminophenazone cyclamate INN

***p*-aminophenylarsonic acid** [see: arsanilic acid]

aminophylline USP, INN, BAN *smooth muscle relaxant; bronchodilator*

Aminoprel capsules (discontinued 1992) OTC *dietary supplement* [multiple amino acids & minerals; vitamins B_6 & C]

aminopromazine INN [also: proquamezine]

aminopterin sodium INN, BAN

4-aminopyridine (*orphan: multiple sclerosis*)

aminopyrine NF [also: aminophenazone]

aminoquin naphthoate [see: pamaquine naphthoate]

aminoquinol INN

aminoquinoline [see: aminoquinol]

4-aminoquinoline [see: chloroquine phosphate]

8-aminoquinoline [see: primaquine phosphate]

aminoquinuride INN

aminorex USAN, INN, BAN *anorexic*

aminosalicylate calcium USP, NF

aminosalicylate potassium USP

aminosalicylate sodium (*p*-aminosalicylate sodium) USP *bacteriostatic; tuberculosis retreatment*

aminosalicylic acid (4-aminosalicylic acid) USP *antibacterial; tuberculostatic;* (*orphan: ulcerative colitis; tuberculosis*)

5-aminosalicylic acid (5-ASA) [see: mesalamine]

aminosalyle sodium [see: aminosalicylate sodium]

aminosidine sulfate [see: paromomycin sulfate]

aminosuccinic acid [see: aspartic acid]

Aminosyn (pH6) 8.5% IV infusion (discontinued 1992) ℞ *total parenteral nutrition; peripheral parenteral* *nutrition* [multiple essential & nonessential amino acids]

Aminosyn II 3.5% in 5% (25%) Dextrose; Aminosyn II 4.25% in 10% (20%, 25%) Dextrose; Aminosyn II 5% in 25% Dextrose IV infusion ℞ *total parenteral nutrition (except 3.5% in 5%); peripheral parenteral nutrition (not 20% and 25%)* [multiple essential & nonessential amino acids; dextrose]

Aminosyn II 3.5% M in 5% Dextrose; Aminosyn II 4.25% M in 10% Dextrose IV infusion ℞ *total parenteral nutrition (4.25% in 10% only); peripheral parenteral nutrition (both)* [multiple essential & nonessential amino acids & electrolytes; dextrose]

Aminosyn 3.5% (5%, 7%, 8.5%, 10%); Aminosyn (pH6) 10%; Aminosyn II 3.5% (5%, 7%, 8.5%, 10%, 15%); Aminosyn-PF 7% (10%) IV infusion ℞ *total parenteral nutrition (except 3.5%); peripheral parenteral nutrition (all)* [multiple essential & nonessential amino acids]

Aminosyn 3.5% M; Aminosyn II 3.5% M IV infusion ℞ *peripheral parenteral nutrition* [multiple essential & nonessential amino acids; electrolytes]

Aminosyn 7% (8.5%) with Electrolytes; Aminosyn II 7% (8.5%, 10%) with Electrolytes IV infusion ℞ *total parenteral nutrition; peripheral parenteral nutrition* [multiple essential & nonessential amino acids; electrolytes]

Aminosyn-HBC 7% IV infusion ℞ *nutritional therapy for high metabolic stress* [multiple branched-chain essential & nonessential amino acids; electrolytes]

Aminosyn-RF 5.2% IV infusion ℞ *nutritional therapy for renal failure* [multiple essential amino acids; arginine]

aminothiazole INN

aminotrate phosphate [see: trolnitrate phosphate]

aminoxaphen [see: aminorex]

aminoxytriphene INN

aminoxytropine tropate HCl [see: atropine oxide HCl]

amiodarone USAN, INN, BAN *ventricular antiarrhythmic*

amiodarone HCl *antiarrhythmic*

Amipaque powder for injection ℞ *parenteral radiopaque agent* [metrizamide]

amiperone INN

amiphenazole INN, BAN

amipizone INN

amipramidine [see: amiloride HCl]

amiprilose INN *anti-inflammatory* [also: amiprilose HCl]

amiprilose HCl USAN *anti-inflammatory* [also: amiprilose]

amiquinsin INN *antihypertensive* [also: amiquinsin HCl]

amiquinsin HCl USAN *antihypertensive* [also: amiquinsin]

amisometradine NF, INN, BAN

amisulpride INN

amiterol INN

Ami-Tex LA long-acting tablets ℞ *decongestant; expectorant* [phenylpropanolamine HCl; guaifenesin]

amithiozone [see: thioacetazone; thiacetazone]

Amitone chewable tablets OTC *antacid* [calcium carbonate]

amitraz USAN, INN, BAN *scabicide*

amitriptyline INN, BAN *antidepressant* [also: amitriptyline HCl]

amitriptyline HCl USP *tricyclic antidepressant* [also: amitriptyline]

amitriptylinoxide INN

amixetrine INN

amlexanox INN

amlodipine INN, BAN *antianginal; antihypertensive* [also: amlodipine besylate]

amlodipine besylate USAN *antianginal; antihypertensive* [also: amlodipine]

amlodipine maleate USAN *antianginal; antihypertensive*

ammoidin [see: methoxsalen]

ammonia [see: ammonia spirit, aromatic]

ammonia N 13 USAN, USP *radioactive diagnostic aid for cardiac and liver imaging*

ammonia solution, strong NF *solvent; source of ammonia*

ammonia spirit, aromatic USP *respiratory stimulant*

ammoniated mercury [see: mercury, ammoniated]

ammonium alum [see: alum, ammonium]

ammonium benzoate USP

ammonium biphosphate *urinary acidifier*

ammonium carbonate NF *source of ammonia*

ammonium chloride USP *acidifier; nonprescription diuretic*

ammonium ichthosulfonate [see: ichthammol]

ammonium mandelate USP

ammonium molybdate USP *dietary molybdenum supplement*

ammonium molybdate tetrahydrate [see: ammonium molybdate]

ammonium phosphate NF *pharmaceutic aid*

ammonium salicylate NF

ammonium valerate NF

ammophyllin [see: aminophylline]

AMO Endosol; AMO Endosol Extra ophthalmic solution ℞ *intraocular irrigating solution* [balanced saline solution]

amobarbital USP, INN *sedative; hypnotic; anticonvulsant* [also: amylobarbitone]

amobarbital sodium USP *hypnotic; sedative; anticonvulsant*

amocaine chloride [see: amolanone HCl]

amocarzine INN

amodiaquine USP, INN, BAN *antiprotozoal*

amodiaquine HCl USP *antimalarial*

Amodopa tablets ℞ *antihypertensive* [methyldopa]

amogastrin INN

amolanone INN

amolanone HCl [see: amolanone]

amonafide INN

Amonidrin tablets OTC *expectorant* [guaifenesin]

Amoni-Opti-E capsules OTC *vitamin supplement* [vitamin E]

amoproxan INN

amopyroquine INN

amorolfine USAN, INN, BAN *antimycotic*

Amosan powder OTC *oral antibacterial* [sodium peroxyborate monohydrate]

amoscanate INN

amosulalol INN

amotriphene [see: aminoxytriphene]

amoxapine USAN, INN, BAN *tricyclic antidepressant*

amoxecaine INN

amoxicillin USAN, USP *bactericidal antibiotic* [also: amoxicilline; amoxycillin]

amoxicillin trihydrate *bactericidal antibiotic*

amoxicilline INN *antibacterial* [also: amoxicillin; amoxycillin]

Amoxil capsules, powder for oral suspension, chewable tablets, pediatric drops ℞ *penicillin-type antibiotic* [amoxicillin trihydrate]

amoxycillin BAN *antibacterial* [also: amoxicillin; amoxicilline]

amoxydramine camsilate INN

amoxydramine camsylate [see: amoxydramine camsilate]

AMP; A$_5$MP (adenosine monophosphate) [see: adenosine phosphate]

amperozide INN, BAN

amphecloral USAN *anorexic* [also: amfecloral]
amphenidone INN
amphetamine BAN *CNS stimulant* [also: amphetamine sulfate; amfetamine]
d-**amphetamine** [see: dextroamphetamine]
(+)-amphetamine [see: dextroamphetamine]
l-**amphetamine** [see: levamphetamine]
(−)-amphetamine [see: levamphetamine]
amphetamine aspartate *CNS stimulant*
amphetamine complex (resin complex of amphetamine & dextroamphetamine) [q.v.]
amphetamine phosphate, dextro [see: dextroamphetamine phosphate]
amphetamine succinate, levo [see: levamphetamine succinate]
amphetamine sulfate USP *CNS stimulant* [also: amfetamine; amphetamine]
amphetamine sulfate, dextro [see: dextroamphetamine sulfate]
Amphocil ℞ *investigational antifungal* [lipid-complex formulation of amphotericin B]
amphocortrin [see: amphomycin]
Amphojel tablets, oral suspension OTC *antacid* [aluminum hydroxide gel]
amphomycin USAN, BAN *antibacterial* [also: amfomycin]
amphotalide INN
amphotericin B USP, INN, BAN *antifungal*
amphotericin B lipid complex (*orphan: cryptococcal meningitis*)
ampicillin USAN, USP, INN, BAN *bactericidal antibiotic*
ampicillin sodium USAN, USP *bactericidal antibiotic*
ampiroxicam INN, BAN

Ampligen *investigational antiviral/immunomodulator;* (*orphan: AIDS*) [poly I: poly C12U]
amprocidum [see: amprolium]
amprolium USP, INN, BAN *coccidiostat for poultry*
amprotropine phosphate
ampyrimine INN
ampyzine INN *CNS stimulant* [also: ampyzine sulfate]
ampyzine sulfate USAN *CNS stimulant* [also: ampyzine]
amquinate USAN, INN *antimalarial*
amrinone USAN, INN, BAN *cardiotonic*
amrinone lactate *cardiac vasodilator*
AMSA; *m*-AMSA (acridinylamine methanesulfon anisidide) [see: amsacrine]
amsacrine USAN, INN, BAN *investigational antineoplastic;* (*orphan: acute adult leukemia*)
Amsidyl (*orphan: acute adult leukemia*) [amsacrine]
Amvisc; Amvisc Plus intraocular injection ℞ *viscoelastic agent for ophthalmic surgery* [sodium hyaluronate]
amyl alcohol, tertiary [see: amylene hydrate]
amyl nitrite USP *vasodilator; antianginal*
amylase [see: alpha amylase]
amylene hydrate NF *solvent*
amylmetacresol INN, BAN
amylobarbitone BAN [also: amobarbital]
amylopectin sulfate, sodium salt [see: sodium amylosulfate]
amylosulfate sodium [see: sodium amylosulfate]
Amytal Sodium Pulvules (capsules), powder for injection (discontinued 1992) ℞ *sedative; hypnotic; anxiolytic; anticonvulsant* [amobarbital sodium]

Amytal tablets (discontinued 1991) ℞ *sedative; hypnotic; anxiolytic* [amobarbital]

Anacin, Aspirin Free film-coated tablets OTC *analgesic; antipyretic* [acetaminophen]

Anacin coated caplets, coated tablets OTC *analgesic; antipyretic; anti-inflammatory* [aspirin; caffeine]

Anacin P.M., Aspirin Free film-coated caplets OTC *analgesic; antipyretic; antihistaminic sleep aid* [acetaminophen; diphenhydramine HCl]

Anacin-3 (name changed to Aspirin Free Anacin in 1992)

Anacin-3, Children's chewable tablets, liquid (discontinued 1993) OTC *analgesic; antipyretic* [acetaminophen]

Anacin-3, Infants' drops (discontinued 1993) OTC *analgesic; antipyretic* [acetaminophen]

Anadrol-50 tablets ℞ *anabolic steroid for anemias* [oxymetholone]

anafebrina [see: aminopyrine]

Anafranil capsules ℞ *treatment of obsessive-compulsive disorders* [clomipramine HCl]

anagestone INN *progestin* [also: anagestone acetate]

anagestone acetate USAN *progestin* [also: anagestone]

anagrelide INN *antithrombotic; (orphan: polycythemia vera; essential thrombocythemia; thrombocytosis)* [also: anagrelide HCl]

anagrelide HCl USAN *antithrombotic* [also: anagrelide]

Ana-Guard injection ℞ *anaphylaxis emergency treatment* [epinephrine]

Anaids tablets ℞ *antacid; sedative* [calcium carbonate; phenobarbital sodium]

anakinra *investigational recombinant interleukin-1 receptor agonist for sepsis and rheumatoid arthritis*

Ana-Kit ℞ *emergency treatment of anaphylaxis* [epinephrine; chlorpheniramine maleate; alcohol pads; tourniquet]

Analbalm emulsion OTC *counterirritant* [methyl salicylate; camphor; menthol]

Analgesia Creme OTC *topical analgesic* [trolamine salicylate]

Analgesic Balm OTC *counterirritant* [methyl salicylate; menthol]

analgesine [see: antipyrine]

Analpram-HC cream ℞ *topical corticosteroid; local anesthetic* [hydrocortisone acetate; pramoxine]

Anamine syrup ℞ *decongestant; antihistamine* [pseudoephedrine HCl; chlorpheniramine maleate]

Anamine T.D. sustained-release capsules ℞ *decongestant; antihistamine* [pseudoephedrine HCl; chlorpheniramine maleate]

ananain *(orphan: enzymatic debridement of severe burns)*

Anaprox; Anaprox DS film-coated tablets ℞ *nonsteroidal anti-inflammatory drug (NSAID); antiarthritic; analgesic* [naproxen sodium]

anarel [see: guanadrel sulfate]

anaritide INN, BAN *antihypertensive; diuretic* [also: anaritide acetate]

anaritide acetate USAN *antihypertensive; diuretic; (orphan: adjunct to renal transplant)* [also: anaritide]

Anaspaz tablets ℞ *anticholinergic; antispasmodic* [hyoscyamine sulfate]

Anatrast paste ℞ *GI contrast radiopaque agent* [barium sulfate]

Anatuss LA tablets ℞ *decongestant; expectorant* [pseudoephedrine HCl; guaifenesin]

Anatuss syrup OTC *decongestant; antitussive; expectorant* [phenylpropanolamine HCl; dextromethorphan hydrobromide; guaifenesin]

Anatuss tablets ℞ *decongestant; antitussive; expectorant; analgesic* [phenylpropanolamine HCl; dextromethorphan hydrobromide; guaifenesin; acetaminophen]

anaxirone INN
anayodin [see: chiniofon]
anazocine INN
anazolene sodium USAN, INN *blood volume and cardiac output test* [also: sodium anoxynaphthonate]
Anbesol, Baby gel OTC *topical oral anesthetic* [benzocaine]
Anbesol, Maximum Strength oral liquid, gel OTC *topical oral anesthetic; antiseptic* [benzocaine; alcohol]
Anbesol oral liquid, gel OTC *topical oral anesthetic; antipruritic/counterirritant; antiseptic* [benzocaine; phenol; alcohol]
ancarolol INN
Ancef powder for IV or IM injection ℞ *cephalosporin-type antibiotic* [cefazolin sodium]
ancitabine INN
Ancobon capsules ℞ *antifungal* [flucytosine]
ancrod USAN, INN, BAN *anticoagulant; (orphan: thrombocytopenia or thrombosis)*
Andoin ointment (discontinued 1991) OTC *moisturizer; emollient* [vitamins A & D; allantoin]
Andozac ℞ *investigational treatment for benign prostatic hyperplasia*
Andro 100; Andro 200 [see: depAndro 100; depAndro 200]
Andro 100 IM injection ℞ *androgen replacement for delayed puberty or breast cancer* [testosterone]
Andro L.A. 200 IM injection ℞ *androgen replacement for delayed puberty or breast cancer* [testosterone enanthate]
Androcur *(orphan: severe hirsutism)* [cyproterone acetate]
Andro-Cyp 100; Andro-Cyp 200 IM injection ℞ *androgen replacement for delayed puberty or breast cancer* [testosterone cypionate]
Andro/Fem IM injection ℞ *estrogen/androgen for menopausal vasomotor symptoms* [estradiol cypionate; testosterone cypionate]
Androgyn [see: depAndrogyn]
Androgyn L.A. IM injection ℞ *estrogen/androgen for menopausal vasomotor symptoms* [estradiol valerate; testosterone enanthate]
Android-5 tablets (discontinued 1991) ℞ *androgen for male hypogonadism, impotence and breast cancer* [methyltestosterone]
Android-10; Android-25 tablets ℞ *androgen for male hypogonadism, impotence and breast cancer* [methyltestosterone]
Android-F tablets (discontinued 1991) ℞ *androgen hormone for male hypogonadism and inoperable breast cancer* [fluoxymesterone]
Androlone-D 200 IM injection ℞ *anabolic steroid for anemia of renal insufficiency* [nandrolone decanoate]
Andronaq-50 injection (discontinued 1991) ℞ *androgen* [testosterone]
Andronaq-LA injection (discontinued 1991) ℞ *androgen* [testosterone cypionate]
Andronate 100; Andronate 200 IM injection ℞ *androgen replacement for delayed puberty or breast cancer* [testosterone cypionate]
Andropository-200 IM injection ℞ *androgen replacement for delayed puberty or breast cancer* [testosterone enanthate]
androstanazole [now: stanozolol]
androstane [see: stanolone; androstanolone]
androstanolone INN [also: stanolone]
androtest P [see: testosterone propionate]
Androvite; Androvite for Men tablets OTC *vitamin/mineral/iron supplement* [multiple vitamins & minerals; iron; folic acid; biotin]
Anectine IV or IM injection, Flo-Pack (powder for injection) ℞ *neu-*

romuscular blocker [succinylcholine chloride]

Anergan 25; Anergan 50 injection ℞ *anthistamine; motion sickness; sleep aid; antiemetic; sedative* [promethazine HCl]

anertan [see: testosterone propionate]

Anestacon solution ℞ *GU mucous membrane anesthetic* [lidocaine HCl]

anesthesin [see: benzocaine]

anesthrone [see: benzocaine]

anethaine [see: tetracaine HCl]

anethole NF *flavoring agent*

aneurine HCl [see: thiamine HCl]

Anexsia 5/500; Anexsia 7.5/650 tablets ℞ *narcotic analgesic* [hydrocodone bitartrate; acetaminophen]

Angio-Conray injection ℞ *parenteral angiography radiopaque agent* [iothalamate sodium]

angiotensin amide USAN, NF, BAN *vasoconstrictor* [also: angiotensinamide]

angiotensinamide INN *vasoconstrictor* [also: angiotensin amide]

Angiovist 282 injection ℞ *parenteral radiopaque agent* [diatrizoate meglumine]

Angiovist 292; Angiovist 370 injection ℞ *parenteral radiopaque agent* [diatrizoate meglumine; diatrizoate sodium]

anhydrohydroxyprogesterone [now: ethisterone]

Anhydron tablets (discontinued 1991) ℞ *diuretic; antihypertensive* [cyclothiazide]

anhydrous lanolin [see: lanolin, anhydrous]

anidoxime USAN, INN, BAN *analgesic*

anilamide INN

anileridine USP, NF, INN, BAN *narcotic analgesic*

anileridine HCl USP *narcotic analgesic*

anilopam INN *analgesic* [also: anilopam HCl]

anilopam HCl USAN *analgesic* [also: anilopam]

anion exchange resin [see: polyamine-methylene resin]

anipamil INN

aniracetam USAN, INN *mental performance enhancer*

anirolac USAN, INN *anti-inflammatory; analgesic*

anisacril INN

anise oil NF

anisindione NF, INN, BAN *anticoagulant*

anisopirol INN

anisopyradamine [see: pyrilamine maleate]

anisotropine methylbromide USAN *peptic ulcer adjunct* [also: octatropine methylbromide]

anisoylated plasminogen streptokinase activator complex (APSAC) [see: anistreplase]

anistreplase USAN, INN, BAN *fibrinolytic; thrombolytic enzyme*

anitrazafen USAN, INN *topical anti-inflammatory*

Anocaine Hemorrhoidal suppositories (discontinued 1992) OTC *topical anesthetic; astringent* [benzocaine; zinc oxide; bismuth subgallate; balsam Peru]

anodynine [see: antipyrine]

anodynon [see: ethyl chloride]

Anodynos DHC tablets ℞ *narcotic analgesic* [hydrocodone bitartrate; acetaminophen]

Anodynos Forte tablets OTC *antihistamine; decongestant; analgesic; antipyretic* [chlorpheniramine maleate; phenylephrine HCl; acetaminophen; salicylamide; caffeine]

Anodynos tablets OTC *analgesic; antipyretic; anti-inflammatory* [aspirin; salicylamide; caffeine]

Anoquan capsules ℞ *analgesic; antipyretic; anti-inflammatory; sedative* [acetaminophen; caffeine; butalbital]

Anorex capsules ℞ *anorexiant* [phendimetrazine tartrate]
anovlar [see: norethindrone & ethinyl estradiol]
Anoxine-AM capsules (discontinued 1991) ℞ *anorexiant* [phentermine HCl]
anoxomer USAN *antioxidant; food additive*
anoxynaphthonate sodium [see: anazolene sodium]
anpirtoline INN
Ansaid tablets ℞ *nonsteroidal anti-inflammatory drug (NSAID); antiarthritic* [flurbiprofen]
Ansamycin (name changed to Mycobutin in 1993)
ansoxetine INN
Anspor capsules, oral suspension (discontinued 1991) ℞ *cephalosporin-type antibiotic* [cephradine]
Answer; Answer 2; Answer Plus; Answer Plus 2; Answer Quick & Simple home test kit OTC *in vitro diagnostic aid for urine pregnancy test*
Answer Ovulation test kit OTC *in vitro diagnostic aid to predict ovulation time*
Antabuse tablets ℞ *deterrent to alcohol consumption* [disulfiram]
antafenite INN
Anta-Gel; Anta-Gel II oral suspension OTC *antacid; antiflatulent* [aluminum hydroxide; magnesium hydroxide; simethicone]
antastan [see: antazoline HCl]
antazoline INN, BAN [also: antazoline HCl]
antazoline HCl USP [also: antazoline]
antazoline phosphate USP *antihistamine*
Antazoline-V eye drops ℞ *topical ocular decongestant/antihistamine* [naphazoline HCl; antazoline phosphate]
antazonite INN
antelmycin INN *anthelmintic* [also: anthelmycin]
anterior pituitary

anthelmycin USAN *anthelmintic* [also: antelmycin]
anthiolimine INN
Anthra-Derm ointment ℞ *topical antipsoriatic* [anthralin]
anthralin USP, NF *antipsoriatic* [also: dithranol]
anthramycin USAN *antineoplastic* [also: antramycin]
anthraquinone of cascara [see: cascara sagrada]
anti pan T lymphocyte monoclonal antibody (*orphan: bone marrow transplants; graft vs. host disease*)
anti-A blood grouping serum USP *in vitro blood testing*
antib [see: thioacetazone; thiacetazone]
anti-B blood grouping serum USP *in vitro blood testing*
anti-B4-blocked ricin (*orphan: leukemia*)
antibason [see: methylthiouracil]
antibiotic 273a₁ [see: paldimycin]
AntibiOtic ear drops, otic suspension ℞ *topical corticosteroidal anti-inflammatory; antibiotic* [polymyxin B sulfate; neomycin sulfate; hydrocortisone]
Antibiotic Ear Solution ℞ *topical corticosteroidal anti-inflammatory; antibiotic* [polymyxin B sulfate; neomycin sulfate; hydrocortisone]
Antibiotic Ear Suspension ℞ *topical corticosteroidal anti-inflammatory; antibiotic* [polymyxin B sulfate; neomycin sulfate; hydrocortisone]
anti-C blood grouping serum [see: blood grouping serum, anti-C]
anti-c blood grouping serum [see: blood grouping serum, anti-c]
anti-CD3 [see: muromonab-CD3]
anticoagulant citrate dextrose (ACD) solution USP *anticoagulant for storage of whole blood and during cardiac surgery*

anticoagulant citrate phosphate dextrose adenine solution USP *anticoagulant for storage of whole blood*

anticoagulant citrate phosphate dextrose solution USP *anticoagulant for storage of whole blood*

anticoagulant heparin solution USP *anticoagulant for storage of whole blood*

anticoagulant sodium citrate solution USP *anticoagulant for plasma and for blood for fractionation*

anticytomegalovirus monoclonal antibodies *(orphan: cytomegalovirus infection in AIDS and organ transplant patients)*

anti-E blood grouping serum [see: blood grouping serum, anti-E]

anti-e blood grouping serum [see: blood grouping serum, anti-e]

antienite INN

antiepilepsirine *(orphan: generalized tonic-clonic epilepsy)*

antiestrogen [see: tamoxifen citrate]

antifebrin [see: acetanilide]

antifolic acid [see: methotrexate]

antihemophilic factor (AHF) USP *antihemophilic*

Antihemophilic Factor (Porcine) Hyate:C powder for IV injection ℞ *antihemophilic* [antihemophilic factor VIII:C]

antihemophilic factor, human [now: antihemophilic factor]

antihemophilic factor, recombinant (rFVIII) *(orphan: hemophilia A)*

antihemophilic factor A [see: antihemophilic factor]

antihemophilic factor B [see: factor IX complex]

antihemophilic globulin (AHG) [see: antihemophilic factor]

antihemophilic human plasma [now: plasma, antihemophilic human]

antihemophilic plasma, human [now: plasma, antihemophilic human]

antiheparin [see: protamine sulfate]

anti-inhibitor coagulant complex *antihemophilic*

anti-J5MAB *(orphan status withdrawn 1993)*

Antilirium IV or IM injection ℞ *anticholinergic antagonist; (orphan: Friedreich's and other ataxias)* [physostigmine salicylate]

antimelanoma antibody XMMME-001-DTPA 111 indium *(orphan: diagnostic imaging for melanoma)*

antimelanoma antibody XMMME-001-RTA *(orphan: stage III melanoma)*

Antiminth oral suspension OTC *anthelmintic* [pyrantel pamoate]

antimony *element (Sb)*

antimony potassium tartrate USP *antischistosomal*

antimony sodium tartrate USP *antischistosomal*

antimony sodium thioglycollate USP

antimony sulfide [see: antimony trisulfide colloid]

antimony trisulfide colloid USAN *pharmaceutic aid*

antimonyl potassium tartrate [see: antimony potassium tartrate]

anti-MY9-blocked ricin *(orphan: myeloid leukemia)*

Anti-My⁹-bR *(orphan: myeloid leukemia)* [blocked ricin conjugated murine MCA myeloid cells (CD-33)]

Antinea cream (discontinued 1992) OTC *topical antifungal; keratolytic* [benzoic acid; salicylic acid]

anti-pellagra vitamin [see: niacin]

anti-pernicious anemia principle [see: cyanocobalamin]

antipyrine USP *analgesic; (orphan: drug-metabolizing capacity tests)* [also: phenazone]

N-antipyrinylnicotinamide [see: nifenazone]

antirabies serum (ARS) USP *passive immunizing agent*

anti-Rh typing serums [now: blood grouping serums]
antiscorbutic vitamin [see: ascorbic acid]
Antispas IM injection ℞ *gastrointestinal antispasmodic* [dicyclomine HCl]
Antispasmodic elixir, tablets ℞ *antispasmodic; sedative* [phenobarbital; hyoscyamine sulfate; atropine sulfate; scopolamine hydrobromide]
antisterility vitamin [see: vitamin E]
Anti-T Lymphocyte Immunotoxin XMMLY-H65-RTA (*orphan: bone marrow transplants; graft vs. host disease*) [anti pan T lymphocyte monoclonal antibody]
anti-TAP-72 immunotoxin (*orphan: metastatic colorectal adenocarcinoma*)
antithrombin III (AT-III) INN, BAN (*orphan: thrombosis and pulmonary emboli; AT-III deficiency*)
antithrombin III, human (*orphan: antithrombin III deficiency; thrombosis*) [see: antithrombin III]
antithrombin III concentrate IV (*orphan: prevent and treat thromboembolism in AT-III deficiency*) [see: antithrombin III]
antithymocyte globulin [see: lymphocyte immune globulin, antithymocyte]
antitoxin botulism equine (ABE) [see: botulism equine antitoxin, trivalent]
α_1-**antitrypsin** [see: alpha$_1$-antitrypsin]
Anti-Tuss syrup OTC *expectorant* [guaifenesin; alcohol]
antivenin (Crotalidae) polyvalent USP *passive immunizing agent*
antivenin (Crotalidae) purified (avian) (*orphan: Crotalidae snake bite*)
antivenin (Latrodectus mactans) USP *passive immunizing agent*
antivenin (Micrurus fulvius) USP *passive immunizing agent*
Antivert; Antivert/25; Antivert/25 Chewable; Antivert/50 tablets ℞ *anticholinergic; antihistamine; antivertigo agent; motion sickness preventative* [meclizine]
antixerophthalmic vitamin [see: vitamin A]
antrafenine INN
antramycin INN *antineoplastic* [also: anthramycin]
Antril ℞ *investigational treatment for sepsis, rheumatoid arthritis, graft versus host disease and leukemia* [anakinra]
Antrizine tablets ℞ *anticholinergic; antihistamine; antivertigo agent; motion sickness preventative* [meclizine]
Antrocol capsules, tablets, elixir ℞ *anticholinergic; sedative* [atropine sulfate; phenobarbital]
Antrypol (available only from the Centers for Disease Control) ℞ *investigational anti-infective for trypanosomiasis and onchocerciasis* [suramin sodium]
Anturane tablets, capsules ℞ *uricosuric for gout* [sulfinpyrazone]
Anucort rectal suppositories (discontinued 1991) ℞ *topical corticosteroidal anti-inflammatory; antipruritic* [hydrocortisone acetate; zinc oxide; bismuth salts]
Anucort-HC rectal suppositories ℞ *topical corticosteroidal anti-inflammatory; antipruritic* [hydrocortisone acetate]
Anugard-H.C. rectal suppositories (discontinued 1991) ℞ *topical corticosteroidal anti-inflammatory; antipruritic* [hydrocortisone acetate; zinc oxide; bismuth salts]
Anumed rectal suppositories OTC *astringent; emollient/protectant* [bismuth subgallate; bismuth resorcin compound; benzyl benzoate; zinc oxide; balsam Peru]
Anumed HC rectal suppositories ℞ *topical corticosteroidal anti-inflammatory; antipruritic* [hydrocortisone acetate; zinc oxide; bismuth salts]

Anuprep HC rectal suppositories ℞ *topical corticosteroidal anti-inflammatory; antipruritic* [hydrocortisone acetate]

Anuprep Hemorrhoidal rectal suppositories OTC *astringent; emollient/protectant* [bismuth subgallate; bismuth resorcin compound; benzyl benzoate; zinc oxide; balsam Peru]

Anusol anorectal ointment OTC *topical anesthetic; antiseptic; astringent* [pramoxine HCl; benzyl benzoate; balsam Peru; zinc oxide]

Anusol rectal suppositories OTC *astringent; emollient/protectant* [bismuth subgallate; bismuth resorcin compound; benzyl benzoate; zinc oxide; balsam Peru]

Anusol-HC 1 ointment ℞ *topical corticosteroid* [hydrocortisone]

Anusol-HC 2.5% cream ℞ *topical corticosteroid* [hydrocortisone]

Anusol-HC rectal suppositories ℞ *topical corticosteroidal anti-inflammatory; antipruritic* [hydrocortisone acetate]

Anxanil film-coated tablets ℞ *anxiolytic* [hydroxyzine HCl]

AOPA (ara-C, Oncovin, prednisone, asparaginase) *chemotherapy protocol*

AOPE (Adriamycin, Oncovin, prednisone, etoposide) *chemotherapy protocol*

Aosept solution OTC *contact lens disinfectant*

AP injection ℞ *diagnosis and treatment of allergies* [epidermal/environmental allergenic extracts]

APAC Improved tablets (discontinued 1991) OTC *analgesic; antipyretic; anti-inflammatory* [aspirin; caffeine]

Apacet chewable tablets OTC *analgesic; antipyretic* [acetaminophen]

apafant INN

apalcillin sodium USAN, INN *antibacterial*

APAP (N-acetyl-p-aminophenol) [see: acetaminophen]

APAP drops, elixir, tablets, chewable tablets, caplets, suppositories OTC *analgesic; antipyretic* [acetaminophen]

Apatate liquid OTC *vitamin supplement* [vitamins B_1, B_6 & B_{12}]

apazone USAN *anti-inflammatory* [also: azapropazone]

APC (AMSA, prednisone, chlorambucil) *chemotherapy protocol*

APC (aspirin, phenacetin & caffeine) [q.v.]

APD (aminohydroxypropylidene diphosphonate) [see: pamidronate disodium]

APE (ara-C, Platinol, etoposide) *chemotherapy protocol*

Aphrodyne tablets ℞ *no approved uses; sympatholytic; mydriatic; aphrodisiac* [yohimbine HCl]

apicillin [see: ampicillin]

apicycline INN

apiquel fumarate [see: aminorex]

A.P.L. powder for injection ℞ *hormone for prepubertal cryptorchidism and hypogonadism* [chorionic gonadotropin]

Aplisol intradermal injection ℞ *tuberculosis skin test* [tuberculin purified protein derivative]

Aplitest single-use intradermal puncture test device ℞ *tuberculosis skin test* [tuberculin purified protein derivative]

aplonidine HCl [see: apraclonidine HCl]

APO (Adriamycin, prednisone, Oncovin) *chemotherapy protocol*

apodol [see: anileridine HCl]

apomorphine BAN *emetic* [also: apomorphine HCl]

apomorphine HCl USP *emetic* [also: apomorphine]

apovincamine INN

APPG (aqueous penicillin G procaine) [see: penicillin G procaine]

Appli-Kit (trademarked form) *ointment and adhesive dosage covers*
Appli-Ruler OTC *dose-determining pads*
Appli-Tape OTC *dosage covers*
apraclonidine INN, BAN *topical adrenergic for glaucoma* [also: apraclonidine HCl]
apraclonidine HCl USAN *topical adrenergic for glaucoma* [also: apraclonidine]
apramycin USAN, INN, BAN *antibacterial*
Aprazone capsules ℞ *uricosuric for gout* [sulfinpyrazone]
Apresazide 25/25; Apresazide 50/50; Apresazide 100/50 capsules ℞ *antihypertensive* [hydralazine HCl; hydrochlorothiazide]
Apresoline HCl tablets, IV or IM injection ℞ *antihypertensive; vasodilator* [hydralazine HCl]
Apresoline-Esidrix tablets (discontinued 1992) ℞ *antihypertensive; diuretic* [hydralazine HCl; hydrochlorothiazide]
aprindine USAN, INN, BAN *antiarrhythmic*
aprindine HCl USAN *antiarrhythmic*
aprobarbital NF, INN *sedative*
Aprodine tablets OTC *decongestant; antihistamine* [pseudoephedrine HCl; triprolidine HCl]
Aprodine with C syrup ℞ *decongestant; antihistamine; antitussive* [pseudoephedrine HCl; triprolidine HCl; codeine phosphate; alcohol]
aprofene INN
aprotinin USAN, INN, BAN *proteinase enzyme inhibitor*
Aprozide 25/25; Aprozide 50/50; Aprozide 100/50 capsules ℞ *antihypertensive* [hydrochlorothiazide; hydralazine HCl]
A.P.S. (aspirin, phenacetin & salicylamide) [q.v.]

APSAC (anisoylated plasminogen streptokinase activator complex) [see: anistreplase]
aptazapine INN *antidepressant* [also: aptazapine maleate]
aptazapine maleate USAN *antidepressant* [also: aptazapine]
aptocaine INN, BAN
apyron [see: magnesium salicylate]
Aqua Gem-E soft capsules OTC *vitamin supplement* [vitamin E]
Aqua-Ban Plus tablets OTC *diuretic* [ammonium chloride; caffeine; ferrous sulfate]
Aqua-Ban tablets OTC *diuretic* [ammonium chloride; caffeine]
Aquabase OTC *ointment base*
Aquacare cream, lotion OTC *moisturizer; emollient; keratolytic* [urea]
Aquacare/HP (name changed to Aquacare in 1990)
Aquachloral Supprettes (suppositories) ℞ *sedative; hypnotic* [chloral hydrate]
aquaday [see: menadione]
aquakay [see: menadione]
AquaMEPHYTON IM or subcu injection ℞ *coagulant; vitamin K deficiency* [phytonadione]
Aquanil lotion OTC *moisturizer; emollient*
Aquaphilic OTC *ointment base*
Aquaphilic with Carbamide OTC *ointment base* [urea]
Aquaphor OTC *ointment base*
Aquaphor Antibiotic ointment OTC *topical antibiotic* [polymyxin B sulfate; bacitracin zinc]
Aquaphyllin syrup ℞ *bronchodilator* [theophylline]
Aqua-Rid tablets (discontinued 1991) OTC *diuretic* [buchu; couch grass; corn silk; hydrangea]
Aquasol A capsules, IM injection ℞ *vitamin deficiency therapy* [vitamin A]
Aquasol A drops OTC *vitamin supplement* [vitamin A]

Aquasol E capsules, drops OTC *vitamin supplement* [vitamin E]

Aquatag tablets (discontinued 1991) ℞ *diuretic; antihypertensive* [benzthiazide]

AquaTar gel OTC *topical antipsoriatic; antiseborrheic* [coal tar extract]

Aquatensen tablets ℞ *diuretic; antihypertensive* [methyclothiazide]

aqueous penicillin G procaine (APPG) [see: penicillin G procaine]

Aquest IM injection ℞ *estrogen replacement therapy; antineoplastic for prostatic and breast cancer* [estrone]

aquinone [see: menadione]

AR-121 *investigational antiviral for AIDS*

ara-A (adenine arabinoside) [see: vidarabine]

ara-AC (azacytosine arabinoside) [see: fazarabine]

arabinofuranosylcytosine [see: cytarabine]

arabinoluranosylcytosine HCl [see: cytarabine HCl]

arabinosyl cytosine [see: cytarabine]

ara-C (cytosine arabinoside) [see: cytarabine]

ara-C + ADR (ara-C, Adriamycin) *chemotherapy protocol*

ara-C + DNR + PRED + MP (ara-C, daunorubicin, prednisolone, mercaptopurine) *chemotherapy protocol*

ara-C + 6-TG (ara-C, thioguanine) *chemotherapy protocol*

arachis oil [see: peanut oil]

ara-C-HU (ara-C, hydroxyurea) *chemotherapy protocol*

ara-cytidine [see: cytarabine]

Aralen HCl IM injection ℞ *antimalarial; amebicide* [chloroquine HCl]

Aralen Phosphate tablets ℞ *antimalarial; amebicide* [chloroquine phosphate]

Aralen Phosphate with Primaquine Phosphate tablets ℞ *malaria prophylaxis* [chloroquine phosphate; primaquine phosphate]

Aramine IV, subcu or IM injection ℞ *vasopressor used in shock* [metaraminol bitartrate]

aranotin USAN, INN *antiviral*

arbaprostil USAN, INN *gastric antisecretory*

arbekacin INN

Arbon Plus tablets OTC *vitamin/mineral/iron supplement* [multiple vitamins & minerals; ferrous fumarate; folic acid; biotin]

Arbon tablets OTC *vitamin/mineral/iron supplement* [multiple vitamins & minerals; ferrous fumarate; folic acid]

arbutamine INN, BAN *cardiac stimulant* [also: arbutamine HCl]

arbutamine HCl USAN *cardiac stimulant* [also: arbutamine]

Arcet tablets ℞ *sedative; analgesic; antipyretic* [butalbital; acetaminophen; caffeine]

arclofenin USAN, INN *hepatic function test*

Arcobee with C capsules OTC *vitamin supplement* [multiple B vitamins; vitamin C]

Arco-Lase chewable tablets OTC *digestive enzymes* [amylase; protease; lipase; cellulase]

Arco-Lase Plus tablets ℞ *digestive enzymes; antispasmodic; sedative* [amylase; protease; lipase; cellulase; hyoscyamine sulfate; atropine sulfate; phenobarbital]

Arcotinic liquid (discontinued 1992) OTC *hematinic* [iron; liver fraction 1; multiple B vitamins; alcohol]

Arcotinic tablets OTC *hematinic* [ferrous fumarate; ferrous sulfate; desiccated liver; vitamin C]

ardacin INN

Arduan powder for IV injection ℞ *neuromuscular blocker* [pipecuronium bromide]

arecoline acetarsone salt [see: drocarbil]
arecoline hydrobromide NF
Aredia IV infusion ℞ *bone resorption suppressant for Paget's disease and hypercalcemia* [pamidronate disodium]
arfalasin INN
arfendazam INN
Arfonad IV infusion ℞ *antihypertensive for hypertensive emergencies* [trimethaphan camsylate]
argatroban INN
Argesic cream OTC *topical analgesic; counterirritant* [methyl salicylate; trolamine]
Argesic-SA tablets ℞ *analgesic; antiinflammatory* [salsalate]
argimesna INN
arginine (L-arginine) USP, INN *nonessential amino acid; ammonia detoxicant; pituitary function test; symbols: Arg, R*
arginine butyrate (orphan: *treatment of beta-hemoglobinopathies and beta-thalassemia*)
arginine glutamate (L-arginine L-glutamate) USAN, BAN *ammonia detoxicant*
arginine HCl USAN, USP *ammonia detoxicant; pituitary (growth hormone) function test*
L-arginine monohydrochloride [see: arginine HCl]
8-L-arginine vasopressin [see: vasopressin]
8-L-argininevasopressin tannate [see: argipressin tannate]
argipressin INN, BAN [also: argipressin tannate]
argipressin tannate USAN *antidiuretic* [also: argipressin]
argiprestocin INN
argon *element* (Ar)
argyn [see: silver protein, mild]
Argyrol S.S. 10% solution OTC *topical mucosal antiseptic* [silver protein, mild]

Argyrol S.S. 20% eye drops ℞ *ophthalmic mucus staining and coagulating agent; topical antiseptic* [silver protein, mild]
arildone USAN, INN *antiviral*
Aristocort; Aristocort A ointment, cream ℞ *topical corticosteroid* [triamcinolone acetonide]
Aristocort Forte IM injection ℞ *glucocorticoid* [triamcinolone diacetate]
Aristocort Intralesional injection ℞ *glucocorticoid* [triamcinolone diacetate]
Aristocort tablets ℞ *glucocorticoid* [triamcinolone]
Aristospan Intra-articular injection ℞ *glucocorticoid* [triamcinolone hexacetonide]
Aristospan Intralesional injection ℞ *glucocorticoid* [triamcinolone hexacetonide]
Arkin Z ℞ *investigational treatment for congestive heart failure*
Arlidin tablets (discontinued 1993) ℞ *vasodilator* [nylidrin HCl]
A.R.M. (Allergy Relief Medicine) caplets OTC *decongestant; antihistamine* [phenylpropanolamine HCl; chlorpheniramine maleate]
Arm-A-Med (delivery system) *nebulizer*
Armour Thyroid tablets ℞ *hypothyroidism; thyroid cancer* [thyroid, desiccated]
arnica *claimed to relieve sprains and bruises (of dubious value)*
arnolol INN
aromatic ammonia spirit [see: ammonia spirit, aromatic]
aromatic cascara fluidextract [see: cascara fluidextract, aromatic]
aromatic cascara sagrada [see: cascara fluidextract, aromatic]
aromatic elixir NF *flavored and sweetened vehicle*
aronixil INN
Aropax (name changed to Paxil in 1992)

arotinolol INN
arprinocid USAN, INN, BAN *coccidiostat*
arpromidine INN
Arrestin IM injection ℞ *anticholinergic; antiemetic* [trimethobenzamide HCl]
ARS (antirabies serum) [q.v.]
arsambide [see: carbarsone]
arsanilic acid INN, BAN *investigational immunomodulator for AIDS*
arseclor [see: dichlorophenarsine HCl]
arsenic *element (As)*
arsenic acid, sodium salt [see: sodium arsenate]
arsenobenzene [see: arsphenamine]
arsenobenzol [see: arsphenamine]
arsenphenolamine [see: arsphenamine]
Arsobal (available only from the Centers for Disease Control) ℞ *investigational anti-infective for trypanosomiasis* [melarsoprol]
arsphenamine USP
arsthinol INN
Artane tablets, elixir, Sequels (sustained-release capsules) ℞ *anticholinergic; antiparkinsonian agent* [trihexyphenidyl HCl]
artegraft USAN *arterial prosthetic aid*
artemether INN
artemisinin INN
arterenol [see: norepinephrine bitartrate]
artesunate INN
Artha-G tablets OTC *analgesic; anti-inflammatory* [salsalate]
ArthriCare, Double Ice gel OTC *counterirritant* [menthol; camphor]
ArthriCare, Odor Free rub OTC *counterirritant* [menthol; methyl nicotinate; capsaicin; aloe]
ArthriCare Daytime Formula (name changed to Odor Free ArthriCare in 1992)
ArthriCare Triple Medicated gel OTC *counterirritant* [methyl salicylate; menthol; methyl nicotinate]

Arthriten tablets OTC *analgesic; antipyretic* [acetaminophen; magnesium salicylate; caffeine]
Arthritis Hot Creme OTC *counterirritant* [methyl salicylate; menthol]
Arthritis Pain Formula Aspirin-Free tablets OTC *analgesic; antipyretic* [acetaminophen]
Arthritis Pain Formula caplets OTC *analgesic; antipyretic; anti-inflammatory; antirheumatic* [aspirin, buffered with magnesium hydroxide and aluminum hydroxide]
Arthropan IM injection ℞ *analgesic; antipyretic; anti-inflammatory; antirheumatic* [choline salicylate]
Arthrotec ℞ *investigational antiarthritic* [diclofenac sodium; misoprostol]
articaine INN [also: carticaine]
Articulose L.A. IM injection ℞ *glucocorticoids* [triamcinolone diacetate]
Articulose-50 IM injection ℞ *glucocorticoids* [prednisolone acetate]
Artificial Tears eye drops, ophthalmic ointment OTC *ocular moisturizer/lubricant*
Artificial Tears Plus eye drops OTC *ocular moisturizer/lubricant*
artilide fumarate USAN *antiarrhythmic*
Arvin (orphan: thrombocytopenia or thrombosis) [ancrod]
AS-101 *investigational immunomodulator; (orphan: AIDS)*
[74]**As** [see: sodium arsenate As 74]
ASA (acetylsalicylic acid) [see: aspirin]
5-ASA (5-aminosalicylic acid) [see: mesalamine]
A.S.A. Enseals (enteric-release tablets), suppositories OTC *analgesic; antipyretic; anti-inflammatory* [aspirin]
Asacol delayed-release tablets ℞ *treatment of active ulcerative colitis, proctosigmoiditis and proctitis* [mesalamine]
Asbron-G Inlay-Tabs (tablets), elixir ℞ *antiasthmatic; bronchodilator; ex-*

pectorant [theophylline sodium glycinate; guaifenesin]

ascorbic acid (L-ascorbic acid) USP, INN, BAN *vitamin C; antiscorbutic; urinary acidifier*

L-ascorbic acid, monosodium salt [see: sodium ascorbate]

L-ascorbic acid 6-palmitate [see: ascorbyl palmitate]

Ascorbicap timed-release capsules OTC *vitamin supplement* [ascorbic acid]

ascorbyl palmitate NF *antioxidant*

Ascriptin; Ascriptin A/D coated tablets OTC *analgesic; antipyretic; anti-inflammatory; antirheumatic* [aspirin, buffered with magnesium hydroxide, aluminum hydroxide, and calcium carbonate]

Asendin tablets ℞ *tricyclic antidepressant* [amoxapine]

aseptichrome [see: merbromin]

A-SHAP (Adriamycin, Solu-Medrol, high-dose ara-C, Platinol) *chemotherapy protocol*

Asmalix elixir ℞ *bronchodilator* [theophylline]

asocainol INN

asparaginase (L-asparaginase) USAN *antineoplastic* [also: colaspase]

asparagine (L-asparagine) *nonessential amino acid; symbols: Asn, N*

L-asparagine amidohydrolase [see: asparaginase]

aspartame USAN, NF, INN, BAN *sweetener*

aspartic acid (L-aspartic acid) USAN, INN *nonessential amino acid; symbols: Asp, D*

aspartocin USAN, INN *antibacterial*

Aspegic ℞ *(orphan: sickle cell crisis)* [lysine acetylsalicylate]

Aspercin; Aspercin Extra tablets OTC *analgesic; anti-inflammatory; antipyretic* [aspirin]

Aspercreme cream OTC *topical analgesic* [trolamine salicylate]

Aspercreme Rub lotion OTC *topical analgesic* [trolamine salicylate]

Aspergum chewing gum tablets OTC *analgesic; antipyretic; anti-inflammatory; antirheumatic* [aspirin]

asperkinase

asperlin USAN *antibacterial; antineoplastic*

Aspermin; Aspermin Extra tablets OTC *analgesic; anti-inflammatory; antipyretic* [aspirin]

aspidosperma USP

aspirin USP, BAN *analgesic; antipyretic; anti-inflammatory; antirheumatic*

aspirin, buffered USP *analgesic; antipyretic; anti-inflammatory; antirheumatic*

aspirin aluminum NF

Aspirin EC enteric-coated tablets OTC *analgesic; antipyretic; anti-inflammatory* [aspirin]

Aspirin Lite Coat tablets OTC *analgesic; antipyretic; anti-inflammatory* [aspirin]

Aspirin with Codeine No. 2, No. 3 & No. 4 tablets ℞ *narcotic analgesic* [codeine phosphate; aspirin]

Aspirin-Free Pain Relief tablets OTC *analgesic; antipyretic* [acetaminophen]

Aspirol (trademarked form) *inhalant*

aspogen [see: dihydroxyaluminum aminoacetate]

aspoxicillin INN

aspro [see: aspirin]

Asproject IM injection (discontinued 1992) ℞ *analgesic; antipyretic; anti-inflammatory; antirheumatic* [sodium thiosalicylate]

astatine *element (At)*

astemizole USAN, INN, BAN *antiallergic; antihistamine*

Astenose ℞ *investigational anticoagulant to block vascular restenosis following cardiac surgery*

AsthmaHaler inhalation aerosol OTC *bronchodilator for bronchial asthma* [epinephrine bitartrate]

Asthmalixir elixir (discontinued 1991) OTC *antiasthmatic; bronchodilator; expectorant; sedative* [theophylline; ephedrine sulfate; guaifenesin; phenobarbital]

AsthmaNefrin solution for inhalation OTC *bronchodilator for bronchial asthma* [racepinephrine]

astifilcon A USAN *hydrophilic contact lens material*

Astramorph PF IV, subcu or IM injection ℞ *narcotic analgesic; preoperative sedative and anxiolytic* [morphine sulfate]

Astroglide gel OTC *vaginal lubricant*

astromicin INN *antibacterial* [also: astromicin sulfate]

astromicin sulfate USAN *antibacterial* [also: astromicin]

AT-III (antithrombin III) [q.v.]

Atabrine HCl tablets ℞ *antimalarial; anthelmintic for giardiasis and cestodiasis* [quinacrine HCl]

atamestane INN

Atarax 100 tablets ℞ *anxiolytic* [hydroxyzine HCl]

Atarax tablets, syrup ℞ *anxiolytic* [hydroxyzine HCl]

atarvet [see: acepromazine]

atenolol USAN, INN, BAN *antiadrenergic (β-receptor)*

Atgam IV infusion ℞ *immunizing agent for allograft rejection* [lymphocyte immune globulin, antithymocyte globulin (equine)]

athyromazole [see: carbimazole]

atipamezole USAN, INN, BAN $α_2$-receptor antagonist

atiprosin INN *antihypertensive* [also: atiprosin maleate]

atiprosin maleate USAN *antihypertensive* [also: atiprosin]

Ativan tablets, IV or IM injection ℞ *anxiolytic* [lorazepam]

atlafilcon A USAN *hydrophilic contact lens material*

ATnativ powder for IV infusion ℞ *(orphan: antithrombin III deficiency; thrombosis)* [antithrombin III, human]

atolide USAN, INN *anticonvulsant*

Atolone tablets ℞ *glucocorticoid* [triamcinolone]

atosiban USAN, INN *oxytocin antagonist*

atovaquone *antiprotozoal*

atracurium besilate INN *skeletal muscle relaxant* [also: atracurium besylate]

atracurium besylate USAN, BAN *skeletal muscle relaxant; neuromuscular blocker* [also: atracurium besilate]

atrimustine INN

Atrocholin tablets (discontinued 1992) OTC *laxative; hydrocholeretic* [dehydrocholic acid]

Atrofed tablets OTC *decongestant; antihistamine* [pseudoephedrine HCl; triprolidine HCl]

Atrohist L.A. sustained-release tablets ℞ *antihistamine; decongestant; anticholinergic* [brompheniramine maleate; phenyltoloxamine citrate; pseudoephedrine HCl; atropine sulfate]

Atrohist Pediatric oral suspension ℞ *pediatric antihistamine and decongestant* [phenylephrine tannate; chlorpheniramine tannate; pyrilamine tannate]

Atrohist Plus sustained-release tablets ℞ *decongestant; antihistamine; anticholinergic* [phenylpropanolamine HCl; phenylephrine HCl; chlorpheniramine maleate; hyoscyamine sulfate; atropine sulfate; scopolamine hydrobromide]

Atrohist Sprinkle sustained-release capsules ℞ *antihistamine; decongestant* [brompheniramine maleate; phenyltoloxamine citrate; phenylephrine HCl]

atromepine INN

Atromid-S capsules ℞ *antihyperlipidemic (cholesterol-lowering)* [clofibrate]

AtroPen auto-injector (automatic IM injection device) ℞ *antidote for organophosphorous or carbamate insecticides* [atropine sulfate; phenol]
atropine USP, BAN *anticholinergic*
Atropine Care 1% eye drops, ophthalmic ointment ℞ *mydriatic; cycloplegic* [atropine sulfate]
atropine methonitrate INN, BAN *anticholinergic* [also: methylatropine nitrate]
atropine methylnitrate [see: methylatropine nitrate]
atropine oxide INN *anticholinergic* [also: atropine oxide HCl]
atropine oxide HCl USAN *anticholinergic* [also: atropine oxide]
atropine propionate [see: prampine]
atropine sulfate USP GI *antispasmodic; bronchodilator; cycloplegic; mydriatic* [also: atropine sulphate]
atropine sulphate BAN *ophthalmic anticholinergic* [also: atropine sulfate]
Atropisol Ophthalmic eye drops ℞ *cycloplegic; mydriatic* [atropine sulfate]
Atrovent inhalation aerosol ℞ *bronchodilator* [ipratropium bromide]
A/T/S topical solution, gel ℞ *topical antibiotic for acne vulgaris* [erythromycin]
Attain liquid OTC *oral nutritional supplement*
attapulgite, activated USP *suspending agent; GI adsorbent*
Attenuvax subcu injection ℞ *measles vaccine* [measles virus vaccine, live attenuated]
[198]**Au** [see: gold Au 198]
augmented betamethasone dipropionate *topical corticosteroid*
Augmentin '125'; Augmentin '250' chewable tablets, powder for oral suspension ℞ *penicillin-type antibiotic* [amoxicillin trihydrate; clavulanate potassium]
Augmentin '250'; Augmentin '500' film-coated tablets ℞ *penicillin-type antibiotic* [amoxicillin trihydrate; clavulanate potassium]
Auralgan Otic ear drops ℞ *topical local anesthetic; analgesic* [benzocaine; antipyrine]
auranofin USAN, INN, BAN *antirheumatic (29% gold)*
Aureomycin ointment OTC *topical antibiotic* [chlortetracycline HCl]
Aureomycin Ophthalmic ointment ℞ *ophthalmic antibiotic* [chlortetracycline HCl]
aureoquin [now: quinetolate]
Auriculin *investigational treatment for acute kidney failure; (orphan: adjunct to renal transplant)* [anaritide acetate]
Aurinol Ear Drops (discontinued 1992) OTC *antibacterial/antifungal* [chloroxylenol; acetic acid; benzalkonium chloride]
Auro Ear Drops OTC *agent to emulsify and disperse ear wax* [carbamide peroxide]
Aurocaine 2 ear drops (discontinued 1992) OTC *antibacterial/antifungal* [boric acid]
Aurocaine Ear Drops OTC *agent to emulsify and disperse ear wax* [carbamide]
Auro-Dri ear drops OTC *antibacterial/antifungal* [boric acid; alcohol]
aurolin [see: gold sodium thiosulfate]
Auromid ear drops (discontinued 1991) ℞ *local anesthetic; analgesic* [benzocaine; antipyrine; glycerin]
auropin [see: gold sodium thiosulfate]
aurosan [see: gold sodium thiosulfate]
aurothioglucose USP *antirheumatic (50% gold)*
aurothioglycanide INN
aurothiomalate disodium [see: gold sodium thiomalate]
aurothiomalate sodium [see: gold sodium thiomalate]
Auroto Otic ear drops ℞ *topical local anesthetic; analgesic* [antipyrine; benzocaine]

Autohaler (delivery form) *breath-activated metered-dose inhaler*
auto-injector (delivery device) *automatic IM injection device*
Autoplex T IV injection or drip ℞ *factor VIII deficiency; correct coagulation deficiency* [anti-inhibitor coagulant complex]
autoprothrombin I [see: factor VII]
autoprothrombin II [see: factor IX]
AV (Adriamycin, vincristine) *chemotherapy protocol*
Avail tablets OTC *vitamin/mineral/iron supplement* [multiple vitamins & minerals; iron; folic acid]
Avalgesic lotion OTC *counterirritant* [methyl salicylate; menthol; camphor; methyl nicotinate; capsicum oleoresin]
AVC vaginal cream, vaginal suppositories ℞ *bacteriostatic* [sulfanilamide]
Aveeno Anti-Itch cream, lotion OTC *topical poison ivy treatment* [calamine; pramoxine HCl; camphor]
Aveeno Cleansing Bar OTC *medicated cleansing bar for acne* [sulfur; salicylic acid; colloidal oatmeal]
Aveeno lotion OTC *moisturizer; emollient* [colloidal oatmeal]
Aveeno Moisturizing cream OTC *moisturizer; emollient*
Aveeno Oilated Bath OTC *bath emollient* [colloidal oatmeal; mineral oil]
Aveeno Regular Bath; Aveeno Shower & Bath OTC *bath emollient* [colloidal oatmeal]
Aventyl HCl Pulvules (capsules) ℞ *tricyclic antidepressant* [nortriptyline HCl]
Aventyl solution ℞ *tricyclic antidepressant* [nortriptyline HCl]
avertin [see: tribromoethanol]
avilamycin USAN, INN, BAN *antibacterial*
avinar [see: uredepa]
Avitene Hemostat fiber, nonwoven web ℞ *topical hemostatic aid in surgery* [microfibrillar collagen hemostat]
Aviva ℞ *investigational treatment for Alzheimer's disease*
avobenzone USAN, INN *sunscreen*
avoparcin USAN, INN, BAN *antibacterial*
AVP (actinomycin D, vincristine, Platinol) *chemotherapy protocol*
avridine USAN, INN *antiviral*
axamozide INN
axerophthol [see: vitamin A]
Axid Pulvules (capsules) ℞ *duodenal ulcer treatment; histamine H$_2$ antagonist* [nizatidine]
Axotal tablets ℞ *analgesic; sedative* [aspirin; butalbital]
Axsain (name changed to Zostrix-HP in 1992)
Aygestin tablets ℞ *progestin; amenorrhea; functional uterine bleeding; endometriosis* [norethindrone acetate]
Ayr Saline nasal mist, nose drops OTC *nasal moisturizer* [sodium chloride (saline)]
5-AZA (5-azacitidine) [see: azacitidine]
azabon USAN, INN *CNS stimulant*
azabuperone INN
azacitidine (5-AZA; 5-AZC) USAN, INN *investigational antineoplastic*
azaclorzine INN *coronary vasodilator* [also: azaclorzine HCl]
azaclorzine HCl USAN *coronary vasodilator* [also: azaclorzine]
azaconazole USAN, INN *antifungal*
azacosterol INN *avian chemosterilant* [also: azacosterol HCl]
azacosterol HCl USAN *avian chemosterilant* [also: azacosterol]
Azactam powder for IV or IM injection ℞ *monobactam-type antibiotic* [aztreonam]
azacyclonol INN, BAN [also: azacyclonol HCl]
azacyclonol HCl NF [also: azacyclonol]

5-azacytosine arabinoside (ara-AC) [see: fazarabine]
5-AZA-2′-deoxycytidine *(orphan: acute leukemia)*
azaftozine INN
azalomycin INN, BAN
azaloxan INN *antidepressant* [also: azaloxan fumarate]
azaloxan fumarate USAN *antidepressant* [also: azaloxan]
azamethonium bromide INN, BAN
azamulin INN
azanator INN *bronchodilator* [also: azanator maleate]
azanator maleate USAN *bronchodilator* [also: azanator]
azanidazole USAN, INN, BAN *antiprotozoal*
azaperone USAN, INN, BAN *antipsychotic*
azapetine BAN
azapetine phosphate [see: azapetine]
azaprocin INN
azapropazone INN, BAN *anti-inflammatory* [also: apazone]
azaquinzole INN
azaribine USAN, INN, BAN *antipsoriatic*
azarole USAN *immunoregulator*
azaserine USAN, INN *antifungal*
azaspirium chloride INN
azastene
azatadine INN, BAN *antihistamine* [also: azatadine maleate]
azatadine maleate USAN, USP *antihistamine* [also: azatadine]
azatepa INN *antineoplastic* [also: azetepa]
azathioprine USP, INN, BAN *immunosuppressive*
azathioprine sodium USP *immunosuppressive*
5-AZC (5-azacitidine) [see: azacitidine]
Azdone tablets ℞ *narcotic analgesic* [hydrocodone bitartrate; aspirin]
azdU (azidouridine) [q.v.]
azelaic acid INN

azelastine INN, BAN *antiallergic; antiasthmatic* [also: azelastine HCl]
azelastine HCl USAN *antiallergic; antiasthmatic* [also: azelastine]
azepexole INN, BAN
azephine [see: azapetine phosphate]
azepinamide [see: glypinamide]
azepindole USAN, INN *antidepressant*
azetepa USAN, BAN *antineoplastic* [also: azatepa]
azetirelin INN
azidamfenicol INN, BAN
azidoamphenicol [see: azidamfenicol]
azidocillin INN, BAN
3′-azido-2′,3′dideoxyuridine *(orphan: AIDS)*
azidothymidine (AZT) [now: zidovudine]
azidouridine (azdU) *investigational antiviral for AIDS*
azimexon INN
azintamide INN
azinthiamide [see: azintamide]
azipramine INN *antidepressant* [also: azipramine HCl]
azipramine HCl USAN *antidepressant* [also: azipramine]
aziridinyl benzoquinone [see: diaziquone]
azithromycin USAN, INN, BAN *macrolide antibacterial antibiotic*
azithromycin dihydrate *macrolide antibiotic*
Azlin IV (discontinued 1991) ℞ *penicillin-type antibiotic* [azlocillin sodium]
azlocillin USAN, INN, BAN *antibacterial*
azlocillin sodium USP *antibacterial*
Azma Aid tablets (discontinued 1991) OTC *antiasthmatic* [theophylline; ephedrine HCl]
Azmacort oral inhalation aerosol ℞ *corticosteroid for bronchial asthma* [triamcinolone acetonide]
Azo Gantanol film-coated tablets ℞ *urinary anti-infective; urinary analgesic*

[sulfamethoxazole; phenazopyridine HCl]

Azo Gantrisin film-coated tablets ℞ *urinary anti-infective; urinary analgesic* [sulfisoxazole; phenazopyridine HCl]

azoconazole [now: azaconazole]

azodisal sodium (ADS) [now: olsalazine sodium]

Azolid tablets, capsules (discontinued 1991) ℞ *antirheumatic* [phenylbutazone]

azolimine USAN, INN *diuretic*

azosemide USAN, INN *diuretic*

Azo-Standard tablets OTC *urinary analgesic* [phenazopyridine HCl]

Azostix reagent strips OTC *in vitro diagnostic aid to estimate the amount of BUN in whole blood*

Azo-Sulfisoxazole tablets ℞ *urinary anti-infective; urinary analgesic* [sulfisoxazole; phenazopyridine HCl]

azotomycin USAN, INN *antineoplastic*

azovan blue BAN *blood volume test* [also: Evans blue]

azovan sodium [see: Evans blue]

AZT (azidothymidine) [now: zidovudine]

AZT-P-ddI *investigational antiviral for AIDS*

aztreonam USAN, USP, INN, BAN *bactericidal antibiotic; monobactam*

Azulfidine EN-tabs enteric-coated tablets ℞ *broad-spectrum bacteriostatic; anti-inflammatory for ulcerative colitis* [sulfasalazine]

Azulfidine tablets, oral suspension ℞ *broad-spectrum bacteriostatic; anti-inflammatory for ulcerative colitis* [sulfasalazine]

azumolene INN *skeletal muscle relaxant* [also: azumolene sodium]

azumolene sodium USAN *skeletal muscle relaxant* [also: azumolene]

azure A carbacrylic resin [see: azuresin]

azuresin NF, BAN

B

B C with Folic Acid Plus tablets ℞ *vitamin/mineral/iron supplement* [multiple vitamins & minerals; ferrous fumarate; folic acid; biotin]

B C with Folic Acid tablets ℞ *vitamin supplement* [multiple B vitamins; vitamin C]

B Complex-150 sustained-release tablets OTC *vitamin supplement* [multiple B vitamins; folic acid; biotin]

B & O Supprettes No. 15A; B & O Supprettes No. 16A suppositories ℞ *narcotic analgesic* [belladonna extract; opium]

B vitamins [see: vitamin B]

B$_1$ (vitamin B$_1$) [see: thiamine HCl]

B$_2$ (vitamin B$_2$) [see: riboflavin]

B$_3$ (vitamin B$_3$) [see: niacin; niacinamide]

B$_5$ (vitamin B$_5$) [see: calcium pantothenate]

B$_6$ (vitamin B$_6$) [see: pyridoxine HCl]

B$_8$ (vitamin B$_8$) [see: adenosine phosphate]

B$_{12}$ (vitamin B$_{12}$) [see: cyanocobalamin]

B$_{12}$ Plus IM injection (discontinued 1991) ℞ *antianemic* [peptonized iron; vitamin B$_{12}$]

B$_{12a}$ (vitamin B$_{12a}$) [see: hydroxocobalamin]

B$_{12b}$ (vitamin B$_{12b}$) [see: hydroxocobalamin]

B-50 soft capsules, tablets, timed-release tablets OTC *vitamin supplement* [multiple B vitamins; folic acid; biotin]

B-100 tablets, timed-release tablets OTC *vitamin supplement* [multiple B vitamins; folic acid; biotin]
B-125; B-150 tablets (discontinued 1992) OTC *vitamin supplement* [multiple B vitamins; folic acid; biotin]
B_c (vitamin B_c) [see: folic acid]
B_t (vitamin B_t) [see: carnitine]
Babee Teething Lotion OTC *topical anesthetic; oral antiseptic; astringent* [benzocaine; cetalkonium chloride; hamamelis water]
Babylax [see: Fleet Babylax]
BAC (benzalkonium chloride) [q.v.]
B-A-C capsules (discontinued 1992) ℞ *analgesic; antipyretic; sedative* [acetaminophen; caffeine; butalbital]
bacampicillin INN, BAN *antibacterial* [also: bacampicillin HCl]
bacampicillin HCl USAN, USP *bactericidal antibiotic* [also: bacampicillin]
Bacarate tablets (discontinued 1991) ℞ *anorexiant* [phendimetrazine tartrate]
BACI ℞ *investigational anti-infective for AIDS*
Bacid capsules OTC *dietary supplement; fever blister treatment; not generally regarded as safe and effective as an antidiarrheal* [Lactobacillus acidophilus; carboxymethylcellulose sodium]
Baciguent ointment OTC *topical antibiotic* [bacitracin]
Baci-IM powder for IM injection ℞ *bactericidal antibiotic* [bacitracin]
bacillus Calmette-Guérin (BCG) vaccine [see: BCG vaccine]
bacitracin USP, INN, BAN *bactericidal antibiotic; (orphan: pseudomembranous enterocolitis)*
bacitracin zinc USP, BAN *bactericidal antibiotic*
bacitracins zinc complex [see: bacitracin zinc]

Bacitrin ointment OTC *topical antibiotic* [bacitracin]
baclofen USAN, USP, INN, BAN *muscle relaxant*
L-baclofen *(orphan: intractable spasticity; trigeminal neuralgia)*
bacmecillinam INN
Bacmin film-coated tablets OTC *vitamin/mineral/iron supplement* [multiple vitamins & minerals; iron; folic acid; biotin]
BACOD (bleomycin, Adriamycin, CCNU, Oncovin, dexamethasone) *chemotherapy protocol*
BACON (bleomycin, Adriamycin, CCNU, Oncovin, nitrogen mustard) *chemotherapy protocol*
BACOP (bleomycin, Adriamycin, cyclophosphamide, Oncovin, prednisone) *chemotherapy protocol*
BACT (BCNU, ara-C, Cytoxan, thioguanine) *chemotherapy protocol*
Bactal Soap liquid (discontinued 1992) OTC *disinfectant/antiseptic* [triclosan]
bacteriostatic sodium chloride [see: sodium chloride]
Bacteriostatic Sodium Chloride Injection ℞ *IV diluent* [0.9% sodium chloride (normal saline)]
Bacticort eye drop suspension ℞ *topical ophthalmic corticosteroidal anti-inflammatory; antibiotic* [hydrocortisone; neomycin sulfate; polymyxin B sulfate]
Bactigen Meningitis Panel slide test ℞ *in vitro diagnostic aid for multiple pathogens*
Bactigen Salmonella-Shigella slide test ℞ *in vitro diagnostic aid for salmonella and shigella*
Bactine Antiseptic Anesthetic aerosol, liquid, spray OTC *topical local anesthetic; antiseptic* [lidocaine HCl; benzalkonium chloride; alcohol]
Bactine First Aid Antibiotic ointment OTC *topical antibiotic* [poly-

myxin B sulfate; neomycin sulfate; bacitracin]

Bactine First Aid Antibiotic Plus Anesthetic ointment OTC *topical antibiotic; topical local anesthetic* [polymyxin B sulfate; neomycin sulfate; bacitracin; diperodon HCl]

Bactine Hydrocortisone; Maximum Strength Bactine cream OTC *topical corticosteroid* [hydrocortisone]

Bactocill capsules, powder for IV or IM injection ℞ *bactericidal antibiotic (penicillinase-resistant penicillin)* [oxacillin sodium]

BactoShield; BactoShield 2 aerosol foam, solution OTC *broad-spectrum antimicrobial; germicidal* [chlorhexidine gluconate; alcohol]

Bactrim DS double strength tablets ℞ *anti-infective; antibacterial* [trimethoprim; sulfamethoxazole]

Bactrim tablets, oral suspension, pediatric suspension, IV infusion ℞ *anti-infective; antibacterial* [trimethoprim; sulfamethoxazole]

Bactroban ointment ℞ *topical antibiotic for impetigo* [mupirocin]

bakeprofen INN

baker's yeast *natural source of protein and B-complex vitamins*

BAL (British antilewisite) [now: dimercaprol]

BAL in Oil deep IM injection ℞ *antidote for arsenic, gold, lead and mercury poisoning* [dimercaprol]

Balanced B-100 tablets (discontinued 1992) OTC *vitamin B supplement* [multiple B vitamins; folic acid; biotin; inositol]

Baldex eye drops, ophthalmic ointment ℞ *ophthalmic topical corticosteroidal anti-inflammatory* [dexamethasone sodium phosphate]

balipramine BAN [also: depramine]

Balmex Baby powder OTC *topical diaper rash treatment* [zinc oxide; balsam Peru; corn starch]

Balmex Emollient lotion OTC *moisturizer; emollient*

Balmex ointment OTC *moisturizer; emollient; astringent; antiseptic* [peruvian balsam; zinc oxide; bismuth subnitrate]

Balneol Perianal Cleansing lotion OTC *emollient/protectant*

Balnetar bath oil OTC *antipsoriatic; antiseborrheic; antipruritic; emollient* [coal tar; lanolin]

balsalazide INN, BAN

balsam Peru [see: peruvian balsam]

balsan [see: peruvian balsam]

bamaluzole INN

bambermycin INN, BAN *antibacterial* [also: bambermycins]

bambermycins USAN *antibacterial* [also: bambermycin]

bambuterol INN

bamethan INN, BAN *vasodilator* [also: bamethan sulfate]

bamethan sulfate USAN *vasodilator* [also: bamethan]

bamifylline INN, BAN *bronchodilator* [also: bamifylline HCl]

bamifylline HCl USAN *bronchodilator* [also: bamifylline]

bamipine INN, BAN

bamnidazole USAN, INN *antiprotozoal (Trichomonas)*

BAMON (bleomycin, Adriamycin, methotrexate, Oncovin, nitrogen mustard) *chemotherapy protocol*

Banacid tablets OTC *antacid* [magnesium hydroxide; aluminum hydroxide; magnesium trisilicate]

Banadyne-3 solution OTC *topical oral anesthetic; counterirritant; antiseptic* [lidocaine; menthol; alcohol]

Banalg Hospital Strength lotion OTC *counterirritant* [methyl salicylate; menthol]

Banalg lotion OTC *counterirritant* [methyl salicylate; camphor; menthol]

Bancap capsules ℞ *analgesic; antipyretic; sedative* [acetaminophen; caffeine; butalbital]
Bancap HC capsules ℞ *narcotic analgesic* [hydrocodone bitartrate; acetaminophen]
bandage, adhesive USP *surgical aid*
bandage, gauze USP *surgical aid*
Banesin tablets OTC *analgesic; antipyretic* [acetaminophen]
Banex liquid ℞ *decongestant; antihistamine; expectorant* [phenylpropanolamine HCl; phenylephrine HCl; guaifenesin]
Banflex IV or IM injection ℞ *skeletal muscle relaxant* [orphenadrine citrate]
Bangesic liniment OTC *counterirritant* [menthol; camphor; methyl salicylate; eucalyptus oil]
banocide [see: diethylcarbamazine citrate]
Banophen capsules, caplets ℞/OTC *antihistamine; motion sickness preventative; sleep aid; antiparkinsonian* [diphenhydramine HCl]
BanSmoke gum OTC *smoking deterrent* [benzocaine]
Banthīne tablets ℞ *anticholinergic; peptic ulcer treatment adjunct* [methantheline bromide]
Bantron tablets OTC *smoking deterrent* [lobeline sulfate alkaloids; tribasic calcium phosphate; magnesium carbonate]
baquiloprim INN, BAN
Barbased tablets, elixir (discontinued 1992) ℞ *sedative; hypnotic* [butabarbital sodium]
barbenyl [see: phenobarbital]
barbexaclone INN
Barbidonna; Barbidonna No. 2 tablets, elixir ℞ *anticholinergic; sedative* [atropine sulfate; scopolamine hydrobromide; hyoscyamine hydrobromide; phenobarbital]
barbiphenyl [see: phenobarbital]

Barbita sugar-coated tablets ℞ *barbiturate sedative; hypnotic* [phenobarbital]
barbital NF, INN [also: barbitone]
barbital, soluble [now: barbital sodium]
barbital sodium NF, INN [also: barbitone sodium]
barbitone BAN [also: barbital]
barbitone sodium BAN [also: barbital sodium]
Barc liquid OTC *pediculicide* [pyrethrins; piperonyl butoxide; petroleum distillate]
Baricon powder for suspension ℞ *GI contrast radiopaque agent* [barium sulfate]
Baridium tablets OTC *urinary analgesic* [phenazopyridine HCl]
barium *element (Ba)*
barium hydroxide lime USP *carbon dioxide absorbent*
barium sulfate USP *GI radiopaque medium*
barmastine USAN, INN *antihistaminic*
Barobag suspension (discontinued 1993) ℞ *GI contrast radiopaque agent* [barium sulfate]
Baro-cat suspension ℞ *GI contrast radiopaque agent* [barium sulfate; sorbitol]
Baroflave powder ℞ *GI contrast radiopaque agent* [barium sulfate]
Barophen elixir ℞ *anticholinergic; sedative* [phenobarbital; hyoscyamine sulfate; atropine sulfate; scopolamine hydrobromide]
Baros effervescent granules ℞ *GI contrast radiopaque agent* [sodium bicarbonate; tartaric acid; simethicone]
barosmin [see: diosmin]
Barosperse powder for suspension ℞ *GI contrast radiopaque agent* [barium sulfate]
Barotrast oral suspension ℞ *GI contrast medium* [barium sulfate]
Barseb HC Scalp lotion (discontinued 1991) ℞ *topical corticosteroid;*

antiseborrheic; antiseptic [hydrocortisone; salicylic acid]
Barseb Thera-Spray (discontinued 1991) ℞ *topical corticosteroid; antiseborrheic; antiseptic* [hydrocortisone; salicylic acid; benzalkonium chloride]
barucainide INN
BAS (benzyl analogue of serotonin) [see: benanserin HCl]
Basaljel capsules, tablets, suspension OTC *antacid* [basic aluminum carbonate]
basic aluminum acetate [see: aluminum subacetate]
basic aluminum aminoacetate [see: dihydroxyaluminum aminoacetate]
basic aluminum carbonate [see: aluminum carbonate, basic]
basic aluminum chloride [see: aluminum sesquichlorohydrate]
basic aluminum glycinate [see: dihydroxyaluminum aminoacetate]
basic bismuth carbonate [see: bismuth subcarbonate]
basic bismuth gallate [see: bismuth subgallate]
basic bismuth nitrate [see: bismuth subnitrate]
basic bismuth potassium bismuthotartrate [see: bismuth potassium tartrate]
basic bismuth salicylate [see: bismuth subsalicylate]
basic fuchsin [see: fuchsin, basic]
basic zinc acetate [see: zinc acetate, basic]
Basis Glycerin Soap; Basis Superfatted Soap bar (discontinued 1992) OTC *therapeutic skin cleanser*
batanopride INN *antiemetic* [also: batanopride HCl]
batanopride HCl USAN *antiemetic* [also: batanopride]
batelapine INN *antipsychotic* [also: batelapine HCl]
batelapine maleate USAN *antipsychotic* [also: batelapine]

batilol INN
batroxobin INN
batyl alcohol [see: batilol]
batylol [see: batilol]
Baumodyne ointment, gel (discontinued 1992) OTC *counterirritant* [methyl salicylate; menthol; eucalyptus oil; methylparaben; butylparaben]
BAVIP (bleomycin, Adriamycin, vinblastine, imidazole carboxamide, prednisone) *chemotherapy protocol*
baxitozine INN
Bayer, Therapy enteric-coated delayed-release caplets OTC *analgesic; antipyretic; anti-inflammatory; antirheumatic* [aspirin]
Bayer 205 (available only from the Centers for Disease Control) ℞ *investigational anti-infective for trypanosomiasis and onchocerciasis* [suramin sodium]
Bayer 2502 (available only from the Centers for Disease Control) ℞ *investigational anti-infective for Chagas disease* [nifurtimox]
Bayer Aspirin, Genuine; Maximum Bayer Aspirin film-coated tablets, film-coated caplets OTC *analgesic; antipyretic; anti-inflammatory; antirheumatic* [aspirin]
Bayer Children's Aspirin chewable tablets OTC *analgesic; antipyretic; anti-inflammatory; antirheumatic* [aspirin]
Bayer Plus caplets OTC *analgesic; antipyretic; anti-inflammatory; antirheumatic* [aspirin, buffered with calcium carbonate, magnesium carbonate and magnesium oxide]
Bayer Select Headache caplets OTC *analgesic; antipyretic* [acetaminophen; caffeine]
Bayer Select Menstrual caplets OTC *analgesic; antipyretic; diuretic* [acetaminophen; pamabrom]

Bayer Select Night Time Pain Relief caplets OTC *analgesic; antipyretic; antihistaminic sleep aid* [acetaminophen; diphenhydramine HCl]

Bayer Select Pain Relief Formula caplets OTC *nonsteroidal anti-inflammatory drug (NSAID); analgesic* [ibuprofen]

Bayer Select Sinus Pain Relief caplets OTC *analgesic; antipyretic; decongestant* [acetaminophen; pseudoephedrine HCl]

Bayer Timed Release, 8-Hour caplets OTC *analgesic; antipyretic; anti-inflammatory; antirheumatic* [aspirin]

Baylocaine 2% Viscous; Baylocaine 4% solution ℞ *topical anesthetic for mouth and pharynx* [lidocaine HCl]

Baypress ℞ *investigational antihypertensive; calcium channel blocker* [nitrendipine]

bazinaprine INN

B-Between capsules OTC *vitamin supplement* [multiple B vitamins]

BBVP-M (BCNU, bleomycin, VePesid, prednisone, methotrexate) *chemotherapy protocol*

B_c (vitamin B_c) [see: folic acid]

BC Cold Powder Non-Drowsy Formula packets OTC *analgesic; antipyretic; anti-inflammatory; decongestant* [aspirin; phenylpropanolamine HCl]

BC Multi Symptom Cold Powder packets OTC *analgesic; antipyretic; anti-inflammatory; decongestant; antihistamine* [aspirin; phenylpropanolamine HCl; chlorpheniramine maleate]

BC tablets, powder OTC *analgesic; antipyretic; anti-inflammatory* [aspirin; salicylamide; caffeine]

BCAA (branched-chain amino acids) *(orphan: amyotrophic lateral sclerosis)* [see: isoleucine; leucine; valine]

BCAVe; B-CAVe (bleomycin, CCNU, Adriamycin, Velban) *chemotherapy protocol*

BCD (bleomycin, cyclophosphamide, dactinomycin) *chemotherapy protocol*

B-C-E & Zinc tablets (discontinued 1993) OTC *vitamin/zinc supplement* [vitamin E; vitamin C; multiple B vitamins; zinc]

BCG vaccine (bacillus Calmette-Guérin) USP *active bacterin for tuberculosis*

B-CHOP (bleomycin, Cytoxin, hydroxydaunomycin, Oncovin, prednisone) *chemotherapy protocol*

BCMF (bleomycin, cyclophosphamide, methotrexate, fluorouracil) *chemotherapy protocol*

BCNU (bis-chloroethyl-nitrosourea) [see: carmustine]

B-Compleet tablets OTC *vitamin supplement* [multiple B vitamins; vitamin C]

B-Compleet-50; B-Compleet-100 cellulose-coated caplet OTC *vitamin supplement* [multiple B vitamins]

B-Complex "50"; B-Complex "100" tablets (discontinued 1992) OTC *vitamin B supplement* [multiple B vitamins; folic acid; inositol; biotin; choline bitartrate]

BCOP (BCNU, cyclophosphamide, Oncovin, prednisone) *chemotherapy protocol*

BCP (BCNU, cyclophosphamide, prednisone) *chemotherapy protocol*

BC-Vite tablets OTC *vitamin supplement* [multiple B vitamins; vitamin C]

BCVP (BCNU, cyclophosphamide, vincristine, prednisone) *chemotherapy protocol*

BCVPP (BCNU, cyclophosphamide, vinblastine, procarbazine, prednisone) *chemotherapy protocol*

BCX-34 ℞ *investigational agent for psoriasis and cutaneous T-cell lymphoma*

B-D glucose chewable tablets OTC *glucose elevating agent* [glucose]
B-DOPA (bleomycin, DTIC, Oncovin, prednisone, Adriamycin) *chemotherapy protocol*
BEAC (BCNU, etoposide, ara-C, cyclophosphamide) *chemotherapy protocol*
Beano drops OTC *digestive aid* [alpha-D-galactosidase enzyme]
Bebulin VH ℞ *investigational coagulant for hemophilia B* [factor IX complex]
BE-C 800 with Iron tablets OTC *vitamin/iron supplement* [vitamin E; vitamin C; multiple B vitamins; iron]
becanthone HCl USAN *antischistosomal* [also: becantone]
becantone INN *antischistosomal* [also: becanthone HCl]
becantone HCl [see: becanthone HCl]
Because vaginal foam OTC *spermicidal contraceptive* [nonoxynol 9]
beclamide INN, BAN
beclobrate INN, BAN
beclometasone INN *corticosteroidal inhalant for asthma; intranasal steroid* [also: beclomethasone dipropionate; beclomethasone]
beclomethasone BAN *corticosteroidal inhalant for asthma; intranasal steroid* [also: beclomethasone dipropionate; beclometasone]
beclomethasone dipropionate USAN, USP *corticosteroidal inhalant for asthma; intranasal steroid* [also: beclometasone; beclomethasone]
beclotiamine INN
Beclovent oral inhalation aerosol ℞ *corticosteroid for bronchial asthma* [beclomethasone dipropionate]
Becomject-100 injection ℞ *parenteral vitamin therapy* [multiple B vitamins]
Beconase AQ nasal spray ℞ *intranasal steroidal anti-inflammatory* [beclomethasone dipropionate]

Beconase nasal inhalation aerosol ℞ *intranasal steroidal anti-inflammatory* [beclomethasone dipropionate]
Becotin Pulvules (discontinued 1991) OTC *vitamin B supplement* [multiple B vitamins]
Becotin with C Pulvules (discontinued 1991) OTC *vitamin supplement* [multiple B vitamins; vitamin C]
beechwood creosote [see: creosote carbonate]
Beelith tablets OTC *dietary supplement* [vitamin B_6; magnesium oxide]
Beepen-VK tablets, powder for oral solution ℞ *bactericidal antibiotic* [penicillin V potassium]
Beesix IM or IV injection ℞ *vitamin deficiency therapy; antidote to isoniazid poisoning* [pyridoxine HCl]
Bee-T-Vites film-coated tablets OTC *vitamin supplement* [multiple B vitamins; vitamin C]
Bee-Zee tablets OTC *vitamin/zinc supplement* [multiple vitamins; zinc]
befiperide INN
befunolol INN
befuraline INN
behepan [see: cyanocobalamin]
bekanamycin INN
belarizine INN
Beldin syrup (discontinued 1991) OTC *antitussive* [diphenhydramine HCl]
belfosdil USAN, INN *antihypertensive; calcium channel blocker*
Belganyl (available only from the Centers for Disease Control) ℞ *investigational anti-infective for trypanosomiasis and onchocerciasis* [suramin sodium]
Belix elixir OTC *antitussive* [diphenhydramine HCl]
Belladenal tablets (discontinued 1991) ℞ *anticholinergic; sedative* [belladonna extract; phenobarbital]
Belladenal-S tablets (discontinued 1991) ℞ *anticholinergic; sedative* [belladonna extract; phenobarbital]

belladonna extract USP GI/GU *anticholinergic/antispasmodic; antiparkinsonian*

Bellafoline tablets ℞ *GI anticholinergic; antispasmodic; antiparkinsonian agent* [belladonna extract]

Bell/ans tablets OTC *antacid* [sodium bicarbonate]

Bellergal-S tablets ℞ *anticholinergic; sedative* [belladonna extract; phenobarbital; ergotamine tartrate; tartrazine]

beloxamide USAN, INN *antihyperlipoproteinemic*

Bel-Phen-Ergot S tablets ℞ *analgesic specific for migraine; sedative* [phenobarbital; ergotamine tartrate; belladonna alkaloids]

bemarinone INN *cardiotonic; positive inotropic; vasodilator* [also: bemarinone HCl]

bemarinone HCl USAN *cardiotonic; positive inotropic; vasodilator* [also: bemarinone]

bemegride USP, INN, BAN

bemesetron USAN, INN *antiemetic*

bemetizide INN, BAN

Beminal 500 tablets OTC *vitamin supplement* [multiple B vitamins; vitamin C]

Beminal Stress Plus with Iron tablets (discontinued 1991) OTC *antianemic* [ferrous fumarate; vitamin E; multiple B vitamins; sodium ascorbate; folic acid]

bemitradine USAN, INN *antihypertensive; diuretic*

bemoradan USAN, INN *cardiotonic*

Bemote capsules, tablets (discontinued 1991) ℞ *gastrointestinal antispasmodic* [dicyclomine HCl]

BEMP (bleomycin, Eldisine, mitomycin, Platinol) *chemotherapy protocol*

benactyzine INN, BAN

benactyzine HCl *mild antidepressant; anticholinergic*

Bena-D 10; Bena-D 50 injection ℞ *antihistamine; motion sickness preventative; sleep aid; antiparkinsonian* [diphenhydramine HCl]

Benadryl; Benadryl 2% cream, spray OTC *topical antihistamine* [diphenhydramine HCl]

Benadryl capsules, tablets, Kapseals (capsules), elixir, injection ℞/OTC *antihistamine; motion sickness preventative; sleep aid; antiparkinsonian* [diphenhydramine HCl]

Benadryl Cold liquid OTC *decongestant; antihistamine; analgesic* [pseudoephedrine HCl; diphenhydramine HCl; acetaminophen; alcohol]

Benadryl Decongestant elixir OTC *decongestant; antihistamine* [pseudoephedrine HCl; diphenhydramine HCl]

Benadryl Decongestant Kapseals (capsules), film-coated tablets (discontinued 1993) OTC *decongestant; antihistamine* [pseudoephedrine HCl; diphenhydramine HCl]

Benadryl Plus film-coated tablets OTC *decongestant; antihistamine; analgesic* [pseudoephedrine HCl; diphenhydramine HCl; acetaminophen]

Benadryl Plus Night-Time (name changed to Benadryl Cold in 1992)

benafentrine INN

Benahist 10; Benahist 50 injection ℞ *antihistamine; motion sickness preventative; sleep aid; antiparkinsonian* [diphenhydramine HCl]

Ben-Allergin-50 injection ℞ *antihistamine; motion sickness preventative; sleep aid; antiparkinsonian* [diphenhydramine HCl]

benanserin HCl

benapen [see: benethamine penicillin]

benaprizine INN *anticholinergic* [also: benapryzine HCl; benapryzine]

benaprizine HCl [see: benapryzine HCl]

benapryzine BAN *anticholinergic* [also: benapryzine HCl; benaprizine]
benapryzine HCl USAN *anticholinergic* [also: benaprizine; benapryzine]
Ben-Aqua 5; Ben-Aqua 10 lotion, gel OTC *topical keratolytic for acne* [benzoyl peroxide]
benaxibine INN
benazepril INN, BAN *antihypertensive; angiotensin-converting enzyme inhibitor* [also: benazepril HCl]
benazepril HCl USAN *antihypertensive; angiotensin-converting enzyme inhibitor* [also: benazepril]
benazeprilat USAN, INN *angiotensin-converting enzyme inhibitor*
bencianol INN
bencisteine INN
benclonidine INN
bencyclane INN [also: bencyclane fumarate]
bencyclane fumarate [also: bencyclane]
bendacalol mesylate USAN *antihypertensive*
bendamustine INN
bendazac USAN, INN *anti-inflammatory* [also: bindazac]
bendazol INN
benderizine INN
bendrofluazide BAN [also: bendroflumethiazide]
bendroflumethiazide USP, INN *diuretic; antihypertensive* [also: bendrofluazide]
Benegyn vaginal cream ℞ *bacteriostatic; antiseptic; vulnerary* [sulfanilamide; aminacrine HCl; allantoin]
Benemid film-coated tablets ℞ *uricosuric for gout* [probenecid]
benethamine penicillin INN, BAN
benexate INN
benfluorex INN
benfosformin INN
benfotiamine INN
benfurodil hemisuccinate INN
bengal gelatin [see: agar]

Ben-Gay gel, lotion (discontinued 1992) OTC *counterirritant* [methyl salicylate; menthol]
Ben-Gay Original ointment OTC *counterirritant* [methyl salicylate; menthol]
Ben-Gay Regular Strength; Ben-Gay Extra Strength cream OTC *counterirritant* [methyl salicylate; menthol]
Ben-Gay Ultra Strength cream OTC *counterirritant* [methyl salicylate; menthol; camphor]
Ben-Gay Vanishing Scent gel OTC *counterirritant* [menthol; camphor]
benhepazone INN
benidipine INN
benmoxin INN
Benoject-10; Benoject-50 injection ℞ *antihistamine; motion sickness preventative; sleep aid; antiparkinsonian* [diphenhydramine HCl]
benolizime INN
Benoquin cream ℞ *depigmenting agent for vitiligo* [monobenzone]
benorilate INN [also: benorylate]
benorterone USAN, INN *antiandrogen*
benorylate BAN [also: benorilate]
benoxafos INN
benoxaprofen USAN, INN, BAN *anti-inflammatory; analgesic*
benoxinate HCl USP *topical anesthetic* [also: oxybuprocaine]
Benoxyl 5; Benoxyl 10 lotion OTC *keratolytic for acne* [benzoyl peroxide]
benpenolisin INN
benperidol USAN, INN, BAN *antipsychotic*
benproperine INN
benrixate INN
bensalan USAN, INN *disinfectant*
benserazide USAN, INN, BAN *decarboxylase inhibitor*
bensuldazic acid INN, BAN
Bensulfoid cream OTC *topical acne treatment* [sulfur; resorcinol; alcohol]

Bensulfoid lotion (discontinued 1991) OTC *topical acne treatment* [sulfur; zinc oxide; thymol; methyl salicylate; alcohol]
Bensulfoid powder (discontinued 1991) R *antibacterial; exfoliant* [highly reactive sulfur fused onto colloidal bentonite]
Bensulfoid tablets R *antibacterial; exfoliant* [sulfur]
bensylyte HCl [see: phenoxybenzamine HCl]
bentazepam USAN, INN *sedative*
bentemazole INN
bentiamine INN
bentipimine INN
bentiromide USAN, INN, BAN *pancreas function test*
bentonite NF *suspending agent*
Bentyl capsules, tablets, IM injection, syrup R *gastrointestinal antispasmodic* [dicyclomine HCl]
benurestat USAN, INN *urease enzyme inhibitor*
Benylin Cough Syrup OTC *antitussive; antihistamine* [diphenhydramine HCl]
Benylin Decongestant liquid OTC *decongestant; antihistamine* [pseudoephedrine HCl; diphenhydramine HCl; alcohol]
Benylin DM syrup OTC *antitussive* [dextromethorphan hydrobromide]
Benylin Expectorant liquid OTC *antitussive; expectorant* [dextromethorphan hydrobromide; guaifenesin; alcohol]
Benza solution OTC *topical antiseptic* [benzalkonium chloride]
Benzac 5; Benzac 10; Benzac AC; Benzac W 2½; Benzac W 5; Benzac W 10 gel R *topical keratolytic for acne* [benzoyl peroxide]
Benzac AC Wash; Benzac W Wash 5; Benzac W Wash 10 liquid R *topical keratolytic for acne* [benzoyl peroxide]

5 Benzagel; 10 Benzagel gel R *keratolytic for acne* [benzoyl peroxide]
benzaldehyde NF *flavoring agent*
benzalkonium chloride (BAC) NF, INN, BAN *preservative; bacteriostatic antiseptic; surfactant/wetting agent*
Benzamycin gel R *topical antibiotic and keratolytic for acne vulgaris* [erythromycin; benzoyl peroxide]
benzaprinoxide INN
benzarone INN
Benzashave shaving cream R *topical keratolytic for acne vulgaris* [benzoyl peroxide]
benzathine benzylpenicillin INN *bactericidal antibiotic* [also: penicillin G benzathine; benzathine penicillin]
benzathine penicillin BAN *bactericidal antibiotic* [also: penicillin G benzathine; benzathine benzylpenicillin]
benzathine penicillin G [see: penicillin G benzathine]
benzatropine INN *antiparkinsonian; anticholinergic* [also: benztropine mesylate; benztropine]
benzatropine mesylate [see: benztropine mesylate]
benzazoline HCl [see: tolazoline HCl]
benzbromarone USAN, INN, BAN *uricosuric*
benzchinamide [see: benzquinamide]
benzchlorpropamide [see: beclamide]
Benzedrex inhaler R *nasal decongestant* [propylhexedrine]
benzene ethanol [see: phenylethyl alcohol]
benzene hexachloride, gamma [now: lindane]
benzeneacetic acid, sodium salt [see: sodium phenylacetate]
1,3-benzenediol [see: resorcinol]
benzenemethanol [see: benzyl alcohol]
benzestrofol [see: estradiol benzoate]
benzestrol USP, INN, BAN
benzethacil [see: penicillin G benzathine]

benzethidine INN, BAN
benzethonium chloride USP, INN, BAN *topical anti-infective; preservative*
benzetimide INN *anticholinergic* [also: benzetimide HCl]
benzetimide HCl USAN *anticholinergic* [also: benzetimide]
benzfetamine INN [also: benzphetamine HCl; benzphetamine]
benzhexol BAN *anticholinergic; antiparkinsonian* [also: trihexyphenidyl HCl; trihexyphenidyl]
N-benzhydryl-N-methylpiperazine [see: cyclizine HCl]
benzilonium bromide USAN, INN, BAN *anticholinergic*
2-benzimidazolepropionic acid [see: procodazole]
benzindamine HCl [see: benzydamine HCl]
benzindopyrine INN *antipsychotic* [also: benzindopyrine HCl]
benzindopyrine HCl USAN *antipsychotic* [also: benzindopyrine]
benzinoform [see: carbon tetrachloride]
benziodarone INN, BAN
benzmalecene INN
benzmethoxazone [see: chlorthenoxazine]
benznidazole INN
benzoaric acid [see: ellagic acid]
benzoate & phenylacetate (sodium benzoate & sodium phenylacetate) (*orphan: hyperammonemia in urea cycle enzymopathy*)
benzobarbital INN
benzocaine USP, INN, BAN *topical anesthetic; nonprescription diet aid*
benzoclidine INN
Benzocol cream OTC *topical local anesthetic* [benzocaine]
benzoctamine INN, BAN *sedative; muscle relaxant* [also: benzoctamine HCl]

benzoctamine HCl USAN, INN *sedative; muscle relaxant* [also: benzoctamine]
Benzodent oral ointment OTC *topical oral anesthetic; analgesic; antiseptic* [benzocaine; hydroxyquinoline sulfate; eugenol]
benzodepa USAN, INN *antineoplastic*
benzodiazepine HCl [see: medazepam HCl]
benzododecinium chloride INN
Benzodyne ear drops OTC *antibacterial/antifungal* [chloroxylenol; acetic acid; benzalkonium chloride]
benzogynestryl [see: estradiol benzoate]
benzoic acid USP *antifungal; urinary acidifier*
benzoic acid, phenylmethyl ester [see: benzyl benzoate]
benzoic acid, potassium salt [see: potassium benzoate]
benzoic acid, sodium salt [see: sodium benzoate]
benzoin USP *topical protectant*
Benzoin Compound tincture OTC *skin protectant* [benzoin; aloe; alcohol]
benzol [see: benzene]
benzonatate USP, INN, BAN *antitussive*
benzophenone
benzopyrrolate [see: benzopyrronium]
benzopyrronium bromide INN
benzoquinone amidoinohydrazone thiosemicarbazone hydrate [see: ambazone]
benzoquinonium chloride
benzorphanol [see: levophenacylmorphan]
benzosulfinide [see: saccharin]
benzosulphinide sodium [see: saccharin sodium]
benzothiozon [see: thioacetazone; thiacetazone]
benzotript INN
benzoxiquine USAN, INN *antiseptic/disinfectant*

benzoxonium chloride INN
benzoyl *p*-aminosalicylate (B-PAS) [see: benzoylpas calcium]
benzoyl peroxide USAN, USP *keratolytic*
***m*-benzoylhydratropic acid** [see: ketoprofen]
benzoylmethylecgonine [see: cocaine]
benzoylpas calcium USAN, USP *antibacterial; tuberculostatic* [also: calcium benzamidosalicylate]
benzoylsulfanilamide [see: sulfabenzamide]
benzoylthiamindisulfide [see: bisbentiamine]
benzoylthiaminmonophosphate [see: benfotiamine]
benzphetamine BAN [also: benzphetamine HCl; benzfetamine]
benzphetamine chloride [see: benzphetamine HCl]
benzphetamine HCl NF *anorexiant; CNS stimulant* [also: benzfetamine; benzphetamine]
benzpiperylon [see: benzpiperylone]
benzpiperylone INN
benzpyrinium bromide NF, INN
benzquercin INN
benzquinamide USAN, INN, BAN *postanesthesia antinauseant and antiemetic*
benzthiazide USP, INN, BAN *diuretic; antihypertensive*
benztropine BAN *antiparkinsonian; anticholinergic* [also: benztropine mesylate; benzatropine]
benztropine mesylate USP *antiparkinsonian; anticholinergic* [also: benzatropine; benztropine]
benztropine methanesulfonate [see: benztropine mesylate]
benzydamine INN, BAN *analgesic; antipyretic; anti-inflammatory* [also: benzydamine HCl]
benzydamine HCl USAN *analgesic; antipyretic; anti-inflammatory* [also: benzydamine]

benzydroflumethiazide [see: bendroflumethiazide]
benzyl alcohol NF, INN *antimicrobial agent; antiseptic; local anesthetic*
benzyl analogue of serotonin (BAS) [see: benanserin HCl]
benzyl antiserotonin [see: benanserin HCl]
benzyl benzoate USP
benzyl carbinol [see: phenylethyl alcohol]
***S*-benzyl thiobenzoate** [see: tibenzate]
benzylamide [see: beclamide]
***N*-benzylanilinoacetamidoxime** [see: cetoxime]
benzyldimethyltetradecylammonium chloride [see: miristalkonium chloride]
benzylhexadecyldimethylammonium [see: cetalkonium]
benzylhexadecyldimethylammonium chloride [see: cetalkonium chloride]
***p*-benzyloxyphenol** [see: monobenzone]
benzylpenicillin INN, BAN *(orphan: penicillin hypersensitivity assessment)*
benzylpenicillin potassium BAN *antibacterial* [also: penicillin G potassium]
benzylpenicillin procaine [see: penicillin G procaine]
benzylpenicillin sodium BAN *antibacterial* [also: penicillin G sodium]
benzylpenicilloic acid [see: benzylpenicillin]
benzylpenicilloyl polylysine USP *penicillin sensitivity test*
benzylpenilloic acid [see: benzylpenicillin]
benzylsulfamide INN
benzylsulfanilamide [see: benzylsulfamide]
BEP (bleomycin, etoposide, Platinol) *chemotherapy protocol*
bepafant INN
bepanthen [see: panthenol]

beperidium iodide INN
bephene oxinaphthoate [see: bephenium hydroxynaphthoate]
bephenium embonate [see: bephenium hydroxynaphthoate]
bephenium hydroxynaphthoate USP, INN, BAN
bepiastine INN
bepridil INN, BAN *vasodilator; calcium channel blocker* [also: bepridil HCl]
bepridil HCl USAN *vasodilator; calcium channel blocker* [also: bepridil]
beractant USAN *pulmonary surfactant; (orphan: neonatal respiratory distress syndrome)*
beraprost USAN, INN *platelet aggregation inhibitor*
beraprost sodium USAN *platelet aggregation inhibitor*
berculon A [see: thioacetazone; thiacetazone]
berkelium *element (Bk)*
bermastine [see: barmastine]
bermoprofen INN
Berocca Plus tablets ℞ *vitamin/mineral/iron supplement* [multiple vitamins & minerals; ferrous fumarate; folic acid; biotin]
Berocca tablets ℞ *vitamin supplement* [multiple B vitamins; vitamin C; folic acid]
Berotec ℞ *investigational bronchodilator; antiasthmatic* [fenoterol hydrobromide]
Berplex Plus tablets ℞ *vitamin/mineral/iron supplement* [multiple vitamins & minerals; ferrous fumarate; folic acid; biotin]
Berplex tablets ℞ *vitamin supplement* [multiple vitamins]
Berubigen injection (discontinued 1991) ℞ *antianemic; vitamin supplement* [cyanocobalamin]
beryllium *element (Be)*
berythromycin USAN, INN *antiamebic; antibacterial*

Besta capsules (discontinued 1993) OTC *vitamin/mineral supplement* [multiple vitamins & minerals]
besulpamide INN
besunide INN
beta carotene USAN, USP *ultraviolet screen; vitamin A precursor* [also: betacarotene]
Beta-2 solution for inhalation ℞ *bronchodilator* [isoetharine HCl]
betacarotene INN *ultraviolet screen* [also: beta carotene]
betacetylmethadol INN, BAN
Betadine aerosol, gauze pads, lubricating gel, cream, mouthwash, ointment, perineal wash, skin cleanser, foam, solution, swab, swabsticks, surgical scrub OTC *broad-spectrum antimicrobial* [povidone-iodine]
Betadine Antiseptic vaginal suppositories, vaginal gel OTC *broad-spectrum antimicrobial* [povidone-iodine]
Betadine Medicated Douche; Betadine Medicated Disposable Douche; Betadine Medicated Premixed Disposable Douche solution OTC *broad-spectrum antimicrobial* [povidone-iodine]
Betadine shampoo OTC *broad-spectrum antimicrobial for dandruff* [povidone-iodine]
beta-estradiol [see: estradiol]
beta-estradiol benzoate [see: estradiol benzoate]
betaeucaine HCl [now: eucaine HCl]
beta-D-galactosidase *digestive enzyme* [see: tilactase]
Betagan Liquifilm eye drops ℞ *antiglaucoma agent (β-blocker)* [levobunolol HCl]
Betagen ointment, solution, surgical scrub OTC *broad-spectrum antimicrobial* [povidone-iodine]
beta-glucocerebrosidase [see: alglucerase]
betahistine INN, BAN *vasodilator* [also: betahistine HCl]

betahistine HCl USAN *vasodilator* [also: betahistine]
beta-hypophamine [see: vasopressin]
betaine HCl USP *electrolyte replenisher*
beta-lactone [see: propiolactone]
Betalin injection (discontinued 1991) ℞ *antianemic; vitamin supplement* [cyanocobalamin]
betameprodine INN, BAN
betamethadol INN, BAN
betamethasone USAN, USP, INN, BAN *glucocorticoid*
betamethasone acetate USP *glucocorticoid*
betamethasone acibutate INN, BAN
betamethasone benzoate USAN, USP, BAN *topical corticosteroid*
betamethasone dipropionate USAN, USP, BAN *topical corticosteroid*
betamethasone dipropionate, augmented *topical corticosteroid*
betamethasone sodium phosphate USP, BAN *glucocorticoid*
betamethasone valerate USAN, USP, BAN *topical corticosteroid*
betamicin INN *antibacterial* [also: betamicin sulfate]
betamicin sulfate USAN *antibacterial* [also: betamicin]
betanaphthol NF
betanidine INN *antihypertensive* [also: bethanidine sulfate; bethanidine]
betanidine sulfate [see: bethanidine sulfate]
Betapace tablets ℞ *antiarrhythmic for life-threatening ventricular arrhythmias (orphan); β-blocker* [sotalol HCl]
Betapen-VK film-coated tablets, powder for oral solution ℞ *bactericidal antibiotic* [penicillin V potassium]
betaprodine INN, BAN
beta-propiolactone [see: propiolactone]
beta-pyridylcarbinol [see: nicotinyl alcohol]

Betaseron ℞ *(orphan: multiple sclerosis; non-A, non-B hepatitis; AIDS)* [interferon beta, recombinant human]
Betatrex cream, ointment, lotion ℞ *topical corticosteroid* [betamethasone valerate]
Beta-Val cream, lotion, ointment ℞ *topical corticosteroid* [betamethasone valerate]
betaxolol INN, BAN *antianginal; antihypertensive; topical antiglaucoma agent* [also: betaxolol HCl]
betaxolol HCl USAN, USP *antianginal; antihypertensive; topical antiglaucoma agent* [also: betaxolol]
betazole INN [also: betazole HCl; ametazole]
betazole HCl USP [also: betazole; ametazole]
betazolium chloride [see: betazole HCl]
bethanechol chloride USP, BAN *cholinergic urinary stimulant* [also: bethanecol chloride]
bethanecol chloride BAN *cholinergic* [also: bethanechol chloride]
bethanidine BAN *antihypertensive* [also: bethanidine sulfate; betanidine]
bethanidine sulfate USAN *antihypertensive; (orphan: primary ventricular fibrillation)* [also: betanidine; bethanidine]
betiatide USAN, INN, BAN *pharmaceutic aid*
Betoptic; Betoptic S Drop-Tainer (eye drops) ℞ *antiglaucoma agent (β-blocker)* [betaxolol HCl]
betoxycaine INN
betoxycaine HCl [see: betoxycaine]
betula oil [see: methyl salicylate]
Betuline lotion OTC *counterirritant* [methyl salicylate; camphor; menthol; peppermint oil]
bevantolol INN, BAN *antianginal; antihypertensive; antiarrhythmic* [also: bevantolol HCl]

bevantolol HCl USAN *antianginal; antihypertensive; antiarrhythmic* [also: bevantolol]

bevonium methylsulphate BAN [also: bevonium metilsulfate]

bevonium metilsulfate INN [also: bevonium methylsulphate]

Bexophene capsules (discontinued 1991) ℞ *narcotic analgesic* [propoxyphene HCl; aspirin; caffeine]

bezafibrate USAN, INN, BAN *antihyperlipoproteinemic*

bezitramide INN, BAN

B.F.I. Antiseptic powder OTC *topical antiseptic* [bismuth-formic-iodide; zinc phenol sulfonate; potassium alum; bismuth subgallate; boric acid; menthol]

BHA (butylated hydroxyanisole) [q.v.]

BHD (BCNU, hydroxyurea, dacarbazine) *chemotherapy protocol*

BHDV; BHD-V (BCNU, hydroxyurea, dacarbazine, vincristine) *chemotherapy protocol*

BHT (butylated hydroxytoluene) [q.v.]

bialamicol INN, BAN *antiamebic* [also: bialamicol HCl]

bialamicol HCl USAN *antiamebic* [also: bialamicol]

biallylamicol [see: bialamicol]

Biamine IM or IV injection (discontinued 1991) ℞ *beriberi treatment* [thiamine HCl]

Biavax II subcu injection ℞ *rubella and mumps vaccine* [rubella & mumps virus vaccine, live]

Biaxin Filmtabs (film-coated tablets) ℞ *macrolide antibiotic* [clarithromycin]

bibenzonium bromide INN, BAN

bibrocathin [see: bibrocathol]

bibrocathol INN

Bicalma chewable tablets OTC *antacid* [calcium carbonate; magnesium trisilicate]

Bichloracetic Acid liquid ℞ *cauterant; keratolytic* [dichloroacetic acid]

bicifadine INN *analgesic* [also: bicifadine HCl]

bicifadine HCl USAN *analgesic* [also: bicifadine]

Bicillin C-R; Bicillin C-R 900/300 IM injection, Tubex (cartridge-needle unit) ℞ *bactericidal antibiotic* [penicillin G benzathine; penicillin G procaine]

Bicillin L-A IM injection, Tubex (cartridge-needle units) ℞ *bactericidal antibiotic* [penicillin G benzathine]

Bicitra solution ℞ *urinary alkalinizing agent* [sodium citrate; citric acid]

biclodil INN *antihypertensive; vasodilator* [also: biclodil HCl]

biclodil HCl USAN *antihypertensive; vasodilator* [also: biclodil]

biclofibrate INN

biclotymol INN

BiCNU powder for IV injection ℞ *antineoplastic for brain tumors, lymphomas and multiple myeloma* [carmustine]

bicozamycin INN

Bicozene cream OTC *topical local anesthetic; antifungal* [benzocaine; resorcinol]

bicyclomycin [see: bicozamycin]

bidimazium iodide INN, BAN

bidisomide USAN, INN *antiarrhythmic*

Biebrich scarlet red [see: scarlet red]

Biebrich scarlet-picroaniline blue

bietamiverine INN

bietamiverine HCl [see: bietamiverine]

bietaserpine INN

bifemelane INN

bifepramide INN

bifeprofen INN

bifluranol INN, BAN

bifonazole USAN, INN, BAN *antifungal*

Bi-K liquid (discontinued 1991) ℞ *potassium supplement* [potassium gluconate; potassium citrate]

bile acids, oxidized [see: dehydrocholic acid]

bile salts *laxative*

Bilezyme tablets ℞ *digestive enzymes* [amylase; protease; dehydrocholic acid; desoxycholic acid]

Bili-Labstix reagent strips OTC *in vitro diagnostic aid for multiple urine products*

Bilivist capsules ℞ *oral cholecystographic radiopaque agent* [ipodate sodium]

Bilopaque capsules ℞ *oral cholecystographic radiopaque agent* [tyropanoate sodium]

Bilron Pulvules (capsules) (discontinued 1992) OTC *choleretic; fat digestive aid* [bile salts]

Biltricide tablets ℞ *anthelmintic* [praziquantel]

bimazol [see: carbimazole]

bimethadol [see: dimepheptanol]

bimethoxycaine lactate

bindazac BAN *anti-inflammatory* [also: bendazac]

binedaline INN

binfloxacin USAN, INN *veterinary antibacterial*

binifibrate INN

biniramycin USAN, INN *antibacterial*

binizolast INN

binodaline [see: binedaline]

binospirone INN *anxiolytic* [also: binospirone mesylate]

binospirone mesylate USAN *anxiolytic* [also: binospirone]

Bio-Acerola C Complex wafers OTC *dietary supplement* [vitamin C; citrus bioflavonoids; rutin]

bioallethrin BAN

Biocadren tablets ℞ *antihypertensive* [timolol maleate]

Biocef capsules, powder for oral suspension ℞ *antibiotic* [cephalexin monohydrate]

Biocult-GC swab test OTC *in vitro diagnostic aid for gonorrhea*

Bioday with Iron tablets OTC *vitamin/iron supplement* [multiple vitamins; iron; folic acid]

Biodel Implant/BCNU biodegradable polymer implant *(orphan: recurrent malignant glioma)* [carmustine]

Biodine Topical 1% solution OTC *broad-spectrum antimicrobial* [povidone-iodine]

Biodine Topical solution OTC *broad-spectrum antimicrobial* [povidone-iodine]

bioflavonoids *vitamin P*

biogastrone [see: carbenoxolone]

biological indicator for dry-heat sterilization USP *sterilization indicator*

biological indicator for ethylene oxide sterilization USP *sterilization indicator*

biological indicator for steam sterilization USP *sterilization indicator*

Biomox powder for oral suspension, capsules ℞ *penicillin-type antibiotic* [amoxicillin trihydrate]

Biomox tablets, powder for oral suspension ℞ *veterinary antibiotic* [amoxicillin]

Biopar Forte tablets (discontinued 1991) ℞ *antianemic; vitamin supplement* [vitamin B_{12}; intrinsic factor; cobalamin]

bioral [see: carbenoxolone]

Bio-Rescue *(orphan: acute iron poisoning)* [dextran; deferoxamine]

bioresmethrin INN

bios I [see: inositol]

bios II [see: biotin]

Biosynject ℞ *(orphan: newborn hemolytic disease; ABO blood incompatability of organ or bone marrow transplants)* [trisaccharides A and B]

Bio-Tab film-coated tablets ℞ *tetracycline-type antibiotic* [doxycycline hyclate]

Biotab tablets OTC *decongestant; antihistamine; analgesic* [phenylpropanolamine HCl; phenyltoloxamine citrate; acetaminophen]

Biotel diabetes test kit OTC *in vitro diagnostic aid for urine glucose*

Biotel kidney test kit OTC *in vitro diagnostic aid for urine hemoglobin, RBCs, and albumin (predictor of kidney diseases)*

Biotel u.t.i. test kit OTC *in vitro diagnostic aid for urine nitrite (predictor of urinary tract infections)*

biotexin [see: novobiocin]

biotin USP, INN *B complex vitamin; vitamin H*

Biotin Forte tablets OTC *vitamin supplement* [multiple B vitamins; vitamin C; folic acid; biotin]

BioTropin ℞ *investigational drug for AIDS*

Bio-tuss C liquid (discontinued 1991) ℞ *antitussive; expectorant* [codeine phosphate; iodinated glycerol]

Biozyme-C ointment (discontinued 1991) ℞ *topical enzyme for biochemical debridement* [collagenase]

BIP (bleomycin, ifosfamide, Platinol) *chemotherapy protocol*

bipenamol INN *antidepressant* [also: bipenamol HCl]

bipenamol HCl USAN *antidepressant* [also: bipenamol]

biperiden USP, INN, BAN *anticholinergic; antiparkinsonian*

biperiden HCl USP, BAN *anticholinergic; antiparkinsonian*

biperiden lactate USP, BAN *anticholinergic; antiparkinsonian*

biphasic insulin [see: insulin, biphasic]

biphenamine HCl USAN *topical anesthetic; antibacterial; antifungal* [also: xenysalate]

Biphetamine 12½; Biphetamine 20 capsules ℞ *CNS stimulant; amphetamine* [dextroamphetamine; amphetamine]

biprofenide [see: bifepramide]

birch oil, sweet [see: methyl salicylate]

biriperone INN

bisacodyl USP, INN, BAN *stimulant laxative*

bisacodyl tannex USAN *laxative*

bisantrene INN *antineoplastic* [also: bisantrene HCl]

bisantrene HCl USAN *antineoplastic* [also: bisantrene]

bisaramil INN

bisatin [see: oxyphenisatin acetate]

bisbendazole INN

bisbentiamine INN

bis-chloroethyl-nitrosourea (BCNU) [see: carmustine]

Bisco-Lax suppositories, enteric-coated tablets OTC *laxative* [bisacodyl]

bisfenazone INN

bisfentidine INN

bishydroxycoumarin [now: dicumarol]

Bismatrol chewable tablets, liquid OTC *antidiarrheal* [bismuth subsalicylate]

bismucatebrol [see: bibrocathol]

bismuth *element (Bi)*

bismuth, milk of USP *antacid; astringent*

bismuth aluminate USAN

bismuth betanaphthol USP

bismuth carbonate USAN

bismuth carbonate, basic [see: bismuth subcarbonate]

bismuth citrate USP

bismuth cream [see: bismuth, milk of]

bismuth gallate, basic [see: bismuth subgallate]

bismuth glycollylarsanilate BAN [also: glycobiarsol]

bismuth hydroxide [see: bismuth, milk of]

bismuth hydroxide nitrate oxide [see: bismuth subnitrate]

bismuth magma [now: bismuth, milk of]
bismuth oxycarbonate [see: bismuth subcarbonate]
bismuth potassium tartrate NF
bismuth sodium triglycollamate USP
bismuth subcarbonate USAN *antacid; GI adsorbent*
bismuth subgallate USAN, USP *antacid; GI adsorbent*
bismuth subnitrate USP *skin protectant*
bismuth subsalicylate (BSS) USAN *antiperistaltic; antacid; GI adsorbent*
bisobrin INN *fibrinolytic* [also: bisobrin lactate]
bisobrin lactate USAN *fibrinolytic* [also: bisobrin]
Bisodol chewable tablets OTC *antacid* [magnesium hydroxide; calcium carbonate]
Bisodol powder OTC *antacid* [sodium bicarbonate; magnesium carbonate]
bisoprolol USAN, INN, BAN *antihypertensive (β-blocker)*
bisoprolol fumarate USAN *antihypertensive (β-blocker)*
bisorcic INN
bisoxatin INN, BAN *laxative* [also: bisoxatin acetate]
bisoxatin acetate USAN *laxative* [also: bisoxatin]
bispyrithione magsulfex USAN *antibacterial; antidandruff; antifungal*
bis-tropamide [now: tropicamide]
bithionol NF, INN, BAN *investigational anti-infective for paragonimiasis and fascioliasis*
bithionolate sodium USAN *topical anti-infective* [also: sodium bitionolate]
bithionoloxide INN
Bitin (available only from the Centers for Disease Control) ℞ *investigational anti-infective for paragonimiasis and fascioliasis* [bithionol]
bitipazone INN

bitolterol INN, BAN *bronchodilator* [also: bitolterol mesylate]
bitolterol mesylate USAN *bronchodilator* [also: bitolterol]
bitoscanate INN
B-Ject-100 injection ℞ *parenteral vitamin therapy* [multiple B vitamins]
black widow spider antivenin [see: antivenin (Latrodectus mactans)]
Black-Draught syrup OTC *laxative* [casanthranol; senna extract]
Black-Draught tablets, granules OTC *laxative* [senna concentrate]
Blairex Hard Contact Lens Cleaner solution OTC *contact lens cleaning solution*
Blairex Sterile Saline aerosol solution OTC *contact lens rinsing and storage solution* [saline solution]
Blanex capsules (discontinued 1991) ℞ *skeletal muscle relaxant; analgesic* [chlorzoxazone; acetaminophen]
blastomycin NF
Blem-Derm cream OTC *acne* [benzoyl peroxide]
Blenoxane powder for IM, IV or subcu injection ℞ *antineoplastic antibiotic* [bleomycin sulfate]
BLEO-COMF (bleomycin, cyclophosphamide, Oncovin, methotrexate, fluorouracil) *chemotherapy protocol*
bleomycin (BLM) INN, BAN *antineoplastic* [also: bleomycin sulfate]
bleomycin sulfate USAN, USP *antineoplastic* [also: bleomycin]
Bleph-10 Liquifilm eye drops ℞ *ophthalmic bacteriostatic* [sodium sulfacetamide]
Bleph-10 S.O.P. ointment ℞ *ophthalmic antibiotic* [sodium sulfacetamide]
Blephamide Liquifilm eye drop suspension ℞ *topical ophthalmic corticosteroidal anti-inflammatory; bacteriostatic* [prednisolone acetate; sodium sulfacetamide]

Blephamide S.O.P. ophthalmic ointment ℞ *topical ophthalmic corticosteroidal anti-inflammatory; bacteriostatic* [prednisolone acetate; sodium sulfacetamide]

Blink-N-Clean solution (discontinued 1992) OTC *contact lens rewetting solution*

Blinx ophthalmic solution OTC *extraocular irrigating solution* [balanced saline solution]

BlisterGard liquid OTC *skin protectant*

Blistex lip ointment OTC *topical antimicrobial; antipruritic; mild anesthetic; vulnerary* [allantoin; liquefied phenol; camphor]

Blistik lip balm OTC *sunscreen; skin protectant* [octyl dimethyl PABA; oxybenzone; dimethicone]

Blis-To-Sol liquid OTC *topical antifungal; keratolytic* [undecylenic acid; salicylic acid]

Blis-To-Sol powder OTC *topical antifungal; keratolytic* [benzoic acid; salicylic acid]

BLM (bleomycin) [q.v.]

Blocadren tablets ℞ *antihypertensive; migraine preventative; β-blocker* [timolol maleate]

blocked ricin conjugated murine monoclonal antibody [see: ricin (blocked) conjugated murine MCA]

blood, whole USP *blood replenisher*

blood, whole human [now: blood, whole]

blood cells, human red [now: blood cells, red]

blood cells, red USP *blood replenisher*

blood group specific substances A, B & AB USP *blood neutralizer*

blood grouping serum, anti-A [see: anti-A blood grouping serum]

blood grouping serum, anti-B [see: anti-B blood grouping serum]

blood grouping serum, anti-C USP *in vitro blood testing*

blood grouping serum, anti-c USP *in vitro blood testing*

blood grouping serum, anti-E USP *in vitro blood testing*

blood grouping serum, anti-e USP *in vitro blood testing*

Blood Nutrients capsule OTC *vitamin/mineral supplement* [multiple vitamins & minerals]

Bluboro powder packets OTC *astringent wet dressing (modified Burow solution)* [aluminum sulfate; calcium acetate]

Blue gel OTC *pediculicide* [pyrethrins; piperonyl butoxide; petroleum distillate]

bluensomycin INN

B-MOPP (bleomycin, nitrogen mustard, Oncovin, procarbazine, prednisone) *chemotherapy protocol*

BMP (BCNU, methotrexate, procarbazine) *chemotherapy protocol*

BMY-45622 *(orphan: ovarian cancer)*

B-Nutron tablets (discontinued 1992) OTC *vitamin/mineral supplement* [multiple vitamins & minerals]

BOAP (bleomycin, Oncovin, Adriamycin, prednisone) *chemotherapy protocol*

Bo-Cal tablets OTC *dietary supplement* [calcium; vitamin D; magnesium]

boforsin [see: colforsin]

bofumustine INN

Boil n Soak solution (discontinued 1992) OTC *contact lens rinsing and storage solution* [preserved saline solution]

Boil-Ease salve OTC *drawing salve for boils* [benzocaine; sulfur; ichthammol; camphor; phenol; juniper tar]

bolandiol INN *anabolic* [also: bolandiol dipropionate]

bolandiol dipropionate USAN *anabolic* [also: bolandiol]

bolasterone USAN, INN *anabolic*

bolazine INN

BOLD (bleomycin, Oncovin, lomustine, dacarbazine) *chemotherapy protocol*
boldenone INN, BAN *anabolic* [also: boldenone undecylenate]
boldenone undecylenate USAN *anabolic* [also: boldenone]
bolenol USAN, INN *anabolic*
bolmantalate USAN, INN, BAN *anabolic*
bolus alba [see: kaolin]
bometolol INN
BOMP (bleomycin, Oncovin, Matulane, prednisone) *chemotherapy protocol*
bone ash [see: calcium phosphate, tribasic]
Bone Meal tablets OTC *dietary supplement* [calcium; phosphorus]
bone powder, purified [see: calcium phosphate, tribasic]
Bonefos (*orphan: increased bone resorption due to malignancy*) [disodium clodronate tetrahydrate]
Bonine chewable tablets OTC *anticholinergic; antihistamine; antivertigo agent; motion sickness preventative* [meclizine]
Bontril PDM tablets ℞ *anorexiant* [phendimetrazine tartrate]
Bontril slow-release capsules ℞ *anorexiant* [phendimetrazine tartrate]
BOP (BCNU, Oncovin, prednisone) *chemotherapy protocol*
BOPAM (bleomycin, Oncovin, prednisone, Adriamycin, mechlorethamine, methotrexate) *chemotherapy protocol*
bopindolol INN
BOPP (BCNU, Oncovin, procarbazine, prednisone) *chemotherapy protocol*
boracic acid [see: boric acid]
borax [see: sodium borate]
boric acid NF *acidifying agent; ocular emollient; antiseptic; astringent*
2-bornanone [see: camphor]
bornaprine INN, BAN

bornaprolol INN
bornelone USAN, INN *ultraviolet screen*
bornyl acetate USAN
borocaptate sodium B 10 USAN *antineoplastic; radioactive agent* [also: sodium borocaptate (^{10}B)]
Borocell ℞ (*orphan: boron neutron capture therapy for glioblastoma multiforme*) [monomercaptoundecahydro-closo-DQ decaborate sodium]
Borofair Otic ear drops ℞ *antibacterial/antifungal* [acetic acid]
Borofax ointment OTC *astringent; antiseptic* [boric acid]
boroglycerin NF
boron *element* (B)
Boropak powder packets OTC *astringent wet dressing (modified Burrow solution)* [aluminum sulfate; calcium acetate]
Boston Cleaner, The solution OTC *contact lens cleaning solution*
Boston Reconditioning Drops OTC *contact lens cleaning and soaking solution*
botiacrine INN
BottomBetter ointment OTC *topical diaper rash treatment*
botulinum toxin, type A (*orphan: blepharospasm and strabismus of dystonia; cervical dystonia; pediatric cerebral palsy*)
botulinum toxin, type B (*orphan: cervical dystonia*)
botulinum toxin, type F (*orphan: spasmodic torticollis; cervical dystonia; essential blepharospasm*)
botulinum toxoid, pentavalent *investigational vaccine*
botulism antitoxin USP *passive immunizing agent*
botulism equine antitoxin, trivalent *passive immunizing agent*
botulism immune globulin (*orphan: infant botulism*)

Bounty Bears chewable tablets OTC *vitamin supplement* [multiple vitamins; folic acid]

Bounty Bears Plus Iron chewable tablets OTC *vitamin/iron supplement* [multiple vitamins; iron; folic acid]

bourbonal [see: ethyl vanillin]

bovine colostrum *(orphan: AIDS-related diarrhea)*

boxidine USAN, INN *antihyperlipoproteinemic*

Boyol salve OTC *topical anti-infective; anesthetic* [ichthammol; benzocaine]

B.P. 5%; B.P. 10% lotion OTC *keratolytic for acne* [benzoyl peroxide]

B.P. Gel 5%; B.P. Gel 10% OTC *keratolytic for acne* [benzoyl peroxide]

B-PAS (benzoyl para-aminosalicylate) [see: benzoylpas calcium]

B-Plex tablets ℞ *vitamin supplement* [multiple B vitamins; vitamin C; folic acid]

BQ tablets OTC *decongestant; antihistamine; analgesic* [phenylpropanolamine HCl; chlorpheniramine maleate; acetaminophen]

BR-96 *investigational antineoplastic* [doxorubicin monoclonal antibody immunoconjugate]

brallobarbital INN

BranchAmin 4% IV infusion ℞ *nutritional therapy for high metabolic stress* [multiple branched-chain essential amino acids]

branched-chain amino acids (BCAA) *(orphan: amyotrophic lateral sclerosis)* [see: isoleucine; leucine; valine]

Brasivol Base OTC *topical acne cleanser* [surfactant cleansing base with neutral soaps]

Brasivol cream OTC *abrasive cleanser for acne* [aluminum oxide]

brazergoline INN

Breathe Free nasal spray OTC *nasal moisturizer* [sodium chloride (saline)]

Breezee Mist Aerosol powder OTC *topical antifungal; anhidrotic* [undecylenic acid; menthol; aluminum chlorhydrate]

brefonalol INN

bremazocine INN

Breonesin capsules OTC *expectorant* [guaifenesin]

brequinar INN *antineoplastic* [also: brequinar sodium]

brequinar sodium USAN *antineoplastic* [also: brequinar]

bretazenil USAN, INN *anxiolytic*

Brethaire oral inhalation aerosol ℞ *bronchodilator* [terbutaline sulfate]

Brethine tablets, IV or subcu injection ℞ *bronchodilator* [terbutaline sulfate]

bretylium tosilate INN *antiadrenergic; antiarrhythmic* [also: bretylium tosylate]

bretylium tosylate USAN, BAN *antiadrenergic; antiarrhythmic* [also: bretylium tosilate]

Bretylol IV or IM injection ℞ *antiarrhythmic* [bretylium tosylate]

Brevibloc IV infusion ℞ *β-blocker for supraventricular tachycardia* [esmolol HCl]

Brevicon tablets ℞ *oral contraceptive* [norethindrone; ethinyl estradiol]

Brevital Sodium powder for IV injection ℞ *general anesthetic* [methohexital sodium]

Brevoxyl gel ℞ *keratolytic for acne* [benzoyl peroxide]

brewer's yeast *natural source of protein and B-complex vitamins*

Brexin-L.A. sustained-release capsules ℞ *antihistamine; decongestant* [chlorpheniramine maleate; pseudoephedrine HCl]

Bricanyl IV or subcu injection, tablets ℞ *bronchodilator* [terbutaline sulfate]

brifentanil HCl USAN *narcotic analgesic*

brimonidine tartrate USAN *ophthalmic adrenergic*

brinaldix [see: clopamide]

brinase INN [also: brinolase]

brindoxime INN
brinolase USAN *fibrinolytic* [also: brinase]
British antilewisite (BAL) [now: dimercaprol]
brivudine INN
brobactam INN
brobenzoxaldine [see: broxaldine]
broclepride INN
brocresine USAN, INN, BAN *histidine decarboxylase inhibitor*
brocrinat USAN, INN *diuretic*
brodimoprim INN
brofaromine INN
Brofed elixir OTC *decongestant; antihistamine* [pseudoephedrine HCl; brompheniramine maleate]
brofezil INN, BAN
brofoxine USAN, INN *antipsychotic*
brolaconazole INN
brolamfetamine INN
Brolene (*orphan: Acanthamoeba keratitis*) [propamidine isethionate]
bromacrylide INN
bromadel [see: carbromal]
bromadoline INN *analgesic* [also: bromadoline maleate]
bromadoline maleate USAN *analgesic* [also: bromadoline]
Bromaline elixir OTC *decongestant; antihistamine* [phenylpropanolamine HCl; brompheniramine maleate]
Bromaline Plus captabs OTC *decongestant; antihistamine; analgesic* [phenylpropanolamine HCl; brompheniramine maleate; acetaminophen]
bromamid INN
Bromanate DC Cough syrup ℞ *decongestant; antihistamine; antitussive* [brompheniramine maleate; phenylpropanolamine HCl; codeine phosphate; alcohol]
Bromanate elixir OTC *decongestant; antihistamine* [brompheniramine maleate; phenylpropanolamine HCl]

Bromanyl syrup ℞ *antihistamine; antitussive* [bromodiphenhydramine HCl; codeine phosphate; alcohol]
bromanylpromide [see: bromamid]
Bromarest DX Cough syrup ℞ *decongestant; antihistamine; antitussive* [pseudoephedrine HCl; brompheniramine maleate; dextromethorphan hydrobromide; alcohol]
Bromatane elixir OTC *antihistamine* [brompheniramine maleate]
Bromatapp elixir OTC *decongestant; antihistamine* [phenylpropanolamine HCl; brompheniramine maleate]
Bromatapp Extended timed-release tablets ℞ *decongestant; antihistamine* [phenylpropanolamine HCl; phenylephrine HCl; brompheniramine maleate]
Bromatapp extended-release tablets ℞/OTC *decongestant; antihistamine* [phenylpropanolamine HCl; brompheniramine maleate]
Bromatol elixir OTC *decongestant; antihistamine* [brompheniramine maleate; phenylpropanolamine HCl]
bromauric acid NF
bromazepam USAN, INN, BAN *minor tranquilizer*
bromazine INN *antihistamine* [also: bromodiphenhydramine HCl; bromodiphenhydramine]
bromazine HCl [see: bromodiphenhydramine HCl]
brombenzonium [see: bromhexine HCl]
bromchlorenone USAN, INN *topical anti-infective*
bromebric acid INN, BAN
bromelain [see: bromelains]
bromelains USAN, INN, BAN *anti-inflammatory*
bromelin [see: bromelains]
bromerguride INN
brometenamine INN
bromethol [see: tribromoethanol]

Bromfed syrup OTC *decongestant; antihistamine* [pseudoephedrine HCl; brompheniramine maleate]

Bromfed timed-release capsules, tablets ℞ *decongestant; antihistamine* [pseudoephedrine HCl; brompheniramine maleate]

Bromfed-DM syrup ℞ *decongestant; antihistamine; antitussive* [pseudoephedrine HCl; brompheniramine maleate; dextromethorphan hydrobromide]

Bromfed-PD timed-release capsules ℞ *pediatric decongestant and antihistamine* [pseudoephedrine HCl; brompheniramine maleate]

bromfenac INN *analgesic* [also: bromfenac sodium]

bromfenac sodium USAN *analgesic* [also: bromfenac]

bromhexine INN, BAN *expectorant; mucolytic;* (*orphan: keratoconjunctivitis sicca of Sjögren syndrome*) [also: bromhexine HCl]

bromhexine HCl USAN *expectorant; mucolytic* [also: bromhexine]

bromindione USAN, INN, BAN *anticoagulant*

bromine *element (Br)*

bromisoval INN [also: bromisovalum]

bromisovalum NF [also: bromisoval]

bromocamphor [see: camphor, monobromated]

bromociclen INN [also: bromocyclen]

bromocriptine USAN, INN, BAN *prolactin enzyme inhibitor*

bromocriptine mesylate USAN, USP *prolactin enzyme inhibitor; antiparkinsonian*

bromocyclen BAN [also: bromociclen]

bromodiethylacetylurea [see: carbromal]

bromodiphenhydramine BAN *antihistamine* [also: bromodiphenhydramine HCl; bromazine]

bromodiphenhydramine HCl USP *antihistamine* [also: bromazine; bromodiphenhydramine]

2-bromo-α-ergocryptine [see: bromocriptine]

bromofenofos INN

bromoform USP

bromofos INN

1-bromoheptadecafluorooctane [see: perflubron]

bromoisovaleryl urea (BVU) [see: bromisovalum]

Bromophen T.D. sustained-release tablets ℞ *decongestant; antihistamine* [phenylpropanolamine HCl; phenylephrine HCl; brompheniramine maleate]

bromophenol blue

bromophin [see: apomorphine HCl]

bromophos [see: bromofos]

bromopride INN

Bromo-Seltzer effervescent granules OTC *antacid; analgesic; antipyretic* [acetaminophen; sodium bicarbonate; citric acid]

bromotheophyllinate aminoisobutanol [see: pamabrom]

bromotheophyllinate pyranisamine [see: pyrabrom]

bromotheophyllinate pyrilamine [see: pyrabrom]

8-bromotheophylline [see: pamabrom]

Bromotuss with Codeine syrup ℞ *antihistamine; antitussive* [bromodiphenhydramine HCl; codeine phosphate; alcohol]

bromovaluree [see: bromisovalum]

11-bromovincamine [see: brovincamine]

bromoxanide USAN, INN *anthelmintic*

bromperidol USAN, INN, BAN *antipsychotic*

bromperidol decanoate USAN *antipsychotic*

Bromphen DC with Codeine Cough syrup ℞ *decongestant; antihis-*

tamine; *antitussive* [phenylpropanolamine HCl; brompheniramine maleate; codeine phosphate; alcohol]

Bromphen DX Cough syrup ℞ *decongestant; antihistamine; antitussive* [pseudoephedrine HCl; brompheniramine maleate; dextromethorphan hydrobromide; alcohol]

Bromphen elixir OTC *decongestant* [brompheniramine maleate]

Bromphen elixir OTC *decongestant; antihistamine* [brompheniramine maleate; phenolpropanolamine HCl]

brompheniramine INN, BAN *antihistamine* [also: brompheniramine maleate]

Brompheniramine Cough syrup OTC *decongestant; antihistamine; antitussive* [phenylpropanolamine HCl; brompheniramine maleate; codeine phosphate; alcohol]

Brompheniramine DC Cough syrup ℞ *decongestant; antihistamine; antitussive* [phenylpropanolamine HCl; brompheniramine maleate; codeine phosphate; alcohol]

brompheniramine maleate USP *antihistamine* [also: brompheniramine]

Brompheril extended-release tablets OTC

Brompton's Cocktail; Brompton's Mixture (refers to any oral narcotic/alcoholic solution containing morphine and either cocaine or a phenothiazine derivative) *prophylaxis for chronic, severe pain*

Bromtapp elixir OTC *antihistamine* [brompheniramine maleate]

bromvalerylurea [see: bromisovalum]

Bronchial capsules ℞ *antiasthmatic; bronchodilator; expectorant* [theophylline; guaifenesin]

Broncho Saline solution OTC *diluent for inhalation bronchodilators; solution for tracheal lavage* [saline solution]

Broncholate CS liquid ℞ *decongestant; antitussive; expectorant* [ephedrine HCl; codeine phosphate; guaifenesin]

Broncholate softgels, syrup ℞ *decongestant; expectorant* [ephedrine HCl; guaifenesin]

Brondecon tablets, elixir ℞ *antiasthmatic; bronchodilator; expectorant* [oxtriphylline; guaifenesin]

Brondelate elixir ℞ *antiasthmatic; bronchodilator; expectorant* [oxtriphylline; guaifenesin]

Bronitin Mist inhalation aerosol OTC *bronchodilator for bronchial asthma* [epinephrine bitartrate]

Bronitin tablets OTC *antiasthmatic; bronchodilator; decongestant; expectorant; antihistamine* [theophylline; ephedrine HCl; guaifenesin; pyrilamine maleate]

Bronkaid Mist inhalation aerosol OTC *bronchodilator for bronchial asthma* [epinephrine nitrate; epinephrine HCl]

Bronkaid tablets OTC *antiasthmatic; bronchodilator; decongestant; expectorant* [theophylline; ephedrine sulfate; guaifenesin]

Bronkephrine subcu or IM injection ℞ *bronchodilator* [ethylnorepinephrine HCl]

Bronkodyl capsules ℞ *bronchodilator* [theophylline]

Bronkolixir elixir OTC *antiasthmatic; bronchodilator; decongestant; expectorant; sedative* [theophylline; ephedrine sulfate; guaifenesin; phenobarbital]

Bronkometer inhalation aerosol ℞ *bronchodilator* [isoetharine mesylate]

Bronkosol solution for inhalation ℞ *bronchodilator* [isoetharine HCl]

Bronkotabs tablets OTC *antiasthmatic; bronchodilator; decongestant; expectorant; sedative* [theophylline; ephedrine sulfate; guaifenesin; phenobarbital]

Bronkotuss Expectorant liquid ℞ *decongestant; antihistamine; expecto-*

rant [ephedrine sulfate; chlorpheniramine maleate; guaifenesin; hydriodic acid; alcohol]
bronopol INN, BAN
broparestrol INN
broperamole USAN, INN *anti-inflammatory*
bropirimine USAN, INN *antineoplastic; antiviral*
broquinaldol INN
brosotamide INN
brosuximide INN
Brotane DX Cough syrup ℞ *antihistamine; antitussive* [pseudoephedrine HCl; brompheniramine maleate; dextromethorphan hydrobromide]
Brotane tablets, elixir OTC *antihistamine* [brompheniramine maleate]
brotianide INN, BAN
brotizolam USAN, INN, BAN *hypnotic*
brovanexine INN
brovincamine INN
broxaldine INN
broxaterol INN
broxitalamic acid INN
broxuridine INN
broxyquinoline INN
brucine sulfate NF
BSS (bismuth subsalicylate) [q.v.]
BSS; BSS Plus ophthalmic solution ℞ *intraocular irrigating solution* [balanced saline solution]
bucainide INN *antiarrhythmic* [also: bucainide maleate]
bucainide maleate USAN *antiarrhythmic* [also: bucainide]
Bucet capsules ℞ *sedative; analgesic* [butalbital; acetaminophen]
bucetin INN, BAN
buchu [see: diosmin]
buciclovir INN
bucillamine INN
bucindolol INN, BAN *antihypertensive* [also: bucindolol HCl]
bucindolol HCl USAN *antihypertensive* [also: bucindolol]
bucladesine INN

Bucladin-S Softabs (chewable tablets) ℞ *anticholinergic; antiemetic; motion sickness preventative* [buclizine HCl]
buclizine INN, BAN *antinauseant; antiemetic; anticholinergic; motion sickness relief* [also: buclizine HCl]
buclizine HCl USAN *antinauseant; antiemetic; anticholinergic* [also: buclizine]
buclosamide INN, BAN
bucloxic acid INN
bucolome INN
bucricaine INN
bucrilate INN *tissue adhesive* [also: bucrylate]
bucromarone USAN, INN *antiarrhythmic*
bucrylate USAN *tissue adhesive* [also: bucrilate]
bucumolol INN
budesonide USAN, INN, BAN *anti-inflammatory*
budipine INN
budotitane INN
budralazine INN
Buf-Bar OTC *medicated cleansing bar for acne* [sulfur; titanium dioxide]
bufenadine [see: bufenadrine]
bufenadrine INN
bufeniode INN
bufetolol INN
bufexamac INN, BAN
bufezolac INN
Buffaprin; Buffaprin Extra tablets OTC *analgesic; anti-inflammatory; antipyretic* [buffered aspirin]
buffered aspirin [see: aspirin, buffered]
Bufferin, Arthritis Strength; Bufferin Extra Strength tablets OTC *analgesic; antipyretic; anti-inflammatory; antirheumatic* [aspirin, buffered with magnesium carbonate and aluminum glycinate]
Bufferin, Tri-Buffered caplets OTC *analgesic; antipyretic; anti-inflammatory; antirheumatic* [aspirin, buffered

with calcium carbonate, magnesium oxide, and magnesium carbonate]

Bufferin, Tri-Buffered tablets (discontinued 1993) OTC *analgesic; antipyretic; anti-inflammatory; antirheumatic* [aspirin, buffered with calcium carbonate, magnesium oxide, and magnesium carbonate]

Bufferin AF Nite Time tablets OTC *antihistaminic sleep aid; analgesic* [diphenhydramine HCl; acetaminophen]

Bufferin coated tablets, coated caplets OTC *analgesic; antipyretic; anti-inflammatory; antirheumatic* [aspirin, buffered with calcium carbonate, magnesium oxide, and magnesium carbonate]

Buffets II tablets OTC *analgesic; antipyretic; anti-inflammatory* [acetaminophen; aspirin; caffeine; aluminum hydroxide]

Buffex tablets OTC *analgesic; antipyretic; anti-inflammatory; antirheumatic* [aspirin, buffered with aluminum glycinate and magnesium carbonate]

Buffinol; Buffinol Extra tablets OTC *analgesic; anti-inflammatory; antipyretic* [buffered aspirin]

bufilcon A USAN *hydrophilic contact lens material*

buflomedil INN, BAN

bufogenin INN

buformin USAN, INN *antidiabetic*

Buf-Oxal 10 gel (discontinued 1991) OTC *topical keratolytic for acne* [benzoyl peroxide]

Buf-Puf Medicated pads OTC *medicated cleansing pad for acne* [salicylic acid; alcohol]

bufrolin INN, BAN

bufuralol INN, BAN

bufylline BAN *diuretic; smooth muscle relaxant* [also: ambuphylline]

Bugs Bunny Children's; Bugs Bunny with Extra C Children's chewable tablets OTC *vitamin supplement* [multiple vitamins; folic acid]

Bugs Bunny Children's Chewable Tablets OTC *vitamin supplement* [multiple vitamins; folic acid]

Bugs Bunny Complete chewable tablets OTC *vitamin/mineral/calcium/iron supplement* [multiple vitamins & minerals; calcium; iron; folic acid; biotin]

Bugs Bunny Plus Iron chewable tablets OTC *vitamin/iron supplement* [multiple vitamins; iron; folic acid]

Bugs Bunny Vitamins and Minerals (name changed to Bugs Bunny Complete in 1993)

bumadizone INN

bumecaine INN

bumepidil INN

bumetanide USAN, USP, INN, BAN *loop diuretic*

bumetrizole USAN, INN *ultraviolet screen*

Bumex tablets, IV or IM injection ℞ *loop diuretic* [bumetanide]

Buminate 5%; Buminate 25% IV infusion ℞ *blood volume expander; shock; burns; hypoproteinemia* [human albumin]

bunaftine INN

bunamidine INN, BAN *anthelmintic* [also: bunamidine HCl]

bunamidine HCl USAN *anthelmintic* [also: bunamidine]

bunamiodyl INN [also: buniodyl]

bunamiodyl sodium [see: bunamiodyl; buniodyl]

bunaprolast USAN, INN *antiasthmatic; 5-lipoxygenase inhibitor*

bunazosin INN

bundlin [now: sedecamycin]

buniodyl BAN [also: bunamiodyl]

bunitrolol INN

bunolol INN *antiadrenergic (β-receptor)* [also: bunolol HCl]

bunolol HCl USAN *antiadrenergic (β-receptor)* [also: bunolol]

buparvaquone INN, BAN

buphenine INN, BAN *peripheral vasodilator* [also: nylidrin HCl]
buphenine HCl [see: nylidrin HCl]
bupicomide USAN, INN *antihypertensive*
bupivacaine INN, BAN *local anesthetic* [also: bupivacaine HCl]
bupivacaine HCl USAN, USP *local anesthetic* [also: bupivacaine]
bupranol [see: bupranolol]
bupranolol INN
Buprenex IV or IM injection ℞ *narcotic agonist-antagonist analgesic* [buprenorphine HCl]
buprenorphine INN, BAN *narcotic agonist-antagonist analgesic* [also: buprenorphine HCl]
buprenorphine HCl USAN *narcotic agonist-antagonist analgesic* [also: buprenorphine]
bupropion BAN *antidepressant* [also: bupropion HCl; amfebutamone]
bupropion HCl USAN *antidepressant* [also: amfebutamone; bupropion]
buquineran INN, BAN
buquinolate USAN, INN *coccidiostat for poultry*
buquiterine INN
buramate USAN, INN *anticonvulsant; antipsychotic*
Burntame topical spray OTC *antiseptic; topical anesthetic* [8-hydroxyquinoline; benzocaine]
burodiline INN
BurOtic ear drops (discontinued 1991) ℞ *antibacterial/antifungal* [acetic acid]
Burow solution [see: aluminum acetate solution]
buserelin INN, BAN *gonad-stimulating principle* [also: buserelin acetate]
buserelin acetate USAN *gonad-stimulating principle* [also: buserelin]
BuSpar tablets ℞ *anxiolytic* [buspirone HCl]
buspirone INN, BAN *minor tranquilizer* [also: buspirone HCl]

buspirone HCl USAN *anxiolytic; minor tranquilizer* [also: buspirone]
busulfan USP, INN *antineoplastic* [also: busulphan]
busulphan BAN *antineoplastic* [also: busulfan]
butabarbital USP *hypnotic; sedative* [also: secbutobarbitone]
butabarbital sodium USP *sedative; hypnotic* [also: secbutabarbital sodium]
butacaine INN, BAN [also: butacaine sulfate]
butacaine sulfate USP [also: butacaine]
Butace capsules ℞ *analgesic; antipyretic; sedative* [acetaminophen; caffeine; butalbital]
butacetin USAN *analgesic; antidepressant*
butacetoluide [see: butanilicaine]
butaclamol INN *antipsychotic* [also: butaclamol HCl]
butaclamol HCl USAN *antipsychotic* [also: butaclamol]
butadiazamide INN
butafosfan INN, BAN
butalamine INN, BAN
Butalan elixir (discontinued 1993) ℞ *sedative; hypnotic* [butabarbital sodium]
butalbital USAN, USP, INN *sedative*
butalgin [see: methadone HCl]
butallylonal NF
butamben USAN, USP *topical anesthetic*
butamben picrate USAN *topical anesthetic*
butamirate INN *antitussive* [also: butamirate citrate; butamyrate]
butamirate citrate USAN *antitussive* [also: butamirate; butamyrate]
butamisole INN *veterinary anthelmintic* [also: butamisole HCl]
butamisole HCl USAN *veterinary anthelmintic* [also: butamisole]
butamiverine [see: butaverine]
butamoxane INN

butamyrate BAN *antitussive* [also: butamirate citrate; butamirate]
butane (*n*-butane) NF *aerosol propellant*
butanilicaine INN, BAN
butanixin INN
butanserin INN
butantrone INN
butaperazine USAN, INN *antipsychotic*
butaperazine maleate USAN *antipsychotic*
butaphyllamine [see: ambuphylline]
butaprost USAN, INN, BAN *bronchodilator*
Butatran tablets (discontinued 1991) ℞ *sedative; hypnotic* [butabarbital sodium]
butaverine INN
butaxamine INN *antidiabetic; antihyperlipoproteinemic* [also: butoxamine HCl; butoxamine]
butaxamine HCl [see: butoxamine HCl]
Butazolidin tablets, capsules (discontinued 1992) ℞ *antirheumatic* [phenylbutazone]
butedronate tetrasodium USAN *bone imaging aid*
butedronic acid INN
butelline [see: butacaine sulfate]
butenemal [see: vinbarbital]
buterizine USAN, INN *peripheral vasodilator*
Butesin Picrate ointment OTC *topical local anesthetic* [butamben picrate]
butetamate INN [also: butethamate]
butethal NF [also: butobarbitone]
butethamate BAN [also: butetamate]
butethamine HCl NF
butethanol [see: tetracaine]
buthalital sodium INN [also: buthalitone sodium]
buthalitone sodium BAN [also: buthalital sodium]
buthiazide USAN *diuretic; antihypertensive* [also: butizide]

Butibel tablets, elixir ℞ *anticholinergic; sedative* [belladonna extract; butabarbital sodium]
butibufen INN
Buticaps capsules (discontinued 1991) ℞ *sedative; hypnotic* [butabarbital sodium]
butidrine INN
butikacin USAN, INN, BAN *antibacterial*
butilfenin USAN, INN *hepatic function test*
butinazocine INN
butinoline INN
butirosin INN *antibacterial* [also: butirosin sulfate; butirosin sulphate]
butirosin sulfate USAN *antibacterial* [also: butirosin; butirosin sulphate]
butirosin sulphate BAN *antibacterial* [also: butirosin sulfate; butirosin]
Butisol Sodium tablets, elixir ℞ *sedative; hypnotic* [butabarbital sodium]
butixirate USAN, INN *analgesic; antirheumatic*
butizide INN *diuretic; antihypertensive* [also: buthiazide]
butobarbitone BAN [also: butethal]
butobendine INN
butoconazole INN, BAN *antifungal* [also: butoconazole nitrate]
butoconazole nitrate USAN, USP *antifungal* [also: butoconazole]
butocrolol INN
butoctamide INN
butofilolol INN
butonate USAN, INN *anthelmintic*
butopamine USAN, INN *cardiotonic*
butopiprine INN
butoprozine INN *antiarrhythmic; antianginal* [also: butoprozine HCl]
butoprozine HCl USAN *antiarrhythmic; antianginal* [also: butoprozine]
butopyrammonium iodide INN
butopyronoxyl USP
butorphanol USAN, INN, BAN *analgesic; antitussive*

butorphanol tartrate USAN, USP, BAN *narcotic agonist-antagonist analgesic; antitussive*
butoxamine BAN *antidiabetic; antihyperlipoproteinemic* [also: butoxamine HCl; butaxamine]
butoxamine HCl USAN *antidiabetic; antihyperlipoproteinemic* [also: butaxamine; butoxamine]
2-butoxyethyl nicotinate [see: nicoboxil]
butoxylate INN
butoxyphenylacethydroxamic acid [see: bufexamac]
butriptyline INN, BAN *antidepressant* [also: butriptyline HCl]
butriptyline HCl USAN *antidepressant* [also: butriptyline]
butropium bromide INN
butydrine [see: butidrine]
butyl alcohol NF *solvent*
butyl aminobenzoate (butyl p-aminobenzoate) [now: butamben]
butyl p-aminobenzoate picrate [see: butamben picrate]
butyl chloride NF
butyl 2-cyanoacrylate [see: enbucrilate]
butyl DNJ (deoxynojirmycin) [see: deoxynojirmycin]
butyl p-hydroxybenzoate [see: butylparaben]
butyl methoxydibenzoylmethane [see: avobenzone]
butylated hydroxyanisole (BHA) NF, BAN *antioxidant*
butylated hydroxytoluene (BHT) NF, BAN *antioxidant*
α-**butylbenzyl alcohol** [see: fenipentol]

1-butylbiguanide [see: buformin]
butylmesityl oxide [see: butopyronoxyl]
butylparaben NF *antifungal agent*
butylphenamide
butylphenylsalicylamide [see: butylphenamide]
Butyn dental ointment (discontinued 1991) OTC [butacaine sulfate]
butynamine INN
butyrylcholesterinase (*orphan: reduction and clearance of serum cocaine levels*)
butyrylperazine [see: butaperazine]
butyvinyl [see: vinylbital]
buzepide metiodide INN
BVAP (BCNU, vincristine, Adriamycin, prednisone) *chemotherapy protocol*
BVCPP (BCNU, vinblastine, cyclophosphamide, procarbazine, prednisone) *chemotherapy protocol*
BVDS (bleomycin, Velban, doxorubicin, streptozocin) *chemotherapy protocol*
BVPP (BCNU, vincristine, procarbazine, prednisone) *chemotherapy protocol*
BVU (bromoisovaleryl urea) [see: bromisovalum]
BW 12C (*orphan: sickle cell disease*)
BW B759U (DHPG) (*orphan status withdrawn 1993*)
Byclomine capsules, tablets ℞ *gastrointestinal antispasmodic* [dicyclomine HCl]
Bydramine Cough Syrup OTC *antihistamine; antitussive* [diphenhydramine HCl]

C

C (vitamin C) [see: ascorbic acid]
C & E softgels OTC *vitamin supplement* [vitamins C & E]
C Factors "1000" Plus tablets OTC *dietary supplement* [vitamin C; citrus & rose hips bioflavonoids; rutin; hesperidin complex]
C Speridin sustained-release tablets OTC *dietary supplement* [ascorbic acid; hesperidin; lemon bioflavonoids]
C vitamin [see: ascorbic acid]
C1-inhibitor (*orphan: prevent angioedema*)
566C80 (*orphan: prevent and treat AIDS-related Pneumocystis carinii pneumonia*)
⁴⁵Ca [see: calcium chloride Ca 45]
⁴⁷Ca [see: calcium chloride Ca 47]
cabastine INN
cabergoline INN
cabis bromatum [see: bibrocathol]
CABOP; CA-BOP (Cytoxin, Adriamycin, bleomycin, Oncovin, prednisone) *chemotherapy protocol*
CABS (CCNU, Adriamycin, bleomycin, streptozocin) *chemotherapy protocol*
cabufocon A USAN *hydrophobic contact lens material*
cabufocon B USAN *hydrophobic contact lens material*
CAC (cisplatin, ara-C, caffeine) *chemotherapy protocol*
cactinomycin USAN, INN *antineoplastic* [also: actinomycin C]
CAD (cyclophosphamide, Adriamycin, dacarbazine) *chemotherapy protocol*
CAD (cytarabine [and] daunorubicin) *chemotherapy protocol*
cade oil [see: juniper tar]
cadexomer INN
cadexomer iodine USAN, BAN *antiseptic; antiulcerative*
cadmium *element* (Cd)

cadralazine INN, BAN
CAE (cyclophosphamide, Adriamycin, etoposide) *chemotherapy protocol*
CAF (cyclophosphamide, Adriamycin, fluorouracil) *chemotherapy protocol*
cafaminol INN
Cafatine PB suppositories (discontinued 1991) ℞ *migraine treatment; vasoconstrictor; anticholinergic; sedative* [ergotamine tartrate; caffeine; belladonna extract; pentobarbital]
Cafatine suppositories ℞ *migraine-specific vasoconstrictor* [ergotamine tartrate; caffeine]
Cafatine tablets (discontinued 1991) ℞ *migraine treatment; vasoconstrictor* [ergotamine tartrate; caffeine]
Cafatine-PB tablets ℞ *migraine treatment; vasoconstrictor; anticholinergic; sedative* [ergotamine tartrate; caffeine; sodium pentobarbital; belladonna extract]
cafedrine INN, BAN
Cafergot P-B suppositories (discontinued 1991) ℞ *migraine treatment; vasoconstrictor; anticholinergic; sedative* [ergotamine tartrate; caffeine; belladonna extract; pentobarbital]
Cafergot tablets, suppositories ℞ *migraine treatment; vasoconstrictor* [ergotamine tartrate; caffeine]
Cafermine PB suppositories (discontinued 1991) ℞ *migraine treatment; vasoconstrictor; anticholinergic; sedative* [ergotamine tartrate; caffeine; belladonna extract; pentobarbital]
Cafetrate P-B suppositories (discontinued 1991) ℞ *migraine treatment; vasoconstrictor; anticholinergic; sedative* [ergotamine tartrate; caffeine; belladonna extract; pentobarbital]
Cafetrate suppositories ℞ *migraine-specific vasoconstrictor* [ergotamine tartrate; caffeine]

73

Cafetrate tablets (discontinued 1991) ℞ *migraine treatment; vasoconstrictor* [ergotamine tartrate; caffeine]

Caffedrine timed-release tablets, timed-release capsules OTC *CNS stimulant; analeptic* [caffeine]

caffeine USP, BAN *diuretic; CNS stimulant; (orphan: apnea of prematurity)*

caffeine, citrated NF

caffeine monohydrate [see: caffeine, citrated]

CAFP (cyclophosphamide, Adriamycin, fluorouracil, prednisone) *chemotherapy protocol*

CAFTH (cyclophosphamide, Adriamycin, fluorouracil, tamoxifen, Halotestin) *chemotherapy protocol*

CAFVP (cyclophosphamide, Adriamycin, fluorouracil, vincristine, prednisone) *chemotherapy protocol*

Caine-1; Caine-2 injection (discontinued 1991) ℞ *injectable local anesthetic* [lidocaine HCl]

Cal Carb-HD powder OTC *calcium supplement* [calcium carbonate]

Caladryl Clear lotion OTC *topical antihistamine; astringent; antiseptic* [diphenhydramine HCl; zinc oxide; alcohol]

Caladryl cream, lotion, spray OTC *topical antihistamine; astringent; antipruritic/anesthetic* [diphenhydramine HCl; calamine; camphor]

Cala-gen lotion OTC *topical antihistamine; antipruritic/anesthetic* [diphenhydramine HCl; camphor]

Calamatum spray OTC *topical poison ivy treatment* [calamine; zinc oxide; menthol; camphor; benzocaine]

calamine USP *topical protectant; astringent*

Calamox ointment OTC *topical poison ivy treatment* [calamine]

Calamycin lotion OTC *topical antihistamine; astringent; anesthetic* [pyrilamine maleate; zinc oxide; calamine; benzocaine; chloroxylenol]

Calan film-coated tablets ℞ *antianginal; antiarrhythmic; antihypertensive* [verapamil HCl]

Calan SR film-coated sustained-release caplets ℞ *antihypertensive* [verapamil HCl]

Cal-Bid tablets (discontinued 1992) OTC *dietary supplement* [calcium; vitamins C & D]

Calbonate chewable tablets OTC *antacid* [calcium carbonate]

Calcet Plus tablets OTC *vitamin/calcium/iron supplement* [multiple vitamins; calcium; iron; folic acid]

Calcet tablets OTC *dietary supplement* [calcium; vitamin D]

Calcibind powder ℞ *to reduce hypercalciuria and prevent stone formation* [cellulose sodium phosphate]

CalciCaps; Super CalciCaps tablets OTC *dietary supplement* [dibasic calcium phosphate; calcium gluconate; calcium carbonate; vitamin D]

CalciCaps with Iron tablets OTC *dietary supplement* [dibasic calcium phosphate; calcium gluconate; calcium carbonate; vitamin D; ferrous gluconate]

Calci-Chew chewable tablets OTC *calcium supplement* [calcium carbonate]

Calciday-667 tablets OTC *calcium supplement* [calcium carbonate]

calcidiol [see: calcifediol]

Calcidrine syrup ℞ *antitussive; expectorant* [codeine; calcium iodide; alcohol]

calcifediol USAN, USP, INN *calcium regulator*

calciferol [now: ergocalciferol]

Calciferol Drops OTC *vitamin supplement* [ergocalciferol]

Calciferol tablets, IM injection ℞ *vitamin deficiency therapy* [ergocalciferol (vitamin D_2)]

Calcijex injection ℞ *treatment of hypocalcemia in dialysis patients; decreases severity of psoriatic lesions* [calcitriol]

Calcilac tablets OTC *antacid* [calcium carbonate; glycine]
Calcimar subcu or IM injection ℞ *calcium regulator* [calcitonin (salmon)]
Calci-Mix capsules OTC *calcium supplement* [calcium carbonate]
Calciparine IV or deep subcu injection ℞ *anticoagulant* [heparin calcium]
calcipotriene USAN *antipsoriatic* [also: calcipotriol]
calcipotriol INN *antipsoriatic* [also: calcipotriene]
calcitonin (human) USAN, INN, BAN *calcium regulator; (orphan: Paget's disease of bone; osteitis deformans)*
calcitonin (salmon) USAN, INN, BAN *calcium regulator; (orphan: Paget's disease of bone; osteitis deformans)*
calcitriol USAN, INN, BAN *calcium regulator*
calcium *element (Ca)*
calcium, oyster shell [see: calcium carbonate]
Calcium 600 + D tablets OTC *dietary supplement* [calcium; vitamin D]
Calcium 600 tablets OTC *dietary supplement* [calcium carbonate]
Calcium 600 with Vitamin D tablets OTC *dietary supplement* [calcium; vitamin D]
calcium acetate USP *buffering agent; (orphan: hyperphosphatemia of end-stage renal failure)*
calcium aminacyl B-PAS (benzoyl para-aminosalicylate) [see: benzoylpas calcium]
calcium 4-aminosalicylate trihydrate [see: aminosalicylate calcium]
calcium amphomycin [see: amphomycin]
calcium ascorbate *vitamin C; antiscorbutic*
calcium benzamidosalicylate INN, BAN *antibacterial; tuberculostatic* [also: benzoylpas calcium]

calcium benzoyl *p*-aminosalicylate (B-PAS) [see: benzoylpas calcium]
calcium benzoylpas [see: benzoylpas calcium]
calcium bis-dioctyl sulfosuccinate [see: docusate calcium]
calcium carbimide INN
calcium carbonate USP *antacid; calcium replenisher; (orphan: hyperphosphatemia of end-stage renal disease)*
calcium carbonate, precipitated [now: calcium carbonate]
calcium carbophil *bulk laxative*
calcium caseinate *dietary supplement; infant formula modifier*
calcium chloride USP *calcium replenisher*
calcium chloride Ca 45 USAN *radioactive agent*
calcium chloride Ca 47 USAN *radioactive agent*
calcium chloride dihydrate [see: calcium chloride]
calcium citrate USP *calcium supplement*
calcium clofibrate INN
calcium cyanamide [see: calcium carbimide]
calcium dioctyl sulfosuccinate [see: docusate calcium]
calcium disodium edathamil [see: edetate calcium disodium]
calcium disodium edetate [see: edetate calcium disodium]
Calcium Disodium Versenate IV, subcu or IM injection ℞ *lead chelation; antidote to lead poisoning and lead encephalopathy* [edetate calcium disodium]
calcium dobesilate INN
calcium doxybensylate [see: calcium dobesilate]
calcium edetate sodium [see: edetate calcium disodium]
calcium EDTA (ethylene diamine tetraacetic acid) [see: edetate calcium disodium]

calcium folinate INN, BAN *antianemic; folate replenisher; antidote to folic acid antagonist* [also: leucovorin calcium]

calcium glubionate USAN, INN *calcium replenisher*

calcium D-glucarate tetrahydrate [see: calcium saccharate]

calcium gluceptate USP *calcium replenisher* [also: calcium glucoheptonate]

calcium glucoheptonate INN *calcium replenisher* [also: calcium gluceptate]

calcium gluconate (calcium D-gluconate) USP *calcium replenisher; (orphan: hydrofluoric acid burns)*

calcium glycerinophosphate [see: calcium glycerophosphate]

calcium glycerophosphate NF

calcium hydroxide USP *astringent*

calcium hydroxide phosphate [see: calcium phosphate, tribasic]

calcium hypophosphite NF

calcium iodide

calcium iododocosanoate [see: iodobehenate calcium]

calcium lactate USP *calcium replenisher*

calcium lactate hydrate [see: calcium lactate]

calcium lactate pentahydrate [see: calcium lactate]

calcium lactobionate USP *calcium supplement*

calcium lactobionate dihydrate [see: calcium lactobionate]

calcium lactophosphate NF

calcium levulate [see: calcium levulinate]

calcium levulinate USP *calcium replenisher*

calcium levulinate dihydrate [see: calcium levulinate]

calcium mandelate USP

calcium oxide [see: lime]

Calcium Oyster Shell tablets OTC *dietary supplement* [calcium carbonate]

calcium pantothenate (calcium D-pantothenate) USP, INN *vitamin B_5; enzyme cofactor* [also: pantothenic acid]

calcium pantothenate, racemic (calcium DL-pantothenate) USP *vitamin; enzyme cofactor*

calcium phosphate, dibasic USP *calcium replenisher; tablet base*

calcium phosphate, monocalcium [see: calcium phosphate, dibasic]

calcium phosphate, tribasic NF *calcium replenisher* [also: durapatite; hydroxyapatite]

calcium polycarbophil USAN, USP *bulk laxative*

calcium polysulfide & calcium thiosulfate [see: lime, sulfurated]

calcium saccharate USP, INN *stabilizer*

calcium silicate NF *tablet excipient*

calcium sodium ferriclate INN *hematinic* [also: ferriclate calcium sodium]

calcium stearate NF *tablet and capsule lubricant*

calcium sulfate NF *tablet and capsule diluent*

calcium tetracemine disodium [see: edetate calcium disodium]

calcium trisodium pentetate INN, BAN *plutonium chelating agent* [also: pentetate calcium trisodium]

calcium undecylenate USAN *antifungal*

CaldeCort aerosol spray OTC *topical corticosteroid* [hydrocortisone]

CaldeCort; CaldeCort Light with Aloe cream OTC *topical corticosteroid* [hydrocortisone acetate]

Calderol capsules ℞ *increase serum calcium levels* [calcifediol]

Caldesene ointment OTC *moisturizer; emollient; astringent; antiseptic* [cod liver oil (vitamins A & D); zinc oxide; lanolin]

Caldesene powder OTC *topical antifungal* [calcium undecylenate]

caldiamide INN *pharmaceutic aid* [also: caldiamide sodium]

caldiamide sodium USAN *pharmaceutic aid* [also: caldiamide]

Calel D tablets OTC *dietary supplement* [calcium carbonate; cholecalciferol]

CALF (cyclophosphamide, Adriamycin, leucovorin calcium, fluorouracil) *chemotherapy protocol*

CALF-E (cyclophosphamide, Adriamycin, leucovorin calcium, fluorouracil, ethinyl estradiol) *chemotherapy protocol*

Calfer-Vite tablets OTC *antianemic* [ferrous fumarate; vitamins A & D; multiple B vitamins; sodium ascorbate]

Calfos-D tablets (discontinued 1991) OTC *dietary supplement* [calcium; vitamin D]

Calglycine chewable tablets OTC *antacid* [calcium carbonate; glycine]

Cal-Guard softgels OTC *calcium supplement* [calcium carbonate]

Calicylic Creme OTC *topical keratolytic; topical analgesic* [salicylic acid; trolamine]

californium *element (Cf)*

calioben [see: calcium iodobehenate]

Calmol 4 rectal cream (discontinued 1991) OTC *astringent* [zinc oxide]

Calmol 4 rectal suppositories OTC *astringent* [cocoa butter; zinc oxide; bismuth subgallate]

Calm-X tablets OTC *anticholinergic; antiemetic; antivertigo agent; motion sickness preventative* [dimenhydrinate]

Cal-Nor injection (discontinued 1992) ℞ *calcium replacement* [calcium glycerophosphate; calcium levulinate]

Calohist lotion OTC *astringent; topical antihistamine; antipruritic* [calamine; diphenhydramine HCl; camphor]

calomel NF

Calphosan IV injection ℞ *calcium replacement* [calcium glycerophosphate; calcium lactate]

Cal-Plus tablets OTC *calcium supplement* [calcium carbonate]

Calpuridin OTC

calteridol INN *pharmaceutic aid* [also: calteridol calcium]

calteridol calcium USAN, BAN *pharmaceutic aid* [also: calteridol]

Caltrate 600 + D tablets OTC *dietary supplement* [calcium carbonate; vitamin D]

Caltrate 600 + Iron/Vitamin D film-coated tablets OTC *dietary supplement* [calcium carbonate; ferrous fumarate; vitamin D]

Caltrate film-coated tablets OTC *calcium supplement* [calcium carbonate]

Caltrate Jr. chewable tablets OTC *calcium supplement* [calcium carbonate]

Caltro tablets OTC *dietary supplement* [calcium]

calusterone USAN, INN *antineoplastic*

CAM (cyclophosphamide, Adriamycin, methotrexate) *chemotherapy protocol*

Cama Arthritis Pain Reliever tablets OTC *analgesic; antipyretic; anti-inflammatory; antirheumatic* [aspirin, buffered with magnesium oxide and aluminum hydroxide]

Camalox chewable tablets (discontinued 1992) OTC *antacid* [magnesium hydroxide; aluminum hydroxide; calcium carbonate]

Camalox oral suspension OTC *antacid* [magnesium hydroxide; aluminum hydroxide; calcium carbonate]

Cam-Ap-Es tablets ℞ *antihypertensive* [hydrochlorothiazide; reserpine; hydralazine HCl]

camazepam INN
CAMB (Cytoxin, Adriamycin, methotrexate, bleomycin) *chemotherapy protocol*
cambendazole USAN, INN, BAN *anthelmintic*
CAMELEON (cytosine arabinoside, methotrexate, Leukovorin, Oncovin) *chemotherapy protocol*
CAMEO (cyclophosphamide, Adriamycin, methotrexate, etoposide, Oncovin) *chemotherapy protocol*
Cameo Oil OTC *bath emollient*
CAMF (cyclophosphamide, Adriamycin, methotrexate, folinic acid) *chemotherapy protocol*
camiglibose USAN *antidiabetic*
camiverine INN
camonagrel INN
camostat INN
CAMP (cyclophosphamide, Adriamycin, methotrexate, procarbazine HCl) *chemotherapy protocol*
camphetamide [see: camphotamide]
Campho-Phenique Antibiotic Plus Pain Reliever ointment OTC *topical antibiotic; local anesthetic* [polymyxin B sulfate; neomycin sulfate; bacitracin zinc; lidocaine]
Campho-Phenique liquid, gel OTC *mild anesthetic; anti-infective; counterirritant* [camphor; phenol; eucalyptus oil]
camphor USP *topical antipruritic; mild local anesthetic; counterirritant*
camphor, monobromated USP
camphorated opium tincture [now: paregoric]
camphorated parachlorophenol [see: parachlorophenol, camphorated]
camphoric acid USP
camphotamide INN
camylofin INN
canbisol INN
candicidin USAN, USP, INN, BAN *antifungal*

Candida extract *diagnosis and treatment of Candida-induced skin infections*
candoxatril BAN
candoxatrilat BAN
Cankaid oral solution (discontinued 1992) OTC *topical oral anti-inflammatory/anti-infective* [carbamide peroxide]
cannabinol INN, BAN *antiemetic; antinauseant*
canrenoate potassium USAN *aldosterone antagonist* [also: canrenoic acid]
canrenoic acid INN, BAN *aldosterone antagonist* [also: canrenoate potassium]
canrenone USAN, INN *aldosterone antagonist*
cantharidin *topical keratolytic*
Cantharone liquid ℞ *topical keratolytic* [cantharidin]
Cantharone Plus ℞ *topical keratolytic* [salicylic acid; podophyllum; cantharidin]
Cantil tablets ℞ *treatment for peptic ulcer* [mepenzolate bromide]
Cantri vaginal cream (discontinued 1992) ℞ *bacteriostatic; antiseptic; vulnerary* [sulfisoxazole; aminacrine HCl; allantoin]
CAO (cyclophosphamide, Adriamycin, Oncovin) *chemotherapy protocol*
CAP (cellulose acetate phthalate) [q.v.]
CAP (cyclophosphamide, Adriamycin, Platinol) *chemotherapy protocol*
CAP (cyclophosphamide, Adriamycin, prednisone) *chemotherapy protocol*
CAP-I (cyclophosphamide, Adriamycin, Platinol) *chemotherapy protocol*
CAP-II (cyclophosphamide, Adriamycin, high-dose Platinol) *chemotherapy protocol*

Capastat Sulfate powder for IM injection R *tuberculostatic* [capreomycin sulfate]
CAP-BOP (cyclophosphamide, Adriamycin, procarbazine, bleomycin, Oncovin, prednisone) *chemotherapy protocol*
Capiscint R *investigational imaging agent for atherosclerotic plaque* [monoclonal antibodies]
Capital with Codeine oral suspension R *narcotic analgesic* [codeine phosphate; acetaminophen]
Capitrol shampoo R *antiseborrheic; antibacterial; antifungal* [chloroxine]
capobenate sodium USAN *antiarrhythmic*
capobenic acid USAN, INN *antiarrhythmic*
Capoten tablets R *antihypertensive; angiotensin-converting enzyme inhibitor* [captopril]
Capozide 25/15; Capozide 50/15; Capozide 25/25; Capozide 50/25 tablets R *antihypertensive* [captopril; hydrochlorothiazide]
CAPPr (cyclophosphamide, Adriamycin, Platinol, prednisone) *chemotherapy protocol*
capreomycin INN, BAN *bactericidal; tuberculosis retreatment* [also: capreomycin sulfate]
capreomycin sulfate USAN, USP *antibacterial; tuberculostatic* [also: capreomycin]
caproxamine INN, BAN
capsaicin *topical analgesic; counterirritant*
capsicum oleoresin *topical analgesic; counterirritant*
Capsulets (trademarked form) *sustained-release caplet*
Captabs (dosage form) *capsule-shaped tablet*
captamine INN *depigmentor* [also: captamine HCl]
captamine HCl USAN *depigmentor* [also: captamine]

captodiame INN, BAN
captodiame HCl [see: captodiame]
captodiamine HCl [see: captodiame]
captopril USAN, USP, INN, BAN *antihypertensive; angiotensin-converting enzyme (ACE) inhibitor*
Captrix cream OTC *topical analgesic* [capsaicin]
capuride USAN, INN *hypnotic*
caracemide USAN, INN *antineoplastic*
Carafate tablets R *treatment for duodenal ulcer* [sucralfate]
caramel NF *coloring agent*
caramiphen INN, BAN
caramiphen edisylate
caramiphen HCl [see: caramiphen]
caraway NF
caraway oil NF
carazolol INN, BAN
carbachol USP, INN, BAN *ophthalmic cholinergic; miotic for surgery; antiglaucoma agent*
carbacholine chloride [see: carbachol]
carbacrylamine resins
carbadipimidine HCl [see: carpipramine dihydrochloride]
carbadox USAN, INN, BAN *antibacterial*
carbaldrate INN
carbamazepine USAN, USP, INN, BAN *analgesic; anticonvulsant*
carbamide [see: urea]
carbamide peroxide USP *topical dental anti-infective*
***N*-carbamoylarsanilic acid** [see: carbarsone]
carbamoylcholine chloride [see: carbachol]
***O*-carbamoylsalicylic acid lactam** [see: carsalam]
carbamylcholine chloride [see: carbachol]
carbamylmethylcholine chloride [see: bethanechol chloride]
carbantel INN *anthelmintic* [also: carbantel lauryl sulfate]

carbantel lauryl sulfate USAN *anthelmintic* [also: carbantel]
carbaril INN [also: carbaryl]
carbarsone USP, INN
carbaryl BAN [also: carbaril]
carbasalate calcium INN *analgesic* [also: carbaspirin calcium]
carbaspirin calcium USAN *analgesic* [also: carbasalate calcium]
carbazeran USAN, INN *cardiotonic*
carbazochrome INN
carbazochrome salicylate INN
carbazochrome sodium sulfonate INN
carbazocine INN
carbenicillin INN, BAN *antibacterial* [also: carbenicillin disodium]
carbenicillin disodium USAN, USP *antibacterial* [also: carbenicillin]
carbenicillin indanyl sodium USAN, USP *bactericidal antibiotic* [also: carindacillin]
carbenicillin phenyl sodium USAN *antibacterial* [also: carfecillin]
carbenicillin potassium USAN *antibacterial*
carbenoxolone INN, BAN *glucocorticoid* [also: carbenoxolone sodium]
carbenoxolone sodium USAN *glucocorticoid* [also: carbenoxolone]
carbenzide INN
carbetapentane citrate NF [also: pentoxyverine]
carbetapentane tannate
carbetimer USAN, INN *antineoplastic*
carbetocin INN, BAN
carbidopa USAN, USP, INN, BAN *decarboxylase inhibitor; antiparkinsonian (used with levodopa)*
carbifene INN *analgesic* [also: carbiphene HCl; carbiphene]
carbimazole INN, BAN
carbinoxamine INN, BAN *antihistamine* [also: carbinoxamine maleate]
Carbinoxamine Compound syrup, pediatric drops ℞ *decongestant; antihistamine; antitussive* [pseudoephedrine HCl; carbinoxamine maleate; dextromethorphan hydrobromide; alcohol]
carbinoxamine maleate USP *antihistamine* [also: carbinoxamine]
carbiphene BAN *analgesic* [also: carbiphene HCl; carbifene]
carbiphene HCl USAN *analgesic* [also: carbifene; carbiphene]
Carbiset tablets ℞ *decongestant; antihistamine* [pseudoephedrine HCl; carbinoxamine maleate]
Carbiset-TR timed-release tablets ℞ *antihistamine; decongestant* [carbinoxamine maleate; pseudoephedrine HCl]
Carbocaine injection ℞ *injectable local anesthetic* [mepivacaine HCl]
Carbocaine with Neo-Cobefrin injection ℞ *injectable local anesthetic* [mepivacaine HCl; levonordefrin]
carbocisteine INN, BAN *mucolytic* [also: carbocysteine]
carbocloral USAN, INN, BAN *hypnotic*
carbocromen INN *coronary vasodilator* [also: chromonar HCl]
carbocysteine USAN *mucolytic* [also: carbocisteine]
Carbodec DM syrup, pediatric drops ℞ *decongestant; antihistamine; antitussive* [pseudoephedrine HCl; carbinoxamine maleate; dextromethorphan hydrobromide; alcohol]
Carbodec tablets, syrup ℞ *decongestant; antihistamine* [pseudoephedrine HCl; carbinoxamine maleate]
Carbodec TR sustained-release tablets ℞ *decongestant; antihistamine* [pseudoephedrine HCl; carbinoxamine maleate]
carbodimid calcium [see: calcium carbimide]
carbofenotion INN [also: carbophenothion]
carbol-fuchsin solution (or paint) USP *antifungal*
carbolic acid [see: phenol]
carbolin [see: carbachol]

carbolonium bromide BAN [also: hexcarbacholine bromide]
carbomer INN, BAN *emulsifying and suspending agent* [also: carbomer 910]
carbomer 1342 NF *emulsifying and suspending agent*
carbomer 910 USAN, NF *emulsifying and suspending agent* [also: carbomer]
carbomer 934 USAN, NF *emulsifying and suspending agent*
carbomer 934P USAN, NF *emulsifying and suspending agent*
carbomer 940 USAN, NF *emulsifying and suspending agent*
carbomer 941 USAN, NF *emulsifying and suspending agent*
carbomycin INN
carbon *element (C)*
carbon, activated
carbon dioxide (CO_2) USP *respiratory stimulant*
carbon tetrachloride NF *solvent*
carbonic acid, calcium salt [see: calcium carbonate]
carbonic acid, dilithium salt [see: lithium carbonate]
carbonic acid, dipotassium salt [see: potassium carbonate]
carbonic acid, disodium salt [see: sodium carbonate]
carbonic acid, magnesium salt [see: magnesium carbonate]
carbonic acid, monopotassium salt [see: potassium bicarbonate]
carbonic acid, monosodium salt [see: sodium bicarbonate]
carbonis detergens, liquor (LCD) [see: coal tar]
carbophenothion BAN [also: carbofenotion]
carboplatin USAN, INN, BAN *antineoplastic*
carboprost USAN, INN, BAN *oxytocic*
carboprost methyl USAN *oxytocic*
carboprost trometanol BAN *oxytocic; prostaglandin-type abortifacient* [also: carboprost trometamine]
carboprost trometamine USAN, USP *oxytocic; prostaglandin-type abortifacient* [also: carboprost trometanol]
carboquone INN
carbose D [see: carboxymethylcellulose sodium]
carbovir *(orphan: AIDS)*
carboxyimamidate [see: carbetimer]
carboxymethylcellulose calcium NF *tablet disintegrant*
carboxymethylcellulose sodium USP *suspending and viscosity-increasing agent; tablet excipient* [also: carmellose; carmellose sodium]
carboxymethylcellulose sodium 12 NF *suspending and viscosity-increasing agent*
carbromal NF, INN
carbubarb INN
carbubarbital [see: carbubarb]
carburazepam INN
carbutamide INN, BAN
carbuterol INN, BAN *bronchodilator* [also: carbuterol HCl]
carbuterol HCl USAN *bronchodilator* [also: carbuterol]
carcainium chloride INN
cardamom seed NF
Cardec-DM syrup, pediatric drops ℞ *decongestant; antihistamine; antitussive* [carbinoxamine maleate; pseudoephedrine HCl; dextromethorphan hydrobromide; alcohol]
Cardec-S syrup ℞ *antihistamine; decongestant* [carbinoxamine maleate; pseudoephedrine HCl]
Cardene capsules ℞ *antianginal; antihypertensive* [nicardipine HCl]
Cardene I.V. injection ℞ *antihypertensive* [nicardipine HCl]
Cardene QD ℞ *investigational once-daily antihypertensive* [nicardipine HCl]
Cardene SR sustained-release capsules ℞ *antihypertensive* [nicardipine HCl]
Cardenz tablets OTC *vitamin/mineral supplement* [multiple vitamins & minerals]

cardiamid [see: nikethamide]
Cardilate oral or sublingual tablets ℞ antianginal [erythrityl tetranitrate]
Cardio-Green powder ℞ in vivo diagnostic aid for cardiac output and hepatic function [indocyanine green]
Cardiolite ℞ cardiac imaging agent [technetium]
Cardi-Omega 3 capsules OTC dietary supplement [omega-3 fatty acids; multiple vitamins & minerals]
cardioplegic solution (calcium chloride, magnesium chloride, potassium chloride, sodium chloride) [q.v.]
Cardioquin tablets ℞ antiarrhythmic [quinidine polygalacturonate]
Cardizem IV injection ℞ for atrial fibrillation or paroxysmal supraventricular tachycardia (PSVT) [diltiazem HCl]
Cardizem SR; Cardizem CD sustained-release capsules ℞ antihypertensive; antianginal [diltiazem HCl]
Cardizem tablets ℞ antianginal [diltiazem HCl]
cardophyllin [see: aminophylline]
Cardura tablets ℞ antihypertensive; antiadrenergic [doxazosin mesylate]
carebastine INN
carena [see: aminophylline]
carfecillin INN, BAN antibacterial [also: carbenicillin phenyl sodium]
carfenazine INN antipsychotic [also: carphenazine maleate; carphenazine]
carfentanil INN narcotic analgesic [also: carfentanil citrate]
carfentanil citrate USAN narcotic analgesic [also: carfentanil]
carfimate INN
Carfin tablets ℞ anticoagulant [warfarin sodium]
cargentos [see: silver protein]
cargutocin INN
carindacillin INN, BAN antibacterial [also: carbenicillin indanyl sodium]
carisoprodol USP, INN, BAN skeletal muscle relaxant

Cari-Tab chewable tablets (discontinued 1992) ℞ pediatric vitamin deficiency and dental caries prevention [vitamins A, C & D; fluoride]
carmantadine USAN, INN antiparkinsonian
carmellose INN suspending agent; tablet excipient [also: carboxymethylcellulose sodium; carmellose sodium]
carmellose sodium BAN suspending agent; tablet excipient [also: carboxymethylcellulose sodium; carmellose]
carmetizide INN
carminomycin HCl [now: carubicin HCl]
carmofur INN
Carmol 10 lotion OTC moisturizer; emollient; keratolytic [urea]
Carmol 20 cream OTC moisturizer; emollient; keratolytic [urea]
Carmol HC cream ℞ topical corticosteroid; moisturizer; emollient [hydrocortisone acetate; urea]
carmoxirole INN
carmustine USAN, INN, BAN antineoplastic; (orphan: polymer implant for recurrent malignant glioma)
Carnation Follow-Up; Carnation GoodStart liquid, powder OTC total or supplementary infant feeding
carnauba wax [see: wax, carnauba]
carnidazole USAN, INN, BAN antiprotozoal
L-carnitine [see: levocarnitine]
carnitine INN vitamin B$_t$
Carnitor tablets, oral solution, IV injection or infusion ℞ carnitine replenisher for deficiency of genetic origin or end-stage renal disease (orphan) [levocarnitine]
carocainide INN
Caroid Laxative tablets (discontinued 1991) OTC laxative [phenolphthalein; cascara sagrada extract]
β-carotene [see: beta carotene]
caroverine INN
caroxazone USAN, INN antidepressant

Carozyme capsules OTC *dietary supplement* [multiple enzymes]
carperidine INN, BAN
carperone INN
carphenazine BAN *antipsychotic* [also: carphenazine maleate; carfenazine]
carphenazine maleate USAN, USP *antipsychotic* [also: carfenazine; carphenazine]
carpindolol INN
carpipramine INN
carpipramine dihydrochloride [see: carpipramine]
carpolene [now: carbomer 934P]
carprazidil INN
carprofen USAN, INN, BAN *nonsteroidal anti-inflammatory drug (NSAID); analgesic; antipyretic*
carpronium chloride INN
Carpuject (delivery system) [prefilled syringe]
carrageenan NF *suspending and viscosity-increasing agent*
Carrisyn ℞ *investigational antiviral/immunomodulator for AIDS* [acemannan]
carsalam INN, BAN
cartazolate USAN, INN *antidepressant*
carteolol INN, BAN *antiadrenergic (β-receptor)* [also: carteolol HCl]
carteolol HCl USAN *antiadrenergic (β-receptor)* [also: carteolol]
carticaine BAN [also: articaine]
Cartrix (delivery system) *prefilled syringes*
Cartrol Filmtabs (film-coated tablets) OTC *antihypertensive; β-blocker* [carteolol HCl]
carubicin INN *antineoplastic* [also: carubicin HCl]
carubicin HCl USAN *antineoplastic* [also: carubicin]
carumonam INN, BAN *antibacterial* [also: carumonam sodium]
carumonam sodium USAN *antibacterial* [also: carumonam]

carvedilol USAN, INN, BAN *antianginal; antihypertensive*
carzelesin USAN *antineoplastic*
carzenide INN
casanthranol USAN, USP *laxative*
cascara fluidextract, aromatic USP *laxative*
cascara sagrada USP *stimulant laxative*
cascara sagrada fluid extract *(orphan: oral drug overdose)*
cascarin [see: casanthranol]
Casec powder OTC *protein supplement* [calcium caseinate]
cassia oil [see: cinnamon oil]
CAST (Color Allergy Screening Test) reagent assay tubes ℞ *in vitro diagnostic aid for immunoglobulin E in serum*
Castaderm liquid OTC *topical antifungal; astringent; antiseptic* [resorcinol; boric acid; acetone; basic fuchsin; phenol; alcohol]
Castel Minus; Castel Plus liquid OTC *topical antifungal* [resorcinol; acetone; basic fuchsin; alcohol]
Castellani Paint solution ℞ *topical antifungal; antibacterial* [basic fuchsin; phenol, resorcinol]
Castellani's paint [see: carbol-fuchsin solution]
Castile soap
castor oil USP *stimulant laxative*
CAT (cytarabine, Adriamycin, thioguanine) *chemotherapy protocol*
Cataflam ℞ *investigational analgesic*
Catapres tablets ℞ *antihypertensive* [clonidine HCl]
Catapres-TTS-1; Catapres-TTS-2; Catapres-TTS-3 transdermal patch ℞ *antihypertensive* [clonidine]
Catarase 1:5,000; Catarase 1:10,000 ophthalmic solution ℞ *enzymatic zonulolytic for intracapsular lens extraction* [chymotrypsin]
Catatrol ℞ *investigational antidepressant; (orphan: cataplexy; narcolepsy)* [viloxazine]

catgut suture [see: absorbable surgical suture]
cathine INN
cathinone INN
cathomycin sodium [see: novobiocin sodium]
Catrix Correction cream OTC *moisturizer; emollient*
CAV (cyclophosphamide, Adriamycin, vinblastine) *chemotherapy protocol*
CAV (cyclophosphamide, Adriamycin, vincristine) *chemotherapy protocol*
CAVe; CA-Ve (CCNU, Adriamycin, vinblastine) *chemotherapy protocol*
CAVP16 (cyclophosphamide, Adriamycin, VP-16) *chemotherapy protocol*
Cav-X Fluoride Treatment gel (discontinued 1991) OTC *dental caries preventative* [stannous fluoride]
C-B Time; C-B Time 500 timed-release tablets OTC *vitamin supplement* [multiple B vitamins; vitamin C]
C-B Time liquid (discontinued 1992) OTC *vitamin supplement* [multiple B vitamins; vitamin C]
CBV (cyclophosphamide, BCNU, VePesid) *chemotherapy protocol*
CBV (Cytoxan, BCNU, VP-16-213) *chemotherapy protocol*
CC-Galactosidase *(orphan: Fabry's disease)* [alpha-galactosidase A]
CCM (cyclophosphamide, CCNU, methotrexate) *chemotherapy protocol*
CCNU (chloroethyl-cyclohexyl-nitrosourea) [see: lomustine]
C-Crystals crystals OTC *vitamin supplement* [vitamin C]
CCV-AV (CCNU, cyclophosphamide, vincristine [alternates with] Adriamycin, vincristine) *chemotherapy protocol*

CCVPP (CCNU, cyclophosphamide, Velban, procarbazine, prednisone) *chemotherapy protocol*
CD4, human truncated 369 AA polypeptide *(orphan: AIDS)*
CD4, recombinant soluble human *investigational antiviral; (orphan: AIDS)*
CD4 immunoadhesin [see: CD4 immunoglobulin G, recombinant human]
CD4 immunoglobulin G, recombinant human *(orphan: AIDS)*
CD4-IgG [see: CD4 immunoglobulin G, recombinant human]
CD4-PE40 [see: sCD4-PE40]
CD5-T lymphocyte immunotoxin *(orphan: graft vs. host disease; graft rejection)*
CD-33 [see: ricin (blocked) conjugated murine MCA myeloid cells]
CD-45 monoclonal antibodies *(orphan: organ transplant rejection)*
CD5 Plus ℞ *investigational treatment for graft versus host disease* [monoclonal antibodies]
CdA (2-chloro-2'-deoxyadenosine) [see: cladribine]
CDDP; C-DDP (cis-diamminedichloroplatinum) [see: cisplatin]
CDE (cyclophosphamide, doxorubicin, etoposide) *chemotherapy protocol*
CDP-cholin [see: citicoline]
CEAker *(orphan: detection of tumor foci in colorectal carcinoma)* [indium In 111 murine anti-CEA monoclonal antibody, type ZCE 025]
CEB (carboplatin, etoposide, bleomycin) *chemotherapy protocol*
Cebid Timecelles (sustained-release capsules) OTC *vitamin supplement* [ascorbic acid]
CECA (cisplatin, etoposide, cyclophosphamide, Adriamycin) *chemotherapy protocol*

Ceclor Pulvules (capsules), powder for oral suspension ℞ *cephalosporin-type antibiotic* [cefaclor]
Cecon solution OTC *vitamin supplement* [vitamin C]
Cedax ℞ *investigational oral antibiotic*
Cedilanid-D IV or IM injection (discontinued 1993) ℞ *increase cardiac output; antiarrhythmic* [deslanoside]
CeeNu capsules, dose pack (two 100 mg + two 40 mg + two 10 mg capsules) ℞ *antineoplastic for brain tumors and Hodgkin's disease* [lomustine]
CEF (cyclophosphamide, epirubicin, fluorouracil) *chemotherapy protocol*
cefacetrile INN *antibacterial* [also: cephacetrile sodium]
cefacetrile sodium [see: cephacetrile sodium]
cefaclor USAN, USP, INN, BAN *bactericidal antibiotic*
cefadroxil USAN, USP, INN, BAN *bactericidal antibiotic*
Cefadyl powder for IV or IM injection ℞ *cephalosporin-type antibiotic* [cephapirin sodium]
cefalexin INN *bactericidal antibiotic* [also: cephalexin]
cefaloglycin INN *antibacterial* [also: cephaloglycin]
cefalonium INN [also: cephalonium]
cefaloram INN [also: cephaloram]
cefaloridine INN *antibacterial* [also: cephaloridine]
cefalotin INN *bactericidal antibiotic* [also: cephalothin sodium; cephalothin]
cefalotin sodium [see: cephalothin sodium]
cefamandole USAN, INN *antibacterial* [also: cephamandole]
cefamandole nafate USAN, USP *bactericidal antibiotic* [also: cephamandole nafate]
cefamandole sodium USP *antibacterial*

Cefanex capsules ℞ *cephalosporin-type antibiotic* [cephalexin monohydrate]
cefaparole USAN, INN *antibacterial*
cefapirin INN, BAN *antibacterial* [also: cephapirin sodium]
cefapirin sodium [see: cephapirin sodium]
cefatrizine USAN, INN, BAN *antibacterial*
cefazaflur INN *antibacterial* [also: cefazaflur sodium]
cefazaflur sodium USAN *antibacterial* [also: cefazaflur]
cefazedone INN, BAN
cefazolin USP, INN *systemic antibacterial* [also: cephazolin]
cefazolin sodium USAN, USP *bactericidal antibiotic* [also: cephazolin sodium]
cefbuperazone USAN, INN *antibacterial*
cefcanel INN
cefcanel daloxate INN
cefdinir USAN, INN *antibacterial*
cefedrolor INN
cefempidone INN, BAN
cefepime USAN, INN *antibacterial*
cefetamet USAN, INN *veterinary antibacterial*
cefetecol USAN, INN, BAN *antibacterial*
cefetrizole INN
cefivitril INN
cefixime USAN, USP, INN, BAN *bactericidal antibiotic*
Cefizox powder for IV or IM injection ℞ *cephalosporin-type antibiotic* [ceftizoxime sodium]
cefmenoxime INN *antibacterial* [also: cefmenoxime HCl]
cefmenoxime HCl USAN, USP *antibacterial* [also: cefmenoxime]
cefmepidium chloride INN
cefmetazole INN *antibacterial* [also: cefmetazole sodium]
cefmetazole sodium USAN *bactericidal antibiotic* [also: cefmetazole]
cefminox INN

Cefobid powder for IV or IM injection ℞ *cephalosporin-type antibiotic* [cefoperazone sodium]
cefodizime INN
Cefol Filmtabs (film-coated tablets) ℞ *vitamin supplement* [multiple vitamins; folic acid]
cefonicid INN, BAN *antibacterial* [also: cefonicid monosodium]
cefonicid monosodium USAN *antibacterial* [also: cefonicid]
cefonicid sodium USAN, USP *bactericidal antibiotic*
cefoperazone INN, BAN *antibacterial* [also: cefoperazone sodium]
cefoperazone sodium USAN, USP *bactericidal antibiotic* [also: cefoperazone]
ceforanide USAN, USP, INN, BAN *bactericidal antibiotic*
Cefotan powder for IV or IM injection ℞ *cephalosporin-type antibiotic* [cefotetan disodium]
cefotaxime INN, BAN *antibacterial* [also: cefotaxime sodium]
cefotaxime sodium USAN, USP *bactericidal antibiotic* [also: cefotaxime]
cefotetan USAN, INN, BAN *antibacterial*
cefotetan disodium USAN, USP *bactericidal antibiotic*
cefotiam INN, BAN *antibacterial* [also: cefotiam HCl]
cefotiam HCl USAN *antibacterial* [also: cefotiam]
cefoxazole INN [also: cephoxazole]
cefoxitin USAN, INN, BAN *antibacterial*
cefoxitin sodium USAN, USP, BAN *bactericidal antibiotic*
cefpimizole USAN, INN *antibacterial*
cefpimizole sodium USAN *antibacterial*
cefpiramide USAN, INN *antibacterial*
cefpiramide sodium USAN *antibacterial*
cefpirome INN *antibacterial* [also: cefpirome sulfate]
cefpirome sulfate USAN *antibacterial* [also: cefpirome]
cefpodoxime INN, BAN *bactericidal antibiotic* [also: cefpodoxime proxetil]
cefpodoxime proxetil USAN *bactericidal antibiotic* [also: cefpodoxime]
cefprozil USAN, INN *antibacterial*
cefprozil monohydrate
cefquinome INN
cefradine INN *bactericidal antibiotic* [also: cephradine]
cefrotil INN
cefroxadine USAN, INN *antibacterial*
cefsulodin INN, BAN *antibacterial* [also: cefsulodin sodium]
cefsulodin sodium USAN *antibacterial* [also: cefsulodin]
cefsumide INN
ceftazidime USAN, USP, INN, BAN *bactericidal antibiotic*
cefteram INN
ceftezole INN
ceftibuten USAN, INN, BAN *antibacterial*
Ceftin tablets ℞ *cephalosporin-type antibiotic* [cefuroxime axetil]
ceftiofur INN, BAN *veterinary antibacterial* [also: ceftiofur HCl]
ceftiofur HCl USAN *veterinary antibacterial* [also: ceftiofur]
ceftiofur sodium USAN *veterinary antibacterial*
ceftiolene INN
ceftioxide INN
ceftizoxime INN, BAN *bactericidal antibiotic* [also: ceftizoxime sodium]
ceftizoxime sodium USAN, USP *bactericidal antibiotic* [also: ceftizoxime]
ceftriaxone INN, BAN *bactericidal antibiotic* [also: ceftriaxone sodium]
ceftriaxone sodium USAN, USP *bactericidal antibiotic* [also: ceftriaxone]
cefuracetime INN, BAN

cefuroxime USAN, INN, BAN *bactericidal antibiotic*
cefuroxime axetil USAN, USP, BAN *bactericidal antibiotic*
cefuroxime pivoxetil USAN *bactericidal antibiotic*
cefuroxime sodium USP, BAN *bactericidal antibiotic*
cefuzonam INN
Cefzil film-coated tablets, powder for oral suspension ℞ *cephalosporin-type antibiotic* [cefprozil]
Celestone Phosphate IV, IM injection ℞ *glucocorticoids* [betamethasone sodium phosphate]
Celestone Soluspan intrabursal, intra-articular, intralesional injection ℞ *glucocorticoids* [betamethasone sodium phosphate; betamethasone acetate]
Celestone tablets, syrup ℞ *glucocorticoids* [betamethasone]
celiprolol INN, BAN *antiadrenergic (β-receptor)* [also: celiprolol HCl]
celiprolol HCl USAN *antiadrenergic (β-receptor)* [also: celiprolol]
cellacefate INN *tablet-coating agent* [also: cellulose acetate phthalate; cellacephate]
cellacephate BAN *tablet-coating agent* [also: cellulose acetate phthalate; cellacefate]
Cellufresh eye drops OTC *ocular moisturizer/lubricant* [carboxymethylcellulose sodium]
cellulase USAN *digestive enzyme*
cellulolytic enzyme [see: cellulase]
cellulose, absorbable [see: cellulose, oxidized]
cellulose, ethyl ester [see: ethylcellulose]
cellulose, hydroxypropyl methyl ether [see: hydroxypropyl methylcellulose]
cellulose, microcrystalline NF *tablet and capsule diluent* [also: dispersible cellulose]
cellulose, oxidized USP *local hemostatic*
cellulose, oxidized regenerated USP *local hemostatic*
cellulose, sodium carboxymethyl [see: carboxymethylcellulose sodium]
cellulose acetate NF *tablet-coating agent; insoluble polymer membrane*
cellulose acetate butyrate [see: cabufocon A; cabufocon B]
cellulose acetate dibutyrate [see: porofocon A; porofocon B]
cellulose acetate phthalate (CAP) NF *tablet-coating agent* [also: cellacefate; cellacephate]
cellulose carboxymethyl ether, sodium salt [see: carboxymethylcellulose sodium]
cellulose diacetate [see: cellulose acetate]
cellulose dihydrogen phosphate, disodium salt [see: cellulose sodium phosphate]
cellulose disodium phosphate [see: cellulose sodium phosphate]
cellulose ethyl ether [see: ethylcellulose]
cellulose gum, modified [now: croscarmellose sodium]
cellulose methyl ether [see: methylcellulose]
cellulose nitrate [see: pyroxylin]
cellulose sodium phosphate (CSP) USAN, USP *antiurolithic*
cellulosic acid [see: cellulose, oxidized]
Celluvisc solution OTC *ophthalmic lubricant* [carboxymethylcellulose sodium]
celmoleukin INN *immunostimulant*
Celontin Kapseals (capsules) ℞ *anticonvulsant* [methsuximide]
celucloral INN, BAN
Cel-U-Jec IV, IM injection ℞ *glucocorticoids* [betamethasone sodium phosphate]

CEM (cytosine arabinoside, etoposide, methotrexate) *chemotherapy protocol*

Cemill 500; Cemill 1000 sustained-release tablets OTC *vitamin supplement* [ascorbic acid]

Cemill plus Bioflavonoids tablets OTC *vitamin supplement* [ascorbic acid; bioflavonoids; rutin]

Cenafed Plus tablets OTC *decongestant; antihistamine* [pseudoephedrine HCl; tripolidine HCl]

Cenafed syrup OTC *nasal decongestant* [pseudoephedrine HCl]

Cenafed tablets (discontinued 1993) OTC *nasal decongestant* [pseudoephedrine HCl]

Cena-K liquid ℞ *potassium supplement* [potassium chloride]

Cenocort A-40 injection ℞ *corticosteroid* [triamcinolone acetonide]

Cenocort Forte injection ℞ *corticosteroid* [triamcinolone diacetate]

Cenolate IV, IM, or subcu injection ℞ *antiscorbutic* [sodium ascorbate]

Centara ℞ *investigational antiarthritic* [monoclonal antibodies]

Center-Al suspension for subcutaneous injection ℞ *allergic hyposensitization therapy* [allergenic extracts, alum precipitated]

CenTNF ℞ *investigational treatment for sepsis* [monoclonal antibodies]

CentoRx ℞ *investigational treatment for blood clot-related disorders* [monoclonal antibodies]

Centovir (*orphan: prophylaxis and treatment of CMV in bone marrow transplants*) [human IgM monoclonal antibody (C-58) to cytomegalovirus (CMV)]

Centoxin (*orphan: gram-negative bacteremia in endotoxin shock*) [nebacumab]

Centrafree tablets OTC *antianemic* [ferrous fumarate; multiple vitamins]

Centrax capsules, tablets ℞ *anxiolytic* [prazepam]

centrazene [see: simtrazene]

centrophenoxine [see: meclofenoxate]

Centrovite Advanced Formula tablets OTC *vitamin/mineral/iron supplement* [multiple vitamins & minerals; ferrous fumarate; folic acid; biotin]

Centrovite Jr. tablets OTC *vitamin/mineral/iron supplement* [multiple vitamins & minerals; ferrous fumarate; folic acid]

Centrum, Advanced Formula liquid OTC *vitamin/mineral/iron supplement* [multiple vitamins & minerals; ferrous fumarate; folic acid; biotin; alcohol]

Centrum Jr. + Extra C; Centrum Jr. + Extra Calcium chewable tablets OTC *vitamin/mineral/calcium/iron supplement* [multiple vitamins & minerals; calcium; iron; folic acid; biotin]

Centrum Jr. + Iron tablets OTC *vitamin/mineral/iron supplement* [multiple vitamins & minerals; iron; folic acid; biotin]

Centrum Silver Gel-Tabs OTC *geriatric vitamin/mineral supplement* [multiple vitamins & minerals; folic acid; biotin]

Centrum tablets OTC *antianemic* [ferrous fumarate; multiple vitamins]

Centurion A-Z tablets OTC *vitamin/mineral/iron supplement* [multiple vitamins & minerals; ferrous fumarate; folic acid; biotin]

Ceo-Two suppository OTC *laxative* [sodium bicarbonate; potassium bitartrate]

CEP (CCNU, etoposide, prednimustine) *chemotherapy protocol*

Cēpacol Anesthetic lozenges OTC *topical anesthetic; oral antiseptic* [cetylpyridinium chloride; benzocaine]

Cēpacol mouthwash/gargle OTC *oral antiseptic* [cetylpyridinium chloride]

Cēpacol Throat lozenges OTC *oral antiseptic* [cetylpyridinium chloride]

Cēpastat Sore Throat lozenges OTC *topical antipruritic/counterirritant; mild local anesthetic* [phenol]

cephacetrile sodium USAN, USP *antibacterial* [also: cefacetrile]

cephalexin USAN, USP, BAN *bactericidal antibiotic* [also: cefalexin]

cephalexin HCl USAN *bactericidal antibiotic*

cephalexin monohydrate *bactericidal antibiotic*

cephaloglycin USAN, USP, BAN *antibacterial* [also: cefaloglycin]

cephalonium BAN [also: cefalonium]

cephaloram BAN [also: cefaloram]

cephaloridine USAN, USP, BAN *antibacterial* [also: cefaloridine]

cephalosporin N [see: adicillin]

cephalothin BAN *bactericidal antibiotic* [also: cephalothin sodium; cefalotin]

cephalothin sodium USAN, USP *bactericidal antibiotic* [also: cefalotin; cephalothin]

cephamandole BAN *antibacterial* [also: cefamandole]

cephamandole nafate BAN *antibacterial* [also: cefamandole nafate]

cephapirin sodium USAN, USP *bactericidal antibiotic* [also: cefapirin]

cephazolin BAN *systemic antibacterial* [also: cefazolin]

cephazolin sodium BAN *systemic antibacterial* [also: cefazolin sodium]

cephoxazole BAN [also: cefoxazole]

cephradine USAN, USP, BAN *bactericidal antibiotic* [also: cefradine]

Cephulac syrup ℞ *prevent and treat portal-systemic encephalopathy* [lactulose]

Ceptaz powder for injection ℞ *antibiotic* [ceftazidime pentahydrate]

ceramide trihexosidase & alpha-galactosidase A (*orphan: Fabry's disease*)

Ceredase IV infusion ℞ (*orphan: enzyme replacement in Gaucher's disease*) [alglucerase]

cerelose [see: glucose]

Cerespan timed-release capsules ℞ *peripheral vasodilator* [papaverine HCl]

cerium *element (Ce)*

cerium oxalate USP

ceronapril USAN, INN *antihypertensive*

Cerose-DM liquid OTC *decongestant; antihistamine; antitussive* [phenylephrine HCl; chlorpheniramine maleate; dextromethorphan hydrobromide; alcohol]

Cerovite tablets OTC *vitamin/mineral/iron supplement* [multiple vitamins & minerals; iron; folic acid; biotin]

Certagen film-coated tablets OTC *vitamin/mineral/iron supplement* [multiple vitamins & minerals; ferrous fumarate; folic acid; biotin]

Certa-Vite Golden tablets OTC *geriatric vitamin/mineral supplement* [multiple vitamins & minerals; folic acid; biotin]

Cerubidine powder for IV injection ℞ *antineoplastic antibiotic for multiple leukemias* [daunorubicin HCl]

ceruletide USAN, INN, BAN *gastric secretory stimulant*

ceruletide diethylamine USAN *gastric secretory stimulant*

Cerumenex ear drops ℞ *agent to emulsify and disperse ear wax* [trolamine polypeptide oleate-condensate]

cesium *element (Cs)*

cesium (^{131}Cs) chloride INN *radioactive agent* [also: cesium chloride Cs 131]

cesium chloride Cs 131 USAN *radioactive agent* [also: cesium (^{131}Cs) chloride]

cetaben INN *antihyperlipoproteinemic* [also: cetaben sodium]

cetaben sodium USAN *antihyperlipoproteinemic* [also: cetaben]

Cetacaine gel, liquid, ointment, aerosol ℞ *topical local anesthetic; antiseptic* [benzocaine; tetracaine HCl; butamben; benzalkonium chloride]

Cetacort lotion ℞ *topical corticosteroid* [hydrocortisone]
cetalkonium *antiseptic*
cetalkonium chloride USAN, INN, BAN *topical anti-infective*
Cetamide ophthalmic ointment ℞ *ophthalmic bacteriostatic* [sodium sulfacetamide]
cetamolol INN *antiadrenergic (β-receptor)* [also: cetamolol HCl]
cetamolol HCl USAN *antiadrenergic (β-receptor)* [also: cetamolol]
Cetane timed-release capsules (discontinued 1992) OTC *vitamin supplement* [ascorbic acid]
Cetaphil cream, lotion OTC *soap-free cleanser*
Cetapred ophthalmic ointment ℞ *topical ophthalmic corticosidal anti inflammatory; bacteriostatic* [prednisolone acetate; sodium sulfacetamide]
cethexonium chloride INN
cetiedil INN *peripheral vasodilator* [also: cetiedil citrate]
cetiedil citrate USAN *peripheral vasodilator; (orphan status withdrawn 1993)* [also: cetiedil]
cetirizine INN, BAN *antihistamine* [also: cetirizine HCl]
cetirizine HCl USAN *antihistamine* [also: cetirizine]
cetobemidone [see: ketobemidone]
cetocycline INN *antibacterial* [also: cetocycline HCl]
cetocycline HCl USAN *antibacterial* [also: cetocycline]
cetofenicol INN *antibacterial* [also: cetophenicol]
cetohexazine INN
cetomacrogol 1000 INN, BAN
cetophenicol USAN *antibacterial* [also: cetofenicol]
cetophenylbutazone [see: kebuzone]
cetostearyl alcohol NF *emulsifying agent*
cetotetrine HCl [now: cetocycline HCl]
cetotiamine INN

cetoxime INN, BAN
cetoxime HCl [see: cetoxime]
cetraxate INN *GI antiulcerative* [also: cetraxate HCl]
cetraxate HCl USAN *GI antiulcerative* [also: cetraxate]
cetrimide INN, BAN
cetrimonium bromide INN *topical antiseptic* [also: cetrimonium chloride]
cetrimonium chloride BAN *topical antiseptic* [also: cetrimonium bromide]
cetyl alcohol NF *emulsifying and stiffening agent*
cetyl esters wax NF *stiffening agent*
cetyldimethylbenzyl ammonium chloride [see: cetalkonium chloride]
cetylpyridinium chloride USP, INN, BAN *topical antiseptic; preservative*
cetyltrimethyl ammonium bromide
Cevalin IV, IM, or subcu injection ℞ *antiscorbutic* [ascorbic acid]
Cevi-Bid timed-release capsules OTC *vitamin supplement* [ascorbic acid]
Cevi-Fer timed-release capsules ℞ *hematinic* [ferrous fumarate; ascorbic acid; folic acid]
Ce-Vi-Sol drops OTC *vitamin supplement* [ascorbic acid]
cevitamic acid [see: ascorbic acid]
cevitan [see: ascorbic acid]
ceylon gelatin [see: agar]
Cezin capsules OTC *vitamin/mineral supplement* [multiple vitamins & minerals]
Cezin-S capsules ℞ *vitamin/mineral supplement* [multiple vitamins & minerals; folic acid]
CFP (cyclophosphamide, fluorouracil, prednisone) *chemotherapy protocol*
CG (chorionic gonadotropin) [see: gonadotropin, chorionic]
C-Gel soft capsules OTC *vitamin supplement* [vitamin C]
CGF (Control Gel Formula) dressing [see: DuoDERM CGF]

CH1VPP; Ch1VPP (chlorambucil, vinblastine, procarbazine, prednisone) *chemotherapy protocol*

CHAD (cyclophosphamide, hexamethylmelamine, Adriamycin, DDP) *chemotherapy protocol*

chalk, precipitated [see: calcium carbonate, precipitated]

Chap Stick lip balm OTC *moisturizer; protectant; emollient* [petrolatum; padimate O; lanolin; isopropyl myristate; cetyl alcohol]

Chap Stick Medicated lip balm OTC *counterirritant; moisturizer; protectant; emollient* [camphor; menthol; phenol]

Chap Stick Petroleum Jelly Plus gel OTC *moisturizer; protectant; emollient* [white petrolatum]

Chap Stick with SUNBLOCK 15 lip balm OTC *moisturizer; protectant; emollient; sunscreen* [petrolatum; padimate O; oxybenzone; cetyl alcohol; lanolin; isopropyl myristate]

Charcoaid liquid OTC *adsorbent poisoning antidote* [activated charcoal]

charcoal *gastric adsorbent/detoxicant; antiflatulent*

charcoal, activated USP *general purpose antidote/adsorbent*

Charcoal Plus tablets OTC *adsorbent; detoxicant; antiflatulent* [activated charcoal; simethicone]

CharcoCaps capsules OTC *adsorbent; detoxicant; antiflatulent* [charcoal]

Chardonna-2 tablets ℞ *anticholinergic; sedative* [belladonna extract; phenobarbital]

chaulmosulfone INN

Chealamide IV infusion ℞ *calcium-lowering agent; antiarrhythmic* [edetate disodium]

Checkmate gel (discontinued 1992) ℞ *topical dental caries preventative* [acidulated phosphate fluoride]

chelafrin [see: epinephrine]

Chelated Magnesium tablets OTC *magnesium supplement* [magnesium amino acid chelate]

Chelated Manganese tablets OTC *manganese supplement* [manganese]

chelen [see: ethyl chloride]

Chemet capsules ℞ *heavy metal chelating agent; (orphan: cystine kidney stones; lead and mercury poisoning)* [succimer]

Chemo-Pin (trademarked form) *chemical-dispensing pin*

Chemstrip 2 GP; Chemstrip 2 LN; Chemstrip 4 the OB; Chemstrip 6; Chemstrip 7; Chemstrip 8; Chemstrip 9; Chemstrip 10 with SG; Chemstrip uGK reagent strips OTC *in vitro diagnostic aid for multiple urine products*

Chemstrip bG reagent strips OTC *in vitro diagnostic aid for blood glucose*

Chemstrip K reagent papers OTC *in vitro diagnostic aid for ketones in the urine*

Chemstrip Micral reagent strips OTC *in vitro diagnostic aid for albumin in the urine*

Chemstrip uG reagent strips OTC *in vitro diagnostic aid for urine glucose*

Chenatal tablets OTC *prenatal vitamin/mineral supplement* [multiple vitamins & minerals]

chenic acid [now: chenodiol]

Chenix tablets ℞ *anticholelithogenic; (orphan: gallstones)* [chenodiol]

chenodeoxycholic acid INN, BAN *anticholelithogenic* [also: chenodiol]

chenodiol USAN *anticholelithogenic; (orphan: gallstones)* [also: chenodeoxycholic acid]

Cheracol D Cough liquid OTC *antitussive; expectorant* [dextromethorphan hydrobromide; guaifenesin; alcohol]

Cheracol Plus liquid OTC *decongestant; antihistamine; antitussive* [phenylpropanolamine HCl; chlorpheniramine maleate; dextromethorphan hydrobromide; alcohol]

Cheracol Sinus sustained-action tablets OTC *decongestant; antitussive* [pseudoephedrine sulfate; dextromethorphan hydrobromide]

Cheracol syrup ℞ *antitussive; expectorant* [codeine phosphate; guaifenesin; alcohol]

Cheralin Expectorant liquid OTC *expectorant* [potassium guaiacolsulfonate; ammonium chloride; antimony potassium tartrate; alcohol]

Cheralin with Codeine liquid ℞ *antitussive; expectorant* [codeine phosphate; potassium guaiacolsulfonate; ammonium chloride; antimony potassium tartrate]

Cherapas tablets (discontinued 1993) ℞ *antihypertensive* [hydrochlorothiazide; reserpine; hydralazine HCl]

cherry juice NF

Chewable C chewable tablets OTC *vitamin supplement* [sodium ascorbate; ascorbic acid]

Chewable Multivitamins with Fluoride tablets ℞ *pediatric vitamin supplement and dental caries preventative* [multiple vitamins; fluoride; folic acid]

Chewable Triple Vitamins with Fluoride tablets ℞ *pediatric vitamin supplement and dental caries preventative* [vitamins A, C & D; fluoride]

Chew-C chewable tablets OTC *vitamin supplement* [sodium ascorbate; ascorbic acid]

Chew-Vites chewable tablets OTC *vitamin supplement* [multiple vitamins; folic acid]

CHEX-UP; ChexUP; Chex-Up (cyclophosphamide, hexamethylmelamine, fluorouracil, Platinol) *chemotherapy protocol*

CHF (cyclophosphamide, hexamethylmelamine, fluorouracil) *chemotherapy protocol*

Chibroxin eye drops ℞ *ophthalmic antibiotic* [norfloxacin]

Chiggerex ointment OTC *topical local anesthetic; counterirritant* [benzocaine; camphor; menthol]

Chigger-Tox liquid OTC *topical local anesthetic* [benzocaine; benzyl benzoate]

Children's Formula Cough Syrup OTC *antitussive; expectorant* [dextromethorphan hydrobromide; guaifenesin]

chillifolinum [see: quillifoline]

chimeric M-T412 (human-murine) IgG monoclonal anti-CD4 (*orphan: multiple sclerosis*)

Chinese gelatin [see: agar]

Chinese isinglass [see: chiniofon]

chinethazone [see: quinethazone]

chiniofon NF, INN

chitosan [see: poliglusam]

CHL + PRED (chlorambucil, prednisone) *chemotherapy protocol*

Chlamydiazyme solid phase immunoassay OTC *in vitro diagnostic aid for Chlamydia trachomatis*

Chlo-Amine chewable tablets ℞ *antihistamine* [chlorpheniramine maleate]

chlophedianol BAN *antitussive* [also: chlophedianol HCl; clofedanol]

chlophedianol HCl USAN *antitussive* [also: clofedanol; chlophedianol]

chlophenadione [see: clorindione]

chloquinate [see: cloquinate]

Chlor-100 injection ℞ *antihistamine; anaphylaxis* [chlorpheniramine maleate]

chloracyzine INN

Chlorafed; Chlorafed HS Timecelles (sustained-release capsules) ℞ *decongestant; antihistamine* [pseudoephedrine HCl; chlorpheniramine maleate]

Chlorafed liquid OTC *decongestant; antihistamine* [pseudoephedrine HCl; chlorpheniramine maleate]

chloral betaine USAN, NF, BAN *sedative* [also: cloral betaine]
chloral hydrate USP, BAN *hypnotic; sedative*
chloral hydrate betaine [see: chloral betaine]
chloralformamide USP
Chloral-Methylol (discontinued 1991) OTC *counterirritant* [methyl salicylate; menthol]
chloralodol INN [also: chlorhexadol]
chloralose (-chloralose) INN
chloralurethane [see: carbocloral]
chlorambucil USP, INN, BAN *antineoplastic*
chloramidobenzol [see: clofenamide]
chloramine [now: chloramine-T]
chloramine-T NF [also: tosylchloramide sodium]
chloramiphene [see: clomiphene citrate]
chloramphenicol USP, INN, BAN *bacteriostatic antibiotic; antirickettsial*
chloramphenicol palmitate USP *antibacterial; antirickettsial*
chloramphenicol pantothenate complex USAN *antibacterial; antirickettsial* [also: cloramfenicol pantotenate complex]
chloramphenicol sodium succinate USP *antibacterial; antirickettsial*
chloranautine [see: dimenhydrinate]
chlorarsen [see: dichlorophenarsine HCl]
Chloraseptic, Children's lozenges OTC *topical anesthetic* [benzocaine]
Chloraseptic, Children's throat spray OTC *topical antipruritic/counterirritant; mild local anesthetic* [phenol]
Chloraseptic lozenges, mouthwash/gargle, throat spray OTC *topical antipruritic/counterirritant; mild local anesthetic* [phenol]
Chlorate tablets OTC *antihistamine* [chlorpheniramine maleate]
chlorazanil INN
chlorazanil HCl [see: chlorazanil]
chlorazodin INN [also: chloroazodin]

chlorazone [see: chloramine-T]
chlorbenzoxamine INN
chlorbenzoxamine HCl [see: chlorbenzoxamine]
chlorbetamide INN, BAN
chlorbutanol [see: chlorobutanol]
chlorbutin [see: chlorambucil]
chlorbutol BAN *antimicrobial agent* [also: chlorobutanol]
chlorcinnazine [see: clocinizine]
chlorcyclizine INN, BAN *antihistamine* [also: chlorcyclizine HCl]
chlorcyclizine HCl USP *antihistamine* [also: chlorcyclizine]
chlordantoin USAN, BAN *antifungal* [also: clodantoin]
chlordiazepoxide USP, INN, BAN *anxiolytic; minor tranquilizer; alcohol withdrawal therapy*
chlordiazepoxide HCl USAN, USP, BAN *sedative*
chlordimorine INN
Chlordrine S.R. sustained-release capsules ℞ *decongestant; antihistamine* [pseudoephedrine HCl; chlorpheniramine maleate]
Chloresium ointment, solution, tablets OTC *vulnerary; wound, fecal and urinary odor control* [chlorophyllin copper complex]
chlorethate [see: clorethate]
chlorethyl [see: ethyl chloride]
chlorfenisate [see: clofibrate]
chlorfenvinphos BAN [also: clofenvinfos]
Chlorgest-HD liquid ℞ *decongestant; antihistamine; antitussive* [phenylephrine HCl; chlorpheniramine maleate; hydrocodone bitartrate]
chlorguanide HCl [see: chloroguanide HCl]
chlorhexadol BAN [also: chloralodol]
chlorhexidine INN, BAN *antimicrobial* [also: chlorhexidine gluconate]
chlorhexidine gluconate USAN *antimicrobial; (orphan: oral mucositis)* [also: chlorhexidine]

chlorhexidine HCl USAN, BAN *topical anti-infective*

chlorhexidine phosphanilate USAN *antibacterial*

chlorimiphenin [see: imiclopazine]

chlorimpiphenine [see: imiclopazine]

chlorinated & iodized peanut oil [see: chloriodized oil]

chlorindanol USAN *spermaticide* [also: clorindanol]

chlorine *element (Cl)*

chloriodized oil USP

chlorisondamine chloride INN, BAN

chlorisondamone chloride [see: chlorisondamine chloride]

chlormadinone INN, BAN *progestin* [also: chlormadinone acetate]

chlormadinone acetate USAN, NF *progestin* [also: chlormadinone]

chlormerodrin NF, INN, BAN

chlormerodrin (^{197}Hg) INN *renal function test; radioactive agent* [also: chlormerodrin Hg 197]

chlormerodrin Hg 197 USAN, USP *renal function test; radioactive agent* [also: chlormerodrin (^{197}Hg)]

chlormerodrin Hg 203 USAN, USP *renal function test; radioactive agent*

chlormeroprin [see: chlormerodrin]

chlormethazanone [see: chlormezanone]

chlormethiazole BAN [also: clomethiazole]

chlormethine INN *antineoplastic* [also: mechlorethamine HCl; mustine]

chlormethine HCl [see: mechlorethamine HCl; mustine]

chlormethylencycline [see: clomocycline]

chlormezanone INN, BAN *mild anxiolytic*

chlormidazole INN, BAN

chlornaphazine INN

chloroacetic acid [see: monochloroacetic, dichloroacetic, or trichloroacetic acid]

chloroazodin USP [also: chlorazodin]

5-chlorobenzoxazolinone [see: chlorzoxazone]

chlorobutanol NF, INN *antimicrobial agent; preservative* [also: chlorbutol]

chlorochine [see: chloroquine]

chlorocresol USAN, NF, INN *antiseptic; disinfectant*

2-chloro-2'-deoxyadenosine (CdA) (*orphan: acute myeloid leukemia; hairy cell leukemia; chronic lymphocytic leukemia*) [also: cladribine]

chlorodeoxylincomycin [see: clindamycin]

chloroethane [see: ethyl chloride]

Chlorofon-F tablets (discontinued 1991) ℞ *skeletal muscle relaxant; analgesic* [chlorzoxazone; acetaminophen]

chloroform NF *solvent*

chloroguanide HCl USP [also: proguanil]

chloroguanide triazine pamoate [see: cycloguanil pamoate]

chloro-iodohydroxyquinoline [see: clioquinol]

chlorolincomycin [see: clindamycin]

chloromethapyrilene citrate [see: chlorothen citrate]

Chloromycetin cream ℞ *broad-spectrum topical antibiotic* [chloramphenicol]

Chloromycetin Hydrocortisone powder for eye drops ℞ *topical ophthalmic corticosteroidal anti-inflammatory; broad-spectrum antibiotic* [hydrocortisone acetate; chloramphenicol]

Chloromycetin Kapseals (capsules) ℞ *broad-spectrum antibiotic* [chloramphenicol]

Chloromycetin Ophthalmic ointment, powder for eye drops ℞ *broad-spectrum antibiotic* [chloramphenicol]

Chloromycetin Otic ear drops ℞ *broad-spectrum antibiotic* [chloramphenicol]

Chloromycetin Palmitate oral suspension ℞ *broad-spectrum antibiotic* [chloramphenicol palmitate]
Chloromycetin Sodium Succinate powder for IV injection ℞ *broad-spectrum antibiotic* [chloramphenicol sodium succinate]
p-**chlorophenol** [see: parachlorophenol]
chlorophenothane NF [also: clofenotane; dicophane]
chlorophenoxamide [see: clefamide]
chlorophenylmercury [see: phenylmercuric chloride]
chlorophyll, water soluble [see: chlorophyllin]
chlorophyll derivatives *vulnerary; reduce malodors from wounds*
chlorophyllin *vulnerary; reduce malodors from wounds*
chlorophyllin copper complex USAN *deodorant*
chloroprednisone INN
chloroprednisone acetate [see: chloroprednisone]
chloroprocaine INN *local anesthetic* [also: chloroprocaine HCl]
chloroprocaine HCl USP *local anesthetic* [also: chloroprocaine]
Chloroptic eye drops ℞ *broad-spectrum antibiotic* [chloramphenicol]
Chloroptic S.O.P. ophthalmic ointment ℞ *broad-spectrum antibiotic* [chloramphenicol]
chloropyramine INN [also: halopyramine]
chloropyrilene INN, BAN [also: chlorothen citrate]
chloroquine USP, INN, BAN *antiamebic; antimalarial*
chloroquine diphosphate [see: chloroquine phosphate]
chloroquine HCl USP *amebicide; antimalarial* [also: chloroquine]
chloroquine phosphate USP, BAN *antimalarial; amebicide; lupus erythematosus suppressant*
chloroserpidine INN

Chloroserpine tablets ℞ *antihypertensive* [chlorothiazide; reserpine]
N-**chlorosuccinimide** [see: succinchlorimide]
chlorothen citrate NF [also: chloropyrilene]
chlorothenium citrate [see: chlorothen citrate]
chlorothenylpyramine [see: chlorothen]
chlorothiazide USP, INN, BAN *diuretic; antihypertensive*
chlorothiazide sodium USAN, USP *diuretic; antihypertensive*
chlorothymol NF
chlorotrianisene USP, INN, BAN *estrogen*
chloroxine USAN *antiseborrheic*
chloroxylenol USP, INN, BAN *bacteriostatic*
chlorozone [see: chloramine-T]
chlorpenthixol [see: clopenthixol]
Chlorphed-LA nasal spray OTC *nasal decongestant* [oxymetazoline HCl]
chlorphenamine INN *antihistamine* [also: chlorpheniramine maleate; chlorpheniramine]
chlorphenamine maleate [see: chlorpheniramine maleate]
chlorphenecyclane [see: clofenciclan]
chlorphenesin INN, BAN *skeletal muscle relaxant* [also: chlorphenesin carbamate]
chlorphenesin carbamate USAN *skeletal muscle relaxant* [also: chlorphenesin]
chlorphenindione [see: clorindione]
chlorpheniramine BAN *antihistamine* [also: chlorpheniramine maleate; chlorphenamine]
chlorpheniramine maleate USP *antihistamine* [also: chlorphenamine; chlorpheniramine]
chlorpheniramine polistirex USAN *antihistamine*
chlorpheniramine tannate

chlorphenoctium amsonate INN, BAN

chlorphenotane [see: chlorophenothane]

chlorphenoxamine INN, BAN [also: chlorphenoxamine HCl]

chlorphenoxamine HCl USP [also: chlorphenoxamine]

chlorphentermine INN, BAN *anorexic* [also: chlorphentermine HCl]

chlorphentermine HCl USAN *anorexic* [also: chlorphentermine]

chlorphenylindandione [see: clorindione]

chlorphthalidone [see: chlorthalidone]

Chlor-Pro 10 injection ℞ *antihistamine* [chlorpheniramine maleate]

Chlorpro tablets OTC *antihistamine* [chlorpheniramine maleate]

chlorprocaine chloride [see: chloroprocaine HCl]

chlorproethazine INN [also: chlorproethazine HCl]

chlorproethazine HCl [also: chlorproethazine]

chlorproguanil INN, BAN

chlorproguanil HCl [see: chlorproguanil]

chlorpromazine USP, INN, BAN *antiemetic; antipsychotic; antidopaminergic; intractable hiccough relief*

chlorpromazine HCl USP, BAN *antiemetic; antipsychotic; intractable hiccough relief*

chlorpropamide USP, INN, BAN *sulfonylurea-type antidiabetic*

chlorprophenpyridamine maleate [see: chlorpheniramine maleate]

chlorprothixene USAN, USP, INN, BAN *antipsychotic*

chlorprothixene HCl *antipsychotic*

chlorprothixene lactate *antipsychotic*

chlorpyrifos BAN

chlorquinaldol INN, BAN

Chlor-Rest tablets OTC *decongestant; antihistamine* [phenylpropanolamine HCl; chlorpheniramine maleate]

Chlorspan-12 timed-release capsules ℞ *antihistamine* [chlorpheniramine maleate]

Chlortab-4 tablets ℞ *antihistamine* [chlorpheniramine maleate]

Chlortab-8 timed-release tablets ℞ *antihistamine* [chlorpheniramine maleate]

chlortalidone INN *diuretic* [also: chlorthalidone]

Chlor-Tel Slocaps (sustained-release capsules) ℞ *antihistamine* [chlorpheniramine maleate]

chlortetracycline INN, BAN *antibacterial antibiotic; antiprotozoal* [also: chlortetracycline bisulfate]

chlortetracycline bisulfate USP *antibacterial; antiprotozoal* [also: chlortetracycline]

chlortetracycline calcium

chlortetracycline HCl USP, BAN *antibacterial antibiotic; antiprotozoal*

chlorthalidone USAN, USP, BAN *diuretic; antihypertensive* [also: chlortalidone]

chlorthenoxazin BAN [also: chlorthenoxazine]

chlorthenoxazine INN [also: chlorthenoxazin]

chlorthiazide [see: chlorothiazide]

chlortrianisestrol [see: chlorotrianisene]

Chlor-Trimeton 4 Hour Relief tablets OTC *decongestant; antihistamine* [pseudoephedrine sulfate; chlorpheniramine maleate]

Chlor-Trimeton 12 Hour Relief sustained-release tablets OTC *decongestant; antihistamine* [pseudoephedrine sulfate; chlorpheniramine maleate]

Chlor-Trimeton Decongestant (name changed to Chlor-Trimeton 4 Hour Relief & 12 Hour Relief in 1992)

Chlor-Trimeton Sinus caplets OTC *decongestant; antihistamine; analgesic* [phenylpropanolamine HCl; chlor-

pheniramine maleate; acetaminophen]
Chlor-Trimeton tablets, Repetabs (repeat-action tablets), syrup, injection OTC *antihistamine; antitussive; anaphylaxis* [chlorpheniramine maleate]
Chlorzone Forte tablets (discontinued 1991) ℞ *skeletal muscle relaxant; analgesic* [chlorzoxazone; acetaminophen]
chlorzoxazone USP, INN, BAN *skeletal muscle relaxant*
chlosudimeprimylum [see: clopamide]
ChlVPP (chlorambucil, vinblastine, procarbazine, prednisone) *chemotherapy protocol*
CHO (cyclophosphamide, hydroxydaunomycin, Oncovin) *chemotherapy protocol*
CHO cells, recombinant [see: CD4, human truncated]
CHOB (cyclophosphamide, hydroxydaunomycin, Oncovin, bleomycin) *chemotherapy protocol*
CHOD (cyclophosphamide, hydroxydaunomycin, Oncovin, dexamethasone) *chemotherapy protocol*
Cholac syrup ℞ *prevent and treat portal-systemic encephalopathy* [lactulose]
cholalic acid [see: dehydrocholic acid]
Cholan-DH tablets (discontinued 1992) OTC *laxative; hydrocholeretic* [dehydrocholic acid]
Cholan-HMB tablets OTC *laxative; hydrocholeretic* [dehydrocholic acid]
Cholebrine tablets ℞ *oral cholecystographic radiopaque agent* [iocetamic acid]
cholecalciferol USP, BAN *vitamin D₃; antirachitic* [also: colecalciferol]
Choledyl delayed-release tablets, pediatric syrup, elixir ℞ *bronchodilator* [oxtriphylline]
Choledyl SA sustained-action tablets ℞ *bronchodilator* [oxtriphylline]

cholera vaccine USP *active bacterin for cholera (Vibrio cholerae)*
cholesterin [see: cholesterol]
cholesterol NF *emulsifying agent*
cholestrin [see: cholesterol]
cholestyramine BAN *bile salts ion-exchange resin; antihyperlipoproteinemic* [also: cholestyramine resin; colestyramine]
cholestyramine resin USP *bile salts ion-exchange resin; antihyperlipoproteinemic* [also: colestyramine; cholestyramine]
cholic acid [see: dehydrocholic acid]
Cholidase tablets OTC *dietary lipotropic with vitamin supplementation* [choline; inositol; vitamins B_6, B_{12} & E]
choline *dietary lipotropic supplement*
choline alfoscerate INN
choline bitartrate NF
choline bromide hexamethylenedicarbamate [see: hexacarbacholine bromide]
choline chloride INN
choline chloride acetate [see: acetylcholine chloride]
choline chloride carbamate [see: carbachol]
choline chloride succinate [see: succinylcholine chloride]
choline dihydrogen citrate NF
choline gluconate INN
choline glycerophosphate [see: choline alfoscerate]
choline magnesium trisalicylate (choline salicylate + magnesium salicylate) [q.v.]
choline perchlorate, nitrate ester [see: nitricholine perchlorate]
choline salicylate USAN, INN, BAN *analgesic; antipyretic; anti-inflammatory; antirheumatic*
choline theophyllinate INN, BAN *bronchodilator* [also: oxtriphylline]
Cholinoid capsules OTC *dietary lipotropic with vitamin supplementation* [choline; inositol; multiple B vita-

mins; vitamin C; lemon bioflavonoids]

Cholografin Meglumine injection ℞ *parenteral cholecystographic and cholangiographic radiopaque agent* [iodipamide meglumine]

Choloxin tablets ℞ *antihyperlipidemic (cholesterol-lowering)* [dextrothyroxine sodium]

Cholybar resin bar ℞ *cholesterol-lowering antihyperlipidemic* [cholestyramine resin]

chondodendron tomentosum [see: tubocurarine chloride]

chondroitin sulfate *ophthalmic surgical aid*

Chooz chewable tablets OTC *antacid* [calcium carbonate]

CHOP (cyclophosphamide, hydroxydaunomycin, Oncovin, prednisone) *chemotherapy protocol*

CHOP-BLEO (cyclophosphamide, hydroxydaunomycin, Oncovin, prednisone, bleomycin) *chemotherapy protocol*

CHOPE (cyclophosphamide, hydroxydaunomycin, Oncovin, prednisone, etoposide) *chemotherapy protocol*

CHOR (cyclophosphamide, hydroxydaunomycin, Oncovin, radiation therapy) *chemotherapy protocol*

Chorex-5; Chorex-10 powder for injection ℞ *hormone for prepubertal cryptorchidism and hypogonadism* [chorionic gonadotropin]

Chorigon powder for injection ℞ *hormone for prepubertal cryptorchidism and hypogonadism* [chorionic gonadotropin]

chorionic gonadotrophin [see: gonadotropin, chorionic]

chorionic gonadotropin (CG) [see: gonadotropin, chorionic]

Choron-10 powder for injection ℞ *hormone for prepubertal cryptorchidism and hypogonadism* [chorionic gonadotropin]

CHP (chlorhexidine phosphanilate) [q.v.]

Christmas factor [see: factor IX complex]

Chromagen gelcaps ℞ *hematinic* [ferrous fumarate; vitamin B_{12} & C; intrinsic factor concentrate]

Chromagen OB capsules (discontinued 1992) OTC *vitamin/mineral/iron supplement* [multiple vitamins & minerals; iron; folic acid]

Chroma-Pak IV injection ℞ *intravenous nutritional therapy* [chromic chloride hexahydrate]

chromargyre [see: merbromin]

chromated albumin [see: albumin, chromated Cr 51 serum]

Chromelin Complexion Blender OTC *skin darkening agent for vitiligo and hypopigmented areas* [dihydroxyacetone]

chromic acid, disodium salt [see: sodium chromate Cr 51]

chromic chloride USP *dietary chromium supplement*

chromic chloride Cr 51 USAN *radioactive agent*

chromic chloride hexahydrate [see: chromic chloride]

chromic phosphate Cr 51 USAN *radioactive agent*

chromic phosphate P 32 USAN, USP *antineoplastic; radioactive agent*

chromium *element (Cr)*

chromium chloride [see: chromic chloride Cr 51]

chromium chloride hexahydrate [see: chromic chloride]

Chromium Chloride IV injection ℞ *intravenous nutritional therapy* [chromic chloride hexahydrate]

Chromium Trace Metal Additive IV injection (discontinued 1991) ℞ *intravenous nutritional therapy* [chromic chloride hexahydrate]

chromocarb INN

chromonar HCl USAN *coronary vasodilator* [also: carbocromen]
Chronotabs (trademarked form) *sustained-action tablet*
Chronulac syrup ℞ *laxative* [lactulose]
chrysazin *(withdrawn from market by FDA)* [see: danthron]
CHVP (cyclophosphamide, hydroxydaunomycin, VM-26, prednisone) *chemotherapy protocol*
Chymex solution ℞ *in vivo pancreatic function test* [bentiromide]
Chymodiactin powder for intradiscal injection ℞ *enzyme for herniated nucleus pulposus* [chymopapain]
chymopapain USAN, INN, BAN *proteolytic enzyme for herniated lumbar discs*
chymotrypsin USP, INN, BAN *proteolytic enzyme; zonulolytic for intracapsular lens extraction*
C.I. acid orange 24 monosodium salt (color index) [see: resorcin brown]
C.I. basic violet 3 (color index) [see: gentian violet]
C.I. basic violet 14 monohydrochloride (color index) [see: fuchsin, basic]
C.I. direct blue 53 tetrasodium salt (color index) [see: Evans blue]
C.I. mordant yellow 5, disodium salt (color index) [see: olsalazine sodium]
ciadox INN
ciamexon INN, BAN
cianergoline INN
cianidanol INN
cianidol [see: cianidanol]
cianopramine INN
ciapilome INN
Ciba Vision Cleaner solution OTC *contact lens surfactant cleaning solution*
Ciba Vision Saline aerosol solution OTC *contact lens rinsing and storage solution* [saline solution]

Cibacalcin subcu or IM injection ℞ *calcium regulator; (orphan: Paget's disease; osteitis deformans)* [calcitonin (human)]
Cibalith-S syrup ℞ *antipsychotic/antimanic* [lithium citrate]
cibenzoline INN, BAN *antiarrhythmic* [also: cifenline]
cicaprost INN
cicarperone INN
ciclacillin INN, BAN *antibacterial* [also: cyclacillin]
ciclactate INN
ciclafrine INN *antihypotensive* [also: ciclafrine HCl]
ciclafrine HCl USAN *antihypotensive* [also: ciclafrine]
ciclazindol USAN, INN, BAN *antidepressant*
cicletanine USAN, INN, BAN *antihypertensive*
ciclindole INN *antidepressant* [also: cyclindole]
cicliomenol INN
ciclobendazole INN, BAN *anthelmintic* [also: cyclobendazole]
ciclofenazine INN *antipsychotic* [also: cyclophenazine HCl]
ciclofenazine HCl [see: cyclophenazine HCl]
cicloheximide INN *antipsoriatic* [also: cycloheximide]
ciclonicate INN
ciclonium bromide INN
ciclopirox INN, BAN *antifungal* [also: ciclopirox olamine]
ciclopirox olamine USAN, USP *antifungal* [also: ciclopirox]
ciclopramine INN
cicloprofen USAN, INN, BAN *anti-inflammatory*
cicloprolol INN *antiadrenergic (β-receptor)* [also: cicloprolol HCl; cycloprolol]
cicloprolol HCl USAN *antiadrenergic (β-receptor)* [also: cicloprolol; cycloprolol]
ciclosidomine INN, BAN

ciclosporin INN *immunosuppressive* [also: cyclosporine; cyclosporin]
ciclotizolam INN, BAN
ciclotropium bromide INN
cicloxilic acid INN
cicloxolone INN, BAN
cicortonide INN
cicrotoic acid INN
cideferron INN
Cidex; Cidex-7; Cidex Plus 28 solution OTC *broad-spectrum antimicrobial* [glutaral]
cidoxepin INN *antidepressant* [also: cidoxepin HCl]
cidoxepin HCl USAN *antidepressant* [also: cidoxepin]
cifenline USAN *antiarrhythmic* [also: cibenzoline]
cifenline succinate USAN *antiarrhythmic*
cifostodine INN
ciglitazone USAN, INN *antidiabetic*
cignolin [see: anthralin]
ciheptolane INN
ciladopa INN, BAN *antiparkinsonian; dopaminergic agent* [also: ciladopa HCl]
ciladopa HCl USAN *antiparkinsonian; dopaminergic agent* [also: ciladopa]
cilastatin INN, BAN *enzyme inhibitor* [also: cilastatin sodium]
cilastatin sodium USAN *enzyme inhibitor* [also: cilastatin]
cilazapril USAN, INN, BAN *antihypertensive; ACE inhibitor*
cilazaprilat INN, BAN
ciliary neurotrophic factor (*orphan: amyotrophic lateral sclerosis*)
ciliary neurotrophic factor, recombinant human (*orphan: spinal and progressive muscular atrophies; amyotrophic and primary lateral scleroses*)
cilobamine INN *antidepressant* [also: cilobamine mesylate]
cilobamine mesylate USAN *antidepressant* [also: cilobamine]
cilofungin USAN, INN *antifungal*
ciloprost [see: iloprost]

cilostamide INN
cilostazol INN
Ciloxan Drop-Tainers (eye drops) ℞ *ophthalmic antibiotic* [ciprofloxacin HCl]
ciltoprazine INN
cilutazoline INN
cimaterol USAN, INN *repartitioning agent*
cimemoxin INN
cimepanol INN
cimetidine USAN, USP, INN, BAN *treatment of GI ulcers; histamine H_2 antagonist*
cimetidine HCl USAN *antagonist to histamine H_2 receptors*
cimetropium bromide INN
cimoxatone INN
cinametic acid INN
cinamolol INN
cinanserin INN *serotonin inhibitor* [also: cinanserin HCl]
cinanserin HCl USAN *serotonin inhibitor* [also: cinanserin]
cinaproxen INN
cincaine chloride [see: dibucaine HCl]
cinchocaine INN, BAN *local anesthetic* [also: dibucaine]
cinchocaine HCl BAN *local anesthetic* [also: dibucaine HCl]
cinchonidine sulfate NF
cinchonine sulfate NF
cinchophen NF, INN, BAN
cinecromen INN
cinepaxadil INN
cinepazet INN, BAN *antianginal* [also: cinepazet maleate]
cinepazet maleate USAN *antianginal* [also: cinepazet]
cinepazic acid INN
cinepazide INN, BAN
cinfenine INN
cinfenoac INN, BAN
cinflumide USAN, INN *muscle relaxant*
cingestol USAN, INN *progestin*
cinitapride INN

cinmetacin INN
cinnamaldehyde NF
cinnamaverine INN
cinnamedrine USAN, INN *smooth muscle relaxant*
cinnamedrine HCl *smooth muscle relaxant*
cinnamic aldehyde [now: cinnamaldehyde]
cinnamon NF
cinnamon oil NF
cinnarizine USAN, INN, BAN *antihistamine*
cinnarizine clofibrate INN
cinnofuradione INN
cinnofuron [see: cinnofuradione]
cinnopentazone INN *anti-inflammatory* [also: cintazone]
cinnopropazone [see: apazone]
Cinobac Pulvules (capsules) ℞ *urinary anti-infective* [cinoxacin]
cinoctramide INN
cinodine HCl USAN *veterinary antibacterial*
cinolazepam INN
cinoquidox INN
cinoxacin USAN, USP, INN, BAN *urinary antibacterial*
cinoxate USAN, USP, INN *ultraviolet screen*
cinoxolone INN, BAN
cinoxopazide INN
cinperene USAN, INN *antipsychotic*
cinprazole INN
cinpropazide INN
Cin-Quin tablets, capsules (discontinued 1992) ℞ *antiarrhythmic* [quinidine sulfate]
cinromide USAN, INN *anticonvulsant*
cintazone USAN *anti-inflammatory* [also: cinnopentazone]
cintramide INN *antipsychotic* [also: cintriamide]
cintriamide USAN *antipsychotic* [also: cintramide]
cinuperone INN
cioteronel USAN, INN *antiandrogen*
ciprafamide INN

Cipralan ℞ *investigational antiarrhythmic* [cifenline succinate]
ciprazafone INN
ciprefadol INN *analgesic* [also: ciprefadol succinate]
ciprefadol succinate USAN *analgesic* [also: ciprefadol]
Cipro film-coated tablets ℞ *broad-spectrum fluoroquinolone-type antibiotic* [ciprofloxacin HCl]
Cipro IV infusion ℞ *broad-spectrum fluoroquinolone-type antibiotic* [ciprofloxacin]
ciprocinonide USAN, INN *adrenocortical steroid*
ciprofibrate USAN, INN, BAN *antihyperlipoproteinemic*
ciprofloxacin USAN, INN, BAN *broad-spectrum bactericidal antibiotic*
ciprofloxacin HCl USAN, USP *broad-spectrum bactericidal antibiotic*
cipropride INN
ciproquazone INN
ciproquinate INN *coccidiostat for poultry* [also: cyproquinate]
ciprostene INN *platelet antiaggregatory agent* [also: ciprostene calcium]
ciprostene calcium USAN *platelet antiaggregatory agent* [also: ciprostene]
ciproximide INN *antipsychotic; antidepressant* [also: cyproximide]
ciramadol USAN, INN *analgesic*
ciramadol HCl USAN *analgesic*
cirazoline INN
Circavite-T tablets OTC *vitamin/mineral/iron supplement* [multiple vitamins & minerals; iron]
cirolemycin USAN, INN *antineoplastic; antibacterial*
cisapride USAN, INN, BAN *peristaltic stimulant*
CISCA; CisCA (cisplatin, cyclophosphamide, Adriamycin) *chemotherapy protocol*
CISCA$_{II}$/VB$_{IV}$ (cisplatin, cyclophosphamide, Adriamycin, vinblas-

tine, bleomycin) *chemotherapy protocol*
cisclomiphene [now: enclomiphene]
cisconazole USAN, INN *antifungal*
***cis*-DDP (diamminedichloroplatinum)** [see: cisplatin]
***cis*-diamminedichloroplatinum (DDP)** [see: cisplatin]
cismadinone INN
cisplatin USAN, USP, INN, BAN *antineoplastic*
***cis*-platinum** [now: cisplatin]
***cis*-platinum II** [now: cisplatin]
13-*cis*-retinoic acid [see: isotretinoin]
cistinexine INN
citalopram INN, BAN
Citanest HCl Forte injection ℞ *injectable local anesthetic for dental procedures* [prilocaine HCl; epinephrine]
Citanest HCl Plain injection ℞ *injectable local anesthetic for dental procedures* [prilocaine HCl]
citatepine INN
citenamide USAN, INN *anticonvulsant*
citenazone INN
citicoline INN
citidoline [see: citicoline]
citiolone INN
Citra pH oral solution OTC *antacid* [sodium citrate]
Citracal 1500 + D tablets (discontinued 1993) OTC *dietary supplement* [calcium citrate; vitamin D]
Citracal Caplets + D OTC *dietary supplement* [calcium citrate; vitamin D]
Citracal Liquitab effervescent tablets OTC *calcium supplement* [calcium citrate]
Citracal tablets OTC *calcium supplement* [calcium citrate]
Citralax effervescent granules OTC *laxative* [magnesium citrate; magnesium sulfate]
citrate dextrose [see: ACD solution]

citrate of magnesia [see: magnesium citrate]
citrate phosphate dextrose [see: anticoagulant citrate phosphate dextrose solution]
citrate phosphate dextrose adenine [see: anticoagulant citrate phosphate dextrose adenine solution]
citrated caffeine [see: caffeine, citrated]
Citrated Caffeine tablets (discontinued 1991) OTC *CNS stimulant; analeptic* [caffeine; citric acid]
citric acid USP *pH adjusting agent*
citric acid, glucono-delta-lactone & magnesium carbonate (*orphan: renal and bladder apatite calculi*)
citric acid, magnesium oxide & sodium carbonate [see: Suby solution G]
citrin [see: bioflavonoids]
Citrocarbonate effervescent granules OTC *antacid* [sodium bicarbonate; sodium citrate]
Citro-Flav 200 capsules OTC *dietary supplement* [citrus bioflavonoids complex]
Citrolith tablets ℞ *urinary alkalinizing agent* [potassium citrate; sodium citrate]
Citro-Nesia solution (discontinued 1993) OTC *laxative* [magnesium citrate]
Citrotein powder OTC *oral nutritional supplement*
citrovorum factor [see: leucovorin calcium]
Citrucel; Citrucel Sugar Free powder OTC *bulk laxative* [methylcellulose]
citrus bioflavonoids [see: bioflavonoids]
Citrus-flav C 500 tablets OTC *dietary supplement* [vitamin C; citrus & acerola bioflavonoids; hesperidin; rutin]

CIVPP (chlorambucil, vinblastine, procarbazine, prednisone) *chemotherapy protocol*
cladribine *antineoplastic; (orphan: hairy cell and chronic lymphocytic leukemias)*
Claforan powder for IV or IM injection, ADD-vantage vials ℞ *cephalosporin-type antibiotic* [cefotaxime sodium]
clamidoxic acid INN, BAN
clamoxyquin BAN *antiamebic* [also: clamoxyquin HCl; clamoxyquine]
clamoxyquin HCl USAN *antiamebic* [also: clamoxyquine; clamoxyquin]
clamoxyquine INN *antiamebic* [also: clamoxyquin HCl; clamoxyquin]
clanfenur INN
clanobutin INN
clantifen INN
claretin-12 [see: cyanocobalamin]
clarithromycin USAN, INN, BAN *macrolide antibacterial antibiotic*
Claritin ℞ *investigational nonsedating antihistamine* [loratadine]
Clarityne (Mexican name for U.S. product Claritin)
clavulanate potassium USAN, USP *β-lactamase inhibitor*
clavulanate potassium & amoxicillin [see: amoxicillin]
clavulanate potassium & ticarcillin [see: ticarcillin disodium]
clavulanic acid INN, BAN
clavulanic acid & amoxicillin [see: amoxicillin]
clavulanic acid & ticarcillin [see: ticarcillin disodium]
clazolam USAN, INN *minor tranquilizer*
clazolimine USAN, INN *diuretic*
clazuril USAN, INN, BAN *coccidiostat for pigeons*
Clean-N-Soak solution OTC *contact lens cleaning and soaking solution*
Clear Away; Clear Away Plantar disc OTC *topical keratolytic* [salicylic acid]
Clear By Design gel OTC *topical keratolytic for acne* [benzoyl peroxide]
Clear Eyes ACR eye drops OTC *topical ocular vasoconstrictor; astringent* [naphazoline HCl; zinc sulfate]
Clear Eyes eye drops OTC *topical ocular vasoconstrictor* [naphazoline HCl]
Clearasil 10%; Clearasil Maximum Strength Acne Treatment lotion, cream OTC *topical keratolytic for acne* [benzoyl peroxide]
Clearasil Adult Care Medicated Blemish Stick OTC *topical acne treatment* [sulfur; resorcinol; titanium dioxide]
Clearasil Antibacterial Soap bar OTC *medicated cleanser for acne* [triclosan; titanium dioxide]
Clearasil Double Clear pads OTC *medicated cleansing pad for acne* [salicylic acid; alcohol]
Clearasil Medicated Astringent liquid OTC *topical acne cleanser* [salicylic acid; alcohol]
Clearblue; Clearblue Easy home test kit OTC *in vitro diagnostic aid for urine pregnancy test*
Clearplan Easy test kit OTC *in vitro diagnostic aid to predict ovulation time*
clebopride USAN, INN *antiemetic*
clefamide INN, BAN
clemastine USAN, BAN *antihistamine*
clemastine fumarate USAN, USP, BAN *antihistamine*
clemeprol INN, BAN
clemizole INN, BAN
clemizole penicillin INN, BAN
clenbuterol INN, BAN
clenpirin INN [also: clenpyrin]
clenpyrin BAN [also: clenpirin]
Clens solution OTC *contact lens cleaning solution*
clentiazem INN *calcium channel antagonist* [also: clentiazem maleate]
clentiazem maleate USAN *calcium channel antagonist* [also: clentiazem]
Cleocin capsules ℞ *lincosamide-type antibiotic; (orphan: AIDS-related*

Pneumocystis carinii pneumonia) [clindamycin HCl]
Cleocin Pediatric granules for oral solution ℞ *lincosamide-type antibiotic* [clindamycin palmitate HCl]
Cleocin Phosphate IV infusion, IM injection ℞ *lincosamide-type antibiotic* [clindamycin phosphate]
Cleocin T gel, topical solution, lotion ℞ *topical antibiotic for acne vulgaris* [clindamycin phosphate]
Cleocin vaginal cream ℞ *antibacterial* [clindamycin phosphate]
Clerz Drops; Clerz 2 solution OTC *contact lens rewetting solution*
cletoquine INN, BAN
Clexane/Lovenox ℞ *investigational antithrombotic for hip and knee surgery* [enoxaparin]
clibucaine INN
clidafidine INN
clidanac INN
clidinium bromide USAN, USP, INN, BAN *peptic ulcer adjunct*
climazolam INN
climbazole INN, BAN
climiqualine INN
clinafloxacin HCl USAN *antibacterial*
clindamycin USAN, INN, BAN *antibiotic; (orphan: AIDS-related Pneumocystis carinii pneumonia)*
clindamycin HCl USP, BAN *bactericidal antibiotic*
clindamycin palmitate HCl USAN, USP *bactericidal antibiotic*
clindamycin phosphate USAN, USP *bactericidal antibiotic*
Clindex capsules ℞ *anticholinergic; anxiolytic* [clidinium bromide; chlordiazepoxide HCl]
Clinicydin ointment (discontinued 1991) OTC *topical antibiotic* [polymyxin B sulfate; neomycin sulfate; bacitracin]
Clinistix reagent strips OTC *in vitro diagnostic aid for urine glucose*
Clinitest tablets OTC *in vitro diagnostic aid for urine glucose*

clinocaine HCl [see: procaine HCl]
clinofibrate INN
clinolamide INN
Clinoril tablets ℞ *nonsteroidal anti-inflammatory drug (NSAID); antiarthritic; analgesic* [sulindac]
Clinoxide capsules ℞ *anticholinergic; anxiolytic* [clidinium bromide; chlordiazepoxide HCl]
clioquinol USP, INN, BAN *topical antibacterial; antifungal*
clioxanide USAN, INN, BAN *anthelmintic*
clipoxamine [see: cliropamine]
Clipoxide capsules ℞ *anticholinergic; anxiolytic* [clidinium bromide; chlordiazepoxide HCl]
cliprofen USAN, INN *anti-inflammatory*
cliropamine INN
Clistin tablets (discontinued 1991) ℞ *antihistamine* [carbinoxamine maleate]
clobamine mesylate [now: cilobamine mesylate]
clobazam USAN, INN, BAN *minor tranquilizer*
clobedolum [see: clonitazene]
clobenoside INN
clobenzepam INN
clobenzorex INN
clobenztropine INN
clobetasol INN, BAN *topical corticosteroidal anti-inflammatory* [also: clobetasol propionate]
clobetasol propionate USAN *topical corticosteroidal anti-inflammatory* [also: clobetasol]
clobetasone INN, BAN *anti-inflammatory* [also: clobetasone butyrate]
clobetasone butyrate USAN *anti-inflammatory* [also: clobetasone]
clobutinol INN
clobuzarit INN, BAN
clocanfamide INN
clocapramine INN
clociguanil INN, BAN
clocinizine INN

clocortolone INN *topical corticosteroid* [also: clocortolone acetate]

clocortolone acetate USAN *topical corticosteroid* [also: clocortolone]

clocortolone pivalate USAN, USP *topical corticosteroid*

clocoumarol INN

Clocream cream OTC *moisturizer; emollient* [cod liver oil (vitamins A & E); cholecalciferol; vitamin A palmitate]

clodacaine INN

clodanolene USAN, INN *skeletal muscle relaxant*

clodantoin INN *antifungal* [also: chlordantoin]

clodazon INN *antidepressant* [also: clodazon HCl]

clodazon HCl USAN *antidepressant* [also: clodazon]

Cloderm cream ℞ *topical corticosteroid* [clocortolone pivalate]

clodoxopone INN

clodronic acid USAN, INN, BAN *calcium regulator*

clofazimine USAN, INN, BAN *bactericidal; tuberculostatic; leprostatic; (orphan: leprosy)*

clofedanol INN *antitussive* [also: chlophedianol HCl; chlophedianol]

clofedanol HCl [see: chlophedianol HCl]

clofenamic acid INN

clofenamide INN

clofenciclan INN

clofenetamine INN

clofenetamine HCl [see: clofenetamine]

clofenotane INN [also: chlorophenothane; dicophane]

clofenoxyde INN

clofenpyride [see: nicofibrate]

clofenvinfos INN [also: chlorfenvinphos]

clofeverine INN

clofexamide INN

clofezone INN

clofibrate USAN, USP, INN, BAN *antihyperlipoproteinemic*

clofibric acid INN

clofibride INN

clofilium phosphate USAN, INN *antiarrhythmic*

clofinol [see: nicofibrate]

cloflucarban USAN *disinfectant* [also: halocarban]

clofluperol INN, BAN *antipsychotic* [also: seperidol HCl]

clofluperol HCl [see: seperidol HCl]

clofoctol INN

cloforex INN

clofurac INN

clogestone INN, BAN *progestin* [also: clogestone acetate]

clogestone acetate USAN *progestin* [also: clogestone]

cloguanamil INN, BAN [also: cloguanamile]

cloguanamile BAN [also: cloguanamil]

clomacran INN, BAN *antipsychotic* [also: clomacran phosphate]

clomacran phosphate USAN *antipsychotic* [also: clomacran]

clomegestone INN *progestin* [also: clomegestone acetate]

clomegestone acetate USAN *progestin* [also: clomegestone]

clometacin INN

clometerone INN *antiestrogen* [also: clometherone]

clometherone USAN *antiestrogen* [also: clometerone]

clomethiazole INN [also: chlormethiazole]

clometocillin INN

Clomid tablets ℞ *ovulation stimulant* [clomiphene citrate]

clomide [see: aklomide]

clomifene INN *gonad-stimulating principle; ovulation stimulant* [also: clomiphene citrate; clomiphene]

clomifenoxide INN

clominorex USAN, INN *anorexic*

clomiphene BAN *gonad-stimulating principle; ovulation stimulant* [also: clomiphene citrate; clomifene]

clomiphene citrate USAN, USP *gonad-stimulating principle; ovulation stimulant* [also: clomifene; clomiphene]

clomipramine INN, BAN *antidepressant* [also: clomipramine HCl]

clomipramine HCl USAN *tricyclic antidepressant; used for obsessive-compulsive disorders* [also: clomipramine]

clomocycline INN, BAN

clomoxir INN

clonazepam USAN, USP, INN, BAN *anticonvulsant*

clonazoline INN

clonidine USAN, INN, BAN *antihypertensive*

clonidine HCl USAN, USP, BAN *antihypertensive; (orphan: epidural analgesia in cancer treatment)*

clonitazene INN, BAN

clonitrate USAN, INN *coronary vasodilator*

clonixeril USAN, INN *analgesic*

clonixin USAN, INN *analgesic*

clopamide USAN, INN, BAN *antihypertensive; diuretic*

clopenthixol USAN, INN, BAN *antipsychotic*

cloperastine INN

cloperidone INN *sedative* [also: cloperidone HCl]

cloperidone HCl USAN *sedative* [also: cloperidone]

clophenoxate [see: meclofenoxate]

clopidogrel INN *investigational preventative for stroke, myocardial ischemia, and peripheral artery disease*

clopidol USAN, INN, BAN *coccidiostat for poultry*

clopimozide USAN, INN *antipsychotic*

clopipazan INN *antipsychotic* [also: clopipazan mesylate]

clopipazan mesylate USAN *antipsychotic* [also: clopipazan]

clopirac USAN, INN, BAN *anti-inflammatory*

cloponone INN, BAN

clopoxide [see: chlordiazepoxide]

clopoxide chloride [see: chlordiazepoxide HCl]

Clopra tablets ℞ *antidopaminergic; antiemetic for chemotherapy; peristaltic* [metoclopramide monohydrochloride monohydrate]

cloprednol USAN, INN, BAN *glucocorticoid*

cloprostenol INN, BAN *prostaglandin* [also: cloprostenol sodium]

cloprostenol sodium USAN *prostaglandin* [also: cloprostenol]

cloprothiazole INN

cloquinate INN, BAN

cloquinozine INN

cloracetadol INN

cloral betaine INN *sedative* [also: chloral betaine]

cloramfenicol pantotenate complex INN *antibacterial; antirickettsial* [also: chloramphenicol pantotenate complex]

cloranolol INN

clorarsen [see: dichlorophenarsine HCl]

clorazepate dipotassium USAN, USP *anxiolytic; minor tranquilizer; alcohol withdrawal relief* [also: dipotassium clorazepate]

clorazepate monopotassium USAN *minor tranquilizer*

clorazepic acid BAN

cloretate INN *sedative; hypnotic* [also: clorethate]

clorethate USAN *sedative; hypnotic* [also: cloretate]

clorexolone USAN, INN, BAN *diuretic*

clorgiline INN [also: clorgyline]

clorgyline BAN [also: clorgiline]

cloricromen INN

cloridarol INN

clorindanic acid INN

clorindanol INN *spermaticide* [also: chlorindanol]
clorindione INN, BAN
clormecaine INN
clorofene INN *disinfectant* [also: clorophene]
cloroperone INN *antipsychotic* [also: cloroperone HCl]
cloroperone HCl USAN *antipsychotic* [also: cloroperone]
clorophene USAN *disinfectant* [also: clorofene]
cloroqualone INN
clorotepine INN
Clorpactin WCS-90 powder for solution OTC *topical antimicrobial* [oxychlorosene sodium]
Clorpactin XCB powder for solution OTC *topical antimicrobial* [oxychlorosene]
clorprenaline INN, BAN *adrenergic; bronchodilator* [also: clorprenaline HCl]
clorprenaline HCl USAN *adrenergic; bronchodilator* [also: clorprenaline]
clorquinaldol [see: chlorquinaldol]
clorsulon USAN, INN *antiparasitic; fasciolicide*
clortermine INN *anorexic* [also: clortermine HCl]
clortermine HCl USAN *anorexic* [also: clortermine]
closantel USAN, INN, BAN *anthelmintic*
closiramine INN *antihistamine* [also: closiramine aceturate]
closiramine aceturate USAN *antihistamine* [also: closiramine]
clostebol INN [also: clostebol acetate]
clostebol acetate BAN [also: clostebol]
Clostridium botulinum toxin [see: botulinum toxin]
Clostridium botulinum toxin, type A (*orphan: essential blepharospasm*)
clothiapine USAN, BAN *antipsychotic* [also: clotiapine]

clothixamide maleate USAN *antipsychotic* [also: clotixamide]
clotiapine INN *antipsychotic* [also: clothiapine]
clotiazepam INN
cloticasone INN, BAN *anti-inflammatory* [also: cloticasone propionate]
cloticasone propionate USAN *anti-inflammatory* [also: cloticasone]
clotioxone INN
clotixamide INN *antipsychotic* [also: clothixamide maleate]
clotixamide maleate [see: clothixamide maleate]
clotrimazole USAN, USP, INN, BAN *broad-spectrum antifungal*
clove oil NF
Cloverine salve OTC *skin protectant*
clovoxamine INN
cloxacepride INN
cloxacillin INN, BAN *antibacterial* [also: cloxacillin benzathine]
cloxacillin benzathine USP *antibacterial* [also: cloxacillin]
cloxacillin sodium USAN, USP *bactericidal antibiotic*
Cloxapen capsules ℞ *bactericidal antibiotic* (*penicillinase-resistant penicillin*) [cloxacillin sodium]
cloxazolam INN
cloxestradiol INN
cloxifenol [see: triclosan]
cloximate INN
cloxiquine INN *antibacterial* [also: cloxyquin]
cloxotestosterone INN
cloxphendyl [see: cloxypendyl]
cloxypendyl INN
cloxyquin USAN *antibacterial* [also: cloxiquine]
clozapine USAN, INN, BAN *sedative; antipsychotic for severe schizophrenia*
Clozaril tablets ℞ *antipsychotic* [clozapine]
Clusivol syrup (discontinued 1992) OTC *vitamin/mineral supplement* [multiple vitamins & minerals]

Clysodrast powder for oral solution ℞ *laxative for pre-procedure bowel prep* [bisacodyl tannex]

C-Max gradual-release tablets OTC *vitamin/mineral supplement* [various minerals; vitamin C]

CMC (carboxymethylcellulose) gum [see: carboxymethylcellulose sodium]

CMC (cyclophosphamide, methotrexate, CCNU) *chemotherapy protocol*

CMC-VAP (cyclophosphamide, methotrexate, CCNU, vincristine, Adriamycin, procarbazine) *chemotherapy protocol*

CMF (cyclophosphamide, methotrexate, fluorouracil) *chemotherapy protocol*

CMF/AV (Cytoxan, methotrexate, fluorouracil, Adriamycin, Oncovin) *chemotherapy protocol*

CMFAVP (cyclophosphamide, methotrexate, fluorouracil, Adriamycin, vincristine, prednisone) *chemotherapy protocol*

CMFP; CMF-P (cyclophosphamide, methotrexate, fluorouracil, prednisone) *chemotherapy protocol*

CMFPT (cyclophosphamide, methotrexate, fluorouracil, prednisone, tamoxifen) *chemotherapy protocol*

CMFPTH (cyclophosphamide, methotrexate, fluorouracil, prednisone, tamoxifen, Halotestin) *chemotherapy protocol*

CMFT (cyclophosphamide, methotrexate, fluorouracil, tamoxifen) *chemotherapy protocol*

CMFVAT (cyclophosphamide, methotrexate, fluorouracil, vincristine, Adriamycin, testosterone) *chemotherapy protocol*

CMFVP (cyclophosphamide, methotrexate, fluorouracil, vincristine, prednisone) *chemotherapy protocol*

CMH (cyclophosphamide, *m*-AMSA, hydroxyurea) *chemotherapy protocol*

C-MOPP (cyclophosphamide, mechlorethamine, Oncovin, procarbazine, prednisone) *chemotherapy protocol*

CMT tablets ℞ *antiarthritic* [choline magnesium trisalicylate]

CMV (cisplatin, methotrexate, vinblastine) *chemotherapy protocol*

CMV MAb ℞ *investigational antiviral for AIDS*

CMV-IGIV (cytomegalovirus immune globulin intravenous) [see: globulin, immune]

CN2 HCl [see: mechlorethamine HCl]

CNOP (cyclophosphamide, Novantrone, Oncovin, prednisone) *chemotherapy protocol*

Co I (coenzyme I) [see: nadide]

Co Tinic IM injection ℞ *antianemic* [ferrous gluconate; multiple B vitamins; procaine]

CO$_2$ (carbon dioxide) [q.v.]

^{57}**Co** [see: cobaltous chloride Co 57]

^{57}**Co** [see: cyanocobalamin Co 57]

^{58}**Co** [see: cyanocobalamin (^{58}Co)]

^{60}**Co** [see: cobaltous chloride Co 60]

^{60}**Co** [see: cyanocobalamin Co 60]

CoAdvil (name changed to Advil Cold & Sinus in 1992)

coagulation factor IX (human) (*orphan: hemophilia B*)

coal tar USP *topical antieczematic; antiseborrheic*

COAP (cyclophosphamide, Oncovin, ara-C, prednisone) *chemotherapy protocol*

Co-APAP tablets OTC *analgesic; antipyretic; antihistamine; decongestant; antitussive* [acetaminophen; chlorpheniramine maleate; pseudoephedrine HCl; dextromethorphan hydrobromide]

COAP-BLEO (cyclophosphamide, Oncovin, ara-C, prednisone, bleomycin) *chemotherapy protocol*

cobalamin concentrate USP *vitamin B_{12}; hematopoietic*

Cobalasine injection (discontinued 1991) ℞ *treatment for varicose veins with stasis dermatitis* [adenosine phosphate]

cobalt *element (Co)*

cobalt-labeled vitamin B_{12} [see: cyanocobalamin Co 57 & Co 60]

cobaltous chloride Co 57 USAN *radioactive agent*

cobaltous chloride Co 60 USAN *radioactive agent*

cobamamide INN

Cobex injection ℞ *antianemic; vitamin supplement* [cyanocobalamin]

cocaine USP, BAN *topical anesthetic for mucous membranes*

cocaine HCl USP *topical anesthetic for mucous membranes*

Cocaine Viscous topical solution ℞ *topical mucosal anesthesia* [cocaine]

cocarboxylase INN [also: co-carboxylase]

co-carboxylase BAN [also: cocarboxylase]

coccidioidin USP *dermal coccidioidomycosis test*

cocculin [see: picrotoxin]

cocoa NF

cocoa butter NF *suppository base; emollient/protectant*

cod liver oil USP, BAN *vitamins A and D source; emollient/protectant*

cod liver oil, nondestearinated NF

codactide INN, BAN

Codafed Expectorant liquid ℞ *decongestant; antitussive; expectorant* [pseudoephedrine HCl; codeine phosphate; guaifenesin; alcohol]

Codalan No. 1, No. 2 & No. 3 tablets (discontinued 1992) ℞ *narcotic analgesic* [codeine phosphate; acetaminophen; aspirin; caffeine]

Codamine syrup, pediatric syrup ℞ *decongestant; antitussive* [hydrocodone bitartrate; phenylpropanolamine HCl]

Codaphen tablets (discontinued 1993) ℞ *analgesic* [acetaminophen; codeine phosphate]

Codegest Expectorant liquid ℞ *decongestant; antitussive; expectorant* [phenylpropanolamine HCl; codeine phosphate; guaifenesin]

Codehist DH elixir ℞ *decongestant; antihistamine; antitussive* [pseudoephedrine HCl; chlorpheniramine maleate; codeine phosphate]

codehydrogenase I [see: nadide]

codeine USP, BAN *antitussive; narcotic analgesic*

codeine phosphate USP, BAN *antitussive; narcotic analgesic*

codeine polistirex USAN *antitussive*

codeine sulfate USP *narcotic analgesic; antitussive*

codelcortone [see: prednisolone]

co-dergocrine mesylate BAN *cognition adjuvant* [also: ergoloid mesylates]

Codiclear DH syrup ℞ *antitussive; expectorant* [hydrocodone bitartrate; guaifenesin]

Codimal A injection ℞ *antihistamine* [brompheniramine maleate]

Codimal capsules, tablets OTC *antihistamine; decongestant; analgesic* [chlorpheniramine maleate; pseudoephedrine HCl; acetaminophen]

Codimal DH syrup ℞ *antitussive; decongestant; antihistamine* [hydrocodone bitartrate; phenylephrine HCl; pyrilamine maleate]

Codimal DM oral solution OTC *antitussive; decongestant; antihistamine* [dextromethorphan hydrobromide; phenylephrine HCl; pyrilamine maleate; alcohol]

Codimal Expectorant oral solution OTC *decongestant; expectorant*

[phenylpropanolamine HCl; guaifenesin]

Codimal L.A.; Codimal L.A. Half extended-release capsules ℞ *antihistamine; decongestant* [chlorpheniramine maleate; pseudoephedrine HCl]

Codimal PH syrup OTC *antitussive; decongestant; antihistamine* [codeine phosphate; phenylephrine HCl; pyrilamine maleate]

codorphone [now: conorphone HCl]

codoxime USAN, INN *antitussive*

Codroxomin IM injection (discontinued 1992) ℞ *antianemic; vitamin supplement* [hydroxocobalamin]

COF/COM (cyclophosphamide, Oncovin, fluorouracil + cyclophosphamide, Oncovin, methotrexate) *chemotherapy protocol*

Coffee Break timed-release caplets (discontinued 1992) OTC *CNS stimulant; analeptic* [caffeine]

coffeine [see: caffeine]

cofisatin INN

cofisatine [see: cofisatin]

cogazocine INN

Cogentin tablets, IV or IM injection ℞ *anticholinergic; antiparkinsonian* [benztropine mesylate]

Co-Gesic tablets ℞ *narcotic analgesic* [hydrocodone bitartrate; acetaminophen]

Cognex ℞ *investigational cognition adjuvant for Alzheimer's disease* [tacrine HCl]

Colabid tablets ℞ *uricosuric for gout* [probenecid; colchicine]

Colace capsules, syrup, drops OTC *stool softener* [docusate sodium]

colaspase BAN *antineoplastic* [also: asparaginase]

Co-Lav powder for oral solution ℞ *pre-procedure bowel evacuant* [polyethylene glycol-electrolyte solution]

Colax tablets OTC *laxative; stool softener* [docusate sodium; phenolphthalein]

ColBenemid tablets ℞ *uricosuric for gout* [probenecid; colchicine]

colchamine [see: demecolcine]

colchicine USP *gout suppressant; (orphan: multiple sclerosis)*

cold cream USP

Cold Relief tablets OTC *decongestant; antihistamine; antitussive; analgesic* [phenylpropanolamine HCl; chlorpheniramine maleate; dextromethorphan hydrobromide; acetaminophen]

Coldrine tablets OTC *decongestant; analgesic* [pseudoephedrine HCl; acetaminophen]

colecalciferol INN *vitamin D_3; antirachitic* [also: cholecalciferol]

Colestid granules ℞ *cholesterol-lowering antihyperlipidemic* [colestipol HCl]

colestipol INN, BAN *antihyperlipoproteinemic; bile acid sequestrant* [also: colestipol HCl]

colestipol HCl USAN, USP *antihyperlipoproteinemic; bile acid sequestrant* [also: colestipol]

colestolone USAN, INN *hypolipidemic*

colestyramine INN *bile salts ion-exchange resin; antihyperlipoproteinemic* [also: cholestyramine resin; cholestyramine]

colestyramine resin [see: cholestyramine resin]

colextran INN

Colfed-A sustained-release capsules ℞ *antihistamine; decongestant* [chlorpheniramine maleate; pseudoephedrine HCl]

colfenamate INN

colforsin USAN, INN *antiglaucoma agent*

colfosceril palmitate USAN, INN, BAN *pulmonary surfactant; (orphan: hyaline membrane disease; respiratory distress syndrome)*

colimecycline INN

colistimethate sodium USAN, USP, INN *bactericidal antibiotic* [also: colistin sulphomethate]

colistin INN, BAN *bactericidal antibiotic* [also: colistin sulfate]
colistin methanesulfonate [see: colistimethate sodium]
colistin sulfate USP *bactericidal antibiotic* [also: colistin]
colistin sulphomethate BAN *bactericidal antibiotic* [also: colistimethate sodium]
collagenase *topical proteolytic enzymes for necrotic tissue debridement*
collodion USP *topical protectant*
colloidal aluminum hydroxide [see: aluminum hydroxide gel]
colloidal oatmeal *demulcent*
colloidal silicon dioxide [see: silicon dioxide, colloidal]
Collyrium Eye Lotion ophthalmic solution (discontinued 1991) OTC *extraocular irrigating solution* [balanced saline solution]
Collyrium for Fresh Eyes ophthalmic solution OTC *extraocular irrigating solution* [balanced saline solution]
Collyrium Fresh ophthalmic solution OTC *extraocular irrigating solution; topical ocular decongestant* [balanced saline solution; tetrahydrozoline]
Collyrium with Tetrahydrozoline eye drops (discontinued 1991) OTC *topical ocular decongestant* [tetrahydrozoline HCl]
ColoCare test kit OTC *in vitro diagnostic aid for fecal occult blood*
Color Allergy Screening Test (CAST) reagent assay tubes ℞ *in vitro diagnostic aid for immunoglobulin E in serum*
Color Ovulation Test kit OTC *in vitro diagnostic aid to predict ovulation time*
Colovage powder for oral solution ℞ *pre-procedure bowel evacuant* [polyethylene glycol-electrolyte solution]
Col-Probenecid tablets ℞ *uricosuric for gout* [probenecid; colchicine]

Colrex troches (discontinued 1991) OTC *topical anesthetic; oral antiseptic* [benzocaine; cetylpyridinium chloride]
Coltab Children's tablets OTC *pediatric decongestant and antihistamine* [phenylephrine HCl; chlorpheniramine maleate]
colterol INN *bronchodilator* [also: colterol mesylate]
colterol mesylate USAN *bronchodilator* [also: colterol]
Coly-Mycin M powder for IV or IM injection ℞ *bactericidal antibiotic* [colistimethate sodium]
Coly-Mycin S Otic suspension ℞ *topical corticosteroidal anti-inflammatory; antibiotic* [hydrocortisone acetate; neomycin sulfate; colistin sulfate]
Coly-Mycin S powder for oral suspension ℞ *bactericidal antibiotic* [colistin sulfate]
Colyte powder for oral solution ℞ *pre-procedure bowel evacuant* [polyethylene glycol-electrolyte solution]
COM (cyclophosphamide, Oncovin, MeCCNU) *chemotherapy protocol*
COM (cyclophosphamide, Oncovin, methotrexate) *chemotherapy protocol*
COMA-A (cyclophosphamide, Oncovin, methotrexate/citrovorum factor, Adriamycin, ara-C) *chemotherapy protocol*
Oncovin, MeCCNU, bleomycin) *chemotherapy protocol*
COMB (Cytoxin, Oncovin, methotrexate, bleomycin) *chemotherapy protocol*
Combipres 0.1; Combipres 0.2; Combipres 0.3 tablets ℞ *antihypertensive* [clonidine HCl; chlorthalidone]
Combistix reagent strips OTC *in vitro diagnostic aid for multiple urine products*

COMe (Cytoxin, Oncovin, methotrexate) *chemotherapy protocol*

COMF (cyclophosphamide, Oncovin, methotrexate, fluorouracil) *chemotherapy protocol*

Comfort eye drops OTC *topical ocular vasoconstrictor* [naphazoline HCl]

Comfort Tears solution OTC *contact lens rewetting solution*

Comfortine ointment OTC *moisturizer; emollient; astringent; antiseptic* [vitamins A & D; lanolin; zinc oxide]

Comhist LA long-acting capsules ℞ *antihistamine; decongestant* [chlorpheniramine maleate; phenyltoloxamine citrate; phenylephrine HCl]

Comhist tablets ℞ *antihistamine; decongestant* [chlorpheniramine maleate; phenyltoloxamine citrate; phenylephrine HCl]

COMLA (cyclophosphamide, Oncovin, methotrexate, leucovorin, ara-C) *chemotherapy protocol*

comosain (*orphan: enzymatic debridement of severe burns*)

COMP (CCNU, Oncovin, methotrexate, procarbazine) *chemotherapy protocol*

COMP (cyclophosphamide, Oncovin, methotrexate, prednisone) *chemotherapy protocol*

Compazine tablets, Spansules (capsules), IV, IM, suppositories, syrup ℞ *antiemetic; tranquilizer* [prochlorperazine maleate]

Compete tablets OTC *vitamin/iron supplement* [multiple vitamins; ferrous gluconate; folic acid]

Compleat Regular Formula; Compleat Modified Formula liquid OTC *enteral nutritional therapy*

Complere tablets OTC *vitamin/mineral supplement* [multiple vitamins, minerals & amino acids]

Complete *investigational contact lens disinfectant*

Complex 15 Face cream OTC *moisturizer; emollient*

Complex 15 Hand & Body cream, lotion OTC *moisturizer; emollient*

Comply liquid OTC *oral nutritional supplement*

compound 42 [see: warfarin]

compound CB3025 [see: melphalan]

compound E [see: cortisone acetate]

compound F [see: hydrocortisone]

compound insulin zinc suspension INN *antidiabetic* [also: insulin zinc]

compound orange spirit [see: orange spirit, compound]

compound Q [see: trichosanthin]

compound S [see: zidovudine]

compound solution of sodium chloride INN *fluid and electrolyte replenisher* [also: Ringer's injection]

compound solution of sodium lactate INN *electrolyte and fluid replenisher; systemic alkalizer* [also: Ringer's injection, lactated]

Compound W liquid, gel OTC *topical keratolytic* [salicylic acid]

Compoz Nighttime Sleep Aid caplet OTC *antihistaminic sleep aid* [diphenhydramine HCl]

Comprecin (name changed to Penetrex in 1991)

compressible sugar [see: sugar, compressible]

Comtrex, Allergy-Sinus caplets, tablets OTC *decongestant; antihistamine; analgesic* [pseudoephedrine HCl; chlorpheniramine maleate; acetaminophen]

Comtrex, Cough Formula liquid OTC *decongestant; antitussive; expectorant; analgesic* [pseudoephedrine HCl; dextromethorphan hydrobromide; guaifenesin; acetaminophen; alcohol]

Comtrex, Day-Night coated caplets (day), coated tablets (night) OTC *decongestant; antitussive; analgesic; antihistamine* [pseudoephedrine HCl; dextromethorphan hydrobromide;

acetaminophen; chlorpheniramine maleate]

Comtrex liquid, tablets, caplets OTC *decongestant; antihistamine; antitussive; analgesic* [pseudoephedrine HCl; chlorpheniramine maleate; dextromethorphan hydrobromide; acetaminophen]

Comtrex Liqui-Gels (liquid-filled capsules) OTC *decongestant; antihistamine; antitussive; analgesic* [phenylpropanolamine HCl; chlorpheniramine maleate; dextromethorphan hydrobromide; acetaminophen]

Conceive Ovulation Predictor 5-day test kit OTC *in vitro diagnostic aid to predict ovulation time*

Concentraid nasal spray, intranasal pipets ℞ *diabetes insipidus; hemophilia A; von Willebrand's disease* [desmopressin acetate]

Concentrated Cleaner solution OTC *contact lens cleaning solution*

Conceptrol Birth Control vaginal cream (discontinued 1991) OTC *spermicidal contraceptive* [nonoxynol 9]

Conceptrol Disposable Contraceptive vaginal gel (discontinued 1991) OTC *spermicidal contraceptive* [nonoxynol 9]

CondomMate vaginal inserts (discontinued 1991) OTC *vaginal lubricant*

Condrin-LA sustained-release capsules ℞ *decongestant; antihistamine* [phenylpropanolamine HCl; chlorpheniramine maleate]

Condylox solution ℞ *topical keratolytic for external genital warts* [podofilox]

conessine INN

conessine hydrobromide [see: conessine]

Conex D.A. tablets OTC *decongestant; antihistamine* [phenylpropanolamine HCl; chlorpheniramine maleate]

Conex lozenges OTC *topical anesthetic; oral antiseptic* [benzocaine; cetylpyridinium chloride]

Conex Plus tablets OTC *decongestant; antihistamine; analgesic* [phenylpropanolamine HCl; chlorpheniramine maleate; acetaminophen]

Conex syrup OTC *decongestant; expectorant* [phenylpropanolamine HCl; guaifenesin]

Conex with Codeine syrup ℞ *decongestant; antitussive; expectorant* [phenylpropanolamine HCl; codeine phosphate; guaifenesin]

confectioner's sugar [see: sugar, confectioner's]

congazone sodium [see: Congo red]

Congespirin for Children chewable tablets OTC *decongestant; analgesic* [phenylephrine HCl; acetaminophen]

Congespirin for Children syrup (discontinued 1991) OTC *antitussive* [dextromethorphan hydrobromide]

Congess JR capsules ℞ *decongestant; expectorant* [pseudoephedrine HCl; guaifenesin]

Congess SR sustained-release capsules ℞ *decongestant; expectorant* [pseudoephedrine HCl; guaifenesin]

Congestac caplets OTC *decongestant; expectorant* [pseudoephedrine HCl; guaifenesin]

Congestant D tablets OTC *decongestant; antihistamine; analgesic* [phenylpropanolamine HCl; chlorpheniramine maleate; acetaminophen]

Congestion Relief, Children's liquid OTC *nasal decongestant* [pseudoephedrine HCl]

Congestion Relief tablets OTC *nasal decongestant* [pseudoephedrine HCl]

Congo red USP

conjugated estrogens [see: estrogens, conjugated]

conorfone INN *analgesic* [also: conorphone HCl]

conorfone HCl [see: conorphone HCl]
conorphone HCl USAN *analgesic* [also: conorfone]
CONPADRI; CONPADRI-I (cyclophosphamide, Oncovin, L-phenylalanine mustard, Adriamycin) *chemotherapy protocol*
Conray 325; Conray 400 injection ℞ *parenteral radiopaque agent* [iothalamate sodium]
Conray; Conray 30; Conray 43 injection ℞ *parenteral radiopaque agent* [iothalamate meglumine]
Consensus Interferon ℞ *investigational antiviral and antineoplastic*
Constant-T sustained-action tablets ℞ *bronchodilator* [theophylline]
Constilac syrup ℞ *laxative* [lactulose]
Constulose syrup ℞ *laxative* [lactulose]
Contac 12 Hour sustained-release capsules, sustained-release caplets OTC *decongestant; antihistamine* [phenylpropanolamine HCl; chlorpheniramine maleate]
Contac Cough & Chest Cold liquid OTC *decongestant; antitussive; expectorant; analgesic* [pseudoephedrine HCl; dextromethorphan hydrobromide; guaifenesin; acetaminophen; alcohol]
Contac Cough Formula liquid OTC *antitussive; expectorant* [dextromethorphan hydrobromide; guaifenesin]
Contac Cough & Sore Throat liquid OTC *antitussive; analgesic* [dextromethorphan hydrobromide; acetaminophen]
Contac Day & Night Cold & Flu caplets OTC *decongestant; antihistamine; antitussive; analgesic* [pseudoephedrine HCl; diphenhydramine HCl; dextromethorphan hydrobromide; acetaminophen]
Contac Jr. Non-Drowsy Cold liquid OTC *decongestant; antitussive; analgesic* [pseudoephedrine HCl; dextromethorphan hydrobromide; acetaminophen]
Contac Maximum Strength Sinus (name changed to Contac Non-Drowsy Formula Sinus in 1991)
Contac Nighttime Cold Medicine liquid (discontinued 1992) OTC *decongestant; antihistamine; antitussive; analgesic* [pseudoephedrine HCl; doxylamine succinate; dextromethorphan hydrobromide; acetaminophen; alcohol]
Contac Non-Drowsy Formula Sinus caplets OTC *decongestant; analgesic* [pseudoephedrine HCl; acetaminophen]
Contac Severe Cold & Flu Hot Medicine powder OTC *decongestant; antihistamine; antitussive; analgesic* [pseudoephedrine HCl; chlorpheniramine maleate; dextromethorphan hydrobromide; acetaminophen]
Contac Severe Cold & Flu Nighttime liquid OTC *decongestant; antihistamine; antitussive; analgesic* [pseudoephedrine HCl; chlorpheniramine maleate; dextromethorphan hydrobromide; acetaminophen; alcohol]
Contac Severe Cold Formula caplets OTC *decongestant; antihistamine; antitussive; analgesic* [phenylephrine HCl; chlorpheniramine maleate; dextromethorphan hydrobromide; acetaminophen]
Contactisol solution (discontinued 1991) OTC *contact lens wetting/soaking solution*
conteben [see: thioacetazone; thiacetazone]
ConTE-Pak-4 IV injection ℞ *intravenous nutritional therapy* [multiple trace elements (metals)]
Contique solution (discontinued 1991) OTC *contact lens wetting solution*
Contrin capsules ℞ *hematinic* [ferrous fumarate; vitamins B_{12} & C; intrinsic factor concentrate; folic acid]

Control timed-release capsules OTC *diet aid* [phenylpropanolamine HCl]

Control-L liquid (discontinued 1993) OTC *lice treatment* [pyrethrins; piperonyl butoxide; petroleum distillate]

Contuss liquid ℞ *decongestant; expectorant* [phenylephrine HCl; phenylpropanolamine HCl; guaifenesin]

Converspaz Improved capsules (discontinued 1991) OTC *digestive enzymes; antispasmodic* [amylase; protease; lipase; cellulase; hyoscyamine sulfate]

Converzyme capsules (discontinued 1991) OTC *digestive enzymes* [amylase; protease; lipase; cellulase]

Cooper's regimen *chemotherapy protocol* [see: CMFVP]

COP [see: creatinolfosfate]

COP (cyclophosphamide, Oncovin, prednisone) *chemotherapy protocol*

COP 1 (copolymer 1) [q.v.]

COPA (Cytoxin, Oncovin, prednisone, Adriamycin) *chemotherapy protocol*

COPA-BLEO (cyclophosphamide, Oncovin, prednisone, Adriamycin, bleomycin) *chemotherapy protocol*

COPAC (CCNU, Oncovin, prednisone, Adriamycin, cyclophosphamide) *chemotherapy protocol*

COPB (cyclophosphamide, Oncovin, prednisone, bleomycin) *chemotherapy protocol*

COP-BLAM (cyclophosphamide, Oncovin, prednisone, bleomycin, Adriamycin, Matulane) *chemotherapy protocol*

COP-BLEO (cyclophosphamide, Oncovin, prednisone, bleomycin) *chemotherapy protocol*

COPE (cyclophosphamide, Oncovin, Platinol, etoposide) *chemotherapy protocol*

Cope tablets OTC *analgesic; antipyretic; anti-inflammatory; antacid* [aspirin; caffeine; magnesium hydroxide; aluminum hydroxide]

Cophene No. 2 sustained-release capsules ℞ *decongestant; antihistamine* [pseudoephedrine HCl; chlorpheniramine maleate]

Cophene XP liquid ℞ *decongestant; antitussive; expectorant* [hydrocodone bitartrate; pseudoephedrine HCl; guaifenesin; alcohol]

Cophene-B subcu or IM injection ℞ *antihistamine; anaphylaxis* [brompheniramine maleate]

Cophene-X capsules ℞ *decongestant; antitussive; expectorant* [phenylephrine HCl; phenylpropanolamine HCl; carbetapentrane citrate; potassium guaiacolsulfonate]

copolymer 1 (COP 1) *(orphan: multiple sclerosis)*

copovithane BAN

COPP (CCNU, Oncovin, procarbazine, prednisone) *chemotherapy protocol*

COPP (cyclophosphamide, Oncovin, procarbazine, prednisone) *chemotherapy protocol*

copper *element (Cu)*

copper chloride dihydrate [see: cupric chloride]

copper gluconate (copper D-gluconate) USP *trace mineral supplement*

copper sulfate pentahydrate [see: cupric sulfate]

Copper Trace Metal Additive IV injection (discontinued 1991) ℞ *intravenous nutritional therapy* [cupric sulfate]

copper 10-undecenoate [see: copper undecylenate]

copper undecylenate USAN

copperhead snake antivenin [see: antivenin (Crotalidae) polyvalent]

Co-Pyronil 2 Pulvules (capsules) OTC *decongestant; antihistamine* [pseudoephedrine HCl; chlorpheniramine maleate]

Co-Q₁₀ soft capsules OTC *dietary supplement* [coenzyme Q₁₀]
Coracin ophthalmic ointment ℞ *topical ophthalmic corticosteroidal anti-inflammatory; antibiotic* [hydrocortisone acetate; neomycin sulfate; bacitracin zinc; polymyxin B sulfate]
coral snake antivenin [see: antivenin (Micrurus fulvius)]
corbadrine INN *adrenergic; vasoconstrictor* [also: levonordefrin]
Cordarone tablets ℞ *antiarrhythmic* [amiodarone HCl]
Cordran ointment, lotion, tape ℞ *topical corticosteroid* [flurandrenolide]
Cordran SP cream ℞ *topical corticosteroid* [flurandrenolide]
Cordran-N cream, ointment (discontinued 1993) ℞ *topical corticosteroid; antibiotic* [flurandrenolide; neomycin sulfate]
Corgard tablets ℞ *antihypertensive; antianginal; β-blocker* [nadolol]
Corgonject-5 powder for injection (discontinued 1991) ℞ *hormone for prepubertal cryptorchidism and hypogonadism* [chorionic gonadotropin]
coriander oil NF
Coricidin 'D' Decongestant; Coricidin Sinus Headache tablets OTC *decongestant; antihistamine; analgesic* [phenylpropanolamine HCl; chlorpheniramine maleate; acetaminophen]
Coricidin Demilets (chewable tablets) OTC *pediatric decongestant, antihistamine and analgesic* [phenylpropanolamine HCl; chlorpheniramine maleate; acetaminophen; saccharin; mannitol]
Coricidin tablets OTC *antihistamine; analgesic* [chlorpheniramine maleate; acetaminophen]
Coridicin Nasal Mist spray (discontinued 1992) OTC *nasal decongestant* [oxymetazoline HCl]
cormed [see: nikethamide]

cormetasone INN *topical anti-inflammatory* [also: cormethasone acetate]
cormetasone acetate [see: cormethasone acetate]
cormethasone acetate USAN *topical anti-inflammatory* [also: cormetasone]
Corn Huskers lotion OTC *moisturizer; emollient*
corn oil NF *solvent; caloric replacement*
Cor-Oticin eye drop suspension (discontinued 1991) ℞ *topical ophthalmic corticosteroidal anti-inflammatory; antibiotic* [hydrocortisone acetate; neomycin sulfate]
corpus luteum extract [see: progesterone]
Corque cream ℞ *topical corticosteroid; antifungal; antibacterial* [hydrocortisone; clioquinol]
Correctol Extra Gentle soft gel capsules OTC *stool softener* [docusate sodium]
Correctol tablets OTC *laxative; stool softener* [yellow phenolphthalein; docusate sodium]
Corsevin M ℞ *investigational agent for coagulation disorders* [monoclonal antibodies]
CortaGel OTC *topical corticosteroid* [hydrocortisone]
Cortaid; Cortaid with Aloe cream, ointment OTC *topical corticosteroid* [hydrocortisone acetate]
Cortaid lotion (discontinued 1993) OTC *topical corticosteroid* [hydrocortisone acetate]
Cortaid pump spray OTC *topical corticosteroid* [hydrocortisone]
Cortatrigen Modified ear drops, otic suspension ℞ *topical corticosteroidal anti-inflammatory; antibiotic* [hydrocortisone; neomycin sulfate; polymyxin B sulfate]
Cort-Dome cream ℞ *topical corticosteroid* [hydrocortisone]
Cort-Dome High Potency rectal suppositories ℞ *topical corticosteroidal*

anti-inflammatory; antipruritic [hydrocortisone acetate]
Cort-Dome lotion (discontinued 1993) ℞ *topical corticosteroid* [hydrocortisone]
Cort-Dome suppositories ℞ *topical corticosteroid for anorectal inflammation* [hydrocortisone acetate]
Cortef Feminine Itch cream OTC *topical corticosteroid* [hydrocortisone acetate]
Cortef tablets, oral suspension ℞ *glucocorticoids* [hydrocortisone]
Cortenema retention enema ℞ *ulcerative colitis* [hydrocortisone]
cortenil [see: desoxycorticosterone acetate]
cortexolone [see: cortodoxone]
Corticaine anorectal cream OTC *topical corticosteroidal anti-inflammatory; antipruritic; anesthetic* [hydrocortisone acetate; dibucaine]
Corticaine cream ℞ *topical corticosteroid* [hydrocortisone acetate]
corticorelin ovine triflutate USAN, INN *corticotropin-releasing hormone; diagnostic aid for Cushing syndrome & adrenocortical insufficiency*
corticotrophin INN, BAN *adrenocorticotropic hormone; glucocorticoid; diagnostic aid* [also: corticotropin]
corticotrophin-zinc hydroxide INN *adrenocorticotropic hormone; glucocorticoid; diagnostic aid* [also: corticotropin zinc hydroxide]
corticotropin USP *adrenocorticotropic hormone; glucocorticoid; diagnostic aid* [also: corticotrophin]
corticotropin, repository USP *adrenocorticotropic hormone; glucocorticoid; diagnostic aid*
corticotropin tetracosapeptide [see: cosyntropin]
corticotropin zinc hydroxide USP *adrenocorticotropic hormone; glucocorticoid; diagnostic aid* [also: corticotrophin-zinc hydroxide]

Cortifoam intrarectal foam aerosol ℞ *ulcerative proctitis* [hydrocortisone acetate]
Cortin cream ℞ *topical corticosteroid; antifungal; antibacterial* [hydrocortisone; clioquinol]
cortisol [see: hydrocortisone]
cortisol 21-acetate [see: hydrocortisone acetate]
cortisol 21-butyrate [see: hydrocortisone butyrate]
cortisol 21-cyclopentanepropionate [see: hydrocortisone cypionate]
cortisol cyclopentylpropionate [see: hydrocortisone cypionate]
cortisol 21-valerate [see: hydrocortisone valerate]
cortisone INN, BAN *glucocorticoid* [also: cortisone acetate]
cortisone acetate USP *glucocorticoid* [also: cortisone]
Cortisporin cream ℞ *topical corticosteroid; antibiotic* [hydrocortisone acetate; neomycin sulfate; polymyxin B sulfate]
Cortisporin eye drop suspension ℞ *topical ophthalmic corticosteroidal anti-inflammatory; antibiotic* [hydrocortisone; neomycin sulfate; polymyxin B sulfate]
Cortisporin ointment ℞ *topical corticosteroid; antibiotic* [hydrocortisone; bacitracin zinc; polymyxin B sulfate]
Cortisporin ophthalmic ointment ℞ *ophthalmic corticosteroidal anti-inflammatory; antibiotic* [hydrocortisone; neomycin sulfate; bacitracin zinc; polymyxin B sulfate]
Cortisporin Otic ear drops, otic suspension ℞ *topical corticosteroidal anti-inflammatory; antibiotic* [hydrocortisone; neomycin sulfate; polymyxin B sulfate]
cortisuzol INN
cortivazol USAN, INN *glucocorticoid*
Cortizone-5; Cortizone-10 ointment, cream OTC *topical corticosteroid* [hydrocortisone]

cortodoxone USAN, INN, BAN *anti-inflammatory*
Cortone Acetate tablets ℞ *glucocorticoids* [cortisone acetate]
Cortril ointment (discontinued 1993) ℞ *topical corticosteroid* [hydrocortisone]
Cortrophin-Zinc IM injection (discontinued 1991) ℞ *steroid* [corticotropin zinc hydroxide]
Cortrosyn powder for injection ℞ *multiple sclerosis; infantile spasms; diagnostic purposes* [cosyntropin]
Corzide 40/5; Corzide 80/5 tablets ℞ *antihypertensive* [nadolol; bendroflumethiazide]
Cosmegen powder for IV injection ℞ *antineoplastic antibiotic* [dactinomycin]
cosmoline [see: petrolatum]
cosyntropin USAN *adrenocorticotropic hormone* [also: tetracosactide; tetracosactrin]
cotarnine chloride NF
cotarnine HCl [see: cotarnine chloride]
Cotazym capsules ℞ *digestive enzymes; antacid* [pancrelipase; calcium carbonate]
Cotazym-S capsules containing enteric-coated spheres ℞ *digestive enzymes* [pancrelipase]
cotinine INN *antidepressant* [also: cotinine fumarate]
cotinine fumarate USAN *antidepressant* [also: cotinine]
Cotrim D.S. double strength tablets ℞ *anti-infective; antibacterial* [sulfamethoxazole; trimethoprim]
Cotrim tablets, pediatric oral suspension ℞ *anti-infective; antibacterial* [sulfamethoxazole; trimethoprim]
co-trimoxazole BAN [also: trimethoprim + sulfamethoxazole]
cotriptyline INN
cotton, purified USP *surgical aid*
cottonseed oil NF *solvent*

Cough Formula liquid OTC *antitussive; antihistamine* [dextromethorphan hydrobromide; chlorpheniramine maleate; alcohol]
Cough Formula with Decongestant liquid OTC *decongestant; antitussive; expectorant* [pseudoephedrine HCl; dextromethorphan hydrobromide; guaifenesin; alcohol]
Coumadin tablets ℞ *anticoagulant* [warfarin sodium]
coumafos INN [also: coumaphos]
coumamycin INN *antibacterial* [also: coumermycin]
coumaphos BAN [also: coumafos]
coumarin NF *anticoagulant*
coumazoline INN
coumermycin USAN *antibacterial* [also: coumamycin]
coumermycin sodium USAN *antibacterial*
coumetarol INN [also: cumetharol]
Counterpain Rub (discontinued 1992) OTC *counterirritant; antiseptic* [methyl salicylate; menthol; eugenol]
Covangesic tablets OTC *decongestant; antihistamine; analgesic* [phenylpropanolamine HCl; phenylephrine HCl; chlorpheniramine maleate; pyrilamine maleate; acetaminophen]
covatin HCl [see: captodiame HCl]
Covicone cream (discontinued 1991) OTC *skin protectant* [dimethicone; nitrocellulose; castor oil]
CP (cyclophosphamide, prednisone) *chemotherapy protocol*
CPA TR extended-release capsules ℞ *decongestant; antihistamine* [phenylpropanolamine HCl; chlorpheniramine maleate]
CPB (cyclophosphamide, Platinol, BCNU) *chemotherapy protocol*
CPC (cyclophosphamide, Platinol, carboplatin) *chemotherapy protocol*
CPI rectal suppositories (discontinued 1992) OTC *astringent; emollient/protectant* [bismuth subgallate; bismuth

resorcin compound; benzyl benzoate; zinc oxide; balsam Peru]
CPM (CCNU, procarbazine, methotrexate) *chemotherapy protocol*
CPOB (cyclophosphamide, prednisone, Oncovin, bleomycin) *chemotherapy protocol*
^{51}**Cr** [see: albumin, chromated Cr 51 serum]
^{51}**Cr** [see: chromic chloride Cr 51]
^{51}**Cr** [see: chromic phosphate Cr 51]
^{51}**Cr** [see: sodium chromate Cr 51]
CRDS (curdlan sulfate) [q.v.]
creatinolfosfate INN
Cremacoat 1 syrup (discontinued 1991) OTC *antitussive* [dextromethorphan hydrobromide]
Creon capsules containing enteric-coated microspheres ℞ *digestive enzymes* [pancreatin]
creosote carbonate USP
Creo-Terpin liquid OTC *antitussive* [dextromethorphan hydrobromide; creosote; terpin hydrate; alcohol]
cresol NF *disinfectant*
cresotamide INN
cresoxydiol [see: mephenesin]
crestomycin sulfate [see: paromomycin sulfate]
Cresylate ear drops ℞ *antibacterial/antifungal* [m-cresyl acetate; alcohol; chlorobutanol]
cresylic acid [see: cresol]
crilanomer INN
crilvastatin USAN, INN *antihyperlipidemic*
crisnatol INN *antineoplastic* [also: crisnatol mesylate]
crisnatol mesylate USAN *antineoplastic* [also: crisnatol]
Criticare HN liquid OTC *complete elemental diet*
croconazole INN
crofilcon A USAN *hydrophilic contact lens material*
cromakalim INN, BAN
cromitrile INN *antiasthmatic* [also: cromitrile sodium]

cromitrile sodium USAN *antiasthmatic* [also: cromitrile]
cromoglicic acid INN *prophylactic antiasthmatic* [also: cromolyn sodium; cromoglycic acid]
cromoglycic acid BAN *prophylactic antiasthmatic* [also: cromolyn sodium; cromoglicic acid]
cromolyn sodium USAN, USP *prophylactic antiasthmatic; (orphan: mastocytosis; vernal keratoconjunctivitis)* [also: cromoglicic acid; cromoglycic acid]
C-Ron; C-Ron Forte tablets (discontinued 1991) OTC *antianemic* [ferrous fumarate; ascorbic acid]
Cronassial *(orphan: retinitis pigmentosa)* [gangliosides, sodium salts]
cronetal [see: disulfiram]
cronidipine INN
cropropamide INN, BAN
croscarmellose INN *tablet disintegrant* [also: croscarmellose sodium]
croscarmellose sodium USAN, NF *tablet disintegrant* [also: croscarmellose]
crospovidone NF *tablet excipient*
cross-linked carboxymethylcellulose sodium [now: croscarmellose sodium]
cross-linked carmellose sodium [see: croscarmellose sodium]
crotaline antivenin [see: antivenin (Crotalidae) polyvalent]
crotamiton USP, INN, BAN *scabicide*
crotetamide INN [also: crotethamide]
crotethamide BAN [also: crotetamide]
crotoniazide INN
crotonylidenisoniazid [see: crotoniazide]
crotoxyfos BAN
crude tuberculin [see: tuberculin, old]
Cruex cream, powder, aerosol powder OTC *topical antifungal* [undecylenic acid; zinc undecylenate]

Cruex powder OTC *topical antifungal* [calcium undecylenate]
crufomate USAN, INN, BAN *veterinary anthelmintic*
cryofluorane INN *aerosol propellant* [also: dichlorotetrafluoroethane]
cryptenamine acetates
cryptosporidium hyperimmune bovine colostrum IgG concentrate (*orphan: cryptosporidium-induced diarrhea in AIDS*)
crystal violet [see: gentian violet]
crystallized trypsin [see: trypsin, crystallized]
Crystamine injection ℞ *antianemic; vitamin supplement* [cyanocobalamin]
Crysti-12 injection ℞ *antianemic; vitamin supplement* [cyanocobalamin]
Crysticillin 300 A.S.; Crysticillin 600 A.S. IM injection ℞ *bactericidal antibiotic* [penicillin G procaine]
Crysti-Liver IM ℞ *antianemic; vitamin supplement* [liver extracts; vitamin B$_{12}$; folic acid]
Crystodigin tablets (discontinued 1991) ℞ *increase cardiac output; antiarrhythmic* [digitoxin]
crystografin [see: meglumine diatriazole]
^{131}**Cs** [see: cesium chloride Cs 131]
C-Solve OTC *lotion base*
C-Solve 2 topical solution ℞ *topical antibiotic for acne vulgaris* [erythromycin]
CSP (cellulose sodium phosphate) [q.v.]
CS-T test kit (discontinued 1992) OTC *in vitro diagnostic aid for fecal occult blood*
CTAB (cetyltrimethyl ammonium bromide)
CTCb (cyclophosphamide, thiotepa, carboplatin) *chemotherapy protocol*
C-Tussin Expectorant liquid (discontinued 1992) ℞ *decongestant; antitussive; expectorant* [pseudoephedrine HCl; codeine phosphate; guaifenesin; alcohol]
Ctx-Plat (cyclophosphamide, Platinol) *chemotherapy protocol*
^{64}**Cu** [see: cupric acetate Cu 64]
Culturette 10 Minute Group A Strep ID throat swab test kit ℞ *in vitro diagnostic test for streptococci*
cumetharol BAN [also: coumetarol]
cupric acetate Cu 64 USAN *radioactive agent*
cupric chloride USP *dietary copper supplement*
cupric sulfate USP *antidote to phosphorus; dietary copper supplement*
Cuprid (name changed to Syprine in 1990)
Cuprimine capsules ℞ *treatment of rheumatoid arthritis, Wilson's disease and cystinuria* [penicillamine]
cuprimyxin USAN, INN *veterinary antibacterial; antifungal*
Cupri-Pak IV injection (discontinued 1992) ℞ *intravenous nutritional therapy* [cupric sulfate]
cuproxoline INN, BAN
curare [see: tubocurarine chloride]
curdlan sulfate (CRDS) *investigational antiviral for AIDS*
Curel Moisturizing cream, lotion OTC *moisturizer; emollient*
curium *element* (Cm)
curral [see: diallybarbituric acid]
Curretab tablets ℞ *progestin; secondary amenorrhea; functional uterine bleeding* [medroxyprogesterone acetate]
Cūtar Bath Oil Emulsion OTC *antipsoriatic; antiseborrheic; antipruritic; emollient* [coal tar; lanolin]
Cūtemol cream OTC *moisturizer; emollient* [allantoin]
Cuticura Acne cream OTC *topical keratolytic for acne* [benzoyl peroxide]
Cuticura Medicated Soap bar OTC *therapeutic skin cleanser*
Cuticura ointment OTC *topical acne treatment* [sulfur; phenol; oxyquinoline]

Cutivate cream, ointment ℞ *topical corticosteroidal anti-inflammatory* [fluticasone propionate]
CV Nutrients soft capsules OTC *dietary supplement* [vitamin E; vitamin C; coenzyme Q_{10}; omega-3 fish oils; multiple minerals; garlic]
CVA (cyclophosphamide, vincristine, Adriamycin) *chemotherapy protocol*
CVA-BMP; CVA + BMP (cyclophosphamide, vincristine, Adriamycin, BCNU, methotrexate, procarbazine) *chemotherapy protocol*
C-VAD; CVAD (cyclophosphamide, vincristine, Adriamycin, dexamethasone) *chemotherapy protocol*
CVB (CCNU, vinblastine, bleomycin) *chemotherapy protocol*
CVBD (CCNU, bleomycin, vinblastine, dexamethasone) *chemotherapy protocol*
CVD (cisplatin, vinblastine, dacarbazine) *chemotherapy protocol*
CVM (cyclophosphamide, vincristine, methotrexate) *chemotherapy protocol*
CVP (cyclophosphamide, vincristine, prednisone) *chemotherapy protocol*
CVPP (CCNU, vinblastine, prednisone, procarbazine) *chemotherapy protocol*
CVPP (cyclophosphamide, Velban, procarbazine, prednisone) *chemotherapy protocol*
CVPP-CCNU (cyclophosphamide, vinblastine, procarbazine, prednisone, CCNU) *chemotherapy protocol*
cyacetacide INN [also: cyacetazide]
cyacetazide BAN [also: cyacetacide]
CyADIC (cyclophosphamide, Adriamycin, DIC) *chemotherapy protocol*
cyamemazine INN
cyamepromazine [see: cyamemazine]

Cyanide Antidote Package ℞ *emergency treatment of cyanide poisoning* [sodium nitrite; sodium thiosulfate; amyl nitrite inhalant]
cyanoacetohydrazide [see: cyacetazide]
cyanocobalamin USP, INN, BAN *vitamin B_{12}; hematopoietic*
cyanocobalamin (^{57}Co) INN *pernicious anemia test; radioactive agent* [also: cyanocobalamin Co 57]
cyanocobalamin (^{58}Co) INN
cyanocobalamin (^{60}Co) INN *pernicious anemia test; radioactive agent* [also: cyanocobalamin Co 60]
cyanocobalamin Co 57 USAN, USP *pernicious anemia test; radioactive agent* [also: cyanocobalamin (^{57}Co)]
cyanocobalamin Co 60 USAN, USP *pernicious anemia test; radioactive agent* [also: cyanocobalamin (^{60}Co)]
Cyanoject injection ℞ *antianemic; vitamin supplement* [cyanocobalamin]
cyclacillin USAN, USP *antibacterial* [also: ciclacillin]
cyclamate calcium NF
cyclamic acid USAN, BAN *non-nutritive sweetener (banned in USA)*
cyclamide [see: glycyclamide]
Cyclan capsules ℞ *peripheral vasodilator* [cyclandelate]
cyclandelate INN, BAN *peripheral vasodilator*
cyclarbamate INN, BAN
cyclazocine USAN, INN *analgesic*
cyclazodone INN
cyclexanone INN
cyclic propylene carbonate [see: propylene carbonate]
cyclindole USAN *antidepressant* [also: ciclindole]
cycliramine INN *antihistamine* [also: cycliramine maleate]
cycliramine maleate USAN *antihistamine* [also: cycliramine]
cyclizine USP, INN, BAN *antihistamine; antiemetic; anticholinergic; motion sickness relief*

cyclizine HCl USP, BAN *antiemetic*
cyclizine lactate USP, BAN *antinauseant*
cyclobarbital NF, INN [also: cyclobarbitone]
cyclobarbital calcium NF
cyclobarbitone BAN [also: cyclobarbital]
cyclobendazole USAN *anthelmintic* [also: ciclobendazole]
cyclobenzaprine INN *muscle relaxant* [also: cyclobenzaprine HCl]
cyclobenzaprine HCl USAN, USP *skeletal muscle relaxant* [also: cyclobenzaprine]
cyclobutoic acid INN
cyclobutyrol INN
cyclocarbothiamine [see: cycotiamine]
Cyclocort ointment, cream, lotion ℞ *topical corticosteroid* [amcinonide]
cyclocoumarol BAN
cyclocumarol [see: cyclocoumarol]
α-cyclodextrin [see: alfadex]
cyclofenil INN, BAN
cyclofilcon A USAN *hydrophilic contact lens material*
cycloguanil embonate INN, BAN *antimalarial* [also: cycloguanil pamoate]
cycloguanil pamoate USAN *antimalarial* [also: cycloguanil embonate]
Cyclogyl eye drops ℞ *cycloplegic; mydriatic* [cyclopentolate HCl]
cyclohexanehexol [see: inositol]
cyclohexanesulfamate dihydrate [see: sodium cyclamate]
cyclohexanesulfamic acid *(banned in USA)* [see: cyclamic acid]
cycloheximide USAN *antipsoriatic* [also: cicloheximide]
p-cyclohexylhydratropic acid [see: hexaprofen]
N-cyclohexyllinoleamide [see: clinolamide]
4-cyclohexyloxybenzoate [see: cyclomethycaine]
1-cyclohexylpropyl carbamate [see: procymate]
N-cyclohexylsulfamic acid *(banned in USA)* [see: cyclamic acid]
cyclomenol INN
cyclomethicone NF *wetting agent*
cyclomethycaine INN, BAN *local anesthetic* [also: cyclomethycaine sulfate]
cyclomethycaine sulfate USP *local anesthetic* [also: cyclomethycaine]
Cyclomydril Ophthalmic eye drops ℞ *mydriatic* [cyclopentolate HCl; phenylephrine HCl]
cyclonium iodide [see: oxapium iodide]
cyclopentamine INN, BAN [also: cyclopentamine HCl]
cyclopentamine HCl USP [also: cyclopentamine]
cyclopentaphene [see: cyclarbamate]
cyclopenthiazide USAN, INN, BAN *antihypertensive*
cyclopentolate INN, BAN *ophthalmic anticholinergic* [also: cyclopentolate HCl]
cyclopentolate HCl USP *ophthalmic anticholinergic; mydriatic; cycloplegic* [also: cyclopentolate]
cyclophenazine HCl USAN *antipsychotic* [also: ciclofenazine]
cyclophosphamide USP, INN, BAN *antineoplastic; immunosuppressive*
cyclopolydimethylsiloxane [see: cyclomethicone]
cyclopregnol INN
cycloprolol BAN *antiadrenergic (β-receptor)* [also: ciclprolol HCl; cicloprolol]
cyclopropane USP, INN *inhalation general anesthetic*
Cyclo-Prostin *(orphan: primary pulmonary hypertension; heparin replacement for hemodialysis)* [epoprostenol]
cyclopyrronium bromide INN
cycloserine USP, INN, BAN *bacteriostatic; tuberculosis retreatment*

L-cycloserine (orphan: Gaucher's disease)
Cyclospasmol capsules ℞ peripheral vasodilator [cyclandelate]
cyclosporin BAN immunosuppressive [also: cyclosporine; ciclosporin]
cyclosporin A [now: cyclosporine]
cyclosporine USAN, USP immunosuppressive; (orphan: keratoconjunctivitis sicca; corneal melting syndrome) [also: ciclosporin; cyclosporin]
cyclothiazide USAN, USP, INN, BAN diuretic; antihypertensive
cyclovalone INN
cycobemin [see: cyanocobalamin]
cycotiamine INN
cycrimine INN, BAN [also: cycrimine HCl]
cycrimine HCl USP [also: cycrimine]
Cycrin tablets ℞ progestin for secondary amenorrhea or functional uterine bleeding [medroxyprogesterone acetate]
cyfluthrin BAN
cyhalothrin BAN
cyheptamide USAN, INN anticonvulsant
cyheptropine INN
CyHOP (cyclophosphamide, Halotestin, Oncovin, prednisone) chemotherapy protocol
Cyklokapron IV injection, tablets ℞ systemic hemostatic; (orphan: angioneurotic edema; coagulopathy) [tranexamic acid]
Cylert tablets, chewable tablets ℞ for attention deficit disorders; CNS stimulant [pemoline]
Cylex; Cylex Sugar-Free throat lozenges OTC oral antiseptic; oral anesthetic [benzocaine; cetylpyridinium chloride]
cymemoxine [see: cimemoxin]
cynarine INN
Cyomin injection ℞ antianemic; vitamin supplement [cyanocobalamin]
cypenamine INN, BAN antidepressant [also: cypenamine HCl]

cypenamine HCl USAN antidepressant [also: cypenamine]
cypothrin USAN veterinary insecticide
cyprazepam USAN, INN sedative
cyprenorphine INN, BAN
cyprenorphine HCl [see: cyprenorphine]
cyprodemanol [see: cyprodenate]
cyprodenate INN
cyproheptadine INN, BAN antihistamine; antipruritic [also: cyproheptadine HCl]
cyproheptadine HCl USP antihistamine; antipruritic [also: cyproheptadine]
cyprolidol INN antidepressant [also: cyprolidol HCl]
cyprolidol HCl USAN antidepressant [also: cyprolidol]
cyproquinate USAN coccidiostat for poultry [also: ciproquinate]
cyproterone INN, BAN antiandrogen [also: cyproterone acetate]
cyproterone acetate USAN antiandrogen; (orphan: severe hirsutism) [also: cyproterone]
cyproximide USAN antipsychotic; antidepressant [also: ciproximide]
cyren A [see: diethylstilbestrol]
cyren B [see: diethylstilbestrol dipropionate]
cyromazine INN, BAN
cystamin [see: methenamine]
cysteamine USAN, BAN antiurolithic; (orphan: nephropathic cystinosis) [also: mercaptamine]
cysteamine HCl USAN antiurolithic; (orphan: nephropathic cystinosis)
cysteine (L-cysteine) INN nonessential amino acid; symbols: Cys, C [also: cysteine HCl]
cysteine HCl (L-cysteine HCl) USP nonessential amino acid [also: cysteine]
L-cysteine HCl monohydrate [see: cysteine HCl]
Cystex tablets ℞ urinary anti-infective; analgesic; acidifier [methenamine;

salicylamide; sodium salicylate; benzoic acid]
cystic fibrosis gene therapy (orphan: cystic fibrosis)
cystic fibrosis transmembrane conductance regulator (orphan: cystic fibrosis)
Cysticide (orphan: neurocysticercosis) [praziquantel]
cystine (L-cystine) USAN amino acid
Cysto-Conray; Cysto-Conray II intracavitary instillation ℞ radiopaque agent [iothalamate meglumine]
cystogen [see: methenamine]
Cystografin; Cystografin Dilute intracavitary instillation ℞ cholecystographic radiopaque agent [diatrizoate meglumine]
Cystospaz tablets ℞ GI anticholinergic; antispasmodic [hyoscyamine sulfate]
Cystospaz-M timed-release capsules ℞ GI anticholinergic; antispasmodic [hyoscyamine sulfate]
CYTABOM (cytarabine, bleomycin, Oncovin, mechlorethamine) chemotherapy protocol
Cytadren tablets ℞ adrenal steroid inhibitor [aminoglutethimide]
cytarabine USAN, USP, INN, BAN antineoplastic; antiviral
cytarabine HCl USAN antiviral
CytoGam powder for IV injection ℞ adjunct to kidney transplants from CMV seropositive donor to CMV seronegative recipient [cytomegalovirus immune globulin, human]
cytomegalovirus immune globulin, human (orphan: primary cytomegalovirus of organ and bone marrow transplants)
cytomegalovirus immune globulin intravenous (CMV-IGIV) [see: globulin, immune]
Cytomel tablets ℞ thyroid hormone therapy [liothyronine sodium]
Cytosar-U powder for subcu, intrathecal or IV injection ℞ antineoplastic for multiple leukemias [cytarabine]
cytosine arabinoside (ara-C) [see: cytarabine]
cytosine arabinoside HCl [now: cytarabine HCl]
Cytotec tablets ℞ prevention of NSAID-induced gastric ulcers [misoprostol]
Cytovene powder for IV infusion ℞ antiviral for cytomegalovirus (orphan: CMV retinitis in AIDS) [ganciclovir sodium]
Cytoxan Lyophilized powder for IV injection ℞ antineoplastic [cyclophosphamide]
Cytoxan tablets, powder for IV injection ℞ antineoplastic [cyclophosphamide]
CY-VA-DACT (Cytoxin, vincristine, Adriamycin, dactinomycin) chemotherapy protocol
CYVADIC; CY-VA-DIC; Cy-VADIC (cyclophosphamide, vincristine, Adriamycin, DIC) chemotherapy protocol
CYVMAD (cyclophosphamide, vincristine, methotrexate, Adriamycin, DTIC) chemotherapy protocol

D

D (vitamin D) [q.v.]
D₂ (vitamin D₂) [see: ergocalciferol]
D-2.5-W; D-5-W; D-10-W; D-20-W; D-25-W; D-30-W; D-40-W; D-50-W; D-60-W; D-70-W ℞ *intravenous nutritional therapy* [dextrose in water]
D₃ (vitamin D₃) [see: cholecalciferol]
D-7.7-W; D-38-W (discontinued 1990) ℞ *intravenous nutritional therapy* [dextrose in water]
D-38.5-W (discontinued 1992) ℞ *intravenous nutritional therapy* [dextrose in water]
DA (daunorubicin, ara-C) *chemotherapy protocol*
D.A. #34 enteric-coated tablets OTC *digestive aid* [pancreatin concentrate; pepsin; ox bile]
D.A. chewable tablets ℞ *antihistamine; decongestant; anticholinergic* [chlorpheniramine maleate; phenylephrine HCl; methscopolamine nitrate]
DAA (dihydroxyaluminum aminoacetate) [q.v.]
dacarbazine USAN, USP, INN, BAN *antineoplastic*
dacemazine INN
dacisteine INN
Dacriose ophthalmic solution OTC *extraocular irrigating solution* [balanced saline solution]
dactinomycin USAN, USP *antineoplastic* [also: actinomycin; actinomycin D]
dacuronium bromide INN, BAN
DADDS (diacetyl diaminodiphenylsulfone) [see: acedapsone]
dagapamil INN
Daily Cleaner solution OTC *contact lens surfactant cleaning solution*
Daily Vitamins liquid OTC *vitamin supplement* [multiple vitamins]
Daily-Key cellulose-coated caplets OTC *vitamin/mineral supplement* [multiple vitamins & minerals; betaine HCl]
Daily-Vite with Iron & Minerals tablets OTC *vitamin/mineral/iron supplement* [multiple vitamins & minerals; iron; folic acid; biotin]
Dairy Ease chewable tablets OTC *digestive aid for lactose intolerance* [lactase enzyme]
Daisy 2 home test kit OTC *in vitro diagnostic aid for urine pregnancy test*
Dakin solution [see: sodium hypochlorite]
Dakrina eye drops OTC *ocular moisturizer/lubricant*
Dalacin T ℞ *investigational topical antiacne agent*
Dalalone D.P. intra-articular, soft tissue, or IM injection ℞ *glucocorticoids* [dexamethasone acetate]
Dalalone intra-articular, intralesional, soft tissue, or IM injection ℞ *glucocorticoids* [dexamethasone sodium phosphate]
Dalalone L.A. intralesional, intra-articular, soft tissue, or IM injection ℞ *glucocorticoids* [dexamethasone acetate]
dalanated insulin [see: insulin, dalanated]
dalbraminol INN
Dalcaine injection ℞ *injectable local anesthetic* [lidocaine HCl]
daledalin INN *antidepressant* [also: daledalin tosylate]
daledalin tosylate USAN *antidepressant* [also: daledalin]
Dalgan IV, subcu or IM injection ℞ *narcotic agonist-antagonist analgesic* [dezocine]
Dallergy sustained-release capsules, tablets, syrup ℞ *decongestant; antihistamine; anticholinergic* [phenylephrine HCl; chlorpheniramine maleate; methscopolamine nitrate]

Dallergy-D sustained-release capsules OTC *decongestant; antihistamine* [pseudoephedrine HCl; chlorpheniramine maleate]

Dallergy-D syrup OTC *decongestant; antihistamine* [phenylephrine HCl; chlorpheniramine maleate]

Dallergy-Jr. sustained-release capsules ℞ *pediatric decongestant and antihistamine* [pseudoephedrine HCl; brompheniramine maleate]

Dalmane capsules ℞ *sedative; hypnotic* [flurazepam HCl]

d-Alpha Gems soft capsules OTC *vitamin supplement* [vitamin E]

daltroban USAN, INN *immunosuppressive*

Damason-P tablets ℞ *narcotic analgesic* [hydrocodone bitartrate; aspirin]

dambose [see: inositol]

dametralast INN

damotepine INN

D-Amp capsules ℞ *penicillin-type antibiotic* [ampicillin trihydrate]

danaproid *investigational therapy for stroke and deep venous thrombosis*

danazol USAN, USP, INN, BAN *anterior pituitary suppressant*

Danazol-NP ℞ *investigational agent for endometriosis, menorrhagia and fibrocystic breast disease* [danazol nanoparticles]

Danex shampoo OTC *antiseborrheic; antibacterial; antifungal* [pyrithione zinc]

daniquidone BAN

danitamon [see: menadione]

danitracen INN

Danocrine capsules ℞ *endometriosis; fibrocystic breast disease; hereditary angioedema* [danazol]

danofloxacin INN *veterinary antibacterial* [also: danofloxacin mesylate]

danofloxacin mesylate USAN *veterinary antibacterial* [also: danofloxacin]

danosteine INN

danthron USP, BAN (*withdrawn from market by FDA*) [also: dantron]

Dantrium capsules, powder for IV injection ℞ *muscle relaxant; (orphan: neuroleptic malignant syndrome)* [dantrolene sodium]

dantrolene USAN, INN, BAN *skeletal muscle relaxant*

dantrolene sodium USAN, BAN *skeletal muscle relaxant (orphan: neuroleptic malignant syndrome)*

dantron INN (*withdrawn from market by FDA*) [also: danthron]

Dapa tablets, capsules OTC *analgesic; antipyretic* [acetaminophen]

Dapacin Cold capsules OTC *decongestant; antihistamine; analgesic* [phenylpropanolamine HCl; chlorpheniramine maleate; acetaminophen]

Dapex-37.5 capsules (discontinued 1992) ℞ *anorexiant* [phentermine HCl]

dapiprazole INN *α-adrenergic blocker; antiglaucoma agent; neuroleptic* [also: dapiprazole HCl]

dapiprazole HCl USAN *α-adrenergic blocker; miotic; neuroleptic* [also: dapiprazole]

dapsone USAN, USP, BAN *bactericidal; leprostatic; herpetiform dermatitis suppressant; (orphan: Pneumocystis carinii)*

daptazole [see: amiphenazole]

daptomycin USAN, INN, BAN *antibacterial*

Daranide tablets ℞ *carbonic anhydrase inhibitors (diuretics)* [dichlorphenamide]

Daraprim tablets ℞ *antimalarial; toxoplasmosis treatment adjunct* [pyrimethamine]

Darbid tablets ℞ *anticholinergic; peptic ulcer treatment adjunct* [isopropamide iodide]

darenzepine INN

Daricon tablets ℞ *adjunctive therapy for peptic ulcer* [oxyphencyclimine HCl]

darodipine USAN, INN *antihypertensive; bronchodilator; vasodilator*

Darvocet-N 50; Darvocet-N 100 tablets ℞ *narcotic analgesic* [propoxyphene napsylate; acetaminophen]

Darvon Compound Pulvules (discontinued 1990) ℞ *narcotic analgesic* [propoxyphene HCl; aspirin; caffeine]

Darvon Compound-65 Pulvules (capsules) ℞ *narcotic analgesic* [propoxyphene HCl; aspirin; caffeine]

Darvon Pulvules (capsules) ℞ *narcotic analgesic* [propoxyphene HCl]

Darvon with A.S.A. Pulvules (discontinued 1990) ℞ *narcotic analgesic* [propoxyphene HCl; aspirin]

Darvon-N tablets, suspension ℞ *narcotic analgesic* [propoxyphene napsylate]

Darvon-N with A.S.A. tablets (discontinued 1990) ℞ *narcotic analgesic* [propoxyphene napsylate; aspirin]

Dasin capsules OTC *analgesic; antipyretic; anti-inflammatory; bronchodilator; emetic* [aspirin; caffeine; atropine sulfate; ipecac]

DAT (daunorubicin, ara-C, thioguanine) *chemotherapy protocol*

Datelliptium ℞ *investigational antineoplastic for breast cancer* [ellipticine]

datelliptium chloride INN

Datril tablets (discontinued 1993) OTC *analgesic; antipyretic* [acetaminophen]

daturine hydrobromide [see: hyoscyamine hydrobromide]

DATVP (daunorubicin, ara-C, thioguanine, vincristine, prednisone) *chemotherapy protocol*

daunomycin [see: daunorubicin HCl; daunorubicin]

daunorubicin (DNR) INN, BAN *antineoplastic* [also: daunorubicin HCl]

daunorubicin HCl USAN, USP *antineoplastic* [also: daunorubicin]

DaunoXome ℞ *investigational antineoplastic for AIDS-related Kaposi sarcoma, colorectal and endometrial cancer* [daunorubicin]

DAVA (desacetyl vinblastine amide) [see: vindesine]

DAVH (dibromodulcitol, Adriamycin, vincristine, Halotestin) *chemotherapy protocol*

davitamon [see: menadione]

Dayalets Filmtabs (film-coated tablets) OTC *vitamin supplement* [multiple vitamins; folic acid]

Dayalets + Iron Filmtabs (film-coated tablets) OTC *vitamin/iron supplement* [multiple vitamins; ferrous sulfate]

DayCare caplets, liquid (name changed to DayQuil in 1992)

Daypro film-coated tablets ℞ *nonsteroidal anti-inflammatory drug (NSAID)* [oxaprozin]

DayQuil LiquiCaps (soft gel capsules), liquid OTC *decongestant; antitussive; expectorant; analgesic* [pseudoephedrine HCl; dextromethorphan hydrobromide; guaifenesin; acetaminophen]

Dayto Himbin tablets ℞ *no approved uses; sympatholytic; mydriatic; aphrodisiac* [yohimbine HCl]

Dayto Sulf vaginal cream ℞ *bacteriostatic* [sulfathiazole; sulfacetamide; sulfabenzamide; urea]

Dayto-Anase tablets OTC *anti-inflammatory* [bromelains]

Day-Vite tablets (discontinued 1993) OTC *vitamin supplement* [multiple vitamins]

dazadrol INN *antidepressant* [also: dazadrol maleate]

dazadrol maleate USAN *antidepressant* [also: dazadrol]

Dazamide tablets ℞ *anticonvulsant; diuretic* [acetazolamide]

dazepinil INN *antidepressant* [also: dazepinil HCl]

dazepinil HCl USAN *antidepressant* [also: dazepinil]

dazidamine INN

dazmegrel USAN, INN, BAN *thromboxane synthetase inhibitor*
dazolicine INN
dazopride INN *peristaltic stimulant* [also: dazopride fumarate]
dazopride fumarate USAN *peristaltic stimulant* [also: dazopride]
dazoquinast INN
dazoxiben INN, BAN *antithrombotic* [also: dazoxiben HCl]
dazoxiben HCl USAN *antithrombotic* [also: dazoxiben]
DBED (dibenzylethylenediamine dipenicillin G) [see: penicillin G benzathine]
DBM (dibromomannitol) [see: mitobronitol]
D&C Brown No. 1 (drugs & cosmetics) [see: resorcin brown]
DC softgels OTC *stool softener* [docusate calcium]
DCA (desoxycorticosterone acetate) [q.v.]
DCF (2'-deoxycoformycin) [see: pentostatin]
DCMP (daunorubicin, cytarabine, mercaptopurine, prednisone) *chemotherapy protocol*
D-Congest M liquid OTC *antitussive; decongestant; expectorant; analgesic; antipyretic* [dextromethorphan hydrobromide; pseudoephedrine HCl; guaifenesin; acetaminophen]
DCV (DTIC, CCNU, vincristine) *chemotherapy protocol*
DDAVP (deamino-D-arginine-vasopressin) [see: desmopressin acetate]
DDAVP injection, nasal spray, rhinal tube ℞ *antidiuretic hormone; (orphan: hemophilia A; von Willebrand's disease)* [desmopressin acetate]
DDC; ddC (dideoxycytidine) [see: zalcitabine]
o,p'-DDD [now: mitotane]
DDI; ddI (dideoxyinosine) [see: didanosine]
DDP; cis-DDP (diamminedichloroplatinum) [see: cisplatin]

DDS (diaminodiphenylsulfone) [now: dapsone]
DDT (dichlorodiphenyltrichloroethane) [see: chlorophenothane]
DDVP (dichlorovinyl dimethyl phosphate) [see: dichlorvos]
DEA (diethanolamine) [q.v.]
deacetyllanatoside C [see: deslanoside]
deadly nightshade leaf [see: belladonna extract]
deanol BAN [also: deanol aceglumate]
deanol aceglumate INN [also: deanol]
deanol acetamidobenzoate
deba [see: barbital]
deboxamet INN
Debrisan beads, paste ℞ *debrider and cleanser for wet wounds* [dextranomer]
debrisoquin sulfate USAN *antihypertensive* [also: debrisoquine]
debrisoquine INN, BAN *antihypertensive* [also: debrisoquin sulfate]
Debrox ear drops OTC *agent to emulsify and disperse ear wax* [carbamide peroxide]
Decabid extended-release tablets (approved by the FDA in 1989, but never released by the manufacturer) ℞ *antiarrhythmic* [indecainide HCl]
Decaderm gel (discontinued 1993) ℞ *topical corticosteroid* [dexamethasone]
Decadron Phosphate cream ℞ *topical corticosteroid* [dexamethasone sodium phosphate]
Decadron Phosphate intra-articular, intralesional, soft tissue or IM injection ℞ *glucocorticoids* [dexamethasone sodium phosphate]
Decadron Phosphate Ocumeter (eye drops), ophthalmic ointment ℞ *ophthalmic corticosteroidal anti-inflammatory* [dexamethasone sodium phosphate]
Decadron Phosphate Respihaler (oral inhalation aerosol) ℞ *cortico-*

steroid for bronchial asthma [dexamethasone sodium phosphate]

Decadron Phosphate Turbinaire (nasal inhalation) ℞ *intranasal steroidal anti-inflammatory* [dexamethasone sodium phosphate]

Decadron tablets, elixir ℞ *glucocorticoids* [dexamethasone]

Decadron with Xylocaine soft tissue injection ℞ *glucocorticoids* [dexamethasone sodium phosphate; lidocaine HCl]

Decadron-LA intralesional, intra-articular, soft tissue, or IM injection ℞ *glucocorticoids* [dexamethasone acetate]

Deca-Durabolin IM injection ℞ *anabolic steroid for anemia of renal insufficiency* [nandrolone decanoate]

Decagen tablets OTC *vitamin/mineral/iron supplement* [multiple vitamins & minerals; iron; folic acid; biotin]

Decaject intra-articular, intralesional, soft tissue, or IM injection ℞ *glucocorticoids* [dexamethasone sodium phosphate]

Decaject-L.A. intralesional, intra-articular, soft tissue, or IM injection ℞ *glucocorticoids* [dexamethasone acetate]

DECAL (dexamethasone, etoposide, cisplatin, ara-C, L-asparaginase) *chemotherapy protocol*

decamethonium bromide USP, INN [also: decamethonium iodide]

decamethonium iodide BAN [also: decamethonium bromide]

Decapeptyl injection *(orphan: ovarian carcinoma of epithelial origin)* [triptorelin pamoate]

decapinol [see: delmopinol]

Decaspray aerosol ℞ *topical corticosteroid* [dexamethasone]

decavitamin USP

Decholin tablets OTC *laxative; hydrocholeretic* [dehydrocholic acid]

decicain [see: tetracaine HCl]

decimemide INN

decitabine USAN, INN, BAN *antineoplastic*

decitropine INN

declaben [now: lodelaben]

declenperone USAN, INN *veterinary sedative*

Declomycin capsules, film-coated tablets ℞ *broad-spectrum antibiotic* [demeclocycline HCl]

decloxizine INN

Decofed syrup OTC *nasal decongestant* [pseudoephedrine HCl]

Decohistine DH liquid ℞ *decongestant; antihistamine; antitussive* [pseudoephedrine HCl; chlorpheniramine maleate; codeine phosphate; alcohol]

Decohistine elixir OTC *decongestant; antihistamine* [phenylephrine HCl; chlorpheniramine maleate]

Decolone-50; Decolone-100 injection (discontinued 1990) ℞ [nandrolone decanoate in sesame oil]

De-Comberol IM injection (discontinued 1991) ℞ *menopausal vasomotor symptoms; postpartum breast engorgement* [estradiol cypionate; testosterone cypionate]

decominol INN

Deconal syrup OTC *decongestant; antihistamine* [phenylpropanolamine HCl; phenylephrine HCl; phenyltoloxamine citrate; chlorpheniramine maleate]

Deconamine SR sustained-release capsules ℞ *decongestant; antihistamine* [pseudoephedrine HCl; chlorpheniramine maleate]

Deconamine tablets, syrup ℞ *decongestant; antihistamine* [pseudoephedrine HCl; chlorpheniramine maleate]

Decongestabs sustained-release tablets ℞ *decongestant; antihistamine* [phenylpropanolamine HCl; phenylephrine HCl; chlorpheniramine maleate; phenyltoloxamine citrate]

Decongestant sustained-release tablets ℞ *decongestant; antihistamine* [phenylpropanolamine HCl; phenylephrine HCl; chlorpheniramine maleate; phenyltoloxamine citrate]

Deconsal capsules (discontinued 1989) OTC *decongestant; expectorant* [pseudoephedrine HCl; guaifenesin]

Deconsal II sustained-release tablets ℞ *decongestant; expectorant* [pseudoephedrine HCl; guaifenesin]

Deconsal Sprinkle sustained-release capsules ℞ *decongestant; expectorant* [phenylephrine HCl; guaifenesin]

decoquinate USAN, INN, BAN *coccidiostat for poultry*

Decotan caplets ℞ *decongestant; antihistamine* [phenylephrine tannate; chlorpheniramine tannate; pyrilamine tannate]

dectaflur USAN, INN *dental caries prophylactic*

Decubitex ointment, powder ℞ *decubitus ulcer treatment* [Biebrich scarlet red sulfonated; zinc oxide]

Decylenes ointment OTC *topical antifungal* [undecylenic acid; zinc undecylenate]

deditonium bromide INN

Deep-Down Rub OTC *counterirritant* [methyl salicylate; menthol; camphor]

DEET (diethyltoluamide) [q.v.]

DeFed-60 tablets OTC *nasal decongestant* [pseudoephedrine HCl]

deferoxamine USAN, INN *iron-chelating agent* [also: desferrioxamine]

deferoxamine HCl USAN

deferoxamine mesylate USAN, USP *antidote to iron poisoning; iron-chelating agent* [also: desferrioxamine mesylate]

defibrotide INN, BAN (*orphan: thrombotic thrombocytopenic purpura*)

deflazacort USAN, INN, BAN *anti-inflammatory*

defosfamide INN

defungit sodium salt [see: bensuldazic acid]

Degest 2 eye drops OTC *topical ocular vasoconstrictor* [naphazoline HCl]

Dehist subcu or IM injection ℞ *antihistamine; anaphylaxis* [brompheniramine maleate]

Dehist sustained-release capsules OTC *decongestant; antihistamine* [phenylpropanolamine HCl; chlorpheniramine maleate]

dehydrated alcohol [see: alcohol, dehydrated]

dehydrex (*orphan: recurrent corneal erosion*)

Dehydrex drops ℞ (*orphan: recurrent corneal erosion*)

dehydroacetic acid NF *preservative*

dehydroandrosterone [see: prasterone]

dehydrocholate sodium USP [also: sodium dehydrocholate]

7-dehydrocholesterol, activated [now: cholecalciferol]

dehydrocholic acid USP, INN, BAN *choleretic; laxative*

dehydrocholin [see: dehydrocholic acid]

dehydroemetine INN, BAN *investigational anti-infective for amebiasis and amebic dysentery*

dehydroepiandrosterone (DHEA) *investigational antiviral/immunomodulator for AIDS*

Del Aqua-5; Del Aqua-10 gel OTC *topical keratolytic for acne* [benzoyl peroxide]

Delacort lotion (discontinued 1993) OTC *topical corticosteroid* [hydrocortisone]

Deladiol-40 IM injection ℞ *estrogen replacement therapy; antineoplastic for prostatic cancer* [estradiol valerate in oil]

Deladumone IM injection ℞ *estrogen/androgen for menopausal vasomotor symptoms* [estradiol valerate; testosterone enanthate]

Deladumone OB injection (discontinued 1989) ℞ *menopausal vasomotor symptoms; postpartum breast engorgement* [estradiol valerate; testosterone enanthate]
delanterone INN
Delaprem ℞ *investigational tocolytic agent* [hexoprenaline sulfate]
delapril INN *antihypertensive; angiotensin-converting enzyme inhibitor* [also: delapril HCl]
delapril HCl USAN *antihypertensive; angiotensin-converting enzyme inhibitor* [also: delapril]
Delatest IM injection ℞ *androgen replacement for delayed puberty or breast cancer* [testosterone enanthate]
Delatestryl IM injection ℞ *androgen replacement for delayed puberty or breast cancer* [testosterone enanthate]
Delaxin tablets (discontinued 1989) ℞ *skeletal muscle relaxant* [methocarbamol]
delayed-release aspirin [see: aspirin]
Delcap (trademarked form) *unit dispensing cap*
Delcort cream OTC *topical corticosteroid* [hydrocortisone]
delergotrile INN
Delestrogen IM injection ℞ *estrogen replacement therapy; antineoplastic for prostatic cancer* [estradiol valerate in oil]
delfantrine INN
delfaprazine INN
Delfen Contraceptive vaginal foam OTC *spermicidal contraceptive* [nonoxynol 9]
delmadinone INN, BAN *progestin; antiandrogen; antiestrogen* [also: delmadinone acetate]
delmadinone acetate USAN *progestin; antiandrogen; antiestrogen* [also: delmadinone]
delmetacin INN
delmopinol INN
delnav [see: dioxathion]

delorazepam INN
deloxolone INN
***m*-delphene** [see: diethyltoluamide]
delprostenate INN, BAN
Delsym sustained-action liquid OTC *antitussive* [dextromethorphan polistirex]
Delta-Cortef tablets ℞ *glucocorticoids* [prednisolone]
deltacortone [see: prednisone]
Delta-D tablets OTC *vitamin supplement* [cholecalciferol]
deltafilcon A USAN *hydrophilic contact lens material*
deltafilcon B USAN *hydrophilic contact lens material*
delta-1-hydrocortisone [see: prednisolone]
Deltalin Gelseals (filled elastic capsules) ℞ *vitamin deficiency therapy* [ergocalciferol]
Deltasone tablets ℞ *glucocorticoids* [prednisone]
delta-9-tetrahydrocannabinol (THC) [see: dronabinol]
delta-9-THC (tetrahydrocannabinol) [see: dronabinol]
Deltavac vaginal cream ℞ *bacteriostatic; antiseptic; vulnerary* [sulfanilamide; aminacrine HCl; allantoin]
deltra-stab [see: prednisolone]
Del-Vi-A capsules ℞ *vitamin deficiency therapy* [vitamin A]
Demazin Repetabs (repeat-action tablets), syrup OTC *decongestant; antihistamine* [phenylpropanolamine HCl; chlorpheniramine maleate]
dembrexine INN, BAN
dembroxol [see: dembrexine]
demecarium bromide USP, INN, BAN *antiglaucoma agent; reversible cholinesterase inhibitor miotic*
demeclocycline USP, BAN *antibacterial*
demeclocycline HCl USP, BAN *gram-negative and gram-positive bacteriostatic; antirickettsial*
demecolcine INN, BAN

demecycline USAN, INN *antibacterial*
demegestone INN
demekastigmine bromide [see: demecarium bromide]
demelverine INN
Demerol APAP tablets (discontinued 1992) ℞ *narcotic analgesic* [meperidine HCl; acetaminophen]
Demerol HCl tablets, syrup, IV or IM injection ℞ *narcotic analgesic* [meperidine HCl]
demetacin [see: delmetacin]
11-demethoxyreserpine [see: deserpidine]
demethylchlortetracycline (DMCT) [now: demeclocycline]
demethylchlortetracycline HCl [see: demeclocycline HCl]
***N*-demethylcodeine** [see: norcodeine]
demexiptiline INN
Demi-Regroton tablets ℞ *antihypertensive* [chlorthalidone; reserpine]
democonazole INN
Demolin liniment OTC *topical analgesic* [methyl salicylate; camphor; racemic menthol; mustard oil]
demoxepam USAN, INN *minor tranquilizer*
demoxytocin INN
Demser capsules ℞ *antihypertensive for pheochromocytoma* [metyrosine]
Demulen 1/50; Demulen 1/35 tablets ℞ *oral contraceptive* [ethynodiol diacetate; ethinyl estradiol]
denatonium benzoate USAN, NF, INN, BAN *alcohol denaturant; flavoring agent*
denaverine INN
denbufylline INN, BAN
denipride INN
denofungin USAN *antifungal; antibacterial*
denopamine INN
Denorex shampoo OTC *antiseborrheic; antipsoriatic; antipruritic; antibacterial* [coal tar; menthol; alcohol]

Denov extended-release capsules ℞ *antihistamine; decongestant* [chlorpheniramine maleate; pseudoephedrine HCl]
denpidazone INN
Denquel toothpaste OTC *tooth desensitizer* [potassium nitrate]
dental-type silica [see: silica, dental-type]
Dentamin-C tablets (discontinued 1989) OTC *vitamin/mineral supplement* [vitamins C & D; calcium; magnesium; zinc]
Dentlock powder OTC *denture adhesive*
denyl sodium [see: phenytoin sodium]
denzimol INN
2'-deoxycoformycin (DCF) [see: pentostatin]
deoxycorticosterone acetate [see: desoxycorticosterone acetate]
deoxycorticosterone pivalate [see: desoxycorticosterone pivalate]
deoxycortolone pivalate BAN *salt-regulating adrenocortical steroid* [also: desoxycorticosterone pivalate]
deoxycortone BAN *salt-regulating adrenocortical steroid* [also: desoxycorticosterone acetate; desoxycortone]
deoxyephedrine HCl [see: methamphetamine HCl]
12-deoxyerythromycin [see: berythromycin]
deoxynojirimycin (DNJ) *investigational antiviral for AIDS*
deoxyribonuclease, recombinant human (rhDNase) (orphan: *liquefying expectorant for cystic fibrosis*)
deoxyribonucleic acid (DNA)
Depacin Cold Capsules OTC *decongestant; antihistamine; analgesic* [phenylpropanolamine HCl; chlorpheniramine maleate; acetaminophen]
Depakene capsules ℞ *anticonvulsant* [valproic acid]

Depakene syrup ℞ *anticonvulsant* [valproate sodium]
Depakote delayed-release tablets, sprinkle capsules ℞ *anticonvulsant* [divalproex sodium]
depAndro; depAndro 200 IM injection ℞ *androgen replacement for delayed puberty or breast cancer* [testosterone cypionate]
depAndrogyn IM injection ℞ *estrogen/androgen for menopausal vasomotor symptoms* [estradiol cypionate; testosterone cypionate]
Depen tablets ℞ *treatment of rheumatoid arthritis, Wilson's disease and cystinuria* [penicillamine]
depepsen [see: sodium amylosulfate]
depGynogen IM injection ℞ *hormone for estrogen replacement therapy* [estradiol cypionate in oil]
depMedalone 40; depMedalone 80 intralesional, soft tissue, and IM injection ℞ *glucocorticoids* [methylprednisolone acetate]
Depo-Estradiol Cypionate IM injection ℞ *hormone for estrogen replacement therapy* [estradiol cypionate in oil]
Depogen IM injection ℞ *hormone for estrogen replacement therapy* [estradiol cypionate in oil]
Depoject intralesional, soft tissue, and IM injection ℞ *glucocorticoids* [methylprednisolone acetate]
Depo-Medrol intralesional, soft tissue, and IM injection ℞ *glucocorticoids* [methylprednisolone acetate]
Deponit transdermal patch ℞ *antianginal* [nitroglycerin]
Depopred-40; Depopred-80 intralesional, soft tissue, and IM injection ℞ *glucocorticoids* [methylprednisolone acetate]
Depo-Provera IM injection ℞ *hormonal adjunct for metastatic endometrial and renal carcinoma; long-term injectable contraceptive* [medroxyprogesterone acetate]
Depotest 100; Depotest 200 IM injection ℞ *androgen replacement for delayed puberty or breast cancer* [testosterone cypionate]
Depo-Testadiol IM injection ℞ *estrogen/androgen for menopausal vasomotor symptoms* [estradiol cypionate; testosterone cypionate]
Depotestogen IM injection ℞ *estrogen/androgen for menopausal vasomotor symptoms* [estradiol cypionate; testosterone cypionate]
DEPO-Testosterone IM injection ℞ *androgen replacement for delayed puberty or breast cancer* [testosterone cypionate]
depramine INN [also: balipramine]
Depranol ℞ *(orphan: sickle cell disease)* [OM 401 (drug code–generic name not yet approved)]
deprenyl (L-deprenyl) [see: selegiline HCl]
deprodone INN, BAN
Deproic capsules (discontinued 1989) ℞ [valproic acid]
Deproist Expectorant with Codeine liquid ℞ *decongestant; antitussive; expectorant* [pseudoephedrine HCl; codeine phosphate; guaifenesin; alcohol]
Deprol tablets ℞ *psychotherapeutic agent* [meprobamate; benactyzine HCl]
deprostil USAN, INN *gastric antisecretory*
deptropine INN, BAN
deptropine citrate [see: deptropine]
dequalinium chloride INN, BAN
Dequasine tablets OTC *dietary supplement* [multiple minerals & amino acids; vitamin C]
Derifil tablets OTC *fecal and urinary odor control* [chlorophyllin]
Derma Comb cream ℞ *topical corticosteroid; antifungal* [triamcinolone acetonide; nystatin]
Derma Medicone (name changed to Medicone Derma in 1991)

Derma Scrub cream OTC *hand scrub*
Derma Soap concentrate (discontinued 1989) OTC *antiseptic* [dowicil 200]
Derma Stat aerosol foam OTC *hand scrub*
Derma Viva lotion OTC *moisturizer; emollient*
Dermabase OTC *cream base*
Dermabet cream ℞ *topical corticosteroid* [betamethasone valerate]
Dermacoat solution OTC *topical local anesthetic; antiseptic; counterirritant* [benzocaine; parachlorometaxylenol; menthol]
Dermacort cream, lotion ℞ *topical corticosteroid* [hydrocortisone]
Dermal-Rub balm OTC *counterirritant* [methyl salicylate; camphor; racemic manthol; cajuput oil]
Dermamycin cream OTC *topical antihistamine* [diphenhydramine HCl]
Dermamycin ointment (discontinued 1991) OTC *astringent; antiseptic; anesthetic; antihistamine* [zinc oxide; benzocaine; chloroxylenol; pyrilamine maleate]
Derma-Pax lotion OTC *topical anthistamine; antiseptic; antipruritic* [pyrilamine maleate; chlorpheniramine maleate; alcohol]
Dermaphill ointment (discontinued 1991) OTC *antifungal; counterirritant; antipruritic* [aluminum acetate basic; phenol; menthol; camphor]
Dermarest gel OTC *topical antihistamine; antifungal* [diphenhydramine HCl; resorcinol; aloe; benzalkonium chloride]
Dermarest Plus gel, spray OTC *topical antihistamine; counterirritant* [diphenhydramine HCl; menthol; aloe; benzalkonium chloride]
Dermarex cream (discontinued 1991) ℞ *topical corticosteroid; antifungal; antibacterial; anesthetic* [hydrocortisone; clioquinol; pramoxine]

Dermasept Antifungal liquid spray OTC *antifungal; antiseptic; anesthetic; astringent* [tolnaftate; tannic acid; zinc chloride; benzocaine; methylbenzethonium HCl; undecylenic acid]
Derma-Smoothe/FS oil ℞ *topical corticosteroid; emollient* [fluocinolone acetonide]
Derma-Soft Creme (discontinued 1990) OTC *topical keratolytic* [salicylic acid]
Dermassage lotion (discontinued 1992) OTC *moisturizer; emollient*
dermatol [see: bismuth subgallate]
Dermatol 10 lotion *moisturizer* [urea]
Dermatophytin "O" shallow subcu or intradermal injection ℞ *diagnosis and treatment of oidiomycin (Candida)-induced infections* [Candida albicans extract]
Dermatophytin shallow subcu or intradermal injection ℞ *diagnosis and treatment of Trichophyton-induced skin infections* [Trichophyton rubrum and T. tonsurans extracts]
DermeD cream (discontinued 1992) OTC *moisturizer; emollient* [vitamins A & D]
DermiCort cream, lotion OTC *topical corticosteroid* [hydrocortisone]
Dermidon cream OTC *topical antihistamine; antibacterial; antipruritic; anesthetic* [pyrilamine maleate; phenyltoloxamine citrate; diperodon HCl; benzalkonium chloride; menthol; camphor]
Dermolate Anal-Itch ointment (discontinued 1991) OTC *topical corticosteroidal anti-inflammatory* [hydrocortisone]
Dermolate Anti-Itch aerosol (discontinued 1989) OTC *topical corticosteroidal anti-inflammatory* [hydrocortisone]
Dermolate Anti-Itch cream OTC *topical corticosteroid* [hydrocortisone]

Dermolate Scalp-Itch lotion (discontinued 1989) OTC *topical corticosteroidal anti-inflammatory* [hydrocortisone]

Dermolin liniment OTC *counterirritant; topical antiseptic* [methyl salicylate; camphor; racemic menthol; mustard oil; alcohol]

Dermoplast aerosol spray, lotion OTC *topical local anesthetic* [benzocaine; menthol]

Dermovan OTC *cream base*

Dermprotective Factor (DPF) (trademarked ingredient) *aromatic syrup* [eriodictyon]

Dermtex HC with Aloe cream OTC *topical corticosteroid* [hydrocortisone]

Dermuspray aerosol spray ℞ *topical enzyme for wound debridement* [trypsin; balsam Peru]

derpanicate INN

DES (diethylstilbestrol) [q.v.]

desacetyl vinblastine amide (DAVA) [see: vindesine]

desacetyl-lanatoside C [see: deslanoside]

desaglybuzole [see: glybuzole]

desamino-oxytocin [see: demoxytocin]

desaspidin INN

desciclovir USAN, INN *antiviral*

descinolone INN *glucocorticoid* [also: descinolone acetonide]

descinolone acetonide USAN *glucocorticoid* [also: descinolone]

Desenex foam, soap OTC *topical antifungal* [undecylenic acid]

Desenex liquid (discontinued 1991) OTC *topical antifungal* [undecylenic acid]

Desenex powder, aerosol powder, ointment, cream OTC *topical antifungal* [undecylenic acid; zinc undecylenate]

Desenex spray liquid OTC *topical antifungal* [tolnaftate]

deserpidine INN, BAN *antihypertensive; rauwolfia derivative*

Desferal Mesylate powder for injection ℞ *adjunct treatment for iron intoxication or overload* [deferoxamine mesylate]

desferrioxamine BAN *iron-chelating agent* [also: deferoxamine]

desferrioxamine mesylate BAN *antidote to iron poisoning; iron-chelating agent* [also: deferoxamine mesylate]

desflurane USAN, INN *inhalation general anesthetic*

desglugastrin INN

desipramine INN, BAN *antidepressant* [also: desipramine HCl]

desipramine HCl USAN, USP *tricyclic antidepressant* [also: desipramine]

Desitin ointment OTC *moisturizer; emollient; astringent; antiseptic* [zinc oxide]

deslanoside USP, INN, BAN *cardiotonic; cardiac glycoside*

deslorelin USAN, INN *LHRH agonist; (orphan: precocious puberty)*

desmethylmoramide INN

desmophosphamide [see: defosfamide]

desmopressin INN, BAN *posterior pituitary antidiuretic hormone* [also: desmopressin acetate]

desmopressin acetate USAN *posterior pituitary antidiuretic hormone; (orphan: hemophilia A; von Willebrand's disease)* [also: desmopressin]

desocriptine INN

Desogen tablets ℞ *oral contraceptive* [ethinyl estradiol; desogestrel]

desogestrel USAN, INN, BAN *progestin*

desolone [see: deprodone]

desomorphine INN, BAN

desonide USAN, INN, BAN *topical corticosteroidal anti-inflammatory*

DesOwen ointment, cream, lotion ℞ *topical corticosteroidal anti-inflammatory* [desonide]

desoximetasone USAN, USP, INN *topical corticosteroidal anti-inflammatory* [also: desoxymethasone]

desoxycorticosterone acetate (DCA; DOCA) USP *salt-regulating adrenocortical steroid* [also: desoxycortone; deoxycortone]

desoxycorticosterone pivalate USP *salt-regulating adrenocortical steroid* [also: deoxycortolone pivalate]

desoxycorticosterone trimethylacetate USP

desoxycortone INN *salt-regulating adrenocortical steroid* [also: desoxycorticosterone acetate; deoxycortone]

***l*-desoxyephedrine** *nasal decongestant*

desoxyephedrine HCl [see: methamphetamine HCl]

desoxymethasone BAN *topical corticosteroidal anti-inflammatory* [also: desoximetasone]

Desoxyn Gradumets (sustained-release tablets), tablets ℞ *CNS stimulant* [methamphetamine HCl]

Despec controlled-release capsules ℞ *decongestant; expectorant* [guaifenesin; phenylpropanolamine HCl]

Despec liquid ℞ *decongestant; expectorant* [guaifenesin; phenylpropanolamine HCl; phenylephrine HCl; alcohol]

Desquam-E 2.5; Desquam-E 5; Desquam-E 10 gel ℞ *topical keratolytic for acne* [benzoyl peroxide]

Desquam-X 2.5; Desquam-X 5; Desquam-X 10 gel ℞ *topical keratolytic for acne* [benzoyl peroxide]

Desquam-X 5; Desquam-X 10 wash ℞ *topical keratolytic for acne* [benzoyl peroxide]

de-Stat solution OTC *contact lens cleaning and soaking solution*

de-Stat 3 solution OTC *contact lens cleaning, disinfecting and storage solution*

destradiol [see: estradiol]

Desyrel film-coated tablets, Dividose (multiple-scored tablets) ℞ *antidepressant* [trazodone HCl]

DET (diethyltryptamine)

detajmium bitartrate INN

Detane gel OTC *topical local anesthetic* [benzocaine]

detanosal INN

deterenol INN *ophthalmic adrenergic* [also: deterenol HCl]

deterenol HCl USAN *ophthalmic adrenergic* [also: deterenol]

detigon HCl [see: chlophedianol HCl]

detirelix INN *luteinizing hormone-releasing hormone (LHRH) antagonist* [also: detirelix acetate]

detirelix acetate USAN *luteinizing hormone-releasing hormone (LHRH) antagonist* [also: detirelix]

detomidine INN, BAN *veterinary analgesic; sedative* [also: detomidine HCl]

detomidine HCl USAN *veterinary analgesic; sedative* [also: detomidine]

detorubicin INN

detralfate INN

detrothyronine INN

Detussin Expectorant liquid ℞ *decongestant; antitussive; expectorant* [hydrocodone bitartrate; pseudoephedrine HCl; guaifenesin; alcohol]

Detussin liquid ℞ *antitussive; decongestant* [hydrocodone bitartrate; pseudoephedrine HCl; alcohol]

deuterium oxide USAN *radioactive agent*

devapamil INN

devazepide USAN *cholecystokinin antagonist*

Devrom chewable tablets OTC *antidiarrheal; antacid* [bismuth subgallate]

Dexacen LA-8 injection ℞ *corticosteroid* [dexamethasone acetate]

Dexacen-4 injection ℞ *corticosteroid* [dexamethasone sodium phosphate]

Dexacidin eye drop suspension, ophthalmic ointment ℞ *topical ophthalmic corticosteroidal anti-inflammatory; antibiotic* [dexamethasone; neomycin sulfate; polymyxin B sulfate]

Dex-A-Diet plus Vitamin C timed-release capsules (discontinued 1992)

OTC *diet aid* [phenylpropanolamine HCl; vitamin C]
Dex-A-Diet timed-release capsules, timed-release caplets (discontinued 1992) OTC *diet aid* [phenylpropanolamine HCl]
Dexafed Cough syrup OTC *decongestant; antitussive; expectorant* [phenylephrine HCl; dextromethorphan hydrobromide; guaifenesin]
Dexameth tablets ℞ *glucocorticoids* [dexamethasone]
dexamethasone USP, INN, BAN *topical/ophthalmic corticosteroid*
dexamethasone acefurate USAN, INN *topical steroid*
dexamethasone acetate USAN, USP, BAN *adrenocortical steroid; glucocorticoid*
dexamethasone dipropionate USAN *steroidal anti-inflammatory*
dexamethasone sodium phosphate USP, BAN *topical/intranasal/ophthalmic corticosteroid*
dexamfetamine INN *CNS stimulant* [also: dextroamphetamine; dexamphetamine]
dexamisole USAN, INN *antidepressant*
dexamphetamine BAN *CNS stimulant* [also: dextroamphetamine; dexamfetamine]
Dexamycin ophthalmic ointment ℞ *topical corticosteroid; antibiotic* [dexamethasone; neomycin sulfate; polymyxin B sulfate]
Dexaphen S.A. sustained-release tablets ℞/OTC *decongestant; antihistamine* [pseudoephedrine sulfate; dexbrompheniramine maleate]
Dexasone intra-articular, intralesional, soft tissue, or IM injection ℞ *glucocorticoids* [dexamethasone sodium phosphate]
Dexasone L.A. intralesional, intra-articular, soft tissue, or IM injection ℞ *glucocorticoids* [dexamethasone acetate]

Dexasporin eye drop suspension, ophthalmic ointment ℞ *topical ophthalmic corticosteroidal anti-inflammatory; antibiotic* [dexamethasone; neomycin sulfate; polymyxin B sulfate]
Dexatrim extended-release tablets OTC *diet aid* [phenylpropanolamine HCl]
Dexatrim plus Vitamin C timed-release capsules OTC *diet aid* [phenylpropanolamine HCl; vitamin C]
Dexatrim Pre-Meal timed-release capsules OTC *diet aid* [phenylpropanolamine HCl]
Dexatuss sugar-free syrup OTC *antitussive; expectorant* [dextromethorphan hydrobromide; guaifenesin]
dexbrompheniramine INN, BAN *antihistamine* [also: dexbrompheniramine maleate]
dexbrompheniramine maleate USP *antihistamine* [also: dexbrompheniramine]
Dexchlor extended-release tablets ℞ *antihistamine* [dexchlorpheniramine maleate]
dexchlorpheniramine INN *antihistamine* [also: dexchlorpheniramine maleate]
dexchlorpheniramine maleate USP *antihistamine* [also: dexchlorpheniramine]
dexclamol INN *sedative* [also: dexclamol HCl]
dexclamol HCl USAN *sedative* [also: dexclamol]
Dexedrine elixir (discontinued 1990) ℞ *amphetamine; CNS stimulant* [dextroamphetamine sulfate]
Dexedrine Spansules (sustained-release capsules), tablets ℞ *amphetamine; CNS stimulant* [dextroamphetamine sulfate]
dexetimide USAN, INN, BAN *anticholinergic*
dexetozoline INN

dexfenfluramine INN, BAN *systemic appetite suppressant* [also: dexfenfluramine HCl]
dexfenfluramine HCl USAN *systemic appetite suppressant* [also: dexfenfluramine]
dexibuprofen INN *analgesic; cyclooxygenase inhibitor; anti-inflammatory* [also: dexibuprofen lysine]
dexibuprofen lysine USAN *analgesic; cyclooxygenase inhibitor; anti-inflammatory* [also: dexibuprofen]
deximafen USAN, INN *antidepressant*
dexindoprofen INN
Dexitac timed-release capsules OTC *CNS stimulant; analeptic* [caffeine]
dexivacaine USAN, INN *anesthetic*
dexlofexidine INN
dexmedetomidine USAN, INN, BAN *tranquilizer*
dexnorgestrel acetime [now: norgestimate]
Dexon injection (discontinued 1990) ℞ *glucocorticoids* [dexamethasone sodium phosphate]
Dexon LA injection (discontinued 1990) ℞ *glucocorticoids* [dexamethasone acetate]
Dexone intra-articular, intralesional, soft tissue, or IM injection ℞ *glucocorticoids* [dexamethasone sodium phosphate]
Dexone LA intralesional, intra-articular, soft tissue, or IM injection ℞ *glucocorticoids* [dexamethasone acetate]
Dexone tablets ℞ *glucocorticoids* [dexamethasone]
dexormaplatin USAN, INN *antineoplastic*
DexŌtic eye drops (discontinued 1992) ℞ *ophthalmic topical corticosteroidal anti-inflammatory* [dexamethasone sodium phosphate]
dexoxadrol INN *CNS stimulant; analgesic* [also: dexoxadrol HCl]
dexoxadrol HCl USAN *CNS stimulant; analgesic* [also: dexoxadrol]

dexpanthenol USAN, USP, INN, BAN *cholinergic; antipruritic; postoperative prophylaxis for paralytic ileus*
dexpropranolol HCl USAN *antiarrhythmic; antiadrenergic (β-receptor)* [also: dexpropranolol]
dexproxibutene INN
dexrazoxane USAN, INN, BAN *cardioprotectant; (orphan: doxorubicin-induced cardiomyopathy)*
dexsecoverine INN
dextilidine INN
dextran INN, BAN *blood flow adjuvant; plasma volume extender* [also: dextran 40]
dextran, high molecular weight [see: dextran 70]
dextran, low molecular weight [see: dextran 40]
dextran 1 *dextran adjunct*
dextran 40 USAN *blood flow adjuvant; plasma volume extender* [also: dextran]
dextran 70 USAN *plasma volume extender; viscosity-increasing agent*
dextran 75 USAN *plasma volume extender*
dextran & deferoxamine *(orphan: acute iron poisoning)*
dextran sulfate *investigational antiviral for AIDS; (orphan: cystic fibrosis)*
dextran sulfate, sodium salt, aluminum complex [see: detralfate]
dextran sulfate sodium *(orphan: AIDS)*
dextranomer INN, BAN *wound debrider/cleanser*
dextrates USAN, NF *tablet binder and diluent*
dextriferron NF, INN, BAN
dextrin NF, BAN *suspending agent; tablet binder and diluent*
dextroamphetamine USAN *CNS stimulant* [also: dexamfetamine; dexamphetamine]
dextroamphetamine phosphate USP

dextroamphetamine saccharate CNS stimulant
dextroamphetamine sulfate USP CNS stimulant
dextrobrompheniramine maleate [see: dexbrompheniramine maleate]
dextrochlorpheniramine maleate [see: dexchlorpheniramine maleate]
dextrofemine INN
dextromethorphan USP, INN, BAN antitussive
dextromethorphan hydrobromide USP, BAN antitussive
dextromethorphan polistirex USAN antitussive
dextromoramide INN, BAN
dextromoramide tartrate [see: dextromoramide]
dextro-pantothenyl alcohol [see: dexpanthenol]
dextropropoxiphene chloride [see: propoxyphene HCl]
dextropropoxyphene INN, BAN narcotic analgesic [also: propoxyphene HCl]
dextropropoxyphene HCl BAN [also: propoxyphene HCl]
dextrorphan INN, BAN
dextrose USP fluid and nutrient replenisher; parenteral antihypoglycemic
dextrose excipient NF tablet excipient
5% Dextrose and Electrolyte #48; 5% Dextrose and Electrolyte #75; 10% Dextrose and Electrolyte #48 IV infusion ℞ intravenous nutritional/electrolyte therapy [combined electrolyte solution; dextrose]
38% Dextrose with Electrolyte Pattern T; 50% Dextrose with Electrolytes #2; 50% Dextrose with Electrolytes 60 mEq/L Acetate IV infusion (discontinued 1990) ℞ intravenous nutritional/electrolyte therapy [combined electrolyte solution; dextrose]
50% Dextrose with Electrolyte Pattern A (B; N) IV infusion ℞ intravenous nutritional/electrolyte therapy [combined electrolyte solution; dextrose]
Dextrostix reagent strips OTC in vitro diagnostic aid for blood glucose
dextrothyronine [see: detrothyronine]
dextrothyroxine BAN antihyperlipoproteinemic [also: dextrothyroxine sodium]
dextrothyroxine sodium USAN, USP, INN antihyperlipoproteinemic [also: dextrothyroxine]
Dey-Dose (delivery system) nebulizer
Dey-Lube ophthalmic ointment (discontinued 1992) ℞ ocular moisturizer/lubricant
Dey-Lute (delivery system) nebulizer
Dey-Pak Sodium Chloride 0.45% & 0.9% solution OTC for respiratory therapy and tracheal lavage [sodium chloride]
Dey-Pak Sodium Chloride 3% & 10% solution ℞ for inducing sputum production for specimen collection [sodium chloride]
Dey-Vial Sodium Chloride 0.9% solution OTC for respiratory therapy and trachial lavage [sodium chloride]
dezaguanine USAN, INN antineoplastic
dezaguanine mesylate USAN antineoplastic
dezinamide investigational antiepileptic
dezocine USAN, INN narcotic analgesic
Dezone injection (discontinued 1989) ℞ glucocorticoids [dexamethasone sodium phosphate]
d-Film gel OTC contact lens cleaning gel
DFMO (difluoromethylornithine) [see: eflornithine]
DFMO (difluoromethylornithine) HCl [see: eflornithine HCl]
DFMO-MGBG chemotherapy protocol [see: DFMO; MGBG]
DFP (diisopropyl flurophosphate) [see: isoflurophate]

DFV (DDP, fluorouracil, VePesid) *chemotherapy protocol*
DHA (docosahexaenoic acid) [see: doconexent; icosapent; omega-3 marine triglycerides]
DHAP (dexamethasone, high-dose ara-C, Platinol) *chemotherapy protocol*
DHC Plus ℞ *investigational analgesic*
DHE (dihydroergotamine) [see: dihydroergotamine mesylate]
D.H.E. 45 IV or IM injection ℞ *migraine prophylaxis or treatment* [dihydroergotamine mesylate]
DHEA (dehydroepiandrosterone) [q.v.]
DHPG (dihydroxy propoxymethyl guanine) [see: ganciclovir]
DHS Tar liquid shampoo, gel shampoo OTC *antiseborrheic; antipsoriatic; antipruritic; antibacterial* [coal tar]
DHS Zinc shampoo OTC *antiseborrheic; antibacterial; antifungal* [pyrithione zinc]
DHT (dihydrotachysterol) [q.v.]
DHT (dihydrotestosterone) [see: stanolone; androstanolone]
DHT tablets, Intensol (concentrated oral solution) ℞ *antihypocalcemic for tetany* [dihydrotachysterol]
Diaβeta (or DiaBeta) tablets ℞ *antidiabetic* [glyburide]
Diabinese tablets ℞ *antidiabetic* [chlorpropamide]
diacerein INN
diacetamate INN, BAN
diacetolol INN, BAN *antiadrenergic (β-receptor)* [also: diacetolol HCl]
diacetolol HCl USAN *antiadrenergic (β-receptor)* [also: diacetolol]
diacetoxyphenylisatin [see: oxyphenisatin acetate]
diacetoxyphenyloxindol [see: oxyphenisatin acetate]
diacetrizoate sodium [see: diatrizoate sodium]
diacetyl diaminodiphenylsulfone (DADDS) [see: acedapsone]

diacetylated monoglycerides NF *plasticizer*
diacetylcholine chloride [see: succinylcholine chloride]
diacetyl-dihydroxydiphenylisatin [see: oxyphenisatin acetate]
diacetyldioxphenylisatin [see: oxyphenisatin acetate]
diacetylmorphine HCl USP *(heroin; banned in USA)* [also: diamorphine]
diacetylmorphine salts *(heroin; banned in USA)*
diacetylsalicylic acid [see: dipyrocetyl]
diacetyltannic acid [see: acetyltannic acid]
diacetylthiamine [see: acetiamine]
Diachlor tablets ℞ *diuretic* [chlorothiazide]
diagniol [see: sodium acetrizoate]
Dia-Kit ℞ *allergic hypersensitivity testing* [allergenic mold extracts]
diallybarbituric acid [see: allobarbital]
diallylbarbituric acid [now: allobarbital]
diallylnortoxiferene dichloride [see: alcuronium chloride]
diallymal [see: allobarbital]
Dialose capsules OTC *stool softener* [docusate potassium]
Dialose Plus capsules OTC *laxative; stool softener* [docusate potassium; casanthranol]
Dialose Plus tablets OTC *laxative; stool softener* [docusate sodium; yellow phenolphthalein]
Dialose tablets OTC *stool softener* [docusate sodium]
Dialume capsules ℞ *antacid* [aluminum hydroxide]
Dialyte Pattern LM solution ℞ *peritoneal dialysis solution* [dextrose; multiple electrolytes]
dia-mer-sulfonamides (sulfadiazine & sulfamerazine) [q.v.]

diamethine [see: dimethyltubocurarinium chloride; dimethyltubocurarine]
diamfenetide INN [also: diamphenethide]
Diamine T.D. timed-release tablets ℞ *anthistamine* [brompheniramine maleate]
diaminedipenicillin G [see: penicillin G benzathine]
diaminodiphenylsulfone (DDS) [now: dapsone]
3,4-diaminopyridine *(orphan: Lambert-Eaton myasthenic syndrome)*
***cis*-diamminedichloroplatinum (DDP)** [see: cisplatin]
diammonium phosphate [see: ammonium phosphate]
diamocaine INN, BAN *local anesthetic* [also: diamocaine cyclamate]
diamocaine cyclamate USAN *local anesthetic* [also: diamocaine]
diamorphine BAN *(heroin; banned in USA)* [also: diacetylmorphine HCl]
Diamox IV injection ℞ *anticonvulsant; diuretic* [acetazolamide sodium]
Diamox tablets, Sequels (sustained-release capsules) ℞ *anticonvulsant; diuretic* [acetazolamide]
diamphenethide BAN [also: diamfenetide]
diampromide INN, BAN
diampron [see: amicarbalide]
diamthazole BAN [also: dimazole]
diamthazole dihydrochloride [see: diamthazole]
Dianeal; Dianeal 137 solution ℞ *peritoneal dialysis solution* [dextrose; multiple electrolytes]
dianeal PD-2 peritoneal dialysis solution with 1.1% amino acids *(orphan: malnourishment of continuous ambulatory peritoneal dialysis)*
Diapa-Kare powder (discontinued 1990) OTC [benzethonium chloride; cornstarch; sodium bicarbonate]

diapamide USAN *diuretic; antihypertensive* [also: tiamizide]
Diaparene Baby cream OTC *topical diaper rash treatment*
Diaparene Cornstarch Baby powder OTC *topical diaper rash treatment* [corn starch; aloe]
Diaparene Cradol liquid OTC *antimicrobial hair dressing* [methylbenzethonium chloride]
Diaparene Diaper Rash ointment OTC *topical diaper rash treatment* [zinc oxide]
Diaparene Medicated powder, cream (discontinued 1993) OTC *topical diaper rash treatment* [methylbenzethonium chloride]
Diaparene Peri-Anal Medicated ointment (discontinued 1993) OTC *topical diaper rash treatment* [methylbenzethonium chloride; zinc oxide]
Diaper Guard ointment OTC *topical diaper rash treatment* [dimethicone; benzalkonium chloride, vitamins A, D & E; zinc oxide]
Diaper Rash ointment OTC *topical diaper rash treatment* [zinc oxide]
diaphene [see: dibromsalan]
diaphenylsulfone [see: dapsone]
Diapid nasal spray ℞ *diabetes insipidus* [lypressin]
Diaqua tablets ℞ *diuretic; antihypertensive* [hydrochlorothiazide]
Diar-Aid tablets OTC *antidiarrheal; GI adsorbent* [activated attapulgite; pectin]
diarbarone INN
Diascan-S reagent strips OTC *in vitro diagnostic aid for blood glucose*
Diasorb tablets, liquid OTC *antidiarrheal; GI adsorbent* [activated attapulgite]
Diastat viscous solution for rectal administration ℞ *(orphan: acute repetitive seizures)* [diazepam]
Diastix reagent strips OTC *in vitro diagnostic aid for urine glucose*
diathymosulfone INN

diatrizoate meglumine USP *GI radiopaque medium* [also: meglumine diatrizoate]
diatrizoate methylglucamine [see: diatrizoate meglumine]
diatrizoate sodium USP *GI radiopaque medium* [also: sodium amidotrizoate; sodium diatrizoate]
diatrizoate sodium I 125 USAN *radioactive agent*
diatrizoate sodium I 131 USAN *radioactive agent*
Diatrizoate-60 injection (discontinued 1990) ℞ [diatrizoate meglumine; diatrizoate sodium]
diatrizoic acid USAN, USP, BAN *radiopaque medium*
Diatrol tablets OTC *antacid; antidiarrheal* [calcium carbonate; pectin]
diaveridine USAN, INN, BAN *antibacterial*
diazacholesterol dihydrochloride [see: azacosterol HCl]
diazepam USAN, USP, INN, BAN *anxiolytic; sedative; skeletal muscle relaxant; (orphan: acute repetitive seizures)*
diazinon BAN [also: dimpylate]
diaziquone USAN, INN *antineoplastic; (orphan: primary brain malignancies; grade III-IV astrocytomas)*
Di-Azo tablets (discontinued 1990) OTC *urinary analgesic* [phenazopyridine HCl]
diazoxide USAN, USP, INN, BAN *emergency antihypertensive; glucose-elevating agent*
dibasic calcium phosphate [see: calcium phosphate, dibasic]
dibasic potassium phosphate [see: potassium phosphate, dibasic]
dibasic sodium phosphate [see: sodium phosphate, dibasic]
dibasol [see: bendazol]
dibazol [see: bendazol]
dibekacin INN, BAN
dibemethine INN
dibencil [see: penicillin G benzathine]

dibencozide [see: cobamamide]
Dibent IM injection ℞ *gastrointestinal antispasmodic* [dicyclomine HCl]
dibenthiamine [see: bentiamine]
dibenzathione [see: sulbentine]
dibenzepin INN, BAN *antidepressant* [also: dibenzepin HCl]
dibenzepin HCl USAN *antidepressant* [also: dibenzepin]
dibenzothiazine [see: phenothiazine]
dibenzothiophene USAN *keratolytic*
dibenzoyl peroxide [see: benzoyl peroxide]
dibenzoylthiamin [see: bentiamine]
dibenzthion [see: sulbentine]
dibenzylethylenediamine dipenicillin G (DBED) [see: penicillin G benzathine]
Dibenzyline capsules ℞ *pheochromocytoma for hypertension and sweating* [phenoxybenzamine HCl]
***N,N*-dibenzylmethylamine** [see: dibemethine]
dibromodulcitol [see: mitolactol]
dibromohydroxyquinoline [see: broxyquinoline]
dibromomannitol (DBM) [see: mitobronitol]
dibromopropamidine BAN [also: dibrompropamidine]
dibrompropamidine INN [also: dibromopropamidine]
dibromsalan USAN, INN *disinfectant*
dibrospidium chloride INN
dibucaine USP *local anesthetic* [also: cinchocaine]
dibucaine HCl USP *local anesthetic* [also: cinchocaine HCl]
dibuprol INN
dibupyrone INN, BAN
dibusadol INN
dibutoline sulfate
DIC (dimethyl imidazole carboxamide) [see: dacarbazine]
Dical CapTabs (capsule-shaped tablets) OTC *dietary supplement* [dibasic calcium phosphate; vitamin D]

dicalcium phosphate [see: calcium phosphate, dibasic]
Dical-D tablets, chewable wafers OTC *dietary supplement* [dibasic calcium phosphate; vitamin D]
dicarbine INN
Dicarbosil chewable tablets OTC *antacid* [calcium carbonate]
dicarfen INN
dichlofenthion BAN
dichloralantipyrine [see: dichloralphenazone]
dichloralphenazone (chloral hydrate + phenazone) BAN *mild sedative*
dichloralpyrine [see: dichloralphenazone]
dichloramine-T NF
dichloranilino imidazolin [see: clonidine HCl]
dichloren [see: mechlorethamine HCl]
dichlorisone INN
dichlorisone acetate [see: dichlorisone]
dichlormethazanone [see: dichlormezanone]
dichlormezanone INN
dichloroacetate sodium (*orphan: congenital lactic acidosis; familial hypercholesterolemia*)
dichloroacetic acid *strong keratolytic/cauterant*
dichlorodifluoromethane NF *aerosol propellant*
dichlorodiphenyl trichloroethane (DDT) [see: chlorophenothane]
dichlorometaxylenol [see: dichloroxylenol]
dichloromethane [see: methylene chloride]
dichlorophen INN, BAN
dichlorophenarsine INN, BAN [also: dichlorophenarsine HCl]
dichlorophenarsine HCl USP [also: dichlorophenarsine]
dichlorotetrafluoroethane NF *aerosol propellant* [also: cryofluorane]

dichlorovinyl dimethyl phosphate (DDVP) [see: dichlorvos]
dichloroxylenol INN, BAN
dichlorphenamide USP, BAN *carbonic anhydrase inhibitor* [also: diclofenamide]
dichlorvos USAN, INN, BAN *anthelmintic*
dichysterol [see: dihydrotachysterol]
diciferron INN
dicirenone USAN, INN *hypotensive; aldosterone antagonist*
Dick test (scarlet fever streptococcus toxin)
diclazuril USAN, INN, BAN *coccidiostat for poultry*
diclofenac INN, BAN *antiarthritic; nonsteroidal anti-inflammatory drug (NSAID); analgesic* [also: diclofenac sodium]
diclofenac sodium USAN *antiarthritic; nonsteroidal anti-inflammatory drug (NSAID); analgesic* [also: diclofenac]
diclofenamide INN *carbonic anhydrase inhibitor* [also: dichlorphenamide]
diclofensine INN
diclofibrate [see: simfibrate]
diclofurime INN
diclometide INN
diclonixin INN
dicloralurea USAN, INN *veterinary food additive*
dicloxacillin USAN, INN, BAN *antibacterial*
dicloxacillin sodium USAN, USP, BAN *bactericidal antibiotic*
dicobalt edetate INN, BAN
dicolinium iodide INN
dicophane BAN [also: chlorophenothane; clofenotane]
dicoumarin [see: dicumarol]
dicoumarol INN [also: dicumarol]
dicresulene INN
dicumarol USAN, USP *anticoagulant* [also: dicoumarol]
dicyclomine BAN *anticholinergic* [also: dicyclomine HCl; dicycloverine]

dicyclomine HCl USP *GI antispasmodic; anticholinergic* [also: dicycloverine; dicyclomine]
dicycloverine INN *anticholinergic* [also: dicyclomine HCl; dicyclomine]
dicycloverine HCl [see: dicyclomine HCl]
dicysteine [see: cystine]
didanosine USAN, INN, BAN *antiviral for AIDS*
didehydrodideoxythymidine [see: stavudine]
Di-Delamine gel, spray OTC *topical antihistamine; bacteriostatic* [diphenhydramine HCl; tripelennamine HCl; benzalkonium chloride; menthol]
2′-3′-dideoxyadenosine *(orphan: AIDS)*
dideoxycytidine (DDC; ddC) [see: zalcitabine]
dideoxyinosine (DDI; ddI) [see: didanosine]
Didrex tablets ℞ *anorexiant* [benzphetamine HCl]
Didronel tablets, IV infusion ℞ *bone resorption suppressant; (orphan: hypercalcemia; metabolic bone disease)* [etidronate disodium]
didrovaltrate INN
didroxane [see: dichlorophen]
dieldrin INN, BAN
diemal [see: barbital]
dienestrol USP, INN *estrogen* [also: dienoestrol]
dienoestrol BAN *estrogen* [also: dienestrol]
dienogest INN
Diet Ayds candy OTC *decrease taste perception of sweetness* [benzocaine]
Diet-Aid Plus Vitamin C timed-release capsules (discontinued 1992) OTC *diet aid* [phenylpropanolamine HCl; vitamin C]
Diet-Aid timed-release capsules (discontinued 1992) OTC *diet aid* [phenylpropanolamine HCl]

dietamiphylline [see: etamiphyllin]
dietamiverine HCl [see: bietamiverine HCl]
diethadione INN, BAN
diethanolamine NF *alkalizing agent*
diethazine INN, BAN
diethazine HCl [see: diethazine]
diethyl phthalate NF *plasticizer*
diethylamine *p*-aminobenzenestibonate [see: stibosamine]
3-diethylaminobutyranilide [see: octacaine]
diethylbarbiturate monosodium [see: barbital sodium]
diethylbarbituric acid [see: barbital]
diethylcarbamazine INN, BAN *anthelmintic* [also: diethylcarbamazine citrate]
diethylcarbamazine citrate USP *anthelmintic* [also: diethylcarbamazine]
diethylcarbamazine dihydrogen citrate [see: diethylcarbamazine citrate]
diethyldithiocarbamate *investigational immunomodulator; (orphan: AIDS)*
diethyldixanthogen [see: dixanthogen]
diethylenediamine citrate [see: piperazine citrate]
diethylenetriamine pentaacetic acid (DTPA) [see: pentetic acid]
***N,N*-diethyllysergamide** [see: lysergide]
diethylmalonylurea [see: barbital]
diethylmalonylurea sodium [see: barbital sodium]
***N,N*-diethylnicotinamide** [see: nikethamide]
diethylpropion BAN *anorexiant* [also: diethylpropion HCl; amfepramone]
diethylpropion HCl USP *anorexiant; CNS stimulant* [also: amfepramone; diethylpropion]
diethylstilbestrol (DES) USP, INN *estrogen* [also: stilboestrol]
diethylstilbestrol diphosphate USP *antineoplastic; estrogen* [also: fosfestrol]
diethylstilbestrol dipropionate NF

***p*-diethylsulfamoylbenzoic acid** [see: etebenecid; ethebenecid]
diethylthiambutene INN, BAN
diethyltoluamide (DEET) USP, BAN *arthropod repellent*
diethyltryptamine (DET)
***N,N*-diethylvanillamide** [see: ethamivan]
dietifen INN
dietroxine [see: diethadione]
Dieutrim T.D. timed-release capsules OTC *diet aid; decrease perception of sweetness* [phenylpropanolamine HCl; benzocaine]
diexanthogen [see: dixanthogen]
difebarbamate INN
difemerine INN [also: difemerine HCl]
difemerine HCl [also: difemerine]
difemetorex INN
difenamizole INN
difencloxazine INN
difencloxazine HCl [see: difencloxazine]
difenidol INN *antiemetic; antivertigo* [also: diphenidol]
difenoximide INN *antiperistaltic* [also: difenoximide HCl]
difenoximide HCl USAN *antiperistaltic* [also: difenoximide]
difenoxin USAN, INN, BAN *antiperistaltic*
difenoxin HCl *antiperistaltic*
difetarsone INN, BAN
difeterol INN
diflorasone INN, BAN *topical corticosteroidal anti-inflammatory* [also: diflorasone diacetate]
diflorasone diacetate USAN, USP *topical corticosteroidal anti-inflammatory* [also: diflorasone]
difloxacin INN *anti-infective; DNA gyrase inhibitor* [also: difloxacin HCl]
difloxacin HCl USAN *anti-infective; DNA gyrase inhibitor* [also: difloxacin]
difluanazine INN *CNS stimulant* [also: difluanine HCl]

difluanazine HCl [see: difluanine HCl]
difluanine HCl USAN *CNS stimulant* [also: difluanazine]
Diflucan tablets, IV infusion ℞ *systemic antifungal* [fluconazole]
diflucortolone USAN, INN, BAN *glucocorticoid*
diflucortolone pivalate USAN *glucocorticoid*
diflumidone INN, BAN *anti-inflammatory* [also: diflumidone sodium]
diflumidone sodium USAN *anti-inflammatory* [also: diflumidone]
diflunisal USAN, USP, INN, BAN *anti-inflammatory; analgesic; antipyretic; antiarthritic; antirheumatic*
difluoromethylornithine (DFMO) [see: eflornithine]
difluoromethylornithine HCl [see: eflornithine HCl]
difluprednate USAN, INN *anti-inflammatory*
difolliculin [see: estradiol benzoate]
diftalone USAN, INN *anti-inflammatory*
digalloyl trioleate USAN
Di-Gel, Advanced Formula chewable tablets OTC *antacid; antiflatulent* [magnesium hydroxide; calcium carbonate; simethicone]
Di-Gel liquid OTC *antacid; antiflatulent* [aluminum hydroxide; magnesium hydroxide; simethicone]
Digestalin tablets (discontinued 1992) OTC *digestive enzymes; antiflatulent; antacid; antidiarrheal* [pancreatin; papain; pepsin; activated charcoal; bismuth subsalicylate; berberis; hydrastis]
Digestamic #2 tablets (discontinued 1991) OTC *digestive enzymes; antispasmodic* [amylase; protease; lipase; papain; hyoscyamine sulfate]
Digestant II tablets OTC *digestive enzymes* [pepsin; pancreatin; bile salts]
Digestex tablets (discontinued 1991) OTC *digestive enzymes; gastric acidi-*

fier [pancreatin; pepsin; ox bile extract; micozyme; betaine HCl]
Digestozyme tablets ℞ *digestive enzymes; laxative* [pancreatin; pepsin; dehydrocholic acid]
Digibind IV injection ℞ *(orphan: antidote to digitalis/digitoxin overdose)* [digoxin immune Fab]
Digidote ℞ *(orphan: antidote to digitalis/digitoxin overdose)* [digoxin immune Fab]
digitalis USP *cardiotonic*
digitalis glycosides mixture *(not manufactured since 1985)*
digitoxin USP, INN, BAN *cardiotonic; cardiac glycoside*
digitoxin, acetyl [see: acetyldigitoxin]
α-digitoxin monoacetate [see: acetyldigitoxin]
digitoxoside [see: digitoxin]
digoxin USP, INN, BAN *cardiotonic; cardiac glycoside*
digoxin antibody [see: digoxin immune Fab]
digoxin immune Fab *(orphan: digitalis/digitoxin intoxication)*
dihematoporphyrin ethers *(orphan: bladder carcinoma; esophageal carcinoma)*
dihexyverine INN *anticholinergic* [also: dihexyverine HCl]
dihexyverine HCl USAN *anticholinergic* [also: dihexyverine]
Dihistine DH liquid OTC *antitussive; decongestant; antihistamine* [codeine phosphate; pseudoephedrine HCl; chlorpheniramine maleate; alcohol]
Dihistine elixir OTC *decongestant; antihistamine* [phenylephrine HCl; chlorpheniramine maleate]
Dihistine Expectorant liquid ℞ *decongestant; antitussive; expectorant* [codeine phosphate; pseudoephedrine HCl; guaifenesin; alcohol]
dihydan soluble [see: phenytoin sodium]
dihydralazine INN, BAN

dihydralazine sulfate [see: dihydralazine]
Dihydrex injection (discontinued 1990) ℞ *antihistamine; motion sickness preventative; sleep aid; antiparkinsonian* [diphenhydramine HCl]
dihydrobenzthiazide [see: hydrobentizide]
dihydrocodeine INN, BAN *analgesic* [also: dihydrocodeine bitartrate]
dihydrocodeine bitartrate USP *analgesic* [also: dihydrocodeine]
dihydrocodeinone bitartrate [see: hydrocodone bitartrate]
dihydroergocornine [see: ergoloid mesylates]
dihydroergocristine [see: ergoloid mesylates]
dihydroergocryptine [see: ergoloid mesylates]
dihydroergotamine (DHE) INN, BAN *antiadrenergic; anticoagulant; rapid control of migraines* [also: dihydroergotamine mesylate]
dihydroergotamine mesylate USAN, USP *antiadrenergic; anticoagulant; rapid control of migraines* [also: dihydroergotamine]
dihydroergotamine methanesulfonate [see: dihydroergotamine mesylate]
dihydroergotoxine mesylate [now: ergoloid mesylates]
dihydroergotoxine methanesulfonate [now: ergoloid mesylates]
dihydroethaverine [see: drotaverine]
dihydrofollicular hormone [see: estradiol]
dihydrofolliculine [see: estradiol]
dihydrogenated ergot alkaloids [now: ergoloid mesylates]
dihydrohydroxycodeinone [see: oxycodone]
dihydrohydroxycodeinone HCl [see: oxycodone HCl]
dihydroisoperparine [see: drotaverine]

dihydromorphinone HCl [now: hydromorphone HCl]
dihydroneopine [see: dihydrocodeine bitartrate]
dihydrostreptomycin (DST) INN *antibacterial* [also: dihydrostreptomycin sulfate]
dihydrostreptomycin sulfate USP *antibacterial* [also: dihydrostreptomycin]
dihydrostreptomycin-streptomycin [see: streptoduocin]
dihydrotachysterol (DHT) USP, INN, BAN *calcium regulator; vitamin D_1*
dihydrotestosterone [see: stanolone; androstanolone]
dihydrotheelin [see: estradiol]
dihydroxy(stearato)aluminum [see: aluminum monostearate]
dihydroxy propoxymethyl guanine (DHPG) [see: gancyclovir]
dihydroxyacetone *skin darkener for vitiligo and hypopigmented areas*
dihydroxyaluminum aminoacetate (DAA) USP *antacid*
dihydroxyaluminum sodium carbonate USP *antacid*
dihydroxyanthranol [see: anthralin]
dihydroxyanthraquinone *(withdrawn from market)* [see: danthron]
1,25-dihydroxycholecalciferol [see: calcitriol]
24,25-dihydroxycholecalciferol *(orphan: uremic osteodystrophy)*
dihydroxyestrin [see: estradiol]
dihydroxyfluorane [see: fluorescein]
dihydroxyphenylalanine (DOPA) [see: levodopa]
dihydroxyphenylisatin [see: oxyphenisatin acetate; oxyphenisatine]
dihydroxyphenyloxindol [see: oxyphenisatin acetate; oxyphenisatine]
dihydroxyprogesterone acetophenide [see: algestone acetophenide]
dihydroxypropyl theophylline [see: dyphylline]
diiodobuphenine [see: bufeniode]

diiodohydroxyquin [now: iodoquinol]
diiodohydroxyquinoline INN, BAN *antiamebic* [also: iodoquinol]
diisopromine INN
diisopromine HCl [see: diisopromine]
diisopropanolamine NF *alkalizing agent*
diisopropyl flurophosphate (DFP) [see: isoflurophate]
diisopropyl flurophosphonate [see: isoflurophate]
diisopropyl phosphorofluoridate [see: isoflurophate]
2,6-diisopropylphenol [see: propofol]
Dilacor XR sustained-release capsules ℞ *antihypertensive* [diltiazem HCl]
Dilantin Infatabs (chewable tablets) ℞ *anticonvulsant* [phenytoin]
Dilantin IV or IM injection, Steri-Dose syringes, Steri-Vials, Kapseals (capsules) ℞ *anticonvulsant* [phenytoin sodium]
Dilantin with Phenobarbital Kapseals (capsules) ℞ *anticonvulsant; sedative* [phenytoin sodium; phenobarbital]
Dilantin-30 Pediatric; Dilantin-125 oral suspension ℞ *anticonvulsant* [phenytoin]
Dilatrate-SR sustained-release capsules ℞ *antianginal* [isosorbide dinitrate]
Dilaudid Cough Syrup ℞ *narcotic antitussive; narcotic analgesic; expectorant* [hydromorphone HCl; guaifenesin; alcohol]
Dilaudid subcu or IM injection, tablets, suppositories ℞ *narcotic analgesic* [hydromorphone HCl]
Dilaudid-HP subcu or IM injection ℞ *narcotic analgesic* [hydromorphone HCl]
dilazep INN
dilevalol INN, BAN *antihypertensive; antiadrenergic (β-receptor)* [also: dilevalol HCl]

dilevalol HCl USAN *antihypertensive; antiadrenergic (β-receptor)* [also: dilevalol]
dilithium carbonate [see: lithium carbonate]
dilmefone INN
Dilocaine injection ℞ *injectable local anesthetic* [lidocaine HCl]
Dilomine IM injection (discontinued 1990) ℞ *gastrointestinal antispasmodic* [dicyclomine HCl]
Dilone tablets (discontinued 1990) ℞ [phenyltoloxamine citrate; acetaminophen; caffeine]
Dilor 200; Dilor 400 tablets ℞ *bronchodilator* [dyphylline]
Dilor elixir, injection ℞ *bronchodilator* [dyphylline]
Dilor-G tablets, liquid ℞ *antiasthmatic; bronchodilator; expectorant* [dyphylline; guaifenesin]
diloxanide INN, BAN
diloxanide furoate *investigational anti-infective for amebiasis*
diltiazem INN, BAN *coronary vasodilator; calcium channel blocker* [also: diltiazem HCl]
diltiazem HCl USAN, USP *coronary vasodilator; calcium channel blocker* [also: diltiazem]
diluted acetic acid [see: acetic acid, diluted]
diluted alcohol [see: alcohol, diluted]
diluted hydrochloric acid [see: hydrochloric acid, diluted]
diluted sodium hypochlorite [see: sodium hypochlorite, diluted]
dimabefylline INN
Dimacid chewable tablets OTC *antacid* [calcium carbonate; magnesium carbonate]
Dimacol film-coated caplets OTC *expectorant; decongestant; antitussive* [guaifenesin; pseudoephedrine HCl; dextromethorphan hydrobromide]
Dimacol liquid (discontinued 1989) OTC *expectorant; decongestant; antitussive* [guaifenesin; pseudoephedrine HCl; dextromethorphan hydrobromide]
dimantine INN *anthelmintic* [also: dymanthine HCl]
dimantine HCl INN [also: dymanthine HCl]
Dimaphen Release-Tabs (timed-release tablets), elixir OTC *decongestant; antihistamine* [phenylpropanolamine HCl; brompheniramine maleate]
Dimaphen S.A. sustained-release tablets ℞ *decongestant; antihistamine* [phenylpropanolamine HCl; phenylephrine HCl; brompheniramine maleate]
Dimaphen-OTC tablets OTC *decongestant; antihistamine* [phenylpropanolamine HCl; brompheniramine maleate]
dimazole INN [also: diamthazole]
dimazole dihydrochloride [see: dimazole; diamthazole]
dimecamine INN
dimecolonium iodide INN
dimecrotic acid INN
dimedrol [see: diphenhydramine HCl]
dimefadane USAN, INN *analgesic*
dimefilcon A USAN *hydrophilic contact lens material*
dimefline INN, BAN *respiratory stimulant* [also: dimefline HCl]
dimefline HCl USAN *respiratory stimulant* [also: dimefline]
dimefocon A USAN *hydrophobic contact lens material*
dimekolin [see: dimecolonium iodide]
dimelazine INN
dimelin [see: dimecolonium iodide]
dimemorfan INN
dimenhydrinate USP, INN, BAN *antiemetic; anticholinergic; antivertigo; motion sickness prophylaxis*
dimenoxadol INN [also: dimenoxadole]
dimenoxadole BAN [also: dimenoxadol]
dimepheptanol INN, BAN

dimepranol INN *immunomodulator* [also: dimepranol acedoben]
dimepranol acedoben USAN *immunomodulator* [also: dimepranol]
dimepregnen INN, BAN
dimepropion BAN [also: metamfepramone]
dimeprozan INN
dimeprozinum [see: dimeprozan]
dimercaprol USP, INN *antidote to arsenic, gold and mercury poisoning*
dimercaptopropanol [see: dimercaprol]
2,3-dimercaptosuccinic acid (DMSA) [see: succimer]
dimesna INN
dimesone INN, BAN
Dimetabs tablets ℞ *anticholinergic; antiemetic; antivertigo agent; motion sickness preventative* [dimenhydrinate]
dimetacrine INN
dimetamfetamine INN
Dimetane Decongestant caplets, elixir OTC *antihistamine; decongestant* [phenylephrine maleate; brompheniramine maleate]
Dimetane tablets, elixir, Extentabs (long-acting tablets) OTC *antihistamine* [brompheniramine maleate]
Dimetane-DC Cough syrup ℞ *decongestant; antihistamine; antitussive* [phenylpropanolamine HCl; brompheniramine maleate; codeine phosphate; alcohol]
Dimetane-DX Cough syrup ℞ *decongestant; antihistamine; antitussive* [pseudoephedrine HCl; brompheniramine maleate; dextromethorphan hydrobromide; alcohol]
Dimetapp 4-Hour Liqui-Gels capsules OTC *antihistamine; decongestant* [brompheniramine maleate; phenylpropanolamine HCl]
Dimetapp Cold & Allergy chewable tablets OTC *antihistamine; decongestant* [brompheniramine maleate; phenylpropanolamine HCl]

Dimetapp Cold & Flu film-coated caplets OTC *antihistamine; decongestant; analgesic* [acetaminophen; phenylpropanolamine HCl; brompheniramine maleate]
Dimetapp DM elixir OTC *antihistamine; decongestant; antitussive* [brompheniramine maleate; phenylpropanolamine HCl; dextromethorphan hydrobromide]
Dimetapp Plus (name changed to Dimetapp Cold & Flu in 1992)
Dimetapp Sinus caplets OTC *decongestant; analgesic* [pseudoephedrine HCl; ibuprofen]
Dimetapp tablets, elixir, Extentabs (long-acting tablets) OTC *antihistamine; decongestant* [brompheniramine maleate; phenylpropanolamine HCl]
dimethadione USAN, INN *anticonvulsant*
dimethazan
dimethazine [see: mebolazine]
dimethicone USAN, NF, BAN *lubricant and hydrophobing agent; soft tissue prosthetic aid* [also: dimeticone]
dimethicone 350 USAN *soft tissue prosthetic aid*
dimethindene BAN *antihistamine* [also: dimethindene maleate; dimetindene]
dimethindene maleate USP *antihistamine* [also: dimetindene; dimethindene]
dimethiodal sodium INN
dimethisoquin BAN [also: dimethisoquin HCl; quinisocaine]
dimethisoquin HCl USAN [also: quinisocaine; dimethisoquin]
dimethisterone USAN, NF, INN, BAN *progestin*
dimetholizine INN
dimethothiazine BAN *serotonin inhibitor* [also: fonazine mesylate; dimetotiazine]
dimethoxanate INN, BAN

dimethoxanate HCl [see: dimethoxanate]
dimethoxyphenyl penicillin sodium [see: methicillin sodium]
dimethpyridene maleate [see: dimethindene maleate]
dimethyl ketone [see: acetone]
dimethyl phthalate USP
dimethyl polysiloxane [see: dimethicone]
dimethyl sulfoxide (DMSO) USAN, USP, INN *topical anti-inflammatory; solvent; (orphan status withdrawn 1993)* [also: dimethyl sulphoxide]
dimethyl sulphoxide BAN *topical anti-inflammatory; solvent* [also: dimethyl sulfoxide]
dimethyl triazeno imidazole carboxamide (DIC; DTIC) [see: dacarbazine]
dimethylaminophenazone [see: aminopyrine]
dimethylcysteine [see: penicillamine]
dimethylglycine HCl
dimethylhexestrol [see: methestrol]
1,5-dimethylhexylamine [see: octodrine]
5,5-dimethyl-2,4-oxazolidinedione (DMO) [see: dimethadione]
dimethyloxyquinazine [see: antipyrine]
o,α-dimethylphenethylamine [see: ortetamine]
dimethylsiloxane polymers [see: dimethicone]
dimethylthiambutene INN, BAN
dimethyltryptamine (DMT)
dimethyltubocurarine BAN [also: dimethyltubocurarinium chloride]
dimethyltubocurarine iodide [see: metocurine iodide]
dimethyltubocurarinium chloride INN [also: dimethyltubocurarine]
dimethylxanthine [see: theophylline]
dimeticone INN *lubricant and hydrophobing agent; soft tissue prosthetic aid* [also: dimethicone]

dimetindene INN *antihistamine* [also: dimethindene maleate; dimethindene]
dimetindene maleate [see: dimethindene maleate]
dimetipirium bromide INN
dimetofrine INN
dimetotiazine INN *serotonin inhibitor* [also: fonazine mesylate; dimethothiazine]
dimetridazole INN, BAN
dimevamide INN
dimevamide sulfate [see: dimevamide]
diminazene INN, BAN
dimoxamine HCl USAN *memory adjuvant*
dimoxaprost INN
dimoxyline INN
dimpylate INN [also: diazinon]
dinaline INN
Dinate IV or IM injection ℞ *anticholinergic; antiemetic; antivertigo agent; motion sickness preventative* [dimenhydrinate]
dinazafone INN
diniprofylline INN
dinitolmide INN, BAN
dinitrotoluamide [see: dinitolmide]
dinoprost USAN, INN, BAN *oxytocic; prostaglandin*
dinoprost trometamol BAN *oxytocic; prostaglandin* [also: dinoprost tromethamine]
dinoprost tromethamine USAN *oxytocic; prostaglandin-type abortifacient* [also: dinoprost trometamol]
dinoprostone USAN, INN, BAN *oxytocic; prostaglandin-type abortifacient*
dinsed USAN, INN *coccidiostat for poultry*
Diocto liquid, syrup OTC *stool softener* [docusate sodium]
Diocto-C syrup OTC *laxative; stool softener* [docusate sodium; casanthranol]
Dioctocal soft gelatin OTC *stool softener* [docusate calcium]

Diocto-K capsules OTC *stool softener* [docusate potassium]

Diocto-K Plus capsules OTC *laxative; stool softener* [docusate potassium; casanthranol]

Dioctolose Plus capsules OTC *laxative; stool softener* [docusate potassium; casanthranol]

dioctyl calcium sulfosuccinate [now: docusate calcium]

dioctyl potassium sulfosuccinate [now: docusate potassium]

dioctyl sodium sulfosuccinate (DSS) [now: docusate sodium]

diodone INN [also: iodopyracet]

Dioeze capsules OTC *stool softener* [docusate sodium]

diohippuric acid I 125 USAN *radioactive agent*

diohippuric acid I 131 USAN *radioactive agent*

diolamine [see: diethanolamine]

diolostene [see: methandriol]

dionin [see: ethylmorphine HCl]

Dionosil Oily suspension for intratracheal use ℞ *radiopaque agent* [propyliodone in peanut oil]

diophyllin [see: aminophylline]

diosmin INN

Diostate D tablets OTC *dietary supplement* [calcium; phosphorus; vitamin D]

diotyrosine I 125 USAN *radioactive agent*

diotyrosine I 131 USAN *radioactive agent*

Dioval IM injection (discontinued 1991) ℞ *estrogen replacement therapy; antineoplastic for prostatic cancer* [estradiol valerate]

Dioval XX; Dioval 40 IM injection ℞ *estrogen replacement therapy; antineoplastic for prostatic cancer* [estradiol valerate in oil]

dioxadilol INN

dioxadrol INN *antidepressant* [also: dioxadrol HCl]

dioxadrol HCl USAN *antidepressant* [also: dioxadrol]

***d*-dioxadrol HCl** [see: dexoxadrol HCl]

dioxamate INN, BAN

dioxaphetyl butyrate INN, BAN

dioxathion BAN [also: dioxation]

dioxation INN [also: dioxathion]

dioxethedrin INN

dioxethedrin HCl [see: dioxethedrin]

dioxifedrine INN

dioxindol [see: oxyphenisatin acetate]

dioxyanthranol [see: anthralin]

dioxyanthraquinone *(withdrawn from market)* [see: danthron]

dioxybenzone USAN, USP, INN *ultraviolet screen*

dipalmitoylphosphatidylcholine (DPPC) [see: colfosceril palmitate]

dipalmitoylphosphatidylcholine & phosphatidylglycerol *(orphan: neonatal respiratory distress syndrome)*

diparcol HCl [see: diethazine HCl]

dipegyl [see: niacinamide]

dipenicillin G [see: penicillin G benzathine]

dipenine bromide BAN [also: diponium bromide]

Dipentum capsules ℞ *anti-inflammatory for ulcerative colitis* [olsalazine sodium]

diperodon USP, INN, BAN *topical anesthetic*

diperodon HCl *topical anesthetic*

diphemanil methylsulfate USP *anticholinergic* [also: diphemanil metilsulfate; diphemanil methylsulphate]

diphemanil methylsulphate BAN *anticholinergic* [also: diphemanil methylsulfate; diphemanil metilsulfate]

diphemanil metilsulfate INN *anticholinergic* [also: diphemanil methylsulfate; diphemanil methylsulphate]

Diphen Cough Syrup OTC *antihistamine; antitussive* [diphenhydramine HCl]

Diphenacen-50 injection ℞ *antihistamine* [diphenhydramine HCl]
diphenadione USP, INN, BAN
Diphenadryl elixir, caplets OTC *antihistamine* [diphenhydramine HCl]
diphenan INN
diphenatil [see: diphemanil methylsulfate]
diphenchloxazine HCl [see: difencloxazine HCl]
diphenesenic acid [see: xenyhexenic acid]
Diphenhist Captabs (capsule-shaped tablets), elixir OTC *antihistamine; motion sickness preventative; sleep aid; antiparkinsonian* [diphenhydramine HCl]
diphenhydramine INN, BAN *antihistamine; anticholinergic; antiparkinsonian; motion sickness relief* [also: diphenhydramine citrate]
diphenhydramine citrate USP *antihistamine; anticholinergic; antiparkinsonian; motion sickness relief* [also: diphenhydramine]
diphenhydramine HCl USP, BAN *antihistamine; antitussive; motion sickness prevention; sleep aid*
diphenhydramine theoclate [see: dimenhydrinate]
diphenidol USAN, BAN *antiemetic; antivertigo* [also: difenidol]
diphenidol HCl USAN *antiemetic*
diphenidol pamoate USAN *antiemetic*
diphenmethanil methylsulfate [see: diphemanil methylsulfate]
diphenoxylate INN, BAN *antiperistaltic* [also: diphenoxylate HCl]
diphenoxylate HCl USP *antiperistaltic* [also: diphenoxylate]
diphenylacetylindandione [see: diphenadione]
Diphenylan Sodium capsules ℞ *anticonvulsant* [phenytoin sodium]
diphenylbutazone [see: phenylbutazone]
diphenylhydantoin [now: phenytoin]

diphenylhydantoin sodium [now: phenytoin sodium]
Diphenylin syrup OTC *antitussive* [diphenhydramine HCl]
diphenylisatin [see: oxyphenisatin]
diphenylpyraline INN, BAN *antihistamine* [also: diphenylpyraline HCl]
diphenylpyraline HCl USP *antihistamine* [also: diphenylpyraline]
diphetarsone [see: difetarsone]
diphexamide iodomethylate [see: buzepide metiodide]
diphosphonic acid [see: etidronic acid]
diphosphopyridine nucleotide (DPN) [now: nadide]
diphosphoric acid, tetrasodium salt [see: sodium pyrophosphate]
diphosphothiamin [see: co-carboxylase]
diphoxazide INN
diphtheria antitoxin USP *passive immunizing agent* [also: diphtheria toxoid]
diphtheria equine antitoxin *passive immunizing agent*
diphtheria & tetanus toxoids, adsorbed USP *active immunizing agent*
diphtheria & tetanus toxoids & pertussis vaccine (DTP) USP *active immunizing agent*
diphtheria toxin, diagnostic [now: diphtheria toxin for Schick test]
diphtheria toxin, inactivated diagnostic [now: Schick test control]
diphtheria toxin for Schick test USP *dermal diphtheria immunity test*
diphtheria toxoid USP *active immunizing agent* [also: diphtheria antitoxin]
diphtheria toxoid, adsorbed USP *active immunizing agent*
dipipanone INN, BAN
dipipanone HCl [see: dipipanone]
dipiproverine INN
dipiproverine HCl [see: dipiproverine]

dipivalyl epinephrine (DPE) [now: dipivefrin]
dipivefrin USAN *ophthalmic adrenergic* [also: dipivefrine]
dipivefrin HCl USP *topical antiglaucoma agent*
dipivefrine INN, BAN *ophthalmic adrenergic* [also: dipivefrin]
diponium bromide INN [also: dipenine bromide]
dipotassium carbonate [see: potassium carbonate]
dipotassium clorazepate INN *anxiolytic; minor tranquilizer; alcohol withdrawal relief* [also: clorazepate dipotassium]
dipotassium hydrogen phosphate [see: potassium phosphate, dibasic]
dipotassium phosphate [see: potassium phosphate, dibasic]
dipotassium pyrosulfite [see: potassium metabisulfite]
diprafenone INN
diprenorphine INN, BAN
Diprivan emulsion for IV ℞ *general anesthetic* [propofol]
diprobutine INN, BAN
diprofene INN
diprogulic acid INN
diproleandomycin INN
Diprolene AF cream ℞ *topical corticosteroid* [augmented betamethasone diproprionate]
Diprolene ointment, gel, lotion ℞ *topical corticosteroid* [augmented betamethasone diproprionate]
diprophylline INN, BAN *bronchodilator* [also: dyphylline]
dipropylacetic acid [see: valproic acid]
2-dipropylaminoethyl diphenylthioacetate [see: diprofene]
1,1-dipropylbutylamine [see: diprobutine]
diproqualone INN
Diprosone ointment, cream, lotion, aerosol ℞ *topical corticosteroid* [betamethasone diproprionate]

diproteverine INN, BAN
diprothazine [see: dimelazine]
diprotrizoate sodium USP [also: sodium diprotrizoate]
diproxadol INN
dipyridamole USAN, USP, INN, BAN *coronary vasodilator; "possibly effective" antianginal; antiplatelet agent*
dipyrithione USAN, INN *antibacterial; antifungal*
dipyrocetyl INN
dipyrone USAN, BAN *analgesic; antipyretic* [also: metamizole sodium]
dirithromycin USAN, INN *antibacterial*
disaccharide tripeptide glycerol dipalmitoyl (*orphan: pulmonary and hepatic metastases of colorectal adenocarcinoma*)
Disalcid film-coated tablets, capsules ℞ *analgesic; antipyretic; anti-inflammatory; antirheumatic* [salsalate]
disalicylic acid [see: salsalate]
Disanthrol capsules OTC *laxative; stool softener* [docusate sodium; casanthranol]
Disinfecting Solution OTC *contact lens disinfectant*
Disipal tablets (discontinued 1989) ℞ [orphenadrine HCl]
disiquonium chloride USAN, INN *antiseptic*
Diskets (trademarked form) *dispersible tablets*
Disobrom sustained-release tablets ℞ *decongestant; antihistamine* [pseudoephedrine sulfate; dexbrompheniramine maleate]
disobutamide USAN, INN *antiarrhythmic*
disodium carbenicillin [see: carbenicillin disodium; carbenicillin]
disodium carbonate [see: sodium carbonate]
disodium cefotetan [see: cefotetan disodium]

disodium chromate [see: sodium chromate]
disodium clodronate tetrahydrate *(orphan: increased bone resorption due to malignancy)*
disodium cromoglycate (DSC; DSCG) [see: cromolyn sodium]
disodium dihydrogen methylenediphosphonate [see: medronate disodium]
disodium edathamil [see: edathamil disodium]
disodium edetate BAN *metal-chelating agent* [also: edetate disodium]
disodium ethylenediamine tetraacetate [see: edetate disodium]
disodium hydrogen phosphate [see: sodium phosphate]
disodium hydrogen phosphate heptahydrate [see: sodium phosphate, dibasic]
disodium hydrogen phosphate hydrate [see: sodium phosphate, dibasic]
(disodium) methylene diphosphonate (MDP) [now: medronate disodium]
disodium phosphate [see: sodium phosphate, dibasic]
disodium phosphate heptahydrate [see: sodium phosphate]
disodium phosphonoacetate monohydrate [see: fosfonet sodium]
disodium phosphorofluoridate [see: sodium monofluorophosphate]
disodium pyrosulfite [see: sodium metabisulfite]
disodium silibinin dihemisuccinate *(orphan: Amanita phalloides [mushroom] liver poisoning)*
disodium sulfate decahydrate [see: sodium sulfate]
disodium thiosulfate pentahydrate [see: sodium thiosulfate]
disofenin USAN, INN, BAN *carrier agent in diagnostic tests*
disogluside INN

Disolan capsules OTC *laxative; stool softener* [docusate sodium; phenolphthalein]
Disolan Forte capsules OTC *laxative; stool softener* [docusate sodium; casanthranol; sodium carboxymethylcellulose]
Disonate capsules, syrup, liquid OTC *stool softener* [docusate sodium]
Disophrol Chronotabs (sustained-action tablets), tablets OTC *decongestant; antihistamine* [pseudoephedrine sulfate; dexbrompheniramine maleate]
Disoplex capsules OTC *laxative; stool softener* [docusate sodium; sodium carboxymethylcellulose]
disoprofol [see: propofol]
disopromine HCl [see: diisopromine HCl]
disopyramide USAN, INN, BAN *antiarrhythmic*
disopyramide phosphate USAN, USP, BAN *antiarrhythmic*
Disorine solution for nebulization (discontinued 1991) ℞ *bronchodilator* [isoetharine HCl]
Disotate IV infusion ℞ *calcium-lowering agent; antiarrhythmic* [edetate disodium]
disoxaril USAN, INN *antiviral*
Di-Spaz capsules, IM injection ℞ *gastrointestinal antispasmodic* [dicyclomine HCl]
dispersible cellulose BAN *tablet and capsule diluent* [also: cellulose, microcrystalline]
Dispertab (trademarked form) *delayed-release tablets*
Dispos-A-Med Isoetharine solution for nebulization (discontinued 1991) ℞ *bronchodilator* [isoetharine HCl]
distaquaine [see: penicillin V]
distigmine bromide INN, BAN
disulergine INN
disulfamide INN [also: disulphamide]
disulfiram USP, INN, BAN *deterrent to alcohol consumption*

disulfurous acid, dipotassium salt [see: potassium metabisulfite]
disulfurous acid, disodium salt [see: sodium metabisulfite]
disulphamide BAN [also: disulfamide]
disuprazole INN
Ital slow-release capsules ℞ *appetite suppresant* [phendimetrazine tartrate]
ditazole INN
ditekiren USAN *antihypertensive; renin inhibitor*
ditercalinium chloride INN
dithiazanine BAN [also: dithiazanine iodide]
dithiazanine iodide USP, INN [also: dithiazanine]
dithranol INN, BAN *antipsoriatic* [also: anthralin]
D.I.T.I.-2 vaginal cream ℞ *bacteriostatic; antiseptic; vulnerary* [sulfanilamide; aminacrine HCl; allantoin]
ditiocarb sodium INN
ditiomustine INN
ditolamide INN
ditophal INN, BAN
Ditropan tablets, syrup ℞ *urinary antispasmodic for neurogenic bladder* [oxybutynin chloride]
Diucardin tablets ℞ *diuretic; antihypertensive* [hydroflumethiazide]
Diulo tablets ℞ *diuretic; antihypertensive* [metolazone]
Diupres-250; Diupres-500 tablets ℞ *antihypertensive* [chlorothiazide; reserpine]
Diurese tablets ℞ *diuretic; antihypertensive* [trichlormethiazide]
Diurese-R tablets (discontinued 1991) ℞ *antihypertensive* [trichlormethiazide; reserpine]
Diurigen tablets (discontinued 1993) ℞ *diuretic* [chlorothiazide]
Diurigen with Reserpine tablets (discontinued 1992) ℞ *antihypertensive* [chlorothiazide; reserpine]
Diuril Sodium powder for IV injection ℞ *diuretic* [chlorothiazide]
Diuril tablets, oral suspension ℞ *diuretic* [chlorothiazide]
Diutensen tablets (discontinued 1990) ℞ *antihypertensive* [methyclothiazide; cryptenamine tannate]
Diutensen-R tablets ℞ *antihypertensive* [methyclothiazide; reserpine]
divabuterol INN
divalproex sodium USAN *anticonvulsant* [also: valproate semisodium; semisodium valproate]
divanilliden cyclohexanone [see: cyclovalone]
divaplon INN
Divide-Tabs (trademarked form) *scored tablets*
Dividose (trademarked form) *multiple-scored tablets*
diviminol [see: viminol]
divinyl ether [see: vinyl ether]
divinyl oxide [see: vinyl ether]
dixamone bromide [see: methantheline bromide]
dixanthogen INN
dixarit [see: clonidine]
dizatrifone INN
Dizmiss chewable tablets OTC *anticholinergic; antivertigo agent; motion sickness preventative* [meclizine]
dizocilpine INN *neuroprotective* [also: dizocilpine maleate]
dizocilpine maleate USAN *neuroprotective* [also: dizocilpine]
Dizymes enteric-coated tablets OTC *digestive enzymes* [pancreatin]
DM Cough Syrup OTC *antitussive* [dextromethorphan hydrobromide]
DMCT (demethylchlortetracycline) [see: demeclocycline]
D-Med 80 intralesional, soft tissue, and IM injection ℞ *glucocorticoids* [methylprednisolone acetate]
DMG tablets OTC *dietary supplement* [calcium gluconate; dimethylglycine HCl]
DML Forte cream OTC *moisturizer; emollient*
DML lotion OTC *moisturizer; emollient*

DMO (dimethyl oxazolidinedione)
[see: dimethadione]
DMSA (dimercaptosuccinic acid)
[see: succimer]
DMSO (dimethyl sulfoxide) [q.v.]
DMT (dimethyltryptamine)
DNA (deoxyribonucleic acid)
DNase (name changed to Pulmozyme in 1993)
DNJ (deoxynojirmycin) [q.v.]
DNR (daunorubicin) [q.v.]
Doan's Backache Spray (discontinued 1992) OTC *counterirritant; topical antiseptic* [methyl salicylate; menthol; methyl nicotinate; isopropyl alcohol]
Doan's Pills tablets OTC *analgesic; antirheumatic* [magnesium salicylate]
DOAP (daunorubicin, Oncovin, ara-C, prednisone) *chemotherapy protocol*
DOB Bath and Shower Oil (discontinued 1990) OTC *bath emollient*
Dobell's mouthwash/gargle (discontinued 1991) OTC *oral antiseptic* [phenol]
dobupride INN
dobutamine USAN, INN, BAN *cardiotonic; vasopressor for shock*
dobutamine HCl USAN, USP, BAN *cardiotonic*
dobutamine lactobionate USAN *cardiotonic*
dobutamine tartrate USAN *cardiotonic*
Dobutrex IV infusion ℞ *vasopressor used in shock* [dobutamine]
DOCA (desoxycorticosterone acetate) [q.v.]
docarpamine INN
docebenone USAN, INN *5-lipoxygenase inhibitor*
doconazole USAN, INN *antifungal*
doconexent INN [also: icosapent; omega-3 marine triglycerides]
docosahexaenoic acid (DHA) [see: doconexent; icosapent; omega-3 marine triglycerides]

Doctar shampoo OTC *antiseborrheic; antipsoriatic; antipruritic; antibacterial* [coal tar]
Dr. Caldwell Senna Laxative liquid OTC *laxative* [senna concentrate]
Dr. Hand's lotion, gel OTC *analgesic for teething*
Docucal-P softgels OTC *laxative; stool softener* [docusate calcium; phenolphthalein]
docusate calcium USAN, USP *stool softener*
docusate potassium USAN, USP *stool softener*
docusate sodium USAN, USP, BAN *stool softener; surfactant/wetting agent* [also: sodium dioctyl sulfosuccinate]
dodeclonium bromide INN
2-dodecylisoquinolinium bromide [see: lauryl isoquinolinium bromide]
dofamium chloride INN, BAN
Dofus capsules OTC *dietary supplement* [Lactobacillus acidophilus]
DOK capsules, syrup, liquid OTC *stool softener* [docusate sodium]
Doktors drops, solution (discontinued 1990) OTC *nasal decongestant* [phenylephrine HCl]
Doktors spray (discontinued 1992) OTC *nasal decongestant* [phenylephrine HCl]
Dolacet capsules ℞ *narcotic analgesic* [hydrocodone bitartrate; acetaminophen]
Dolanex elixir OTC *analgesic; antipyretic* [acetaminophen]
dolantal [see: meperidine HCl]
dolantin [see: meperidine HCl]
dolasetron INN *antiemetic; antimigraine* [also: dolasetron mesylate]
dolasetron mesylate USAN *antiemetic; antimigraine* [also: dolasetron]
Dolene AP-65 tablets (discontinued 1992) ℞ *narcotic analgesic* [propoxyphene HCl; acetaminophen]
Dolene capsules ℞ *narcotic analgesic* [propoxyphene HCl; acetaminophen]

Dolfen tablets ℞ *narcotic analgesic* [hydrocodone bitartrate; acetaminophen]

doliracetam INN

Dolobid tablets ℞ *analgesic; antiarthritic; antirheumatic; anti-inflammatory; antipyretic* [diflunisal]

Dolomite tablets OTC *mineral supplement* [calcium; magnesium]

Dolophine HCl tablets, subcu or IM injection ℞ *narcotic analgesic; narcotic addiction detoxicant* [methadone HCl]

dolosal [see: meperidine HCl]

Dolprn #3 tablets (discontinued 1990) ℞ *narcotic analgesic; antacid* [codeine phosphate; acetaminophen; aspirin; magnesium hydroxide; aluminum hydroxide]

Dolsed tablets ℞ *urinary anti-infective; analgesic; antispasmodic; acidifier* [methenamine; phenyl salicylate; atropine sulfate; methylene blue; hyoscyamine; benzoic acid]

dolvanol [see: meperidine HCl]

domazoline INN *anticholinergic* [also: domazoline fumarate]

domazoline fumarate USAN *anticholinergic* [also: domazoline]

Domeboro Otic [see: Otic Domeboro]

Domeboro powder packets, effervescent tablets OTC *astringent wet dressing (modified Burow solution)* [aluminum sulfate; calcium acetate]

Dome-Paste medicated gauze bandage OTC *protection and support of extremities* [zinc oxide; calamine; gelatin]

domestrol [see: diethylstilbestrol]

domibrom [see: domiphen bromide]

domiodol USAN, INN *mucolytic*

domiphen bromide USAN, BAN *topical anti-infective*

domipizone INN

Dommanate IV or IM injection ℞ *anticholinergic; antiemetic; antivertigo agent; motion sickness preventative* [dimenhydrinate]

Domol Bath and Shower Oil OTC *bath emollient*

domoprednate INN

domoxin INN

domperidone USAN, INN, BAN *antiemetic*

Donatussin DC syrup ℞ *decongestant; antitussive; expectorant* [phenylephrine HCl; hydrocodone bitartrate; guaifenesin]

Donatussin drops ℞ *pediatric decongestant, antihistamine and expectorant* [phenylephrine HCl; chlorpheniramine maleate; guaifenesin]

Donatussin syrup ℞ *decongestant; antihistamine; antitussive; expectorant* [phenylephrine HCl; chlorpheniramine maleate; dextromethorphan hydrobromide; guaifenesin]

Dondril tablets OTC *decongestant; antihistamine; antitussive* [phenylephrine HCl; chlorpheniramine maleate; dextromethorphan hydrobromide]

donetidine USAN, INN, BAN *antagonist to histamine H_2 receptors*

Donnagel liquid, chewable tablets OTC *antidiarrheal; GI adsorbent* [attapulgite]

Donnagel oral suspension (discontinued 1992) OTC *GI adsorbent; antidiarrheal* [kaolin; pectin; hyoscyamine sulfate; atropine sulfate; scopolamine hydrobromide]

Donnagel-PG liquid ℞ *GI adsorbent; not generally regarded as safe and effective as an antidiarrheal* [opium; kaolin; pectin; hyoscyamine sulfate; atropine sulfate; scopolamine hydrobromide]

Donnamar tablets ℞ *anticholinergic; antispasmodic* [hyoscyamine sulfate]

Donnamor elixir ℞ *anticholinergic; sedative* [atropine sulfate; scopolamine hydrobromide; hyoscyamine hydrobromide; phenobarbital]

Donnapectolin-PG liquid ℞ *GI adsorbent; not generally regarded as safe and effective as an antidiarrheal* [opium; kaolin; pectin; hyoscyamine sulfate; atropine sulfate; scopolamine hydrobromide]

Donnapine tablets ℞ *anticholinergic; sedative* [atropine sulfate; scopolamine hydrobromide; hyoscyamine hydrobromide; phenobarbital]

Donna-Sed elixir ℞ *anticholinergic; sedative* [atropine sulfate; scopolamine hydrobromide; hyoscyamine hydrobromide; phenobarbital]

Donnatal capsules, tablets, elixir, Extentabs (extended-release tablets) ℞ *anticholinergic; sedative* [atropine sulfate; scopolamine hydrobromide; hyoscyamine sulfate; phenobarbital]

Donnatal No. 2 tablets ℞ *anticholinergic; sedative* [atropine sulfate; scopolamine hydrobromide; hyoscyamine sulfate; phenobarbital]

Donnazyme tablets ℞ *digestive enzymes* [pancreatin]

Donphen tablets (discontinued 1991) ℞ *anticholinergic; sedative* [atropine sulfate; scopolamine hydrobromide; hyoscyamine hydrobromide; phenobarbital]

L-dopa [see: levodopa]

DOPA (dihydroxyphenylalanine) [see: levodopa]

dopamantine USAN, INN *antiparkinsonian*

dopamine INN, BAN *adrenergic* [also: dopamine HCl]

dopamine HCl USAN, USP *adrenergic; vasopressor for shock* [also: dopamine]

Dopar capsules ℞ *antiparkinsonian* [levodopa]

Dopastat IV ℞ *vasopressor used in shock* [dopamine HCl]

dopexamine USAN, INN, BAN *cardiovascular agent*

dopexamine HCl USAN, BAN *cardiovascular agent*

Dopram IV injection or infusion ℞ *CNS stimulant; analeptic; adjunct to postanesthesia "stir-up"* [doxapram HCl]

dopropidil INN

doqualast INN

Doral tablets ℞ *sedative; hypnotic* [quazepam]

dorastine INN *antihistamine* [also: dorastine HCl]

dorastine HCl USAN *antihistamine* [also: dorastine]

Dorcol Children's Cough syrup OTC *decongestant; antitussive; expectorant* [pseudoephedrine HCl; dextromethorphan hydrobromide; guaifenesin]

Dorcol Children's Decongestant liquid OTC *nasal decongestant* [pseudoephedrine HCl]

Dorcol Children's Fever & Pain Reducer liquid OTC *analgesic; antipyretic* [acetaminophen]

Dorcol Pediatric Cold Formula liquid OTC *pediatric decongestant and antihistamine* [pseudoephedrine HCl; chlorpheniramine maleate]

doreptide INN

doretinel USAN, INN *antikeratinizing agent*

Doriden tablets (discontinued 1990) ℞ *sedative; hypnotic* [glutethimide]

Dormarex capsules OTC *antihistaminic sleep aid* [pyrilamine maleate]

Dormarex 2 tablets OTC *antihistaminic sleep aid; motion sickness preventative* [diphenhydramine HCl]

dormethan [see: dextromethorphan hydrobromide]

Dormin capsules OTC *antihistaminic sleep aid* [diphenhydramine HCl]

dormiral [see: phenobarbital]

dormonal [see: barbital]

Doryx capsules ℞ *tetracycline-type antibiotic* [doxycycline hyclate]

dorzolamide HCl USAN *carbonic anhydrase inhibitor*

DOS softgels OTC *stool softener* [docusate sodium]
Dosepak (trademarked form) *unit of use package*
dosergoside INN
Dosette (trademarked form) *injectable unit-of-use system (vials, ampules, syringes, etc.)*
Dospan (trademarked form) *controlled-release tablets*
Doss 300 capsules (discontinued 1989) OTC [docusate sodium]
dosulepin INN *antidepressant* [also: dothiepin HCl; dothiepin]
dosulepin HCl [see: dothiepin HCl]
dotarizine INN
dotefonium bromide INN
dothiepin BAN *antidepressant* [also: dothiepin HCl; dosulepin]
dothiepin HCl USAN *antidepressant* [also: dosulepin; dothiepin]
Double Ice ArthriCare [see: ArthriCare, Double Ice]
doxacurium chloride USAN, INN, BAN *neuromuscular blocker; muscle relaxant*
doxaminol INN
doxapram INN, BAN *respiratory stimulant* [also: doxapram HCl]
doxapram HCl USAN, USP *respiratory stimulant; analeptic* [also: doxapram]
doxaprost USAN, INN *bronchodilator*
doxate [see: docusate sodium]
doxazosin INN, BAN *antihypertensive* [also: doxazosin mesylate]
doxazosin mesylate USAN *antihypertensive; α_1-adrenergic blocker* [also: doxazosin]
doxefazepam INN
doxenitoin INN
doxepin INN, BAN *antidepressant* [also: doxepin HCl]
doxepin HCl USAN, USP *tricyclic antidepressant; anxiolytic* [also: doxepin]
doxibetasol INN [also: doxybetasol]

Doxidan capsules OTC *laxative; stool softener* [docusate calcium; phenolphthalein]
doxifluridine INN
Doxil ℞ *investigational antineoplastic for AIDS-related Kaposi sarcoma, leukemia, breast and ovarian cancers* [liposome formulation of doxorubicin]
Doxinate capsules, solution OTC *stool softener* [docusate sodium]
doxofylline USAN, INN *bronchodilator*
doxorubicin USAN, INN, BAN *antineoplastic*
doxorubicin HCl USP *antineoplastic*
doxpicodin HCl [now: doxpicomine HCl]
doxpicomine INN *analgesic* [also: doxpicomine HCl]
doxpicomine HCl USAN *analgesic* [also: doxpicomine]
Doxy 100; Doxy 200 powder for IV injection ℞ *tetracycline-type antibiotic* [doxycycline hyclate]
Doxy Caps capsules ℞ *tetracycline-type antibiotic* [doxycycline hyclate]
Doxy Tabs tablets ℞ *tetracycline-type antibiotic* [doxycycline hyclate]
doxybetasol BAN [also: doxibetasol]
Doxychel Hyclate capsules, tablets, powder for IV injection ℞ *tetracycline-type antibiotic* [doxycycline hyclate]
doxycycline USAN, USP, INN, BAN *bacteriostatic; antirickettsial; malaria prophylaxis*
doxycycline calcium USP *antibacterial; antiprotozoal*
doxycycline fosfatex USAN, BAN *antibacterial*
doxycycline hyclate USP *antibacterial*
doxylamine INN, BAN *antihistamine* [also: doxylamine succinate]
doxylamine succinate USP *antihistamine; sleep aid* [also: doxylamine]

Doxysom Nighttime Sleep-Aid tablets OTC *antihistaminic sleep aid* [doxylamine succinate]

DPE (dipivalyl epinephrine) [now: dipivefrin]

DPF [see: Dermprotective Factor]

DPN (diphosphopyridine nucleotide) [now: nadide]

DPPC (dipalmitoylphosphatidylcholine) [see: colfosceril palmitate]

Dr. Dermi-Heal ointment OTC *antipruritic; astringent; vulnerary* [zinc oxide; allantoin; balsam Peru]

Dramamine IV or IM injection ℞ *antinauseant; antiemetic; antivertigo; motion sickness preventative* [dimenhydrinate]

Dramamine tablets, chewable tablets, liquid OTC *antinauseant; antiemetic; antivertigo; motion sickness preventative* [dimenhydrinate]

Dramamine II tablets OTC *anticholinergic; antihistamine; antivertigo agent; motion sickness preventative* [meclizine]

Dramanate IV or IM injection ℞ *antinauseant; antiemetic; antivertigo; motion sickness preventative* [dimenhydrinate]

dramarin [see: dimenhydrate]

dramedilol INN

Dramilin IV or IM injection ℞ *antinauseant; antiemetic; antivertigo; motion sickness preventative* [dimenhydrinate]

Dramocen IV or IM injection ℞ *antiemetic; motion sickness preventative* [dimenhydrinate]

Dramoject IV or IM injection ℞ *antinauseant; antiemetic; antivertigo; motion sickness preventative* [dimenhydrinate]

dramyl [see: dimenhydrate]

draquinolol INN

Drawitol Drawing Salve ointment OTC *topical local anesthetic; antiseptic; antibacterial* [diperodon HCl; benzalkonium chloride; carbolic acid; ichthammol; thymol; camphor; juniper tar]

drazidox INN

Drest gel (discontinued 1989) OTC *antiseptic hair dressing* [benzalkonium chloride; alcohol]

dribendazole USAN, INN *anthelmintic*

dricol [see: amidephrine]

Dri/Ear ear drops OTC *antibacterial/antifungal* [boric acid; alcohol]

dried aluminum hydroxide gel [see: aluminum hydroxide gel, dried]

dried basic aluminum carbonate [see: aluminum carbonate, basic]

dried ferrous sulfate [see: ferrous sulfate, dried]

dried yeast [see: yeast, dried]

drinidene USAN, INN *analgesic*

Drisdol capsules ℞ *vitamin deficiency therapy* [ergocalciferol]

Drisdol Drops OTC *vitamin supplement* [ergocalciferol]

Dristan Allergy caplets OTC *decongestant; antihistamine* [pseudoephedrine HCl; brompheniramine maleate]

Dristan Cold, No Drowsiness coated caplets OTC *decongestant; analgesic* [pseudoephedrine HCl; acetaminophen]

Dristan Cold; Dristan Advanced Formula tablets OTC *decongestant; antihistamine; analgesic* [phenylephrine HCl; chlorpheniramine maleate; acetaminophen]

Dristan Cold & Flu powder OTC *analgesic; antipyretic; decongestant; antihistamine; antitussive* [acetaminophen; pseudoephedrine HCl; chlorpheniramine maleate; dextromethorphan hydrobromide; ascorbic acid]

Dristan Decongestant inhaler OTC *nasal decongestant* [propylhexedrine; camphor; eucalyptol; menthol]

Dristan Juice Mix-In powder OTC *analgesic; antipyretic; decongestant;*

antitussive [acetaminophen; pseudoephedrine HCl; dextromethorphan hydrobromide]

Dristan Long Lasting nasal spray OTC *nasal decongestant* [oxymetazoline HCl]

Dristan nasal spray OTC *nasal decongestant; antihistamine* [phenylephrine HCl; pheniramine maleate]

Dristan Saline Spray OTC *nasal moisturizer* [sodium chloride (saline)]

Dristan Sinus caplets OTC *decongestant; analgesic* [pseudoephedrine HCl; ibuprofen]

Dristan-AF tablets OTC *decongestant; antihistamine; analgesic* [phenylephrine HCl; chlorpheniramine maleate; acetaminophen; caffeine]

Drithocreme; Drithocreme HP 1%; Dritho-Scalp cream ℞ *topical antipsoriatic* [anthralin]

Drixoral Non-Drowsy Formula extended-release tablets OTC *nasal decongestant* [pseudoephedrine sulfate]

Drixoral Plus; Drixoral Sinus extended-release tablets OTC *decongestant; antihistamine; analgesic* [pseudoephedrine sulfate; dexbrompheniramine maleate; acetaminophen]

Drixoral Sustained-Action Tablets OTC *decongestant; antihistamine* [pseudoephedrine sulfate; dexbrompheniramine maleate]

Drixoral syrup OTC *decongestant; antihistamine* [pseudoephedrine sulfate; brompheniramine maleate]

Drize sustained-release capsules ℞ *antihistamine; decongestant* [chlorpheniramine maleate; phenylpropanolamine HCl]

drobuline USAN, INN *antiarrhythmic*
drocarbil NF
drocinonide USAN, INN *anti-inflammatory*
droclidinium bromide INN
drocode [see: dihydrocodeine]
drofenine INN

droloxifene INN
drometrizole USAN, INN *ultraviolet screen*
dromostanolone propionate USAN, USP *antineoplastic* [also: drostanolone]
dronabinol USAN, INN *antiemetic for chemotherapy; (orphan: appetite stimulant in AIDS)*
drop chalk [see: calcium carbonate]
Drop-Dose (delivery system) *prefilled eye droppers*
dropempine INN
droperidol USAN, USP, INN, BAN *general anesthetic; antipsychotic*
Dropperettes (delivery system) *prefilled droppers*
droprenilamine USAN, INN *coronary vasodilator*
dropropizine INN, BAN
Drop-Tainers (trademarked form) *eye drops*
drostanolone INN, BAN *antineoplastic* [also: dromostanolone propionate]
drotaverine INN
drotebanol INN, BAN
Drotic ear drops ℞ *topical corticosteroidal anti-inflammatory; antibiotic* [hydrocortisone; neomycin sulfate; polymyxin B sulfate]
droxacin INN *antibacterial* [also: droxacin sodium]
droxacin sodium USAN *antibacterial* [also: droxacin]
droxicainide INN
droxicam INN
droxidopa INN
droxifilcon A USAN *hydrophilic contact lens material*
droxypropine INN, BAN
Dry and Clear Double Strength cream (discontinued 1992) OTC *topical keratolytic for acne* [benzoyl peroxide]
Dry and Clear lotion (discontinued 1992) OTC *topical keratolytic for acne* [benzoyl peroxide]

Dry Eye Therapy eye drops OTC *ocular moisturizer/lubricant*

Drysol solution ℞ *astringent for hyperhidrosis* [aluminum chloride]

Drytex lotion OTC *topical acne cleanser* [salicylic acid; acetone; isopropyl alcohol; methylbenzethonium chloride]

DSC; DSCG (disodium cromoglycate) [see: cromolyn sodium]

d-SEB Gel Skin Cleanser (discontinued 1989) OTC *topical acne cleanser* [parachlorometaxylenol; isopropanol]

DSMC Plus capsules OTC *laxative; stool softener* [docusate potassium; casanthranol]

DSS (dioctyl sodium sulfosuccinate) [now: docusate sodium]

D-S-S capsules OTC *stool softener* [docusate sodium]

D-S-S Plus capsules OTC *laxative; stool softener* [docusate sodium; casanthranol]

DST (dihydrostreptomycin) [q.v.]

DTIC (dimethyl triazeno imidazole carboxamide) [see: dacarbazine]

DTIC-ACT-D (DTIC, actinomycin D) *chemotherapy protocol*

DTIC-Dome IV injection ℞ *antineoplastic for metastatic malignant melanoma and Hodgkin's disease* [dacarbazine]

DTP (diphtheria & tetanus [toxoids] & pertussis [vaccine]) [q.v.]

DTPA (diethylenetriaminepentaacetic acid) [see: pentetic acid]

Duadacin capsules OTC *decongestant; antihistamine; analgesic* [phenylpropanolamine HCl; chlorpheniramine maleate; acetaminophen]

duazomycin USAN, INN *antineoplastic*

duazomycin A [see: duazomycin]

duazomycin B [see: azotomycin]

duazomycin C [see: ambomycin]

ducodal [see: oxycodone]

Dulcagen enteric-coated tablets, suppositories OTC *laxative* [bisacodyl]

Dulcet (trademarked form) *chewable tablets*

Dulcolax Bowel Prep Kit 4 enteric-coated tablets + 1 suppository OTC *pre-procedure bowel evacuant* [bisacodyl]

Dulcolax enteric-coated tablets, suppositories OTC *laxative* [bisacodyl]

Dull-C powder OTC *vitamin supplement* [ascorbic acid]

dulofibrate INN

dulozafone INN

dumorelin INN

duneryl [see: phenobarbital]

DuoCet tablets ℞ *narcotic analgesic* [hydrocodone bitartrate; acetaminophen]

Duo-Cyp IM injection ℞ *estrogen/androgen for menopausal vasomotor symptoms* [estradiol cypionate; testosterone cypionate]

DuoDerm CGF; DuoDerm Extra Thin; DuoDerm Hydroactive adhesive dressings OTC *occlusive wound dressing* [hydrocolloid gel]

DuoDerm Hydroactive paste, granules OTC *wound dressing* [hydrocolloid gel]

DuoFilm liquid, patch OTC *topical keratolytic* [salicylic acid]

duo-Flow solution OTC *contact lens cleaning and soaking solution*

Duo-K liquid ℞ *potassium supplement* [potassium gluconate; potassium chloride]

Duolube ophthalmic ointment OTC *ocular moisturizer/lubricant*

Duo-Medihaler inhalation aerosol ℞ *bronchodilator* [isoproterenol HCl; phenylephrine bitartrate]

duometacin INN

duomycin [see: chlortetracycline HCl]

duoperone INN *neuroleptic* [also: duoperone fumarate]

duoperone fumarate USAN *neuroleptic* [also: duoperone]
DuoPlant for Feet gel ℞ *topical keratolytic* [salicylic acid]
duotal [see: guaiacol carbonate]
Duo-Trach Kit injection (discontinued 1989) ℞ *injectable local anesthetic* [lidocaine HCl]
Duotrate; Duotrate 45 sustained-release capsules ℞ *antianginal* [pentaerythritol tetranitrate]
Duoval PA injection (discontinued 1989) ℞ [estradiol valerate; testosterone enanthate]
Duphalac syrup ℞ *laxative* [lactulose]
Duphrene syrup, tablets (discontinued 1989) OTC [phenylephrine HCl; chlorpheniramine maleate; pyrilamine maleate]
Duphulac syrup ℞ *laxative* [lactulose]
Duplex T shampoo OTC *antiseborrheic; antipsoriatic; antipruritic; antibacterial* [coal tar]
duponol [see: sodium lauryl sulfate]
dupracetam INN
Durabolin IM injection ℞ *anabolic steroid for metastatic breast cancer in women* [nandrolone phenpropionate]
Duracaps (dosage form) *sustained-release capsules*
DURAcare; DURAcare II solution OTC *contact lens surfactant cleaning solution*
Duracid chewable tablets OTC *antacid* [aluminum hydroxide; magnesium carbonate; calcium carbonate]
Duracillin A.S. injection (discontinued 1990) ℞ [penicillin G procaine]
Duradyne DHC tablets ℞ *narcotic analgesic* [hydrocodone bitartrate; acetaminophen]
Duradyne tablets OTC *analgesic; antipyretic; anti-inflammatory* [acetaminophen; aspirin; caffeine]
Dura-Estrin IM injection ℞ *hormone for estrogen replacement therapy* [estradiol cypionate in oil]

Duragen-10 IM injection (discontinued 1992) ℞ *estrogen replacement therapy; antineoplastic for prostatic cancer* [estradiol valerate in oil]
Duragen-20; Duragen-40 IM injection ℞ *estrogen replacement therapy; antineoplastic for prostatic cancer* [estradiol valerate in oil]
Duragesic-25; Duragesic-50; Duragesic-75; Duragesic-100 transdermal patch ℞ *narcotic analgesic* [fentanyl citrate]
Dura-Gest capsules ℞ *decongestant; expectorant* [phenylephrine HCl; phenylpropanolamine HCl; guaifenesin]
Duralex sustained-release capsules ℞ *decongestant; antihistamine* [pseudoephedrine HCl; chlorpheniramine maleate]
Duralone-40; Duralone-80 intralesional, soft tissue, and IM injection ℞ *glucocorticoids* [methylprednisolone acetate]
Duralutin IM injection ℞ *progestin; amenorrhea; functional uterine bleeding* [hydroxyprogesterone caproate]
Duramist Plus nasal spray OTC *nasal decongestant* [oxymetazoline HCl]
Duramorph IV, subcu or IM injection ℞ *narcotic analgesic; preoperative sedative and anxiolytic* [morphine sulfate]
Duranest HCl injection ℞ *injectable local anesthetic* [etidocaine HCl]
Duranest injection ℞ *local anesthesia* [etidocaine HCl]
durapatite USAN *prosthetic aid* [also: calcium phosphate, tribasic; hydroxyapatite]
Durapro (name changed to Daypro in 1992)
Duraquin sustained-release tablets (discontinued 1992) ℞ *antiarrhythmic* [quinidine gluconate]
DuraSite (delivery system) *polymer-based eye drops*

Dura-Tabs (trademarked form) *sustained-release tablets*

Dura-Tap PD prolonged-action capsule ℞ *antihistamine; decongestant* [chlorpheniramine maleate; pseudoephedrine HCl]

Duratears Naturale ophthalmic ointment OTC *ocular moisturizer/lubricant*

Duratest 100; Duratest 200 IM injection ℞ *androgen replacement for delayed puberty or breast cancer* [testosterone cypionate]

Duratestrin IM injection ℞ *estrogen/androgen for menopausal vasomotor symptoms* [estradiol cypionate; testosterone cypionate]

Durathate-200 IM injection ℞ *androgen replacement for delayed puberty or breast cancer* [testosterone enanthate]

Duration nasal spray OTC *nasal decongestant* [oxymetazoline HCl]

Duration nose drops (discontinued 1992) OTC *nasal decongestant* [phenylephrine HCl]

Dura-Vent long-acting tablet ℞ *decongestant; expectorant* [phenylpropanolamine HCl; guaifenesin]

Dura-Vent/A continuous-release capsule ℞ *decongestant; antihistamine* [phenylpropanolamine HCl; chlorpheniramine maleate]

Dura-Vent/DA chewable tablets (name changed to D.A. chewable tablets in 1991)

Dura-Vent/DA sustained-release tablet ℞ *antihistamine; decongestant; anticholinergic* [chlorpheniramine maleate; phenylephrine HCl; methscopolamine nitrate]

Duricef capsules, tablets, oral suspension ℞ *cephalosporin-type antibiotic* [cefadroxil monohydrate]

dusting powder, absorbable USP *surgical glove lubricant*

Duvoid tablets ℞ *postsurgical cholinergic bladder muscle stimulant* [bethanechol chloride]

DV vaginal cream ℞ *atrophic vaginitis; estrogen deficiency in menopause* [dienestrol]

DVB (DDP, vindesine, bleomycin) *chemotherapy protocol*

DVP (daunorubicin, vincristine, prednisone) *chemotherapy protocol*

DVPL-ASP (daunorubicin, vincristine, prednisone, L-asparaginase) *chemotherapy protocol*

Dwelle eye drops OTC *ocular moisturizer/lubricant*

Dyazide capsules ℞ *diuretic; antihypertensive* [hydrochlorothiazide; triamterene]

Dycill capsules ℞ *bactericidal antibiotic (penicillinase-resistant penicillin)* [dicloxacillin sodium]

dyclocaine BAN *topical anesthetic* [also: dyclonine HCl; dyclonine]

Dyclone solution ℞ *anesthetic prior to upper GI and respiratory endoscopies* [dyclonine HCl]

dyclonine INN *topical anesthetic* [also: dyclonine HCl; dyclocaine]

dyclonine HCl USP *topical anesthetic* [also: dyclonine; dyclocaine]

dydrogesterone USAN, USP, INN, BAN *progestin*

Dyflex-200 tablets ℞ *bronchodilator* [dyphylline]

Dyflex-400 tablets (discontinued 1993) ℞ *bronchodilator* [dyphylline]

Dyflex-G tablets ℞ *antiasthmatic; expectorant* [dyphylline; guaifenesin]

dyflos BAN *antiglaucoma agent; irreversible cholinesterase inhibitor miotic* [also: isoflurophate]

dylate [see: clonitrate]

Dyline-GG tablets, liquid ℞ *antiasthmatic; bronchodilator; expectorant* [dyphylline; guaifenesin]

dymanthine HCl USAN *anthelmintic* [also: dimantine HCl]

Dymelor tablets ℞ *antidiabetic* [acetohexamide]

Dymenate IV or IM injection ℞ *antinauseant; antiemetic; antivertigo; motion sickness preventative* [dimenhydrinate]

Dynacin capsules ℞ *tetracycline-type antibiotic* [minocycline HCl]

DynaCirc capsules ℞ *antihypertensive* [isradipine]

dynacoryl [see: nikethamide]

Dyna-Hex Skin Cleanser; Dyna-Hex 2 Skin Cleanser liquid OTC *broad-spectrum antimicrobial; germicidal* [chlorhexidine gluconate; alcohol]

dynamine (*orphan: Lambert-Eaton myasthenic syndrome; hereditary motor and sensory neuropathy*)

Dynapen capsules, powder for oral suspension ℞ *bactericidal antibiotic (penicillinase-resistant penicillin)* [dicloxacillin sodium]

dynarsan [see: acetarsone]

dyphylline USP *bronchodilator* [also: diprophylline]

Dyphylline GG elixir OTC *bronchodilator; expectorant* [dyphylline; guaifenesin]

Dyprotex pads OTC *topical diaper rash treatment* [zinc oxide; dimethicone]

Dyrenium capsules ℞ *potassium-conserving diuretic* [triamterene]

Dyrexan-OD sustained-release capsules ℞ *anorexiant* [phendimetrazine tartrate]

Dysport (*orphan: essential blepharospasm*) [Clostridium botulinum toxin, type A]

dysprosium *element* (Dy)

DZAPO (daunorubicin, azacitidine, ara-C, prednisone, Oncovin) *chemotherapy protocol*

E

E-200; E-400; E-1000 softgels OTC *vitamin supplement* [vitamin E]

E5 ℞ *investigational agent for gram-negative sepsis* [H65-RTA monoclonal antibody]

Eaase capsules (discontinued 1993) OTC *dietary supplement* [multiple amino acids, vitamins & minerals]

EACA (epsilon-aminocaproic acid) [see: aminocaproic acid]

EAP (etoposide, Adriamycin, Platinol) *chemotherapy protocol*

Ear-Dry ear drops OTC *antibacterial/antifungal* [boric acid; alcohol]

Ear-Eze ear drops ℞ *topical corticosteroidal anti-inflammatory; antibiotic* [hydrocortisone; neomycin sulfate; polymyxin B sulfate]

Early Detector test kit (discontinued 1991) OTC *in vitro diagnostic aid for fecal occult blood*

Earocol Ear Drops (discontinued 1992) ℞ *local anesthetic; analgesic* [benzocaine; antipyrine; glycerin]

EarSol ear drops OTC *antiseptic* [alcohol; eriodictyon]

EarSol-HC ear drops OTC *topical corticosteroidal anti-inflammatory; antiseptic* [hydrocortisone; alcohol; eriodictyon]

earthnut oil [see: peanut oil]

Easprin enteric-coated delayed-release tablets ℞ *analgesic; antipyretic; anti-inflammatory; antirheumatic* [aspirin]

Easy Eyes tablets (discontinued 1992) OTC *contact lens rinsing and storage* *solution* [sodium chloride for normal saline solution]

EasyClean/GP Daily Cleaner solution (discontinued 1992) OTC *contact lens cleaning solution*

EasyClean/GP Weekly Enzymatic Cleaner solution OTC *contact lens cleaning solution*

E-Base delayed-release enteric-coated caplets and tablets ℞ *macrolide antibiotic* [erythromycin]

ebastine USAN, INN *antihistamine*

ebiratide INN

ebrotidine INN

ebselen INN

ecarazine [see: todralazine]

ecastolol INN

Ecee Plus tablets OTC *vitamin/mineral supplement* [vitamins C & E; zinc sulfate; magnesium sulfate]

ECHO (etoposide, cyclophosphamide, hydroxydaunomycin, Oncovin) *chemotherapy protocol*

echothiophate iodide USP *antiglaucoma agent; irreversible cholinesterase inhibitor miotic* [also: ecothiopate iodide]

ecipramidil INN

eclanamine INN *antidepressant* [also: eclanamine maleate]

eclanamine maleate USAN *antidepressant* [also: eclanamine]

eclazolast USAN, INN *antiallergic; mediator release inhibitor*

Eclipse After Sun lotion (discontinued 1992) OTC *moisturizer; emollient*

ecogramostim BAN

ecomustine INN

econazole USAN, INN, BAN *antifungal*

econazole nitrate USAN, USP, BAN *antifungal*

Econo B & C caplets OTC *vitamin supplement* [multiple B vitamins; vitamin C]

Econopred Ophthalmic; Econopred Plus Drop-Tainers (eye drop suspension) ℞ *ophthalmic topical corticosteroidal anti-inflammatory* [prednisolone acetate]

ecostigmine iodide [see: echothiophate iodide]

ecothiopate iodide INN, BAN *antiglaucoma agent; irreversible cholinesterase inhibitor miotic* [also: echothiophate iodide]

Ecotrin enteric-coated tablets, enteric-coated caplets OTC *analgesic; antipyretic; anti-inflammatory; antiarthritic* [aspirin]

ectylurea BAN

Ed A-Hist long-acting capsules ℞ *decongestant; antihistamine* [phenylephrine HCl; chlorpheniramine maleate]

EDAP (etoposide, dexamethasone, ara-C, Platinol) *chemotherapy protocol*

edathamil [now: edetate calcium disodium]

edathamil calcium disodium [now: edetate calcium disodium]

edathamil disodium [now: edetate disodium]

edatrexate USAN, INN *antineoplastic*

Edecrin Sodium powder for IV injection ℞ *loop diuretic* [ethacrynate sodium]

Edecrin tablets ℞ *loop diuretic* [ethacrynic acid]

edelfosine INN

edetate calcium disodium USAN, USP *heavy metal chelating agent* [also: sodium calcium edetate; sodium calciumedetate]

edetate dipotassium USAN *chelating agent*

edetate disodium USP *chelating agent; preservative; antioxidant* [also: disodium edetate]

edetate sodium USAN *chelating agent*

edetate trisodium USAN *chelating agent*

edetic acid NF, INN, BAN *chelating agent*

edetol USAN, INN *alkalizing agent*
edifolone INN *antiarrhythmic* [also: edifolone acetate]
edifolone acetate USAN *antiarrhythmic* [also: edifolone]
edithamil [see: edetate]
edogestrone INN, BAN
edoxudine USAN, INN *antiviral*
edrofuradene [see: nifurdazil]
edrophone chloride [see: edrophonium chloride]
edrophonium chloride USP, INN, BAN *antidote to curare; myasthenia gravis diagnostic aid*
EDTA (ethylenediaminetetraacetic acid) [see: edetate disodium]
EDTA calcium [see: edetate calcium disodium]
ED-TLC; ED Tuss HC liquid ℞ *decongestant; antihistamine; antitussive* [phenylephrine HCl; chlorpheniramine maleate; hydrocodone bitartrate]
EES (erythromycin ethylsuccinate) [q.v.]
E.E.S. 200 oral suspension ℞ *macrolide antibiotic* [erythromycin ethylsuccinate]
E.E.S. 400 film-coated tablets, oral suspension ℞ *macrolide antibiotic* [erythromycin ethylsuccinate]
E.E.S. granules for oral suspension ℞ *macrolide antibiotic* [erythromycin ethylsuccinate]
Efamol PMS soft gel capsules OTC *dietary supplement* [multiple vitamins & amino acids]
efaroxan INN, BAN
Efed II capsules OTC *decongestant* [phenylpropanolamine HCl]
Efedron Nasal jelly (discontinued 1992) OTC *nasal decongestant* [ephedrine]
E-Ferol ointment (discontinued 1992) OTC *emollient* [vitamin E]
efetozole INN

Effer-K effervescent tablets ℞ *potassium supplement* [potassium bicarbonate; potassium citrate]
Effer-Syllium effervescent powder OTC *bulk laxative* [psyllium hydrocolloid]
Effervescent Potassium effervescent tablets ℞ *potassium supplement* [potassium bicarbonate; potassium citrate]
eflornithine INN, BAN *antineoplastic; antiprotozoal* [also: eflornithine HCl]
eflornithine HCl USAN *antineoplastic; antiprotozoal; (orphan: sleeping sickness; Pneumocystis carinii pneumonia)* [also: eflornithine]
efloxate INN
eflumast INN
Efodine ointment OTC *broad-spectrum antimicrobial* [povidone-iodine]
Efricon Expectorant liquid ℞ *decongestant; antihistamine; antitussive; expectorant* [phenylephrine HCl; chlorpheniramine maleate; codeine phosphate; ammonium chloride; potassium guaiacolsulfonate; sodium citrate]
efrotomycin USAN, INN, BAN *veterinary growth stimulant*
Efudex cream, topical solution ℞ *antineoplastic for actinic keratoses and basal cell carcinomas* [fluorouracil]
E-Gems Plus soft capsules OTC *vitamin supplement* [vitamin E]
E-Gems soft capsules, oil drops, cream, lip balm, shampoo, bar soap OTC *vitamin supplement; topical antioxidant* [vitamin E]
E-Gems with C soft capsules OTC *vitamin supplement* [vitamins E & C]
egtazic acid USAN, INN *pharmaceutic aid*
EHDP (ethane hydroxydiphosphonate) [see: etidronate disodium]
Ehrlich 594 [see: acetarsone]
Ehrlich 606 [see: arsphenamine]

eicosapentaenoic acid (EPA) [see: doconexent; icosapent; omega-3 marine triglycerides]
882 ℞ *investigational antiviral for AIDS*
einsteinium *element (Es)*
elantrine USAN, INN *anticholinergic*
elanzepine INN
Elaqua XX cream (discontinued 1991) OTC *moisturizer; emollient; keratolytic* [urea]
Elase powder, ointment ℞ *topical enzyme for biochemical debridement* [fibrinolysin; desoxyribonuclease]
Elase-Chloromycetin ointment ℞ *topical enzyme for biochemical debridement; antibiotic* [fibrinolysin; desoxyribonuclease; chloramphenicol]
elastofilcon A USAN *hydrophilic contact lens material*
Elavil film-coated tablets, IM injection ℞ *tricyclic antidepressant* [amitriptyline HCl]
elbanizine INN
elcatonin INN
Eldec Kapseals (discontinued 1992) ℞ *vitamin/mineral/iron therapy* [multiple vitamins & minerals; iron; folic acid]
Eldecort ℞ *investigational topical anti-inflammatory drug*
Eldepryl tablets ℞ *(orphan: Parkinson's disease)* [selegiline HCl]
Eldercaps capsules ℞ *vitamin/mineral supplement* [multiple vitamins & minerals; folic acid]
Eldertonic elixir OTC *vitamin/mineral supplement* [multiple B vitamins & minerals]
eldexomer INN
Eldisine ℞ *investigational antineoplastic* [vindesine sulfate]
Eldopaque cream OTC *hyperpigmentation bleaching agent; sunscreen* [hydroquinone in a sunblock base]
Eldopaque-Forte cream ℞ *hyperpigmentation bleaching agent; sunscreen* [hydroquinone in a sunblock base]

Eldoquin cream, lotion OTC *hyperpigmentation bleaching agent* [hydroquinone]
Eldoquin-Forte Sunbleaching cream ℞ *hyperpigmentation bleaching agent* [hydroquinone]
electrocortin [see: aldosterone]
Electrol tablets OTC *sodium-free electrolyte replacement*
eledoisin INN
ELF (etoposide, leucovorin, fluorouracil) *chemotherapy protocol*
elfazepam USAN, INN *veterinary appetite stimulant*
elgodipine INN
Elimite cream ℞ *pediculicide; scabicide* [permethrin]
Elixomin elixir ℞ *bronchodilator* [theophylline]
Elixophyllin capsules, elixir ℞ *bronchodilator* [theophylline]
Elixophyllin SR timed-release capsules ℞ *bronchodilator* [theophylline]
Elixophyllin-GG liquid ℞ *antiasthmatic; bronchodilator; expectorant* [theophylline; guaifenesin]
Elixophyllin-KI liquid ℞ *antiasthmatic; bronchodilator; expectorant* [theophylline; potassium iodide]
ellagic acid INN
ellipticine *investigational antineoplastic for breast cancer*
elliptinium acetate INN, BAN
Elmiron *(orphan: interstitial cystitis)* [sodium pentosan polysulphate]
elmustine INN
elnadipine INN
Elocon ointment, cream, lotion ℞ *topical corticosteroid* [mometasone furoate]
E-Lor film-coated tablets ℞ *narcotic analgesic* [propoxyphene HCl; acetaminophen]
elsamitrucin USAN, INN *antineoplastic*
Elspar powder for IV or IM injection ℞ *antineoplastic adjunct for acute lymphocytic leukemia* [asparaginase]

eltenac INN
eltoprazine INN
elucaine USAN, INN *gastric anticholinergic*
Elyzol Dentalgel ℞ *investigational treatment for periodontitis*
elziverine INN
Emagrin Forte tablets OTC *decongestant; expectorant; analgesic; antipyretic* [phenylephrine HCl; guaifenesin; acetaminophen]
Emagrin tablets OTC *analgesic; antipyretic; anti-inflammatory* [aspirin; salicylamide; caffeine]
embinal [see: barbital sodium]
Embolex injection (discontinued 1991) ℞ *anticoagulant* [heparin sodium; dihydroergotamine]
embramine INN, BAN
embramine HCl [see: embramine]
embutramide INN, BAN
Emcyt capsules ℞ *antineoplastic for prostatic carcinoma* [estramustine phosphate sodium]
emedastine INN
emepronium bromide INN, BAN
emepronium carrageenate BAN
Emergent-Ez Kit ℞ [multiple drugs and devices for emergencies]
Emersal emulsion ℞ *topical antipsoriatic; antiseborrheic* [ammoniated mercury; salicylic acid]
Emete-con IV or IM injection ℞ *postanesthesia antiemetic* [benzoquinamide HCl]
emetine BAN *antiamebic* [also: emetine HCl]
emetine bismuth iodide [see: emetine HCl]
emetine HCl USP *amebicide* [also: emetine]
Emetrol solution OTC *antinauseant; antiemetic* [phosphorated carbohydrate solution]
Emgel gel ℞ *antibiotic for acne* [erythromycin]
emiglitate INN, BAN

emilium tosilate INN *antiarrhythmic* [also: emilium tosylate]
emilium tosylate USAN *antiarrhythmic* [also: emilium tosilate]
Eminase IV injection ℞ *acute MI* [anistreplase]
EM-K 10% liquid (discontinued 1991) ℞ *potassium supplement* [potassium chloride]
Emko; Emko Pre-Fil vaginal foam OTC *spermicidal contraceptive* [nonoxynol 9]
Emla cream ℞ *topical local anesthetic* [lidocaine; prilocaine]
Emollia lotion OTC *moisturizer; emollient*
emonapride INN
emopamil INN
emorfazone INN
Empirin tablets OTC *analgesic; antipyretic; anti-inflammatory; antirheumatic* [aspirin]
Empirin with Codeine No. 2 tablets (discontinued 1992) ℞ *narcotic analgesic* [codeine phosphate; aspirin]
Empirin with Codeine No. 3 & No. 4 tablets ℞ *narcotic analgesic* [codeine phosphate; aspirin]
emtryl [see: dimetridazole]
Emul-O-Balm (discontinued 1992) OTC *counterirritant* [methyl salicylate; camphor; menthol]
emulsifying wax [see: wax, emulsifying]
Emulsoil emulsion OTC *laxative* [castor oil]
E-Mycin enteric-coated tablets ℞ *macrolide antibiotic* [erythromycin]
emylcamate INN, BAN
enalapril INN, BAN *antihypertensive; angiotensin-converting enzyme inhibitor* [also: enalapril maleate]
enalapril maleate USAN, USP *antihypertensive; angiotensin-converting enzyme inhibitor* [also: enalapril]
enalaprilat USAN, USP, INN, BAN *antihypertensive; angiotensin-converting enzyme inhibitor*

enalkiren USAN, INN *antihypertensive; renin inhibitor*

enallynymal sodium [see: methohexital sodium]

enbucrilate INN, BAN

encainide INN, BAN *antiarrhythmic* [also: encainide HCl]

encainide HCl USAN *antiarrhythmic* [also: encainide]

Encare vaginal suppositories OTC *spermicidal contraceptive* [nonoxynol 9]

En-Cebrin Pulvules (capsules) OTC *vitamin/mineral/iron supplement* [multiple vitamins & minerals; iron]

enciprazine INN, BAN *minor tranquilizer* [also: enciprazine HCl]

enciprazine HCl USAN *minor tranquilizer* [also: enciprazine]

enclomifene INN [also: enclomiphene]

enclomiphene USAN [also: enclomifene]

encyprate USAN, INN *antidepressant*

End Lice liquid OTC *pediculicide* [pyrethrins; piperonyl butoxide]

Endafed sustained-release capsules ℞ *antihistamine; decongestant* [pseudoephedrine HCl; brompheniramine maleate]

Endal Expectorant liquid ℞ *decongestant; antitussive; expectorant* [phenylpropanolamine HCl; codeine phosphate; guaifenesin; alcohol]

Endal timed-release tablets ℞ *decongestant; expectorant* [phenylephrine HCl; guaifenesin]

Endal-HD; Endal-HD Plus liquid ℞ *decongestant; antihistamine; antitussive* [phenylephrine HCl; chlorpheniramine maleate; hydrocodone bitartrate]

Endep film-coated tablets ℞ *tricyclic antidepressant* [amitriptyline HCl]

endiemal [see: metharbital]

endixaprine INN

endobenzyline bromide

endocaine [see: pyrrocaine]

endolate [see: meperidine HCl]

Endolor capsules ℞ *analgesic; antipyretic; anti-inflammatory; sedative* [acetaminophen; caffeine; butalbital]

endomide INN

endomycin

Endosol solution (discontinued 1992) ℞ *irrigant for eyes, ears, nose and throat during surgery* [balanced salt solution]

endralazine INN, BAN *antihypertensive* [also: endralazine mesylate]

endralazine mesylate USAN *antihypertensive* [also: endralazine]

Endrate IV infusion ℞ *calcium-lowering agent; antiarrhythmic* [edetate disodium]

endrisone INN *topical ophthalmic anti-inflammatory* [also: endrysone]

endrysone USAN *topical ophthalmic anti-inflammatory* [also: endrisone]

Enduron tablets ℞ *antihypertensive* [methyclothiazide]

Enduronyl; Enduronyl Forte tablets ℞ *antihypertensive* [methyclothiazide; deserpidine]

Enecat concentrated suspension ℞ *GI contrast radiopaque agent* [barium sulfate; sorbitol]

enefexine INN

Ener-B nasal gel OTC *vitamin supplement* [cyanocobalamin]

enestebol INN

Enfamil; Enfamil Premature 20 Formula; Enfamil with Iron liquid, Nursette (prefilled disposable bottle) OTC *total or supplementary infant feeding* [whey protein formula]

Enfamil Human Milk Fortifier packets of powder OTC *supplement to breast milk*

enfenamic acid INN

enflurane USAN, USP, INN, BAN *inhalation general anesthetic*

Engerix-B IM injection ℞ *hepatitis B vaccine* [hepatitis B virus vaccine, recombinant]

Engran-HP tablets (discontinued 1992) OTC *vitamin/mineral/iron supplement* [multiple vitamins & minerals; iron; folic acid]
enhexymal [see: hexobarbital]
eniclobrate INN
enilconazole USAN, INN, BAN *antifungal*
enilospirone INN
enisoprost USAN, INN *antiulcerative; (orphan: organ transplant rejection)*
Enisyl tablets OTC *dietary amino acid supplement* [L-lysine]
Enkaid capsules (discontinued 1991, but with limited availability only to patients who received the drug prior to 9/91) ℞ *antiarrhythmic* [encainide HCl]
Enlon IV or IM injection ℞ *myasthenia gravis treatment; antidote to curare-type overdose* [edrophonium chloride]
Enlon Plus IV or IM injection ℞ *muscle stimulant; neuromuscular blocker antagonist* [edrophonium chloride; atropine sulfate]
enloplatin USAN, INN *antineoplastic*
ENO powder OTC *antacid* [sodium tartrate; sodium citrate]
enocitabine INN
enolicam INN *anti-inflammatory; antirheumatic* [also: enolicam sodium]
enolicam sodium USAN *anti-inflammatory; antirheumatic* [also: enolicam]
Enomine capsules ℞ *decongestant; expectorant* [phenylpropanolamine HCl; phenylephrine HCl; guaifenesin]
Enomine LA long-acting tablets (discontinued 1992) ℞ *decongestant; expectorant* [phenylpropanolamine HCl; guaifenesin]
Enovid tablets ℞ *progestin; hypermenorrhea; endometriosis* [mestranol; norethynodrel]
Enovil IM injection ℞ *tricyclic antidepressant* [amitriptyline HCl]

enoxacin USAN, INN, BAN *antibacterial*
enoxamast INN
enoxaparin BAN *investigational antithrombotic* [also: enoxaparin sodium]
enoxaparin sodium INN *investigational antithrombotic* [also: enoxaparin]
enoximone USAN, INN, BAN *cardiotonic*
enoxolone INN, BAN
enphenemal [see: mephobarbital]
enpiprazole INN, BAN
enpiroline INN *antimalarial* [also: enpiroline phosphate]
enpiroline phosphate USAN *antimalarial* [also: enpiroline]
enprazepine INN
enprofen [now: furaprofen]
enprofylline USAN, INN *bronchodilator*
enpromate USAN, INN *antineoplastic*
enprostil USAN, INN, BAN *antisecretory; antiulcerative*
enramycin INN
Enrich Liquid with Fiber OTC *total enteral nutrition*
enrofloxacin USAN, INN, BAN *veterinary antibacterial*
Enseals (trademarked form) *enteric-coated tablets*
Ensure; Ensure HN liquid, powder OTC *total enteral nutrition*
Ensure Plus; Ensure HN Plus liquid OTC *oral nutritional supplement*
E.N.T. tablets OTC *antihistamine; decongestant* [brompheniramine maleate; phenylpropanolamine HCl]
EN-tabs (trademarked form) *enteric-coated tablets*
Entero-Test; Entero-Test Pediatric capsules OTC *in vitro diagnostic aid to identify duodenal parasites, upper GI bleeding, pH disorders, and reflux*
Entex capsules, liquid ℞ *decongestant; expectorant* [phenylephrine HCl; phenylpropanolamine HCl; guaifenesin]

Entex LA long-acting tablet ℞ *decongestant; expectorant* [phenylpropanolamine HCl; guaifenesin]

Entex PSE prolonged-action tablets ℞ *decongestant; expectorant* [pseudoephedrine HCl; guaifenesin]

Entolase capsules (discontinued 1991) ℞ *digestive enzymes* [pancrelipase]

Entolase-HP capsules containing enteric-coated microbeads ℞ *digestive enzymes* [pancrelipase]

Entozyme tablets ℞ *digestive enzymes* [pancreatin]

Entri-Pak (dosage form) *liquid-filled pouch*

Entrition; Half-Strength Entrition; Entrition HN; Entrition RDA Entri-Pak (liquid-filled pouch) OTC *oral nutritional supplement*

Entrobar suspension ℞ *GI contrast radiopaque agent* [barium sulfate]

entsufon INN *detergent* [also: entsufon sodium]

entsufon sodium USAN *detergent* [also: entsufon]

Entuss Expectorant liquid ℞ *antitussive; expectorant* [hydrocodone bitartrate; potassium guaiacolsulfonate]

Entuss Expectorant tablets ℞ *antitussive; expectorant* [hydrocodone bitartrate; guaifenesin]

Entuss-D JR. liquid ℞ *pediatric decongestant, antitussive and expectorant* [pseudoephedrine HCl; hydrocodone bitartrate; guaifenesin; alcohol]

Entuss-D tablets, liquid ℞ *decongestant; antitussive; expectorant* [pseudoephedrine HCl; hydrocodone bitartrate; guaifenesin]

Enuclene eye drops OTC *cleaning, wetting and lubricating agent for artificial eyes* [tyloxapol]

Enulose syrup ℞ *prevent and treat portal-systemic encephalopathy* [lactulose]

Enviclusive *semi-occlusive film dressing for use with Envisan*

Envinet *nylon net for use with Envisan*

enviomycin INN

enviradene USAN, INN *antiviral*

Enviro-Stress slow-release tablets OTC *vitamin/mineral supplement* [multiple vitamins & minerals; folic acid]

enviroxime USAN, INN *antiviral*

Envisan Treatment Multipack beads, paste (discontinued 1992) ℞ *debrider and cleanser for wet wounds* [dextranomer]

Enzactin cream (discontinued 1991) OTC *topical antifungal* [triacetin]

Enzobile Improved enteric-coated tablets (discontinued 1992) OTC *digestive enzymes* [pancreatic enzyme concentrate; ox bile extract; cellulase; pepsin]

Enzone cream ℞ *topical corticosteroid; local anesthetic* [hydrocortisone acetate; pramoxine HCl]

Enzyme chewable tablets OTC *digestive enzymes* [amylase; protease; lipase; cellulase]

E.P. Mycin capsules (discontinued 1991) ℞ *tetracycline-type antibiotic* [oxytetracycline HCl]

EPA (eicosapentaenoic acid) [see: doconexent; icosapent; omega-3 marine triglycerides]

epalrestat INN

epanolol INN, BAN

eperisone INN

epervudine INN

ephedrine USP, BAN *bronchodilator; nasal decongestant; vasopressor for shock*

Ephedrine and Amytal Pulvules (capsules) (discontinued 1991) ℞ *decongestant* [ephedrine sulfate; amobarbital]

ephedrine HCl USP, BAN *bronchodilator; nasal decongestant; vasopressor for shock*

ephedrine sulfate USP *bronchodilator; nasal decongestant* [also: ephedrine sulphate]

ephedrine sulphate BAN *bronchodilator; nasal decongestant* [also: ephedrine sulfate]

ephedrine tannate

Epi-C concentrated suspension ℞ *GI contrast radiopaque agent* [barium sulfate]

epicainide INN

epicillin USAN, INN, BAN *antibacterial*

epicriptine INN

Epiderm balm OTC *counterirritant; topical antiseptic* [methyl salicylate; menthol; alcohol]

epidermal growth factor, human *(orphan: wound healing in burns and eye surgery)*

epiestriol INN [also: epioestriol]

Epifoam aerosol foam ℞ *topical corticosteroid; local anesthetic* [hydrocortisone acetate; pramoxine]

Epifrin eye drops ℞ *antiglaucoma agent* [epinephrine HCl]

epilin [see: dietifen]

E-Pilo-1; E-Pilo-2; E-Pilo-3; E-Pilo-4; E-Pilo-6 eye drops ℞ *antiglaucoma agent* [pilocarpine HCl; epinephrine bitartrate]

Epilyt lotion concentrate OTC *moisturizer; emollient*

epimestrol USAN, INN, BAN *anterior pituitary activator*

Epinal eye drops ℞ *antiglaucoma agent* [epinephrine borate]

epinastine INN

epinephran [see: epinephrine]

epinephrine USP, INN *vasoconstrictor; bronchodilator; topical antiglaucoma agent; vasopressor for shock* [also: adrenaline]

epinephrine bitartrate USP *bronchodilator; ophthalmic adrenergic; topical antiglaucoma agent*

epinephrine borate *topical antiglaucoma agent*

epinephrine HCl *nasal decongestant; topical antiglaucoma agent*

epinephryl borate USAN, USP *adrenergic*

epioestriol BAN [also: epiestriol]

EpiPen; EpiPen Jr. auto-injector (automatic IM injection device) ℞ *emergency treatment of anaphylaxis* [epinephrine]

epipropidine USAN, INN *antineoplastic*

epirizole USAN, INN *analgesic; anti-inflammatory*

epiroprim INN

epirubicin INN, BAN *antineoplastic* [also: epirubicin HCl]

epirubicin HCl USAN *antineoplastic* [also: epirubicin]

epitetracycline HCl USP *antibacterial*

epithiazide USAN, BAN *antihypertensive; diuretic* [also: epitizide]

epithioandrostanol [see: epitiostanol]

epitiostanol INN

epitizide INN *antihypertensive; diuretic* [also: epithiazide]

Epitol tablets ℞ *anticonvulsant* [carbamazepine]

Epitrate eye drops (discontinued 1992) ℞ *antiglaucoma agent* [epinephrine bitartrate]

EPlus tablets OTC *vitamin supplement* [multiple vitamins; lemon bioflavonoids]

EPO (epoetin alfa) [q.v.]

EPOCH (etoposide, prednisone, Oncovin, cyclophosphamide, Halotestin) *chemotherapy protocol*

epoetin alfa (EPO) USAN, INN, BAN *antianemic; hematinic; (orphan: anemia of end-stage renal disease, prematurity or HIV)*

epoetin beta USAN, INN, BAN *antianemic; hematinic; (orphan: anemia of end-stage renal disease)*

Epogen IV or subcu injection ℞ *stimulates RBC production; (orphan: anemia of end-stage renal disease or HIV)* [epoetin alfa; human albumin]

epoprostenol USAN, INN *platelet inhibitor; (orphan: pulmonary hyperten-*

sion; heparin replacement in hemodialysis)
epoprostenol & prostacyclin (orphan: pulmonary hypertension; hemodialysis)
epoprostenol sodium USAN, BAN platelet inhibitor
epostane USAN, INN, BAN interceptive
epoxytropine tropate methylbromide [see: methscopolamine bromide]
Eppy/N ½%; Eppy/N 1%; Eppy/N 2% eye drops ℞ antiglaucoma agent [epinephrine borate]
eprazinone INN
Eprex (orphan: anemia of AIDS and ARC) [erythropoietin, recombinant human]
Epromate tablets ℞ analgesic; antipyretic; anti-inflammatory; anxiolytic [aspirin; meprobamate]
eprovafen INN
eproxindine INN
eprozinol INN
epsikapron [see: aminocaproic acid]
epsilon-aminocaproic acid (EACA) [see: aminocaproic acid]
epsiprantel INN, BAN
Epsom salt [see: magnesium sulfate]
e.p.t. home test kit OTC in vitro diagnostic aid for urine pregnancy test
eptaloprost INN
eptamestrol [see: etamestrol]
eptaprost [see: eptaloprost]
eptastatin sodium [see: pravastatin sodium]
eptazocine INN
Equagesic tablets ℞ analgesic; antipyretic; anti-inflammatory; anxiolytic [aspirin; meprobamate]
Equalactin chewable tablets OTC bulk laxative; antidiarrheal [calcium polycarbophil]
Equanil tablets ℞ anxiolytic [meprobamate]
Equazine M tablets ℞ analgesic; antipyretic; anti-inflammatory; anxiolytic [aspirin; meprobamate; tartrazine]

Equilet chewable tablets OTC antacid [calcium carbonate]
equilin USP estrogen
Eramycin film-coated tablets ℞ macrolide antibiotic [erythromycin stearate]
erbium element (Er)
erbulozole USAN, INN antineoplastic adjunct
Ercaf tablets ℞ migraine-specific vasoconstrictor [ergotamine tartrate; caffeine]
Ercatab tablets (discontinued 1991) ℞ migraine treatment; vasoconstrictor [ergotamine tartrate; caffeine]
erdosteine INN
Ergamisol tablets ℞ antineoplastic adjuvant for colon cancer [levamisole HCl]
Ergo Caff tablets (discontinued 1991) ℞ migraine treatment; vasoconstrictor [ergotamine tartrate; caffeine]
ergocalciferol USP, INN, BAN vitamin D_2; antirachitic
ergoloid mesylates USAN, USP cognition adjuvant for age-related mental capacity decline [also: co-dergocrine mesylate]
Ergomar sublingual tablets (discontinued 1991) ℞ agent for migraine; vasoconstrictor [ergotamine tartrate]
ergometrine INN, BAN oxytocic [also: ergonovine maleate]
ergonovine maleate USP oxytocic [also: ergometrine]
Ergostat sublingual tablets ℞ migraine-specific vasoconstrictor [ergotamine tartrate]
ergosterol, activated [see: ergocalciferol]
ergot alkaloids [see: ergoloid mesylates]
ergotamine INN, BAN migraine-specific analgesic [also: ergotamine tartrate]
ergotamine tartrate USP migraine-specific analgesic [also: ergotamine]
ericolol INN

Eridium tablets ℞ *urinary analgesic* [phenazopyridine HCl]
eriodictyon NF
eritrityl tetranitrate INN *coronary vasodilator* [also: erythrityl tetranitrate]
erizepine INN
E-R-O Ear Drops OTC *agent to emulsify and disperse ear wax* [carbamide peroxide]
erocainide INN
Erwinase ℞ *(orphan: acute lymphocytic leukemia)* [erwinia L-asparaginase]
Erwinia L-asparaginase *investigational antineoplastic; (orphan: acute lymphocytic leukemia)*
ERYC delayed-release capsules containing enteric-coated pellets ℞ *macrolide antibiotic* [erythromycin]
Erycette topical solution ℞ *topical antibiotic for acne vulgaris* [erythromycin]
EryDerm topical solution ℞ *topical antibiotic for acne vulgaris* [erythromycin]
Erygel gel ℞ *antibiotic for acne* [erythromycin]
Erymax topical solution ℞ *topical antibiotic for acne vulgaris* [erythromycin]
EryPed 200; EryPed 400 oral suspension ℞ *macrolide antibiotic* [erythromycin ethylsuccinate]
EryPed drops, chewable tablets, granules for oral suspension ℞ *macrolide antibiotic* [erythromycin ethylsuccinate]
Ery-Tab enteric-coated delayed-release tablets ℞ *macrolide antibiotic* [erythromycin]
erythorbic acid
erythrityl tetranitrate USAN, USP *coronary vasodilator; antianginal* [also: eritrityl tetranitrate]
Erythrocin Stearate Filmtabs (film-coated tablets) ℞ *antibiotic* [erythromycin stearate]

erythrol tetranitrate [now: erythrityl tetranitrate]
erythromycin USP, INN, BAN *macrolide bactericidal/bacteriostatic antibiotic*
erythromycin 2'-acetate octadecanoate [see: erythromycin acistrate]
erythromycin 2'-acetate stearate [see: erythromycin acistrate]
erythromycin acistrate USAN, INN *antibacterial*
erythromycin B [see: berythromycin]
erythromycin estolate USAN, USP, BAN *macrolide bactericidal/bacteriostatic antibiotic*
erythromycin ethyl succinate BAN *antibacterial* [also: erythromycin ethylsuccinate]
erythromycin ethylcarbonate USP
erythromycin ethylsuccinate (EES) USP *macrolide bactericidal/bacteriostatic antibiotic* [also: erythromycin ethyl succinate]
erythromycin gluceptate USP *antibacterial*
erythromycin glucoheptonate [see: erythromycin gluceptate]
erythromycin lactobionate USP *macrolide bactericidal/bacteriostatic antibiotic*
erythromycin lauryl sulfate, propionyl [now: erythromycin estolate]
erythromycin monoglucoheptonate [see: erythromycin gluceptate]
erythromycin octadecanoate [see: erythromycin stearate]
erythromycin 2'-propanoate [see: erythromycin propionate]
erythromycin propionate USAN *antibacterial*
erythromycin 2'-propionate dodecyl sulfate [see: erythromycin estolate]
erythromycin propionate lauryl sulfate [now: erythromycin estolate]
erythromycin stearate USP, BAN *macrolide bactericidal/bacteriostatic antibiotic*

erythromycin stinoprate INN
erythropoietin, recombinant human (rEPO) [see: epoetin alfa; epoetin beta]
erythrosine sodium USP *dental disclosing agent*
Eryzole granules for oral suspension ℞ *antibiotic* [erythromycin ethylsuccinate; sulfisoxazole acetyl]
esafloxacin INN
esaprazole INN
esculamine INN
E-Sel soft capsules OTC *vitamin/mineral supplement* [vitamin E; selenium methionine]
eseridine INN
eserine [see: physostigmine]
Eserine Salicylate eye drops ℞ *antiglaucoma agent; reversible cholinesterase inhibitor miotic* [physostigmine salicylate]
Eserine Sulfate ophthalmic ointment ℞ *antiglaucoma agent; reversible cholinesterase inhibitor miotic* [physostigmine sulfate]
esflurbiprofen INN, BAN
Esgic; Esgic-Plus tablets, capsules ℞ *analgesic; antipyretic; anti-inflammatory; sedative* [acetaminophen; caffeine; butalbital]
Esgic with Codeine capsules (discontinued 1991) ℞ *narcotic analgesic; sedative* [codeine phosphate; acetaminophen; caffeine; butalbital]
Esidrix tablets ℞ *diuretic; antihypertensive* [hydrochlorothiazide]
Esimil tablets ℞ *antihypertensive* [hydrochlorothiazide; guanethidine monosulfate]
Eskalith capsules, tablets ℞ *psychotherapeutic* [lithium carbonate]
Eskalith CR controlled-release tablets ℞ *psychotherapeutic* [lithium carbonate]
esmolol INN, BAN *antiadrenergic (β-receptor)* [also: esmolol HCl]
esmolol HCl USAN *antiadrenergic (β-receptor)* [also: esmolol]

E-Solve OTC *lotion base*
E-Solve 2 topical solution ℞ *topical antibiotic for acne vulgaris* [erythromycin]
Esophotrast oral suspension ℞ *esophageal contrast medium* [barium sulfate]
esorubicin INN *antineoplastic* [also: esorubicin HCl]
esorubicin HCl USAN *antineoplastic* [also: esorubicin]
Esotérica Dry Skin Treatment lotion OTC *moisturizer; emollient*
Esotérica Facial; Esotérica Fortified; Esotérica Sunscreen cream OTC *hyperpigmentation bleaching agent; sunscreen* [hydroquinone; padimate O; oxybenzone]
Esotérica Regular; Esotérica Sensitive Skin Formula cream OTC *hyperpigmentation bleaching agent* [hydroquinone]
Esotérica Soap OTC *bath emollient*
E.S.P. oral suspension ℞ *anti-infective; antibacterial* [erythromycin ethylsuccinate; sulfisoxazole acetyl]
Espotabs tablets OTC *laxative* [yellow phenolphthalein]
esproquin HCl USAN *adrenergic* [also: esproquine]
esproquine INN *adrenergic* [also: esproquin HCl]
Estar gel OTC *topical antipsoriatic; antiseborrheic* [coal tar]
estazolam USAN, INN *hypnotic*
Ester-C Plus; Extra Potency Ester-C Plus capsules OTC *dietary supplement* [vitamin C; calcium; various bioflavonoids; rutin]
Ester-C Plus Multi-Mineral capsules OTC *dietary supplement* [vitamin C; multiple minerals; various bioflavonoids; rutin]
esterified estrogens [see: estrogens, esterified]
esterifilcon A USAN *hydrophilic contact lens material*
estilben [see: diethylstilbestrol dipropionate]

Estinyl tablets ℞ *hormone for estrogen replacement therapy or inoperable prostatic and breast cancer* [ethinyl estradiol]
Estivin II eye drops ℞ *topical ocular vasoconstrictor* [naphazoline HCl]
Estivin Ophthalmic eye drops (discontinued 1991) OTC *ocular emollient* [rose petal aqueous infusion]
estomycin sulfate [see: paromomycin sulfate]
Estrace tablets ℞ *estrogen replacement; antineoplastic for prostatic and breast cancer; osteoporosis preventative* [estradiol]
Estrace vaginal cream ℞ *topical estrogen for atrophic vaginitis* [estradiol]
Estra-D IM injection ℞ *hormone for estrogen replacement therapy* [estradiol cypionate in oil]
Estraderm transdermal patch ℞ *estrogen replacement therapy* [estradiol]
estradiol USP, INN *estrogen* [also: oestradiol]
estradiol benzoate USP, INN [also: oestradiol benzoate]
estradiol 17-cyclopentanepropionate [see: estradiol cypionate]
estradiol cypionate USP *estrogen*
estradiol dipropionate NF
estradiol enanthate USAN *estrogen*
estradiol 17-heptanoate [see: estradiol enanthate]
Estradiol L.A.; Estradiol L.A. 20; Estradiol L.A. 40 IM injection ℞ *estrogen replacement therapy; antineoplastic for prostatic cancer* [estradiol valerate]
estradiol monobenzoate [see: estradiol benzoate]
estradiol 17-nicotinate 3-propionate [see: estrapronicate]
estradiol phosphate polymer [see: polyestradiol phosphate]
estradiol 17-undecanoate [see: estradiol undecylate]
estradiol undecylate USAN, INN *estrogen*

estradiol valerate USP, INN *estrogen* [also: oestradiol valerate]
estradiol valerate in oil [see: estradiol valerate]
Estradurin powder for IM injection ℞ *hormonal therapy for inoperable progressing prostatic cancer* [polyestradiol phosphate]
Estra-L 20; Estra-L 40 IM injection ℞ *estrogen replacement therapy; antineoplastic for prostatic cancer* [estradiol valerate in oil]
estramustine USAN, INN, BAN *antineoplastic*
estramustine phosphate sodium USAN, BAN *antineoplastic*
estrapronicate INN
Estratab tablets ℞ *estrogen deficiency; inoperable prostatic and breast cancer* [esterified estrogens]
Estratest; Estratest H.S. tablets ℞ *estrogen/androgen for menopausal vasomotor symptoms* [esterified estrogens; methyltestosterone]
Estra-Testrin IM injection ℞ *estrogen/androgen for menopausal vasomotor symptoms* [estradiol valerate; testosterone enanthate]
estrazinol INN *estrogen* [also: estrazinol hydrobromide]
estrazinol hydrobromide USAN *estrogen* [also: estrazinol]
estriol USP *estrogen* [also: estriol succinate; oestriol succinate]
estriol succinate INN *estrogen* [also: estriol; oestriol succinate]
estrobene [see: diethylstilbestrol]
estrobene DP [see: diethylstilbestrol dipropionate]
Estro-Cyp IM injection ℞ *hormone for estrogen replacement therapy* [estradiol cypionate in oil]
estrofurate USAN, INN *estrogen*
estrogenic substances, conjugated [see: estrogens, conjugated]
estrogenine [see: diethylstilbestrol]
estrogens, conjugated USP *estrogen*
estrogens, esterified USP *estrogen*

Estroject-2 IM injection (discontinued 1992) ℞ *estrogen replacement therapy; antineoplastic for prostatic and breast cancer* [estrone]

Estroject-L.A. IM injection ℞ *hormone for estrogen replacement therapy* [estradiol cypionate in oil]

estromenin [see: diethylstilbestrol]

estrone USP, INN *estrogen* [also: oestrone]

Estrone 5 IM injection ℞ *estrogen replacement therapy; antineoplastic for prostatic and breast cancer* [estrone]

estrone hydrogen sulfate [see: estrone sodium sulfate]

estrone sodium sulfate

Estronol injection (discontinued 1993) ℞ *estrogen replacement therapy; antineoplastic for prostatic and breast cancer* [estrone]

Estronol-LA injection (discontinued 1993) ℞ *estrogen* [estradiol cypionate]

estropipate USP *estrogen*

estropipate sulfate *estrogen*

Estrovis tablets ℞ *hormone for estrogen replacement therapy* [quinestrol]

esuprone INN

etabenzarone INN

etacepride INN

etacrynic acid INN *diuretic* [also: ethacrynic acid]

etafedrine INN, BAN *adrenergic* [also: etafedrine HCl]

etafedrine HCl USAN *adrenergic* [also: etafedrine]

etafenone INN

etafilcon A USAN *hydrophilic contact lens material*

etamestrol INN

etaminile INN

etamiphyllin INN [also: etamiphylline]

etamiphyllin methesculetol [see: metescufylline]

etamiphylline BAN [also: etamiphyllin]

etamivan INN *central and respiratory stimulant* [also: ethamivan]

etamocycline INN

etamsylate INN *hemostatic* [also: ethamsylate]

etanidazole USAN, INN *antineoplastic; hypoxic cell radiosensitizer*

etanterol INN

etaperazine [see: perphenazine]

etaqualone INN

etarotene USAN, INN *keratolytic*

etasuline INN

etazepine INN

etazolate INN *antipsychotic* [also: etazolate HCl]

etazolate HCl USAN *antipsychotic* [also: etazolate]

etebenecid INN [also: ethebenecid]

etenzamide BAN [also: ethenzamide]

eterobarb USAN, INN, BAN *anticonvulsant*

etersalate INN

ethacridine INN [also: ethacridine lactate]

ethacridine lactate [also: ethacridine]

ethacrynate sodium USAN, USP *diuretic*

ethacrynic acid USAN, USP, BAN *loop diuretic* [also: etacrynic acid]

ethambutol INN, BAN *bacteriostatic; primary tuberculostatic* [also: ethambutol HCl]

ethambutol HCl USAN, USP *bacteriostatic; primary tuberculostatic* [also: ethambutol]

ethamivan USAN, USP, BAN *central and respiratory stimulant* [also: etamivan]

Ethamolin IV injection ℞ *sclerosing agent; (orphan: bleeding esophageal varices)* [ethanolamine oleate]

ethamsylate USAN, BAN *hemostatic* [also: etamsylate]

ethanol [see: alcohol]

ethanolamine oleate USAN *sclerosing agent; (orphan: bleeding esophageal varices)* [also: monoethanolamine oleate]

Ethaquin tablets ℞ *peripheral vasodilator* [ethaverine HCl]
Ethatab tablets ℞ *peripheral vasodilator* [ethaverine HCl]
ethaverine INN *peripheral vasodilator*
ethaverine HCl *peripheral vasodilator* [see: ethaverine]
Ethavex-100 tablets ℞ *peripheral vasodilator* [ethaverine HCl]
ethchlorvynol USP, INN, BAN *sedative; hypnotic*
ethebenecid BAN [also: etebenecid]
ethenzamide INN [also: etenzamide]
ether USP *inhalation anesthetic*
ethiazide INN, BAN
ethidium bromide [see: homidium bromide]
ethinamate USP, INN, BAN *sedative; hypnotic*
ethinyl estradiol USP *estrogen; (orphan: Turner syndrome)* [also: ethinylestradiol; ethinyloestradiol]
ethinylestradiol INN *estrogen* [also: ethinyl estradiol; ethinyloestradiol]
ethinyloestradiol BAN *estrogen* [also: ethinyl estradiol; ethinylestradiol]
ethiodized oil USP *radiopaque medium*
ethiodized oil (^{131}I) INN *antineoplastic; radioactive agent* [also: ethiodized oil I 131]
ethiodized oil I 131 USAN *antineoplastic; radioactive agent* [also: ethiodized oil (^{131}I)]
Ethiodol intracavitary instillation ℞ *hysterosalpingographic and lymphographic contrast medium* [ethiodized oil]
ethiofos *(previously used USAN)* [now: amifostine]
ethionamide USAN, USP, INN, BAN *bacteriostatic; tuberculosis retreatment*
ethisterone NF, INN, BAN
Ethmozine film-coated tablets ℞ *antiarrhythmic* [moricizine HCl]
ethodryl [see: diethylcarbamazine citrate]
ethoglucid BAN [also: etoglucid]

ethoheptazine BAN [also: ethoheptazine citrate]
ethoheptazine citrate NF, INN [also: ethoheptazine]
ethohexadiol USP
ethomoxane INN, BAN
ethomoxane HCl [see: ethomoxane]
Ethon tablets ℞ *diuretic; antihypertensive* [methyclothiazide]
ethonam nitrate USAN *antifungal* [also: etonam]
ethopabate BAN
ethopropazine BAN *antiparkinsonian* [also: ethopropazine HCl; profenamine]
ethopropazine HCl USP *antiparkinsonian; anticholinergic* [also: profenamine; ethopropazine]
ethosalamide BAN [also: etosalamide]
ethosuximide USAN, USP, INN, BAN *anticonvulsant*
ethotoin USP, INN, BAN *anticonvulsant*
ethoxarutine [see: ethoxazorutoside]
ethoxazene HCl USAN *analgesic* [also: etoxazene]
ethoxazorutoside INN
ethoxyacetanilide *(withdrawn from market)* [see: phenacetin]
o-**ethoxybenzamide** [see: ethenzamide; etenzamide]
ethoxzolamide USP
Ethrane liquid for vaporization ℞ *inhalation general anesthetic* [enflurane]
ethybenztropine USAN, BAN *anticholinergic* [also: etybenzatropine]
ethyl acetate NF *solvent*
ethyl alcohol (EtOH; ETOH) [now: alcohol]
ethyl aminobenzoate [now: benzocaine]
ethyl 2-benzimidazolecarbamate [see: lobendazole]
ethyl *N*-benzylcyclopropanecarbamate [see: encyprate]
ethyl biscoumacetate NF, INN, BAN

ethyl biscumacetate [see: ethyl biscoumacetate]
ethyl carbamate [now: urethane]
ethyl carfluzepate INN
ethyl cartrizoate INN
ethyl chloride USP *topical anesthetic*
ethyl dibunate USAN, INN, BAN *antitussive*
ethyl dirazepate INN
ethyl ether [see: ether]
ethyl *p*-fluorophenyl sulfone [see: fluoresone]
ethyl *p*-hydroxybenzoate [see: ethylparaben]
ethyl loflazepate INN
ethyl nitrite NF
ethyl oleate NF *vehicle*
ethyl oxide [see: ether]
ethyl vanillin NF *flavoring agent*
ethylcellulose NF *tablet binder*
ethylchlordiphene [see: etofamide]
ethyldicoumarol [see: ethyl biscoumacetate]
ethylene NF *inhalation general anesthesia*
ethylene distearate [see: glycol distearate]
ethylenediamine USP
ethylenediaminetetraacetate [see: edetate disodium]
ethylenediaminetetraacetic acid (EDTA) [see: edetate disodium]
N,N-ethylenediarsanilic acid [see: difetarsone]
ethylenedinitrilotetraacetate disodium [see: edetate disodium]
ethylestrenol USAN, INN *anabolic* [also: ethyloestrenol]
ethylhexanediol [see: ethohexadiol]
2-ethylhexyl diphenyl phosphate [see: octicizer]
ethylhydrocupreine HCl NF
ethylmethylthiambutene INN, BAN
ethylmorphine BAN [also: ethylmorphine HCl]
ethylmorphine HCl NF [also: ethylmorphine]

ethylnorepinephrine HCl USP *bronchodilator*
ethyloestradiol BAN *estrogen* [also: ethinyl estradiol]
ethyloestrenol BAN *anabolic* [also: ethylestrenol]
ethylpapaverine HCl [see: ethaverine HCl]
ethylparaben NF *antifungal agent*
ethylphenacemide [see: pheneturide]
ethylstibamine [see: stibosamine]
2-ethylthioisonicotinamide [see: ethionamide]
ethynerone USAN, INN *progestin*
ethynodiol BAN *progestin* [also: ethynodiol diacetate; etynodiol]
ethynodiol diacetate USAN, USP *progestin* [also: etynodiol; ethynodiol]
Ethyol (*orphan: chemoprotective agent for cisplatin and cyclophosphamide chemotherapy*) [amifostine]
ethypicone INN
ethypropymal sodium [see: probarbital sodium]
etibendazole USAN, INN *anthelmintic*
eticlopride INN
eticyclidine INN
etidocaine USAN, INN, BAN *local anesthetic*
etidocaine HCl *local anesthetic*
etidronate disodium USAN, USP *calcium regulator; pharmaceutic aid;* (*orphan: hypercalcemia; metabolic bone disease*)
etidronate monosodium
etidronate sodium (*this term used only when the form of sodium cannot be more accurately identified*)
etidronate tetrasodium
etidronate trisodium
etidronic acid USAN, INN, BAN *calcium regulator*
etifelmine INN
etifenin USAN, INN, BAN *diagnostic aid*
etifoxin BAN [also: etifoxine]
etifoxine INN [also: etifoxin]

etilamfetamine INN
etilefrine INN
etilefrine pivalate INN
etintidine INN *antagonist to histamine H_2 receptors* [also: etintidine HCl]
etintidine HCl USAN *antagonist to histamine H_2 receptors* [also: etintidine]
etipirium iodide INN
etiproston INN
etiracetam INN
etiroxate INN
etisazole INN, BAN
etisomicin INN, BAN
etisulergine INN
etizolam INN
etobedolum [see: etonitazene]
etocarlide INN
etocrilene INN *ultraviolet screen* [also: etocrylene]
etocrylene USAN *ultraviolet screen* [also: etocrilene]
etodolac USAN, INN, BAN *antiarthritic; nonsteroidal anti-inflammatory drug (NSAID); analgesic* [also: etodolic acid]
etodolic acid INN *antiarthritic; nonsteroidal anti-inflammatory drug (NSAID); analgesic* [also: etodolac]
etodroxizine INN
etofamide INN
etofenamate USAN, INN, BAN *analgesic; anti-inflammatory*
etofenprox INN
etofibrate INN
etoformin INN *antidiabetic* [also: etoformin HCl]
etoformin HCl USAN *antidiabetic* [also: etoformin]
etofuradine INN
etofylline INN
etofylline clofibrate INN *antihyperlipoproteinemic* [also: theofibrate]
etoglucid INN [also: ethoglucid]
EtOH; ETOH (ethyl alcohol) [now: alcohol]
etolorex INN
etolotifen INN
etoloxamine INN
etomidate USAN, INN, BAN *general anesthetic; hypnotic*
etomidoline INN
etomoxir INN
etonam INN *antifungal* [also: ethonam nitrate]
etonam nitrate [see: ethonam nitrate]
etonitazene INN, BAN
etoperidone INN *antidepressant* [also: etoperidone HCl]
etoperidone HCl USAN *antidepressant* [also: etoperidone]
etophylate [see: acepifylline]
etoposide USAN, INN, BAN *antineoplastic*
etoposide phosphate USAN *antineoplastic*
etoprindole INN
etoprine USAN *antineoplastic*
etorphine INN, BAN
etosalamide INN [also: ethosalamide]
etoxadrol INN *anesthetic* [also: etoxadrol HCl]
etoxadrol HCl USAN *anesthetic* [also: etoxadrol]
etoxazene INN *analgesic* [also: ethoxazene HCl]
etoxazene HCl [see: ethoxazene HCl]
etoxeridine INN, BAN
etozolin USAN, INN *diuretic*
etrabamine INN
Etrafon; Etrafon 2–10; Etrafon-A; Etrafon-Forte tablets ℞ *antipsychotic; antidepressant* [perphenazine; amitriptyline HCl]
etretin [see: acitretin]
etretinate USAN, INN, BAN *systemic antipsoriatic*
etryptamine INN, BAN *CNS stimulant* [also: etryptamine acetate]
etryptamine acetate USAN *CNS stimulant* [also: etryptamine]
ETS-2% topical solution ℞ *topical antibiotic for acne vulgaris* [erythromycin]
etybenzatropine INN *anticholinergic* [also: ethybenztropine]

etymemazine INN
etymemazine HCl [see: etymemazine]
etynodiol INN *progestin* [also: ethynodiol diacetate; ethynodiol]
etyprenaline [see: isoetharine]
eucaine HCl NF
Eucalyptamint ointment OTC *analgesic* [menthol]
eucalyptol USAN *topical bacteriostatic antiseptic/germicidal*
eucalyptus oil NF *topical antiseptic*
eucatropine INN, BAN *ophthalmic anticholinergic* [also: eucatropine HCl]
eucatropine HCl USP *ophthalmic anticholinergic* [also: eucatropine]
Eucerin OTC *cream base*
Eucerin Cleansing lotion OTC *cleanser; moisturizer; emollient*
Eucerin cream, lotion OTC *moisturizer; emollient*
eucodal [see: oxycodone]
Eudal-SR sustained-release tablets ℞ *decongestant; expectorant* [pseudoephedrine HCl; guaifenesin]
euflavine [see: acriflavine]
eugenol USP *dental analgesic*
eukadol [see: oxycodone]
Eulexin capsules ℞ *adjunctive hormonal chemotherapy for metastatic prostatic cancer* [flutamide]
euprocin INN *topical anesthetic* [also: euprocin HCl]
euprocin HCl USAN *topical anesthetic* [also: euprocin]
euquinine [see: quinine ethylcarbonate]
Eurax cream, lotion ℞ *scabicide; antipruritic* [crotamiton]
europium *element (Eu)*
Euthroid tablets (discontinued 1992) ℞ *thyroid hormone therapy* [liotrix]
Eutonyl Filmtabs (discontinued 1991) ℞ *antihypertensive* [pargyline HCl]
Eutron Filmtabs (discontinued 1991) ℞ *antihypertensive* [methyclothiazide; pargyline HCl]

EVA (etoposide, vinblastine, Adriamycin) *chemotherapy protocol*
Evac-Q-Kit oral solution + 2 tablets + 2 suppositories OTC *pre-procedure bowel evacuant* [Evac-Q-Mag (q.v.); Evac-Q-Tabs (q.v.); Evac-Q-Sert (q.v.)]
Evac-Q-Kwik Kit oral solution + 2 tablets + 1 suppository OTC *pre-procedure bowel evacuant* [Evac-Q-Mag (q.v.); Evac-Q-Tabs (q.v.); Evac-Q-Kwik suppository (q.v.)]
Evac-Q-Kwik suppositories OTC *laxative* [bisacodyl]
Evac-Q-Mag carbonated oral solution OTC *laxative* [magnesium citrate; citric acid; potassium citrate]
Evac-Q-Sert suppositories OTC *laxative* [sodium bicarbonate; potassium bitartrate]
Evac-Q-Tabs tablets OTC *laxative* [phenolphthalein]
Evac-U-Gen chewable tablets OTC *laxative* [yellow phenolphthalein]
Evac-U-Lax chewable wafers OTC *laxative* [phenolphthalein]
evandamine INN
Evans blue USP *blood volume test* [also: azovan blue]
Everone 100; Everone 200 IM injection ℞ *androgen replacement for delayed puberty or breast cancer* [testosterone enanthate]
E-Vista IM injection ℞ *anxiolytic* [hydroxyzine HCl]
E-Vital cream (discontinued 1992) OTC *moisturizer; emollient; vulnerary* [vitamins E & D; panthenol; allantoin]
E-Vitamin ointment OTC *emollient* [vitamin E; lanolin]
E-Vitamin Succinate capsules OTC *vitamin supplement* [vitamin E]
E-VMAC (escalated methotrexate, vinblastine, Adriamycin, cisplatin) *chemotherapy protocol*
E-VMAC (escalated methotrexate, vinblastine, Adriamycin, cyclo-

phosphamide) *chemotherapy protocol*
exalamide INN
exametazime USAN, INN, BAN *regional cerebral perfusion imaging aid*
exaprolol INN *antiadrenergic (β-receptor)* [also: exaprolol HCl]
exaprolol HCl USAN *antiadrenergic (β-receptor)* [also: exaprolol]
Excedrin, Aspirin Free caplets OTC *analgesic; antipyretic* [acetaminophen; caffeine]
Excedrin, Sinus coated tablets, caplets OTC *decongestant; analgesic* [pseudoephedrine HCl; acetaminophen]
Excedrin caplets, tablets OTC *analgesic; antipyretic; anti-inflammatory* [acetaminophen; aspirin; caffeine]
Excedrin IB tablets, caplets OTC *nonsteroidal anti-inflammatory drug (NSAID); antiarthritic; analgesic* [ibuprofen]
Excedrin P.M. liquid OTC *analgesic; antipyretic; antihistaminic sleep aid* [acetaminophen; diphenhydramine HCl]
Excedrin P.M. tablets, caplets OTC *analgesic; antipyretic; antihistaminic sleep aid* [acetaminophen; diphenhydramine citrate]
Excita Extra condom OTC *spermicidal/barrier contraceptive* [nonoxynol 9]
Exelderm solution, cream ℞ *topical antifungal* [sulconazole nitrate]
exepanol INN
Exidine Skin Cleanser; Exidine-2 Scrub; Exidine-4 Scrub liquid OTC *broad-spectrum antimicrobial; germicidal* [chlorhexidine gluconate; alcohol]
exifone INN
exiproben INN
Ex-Lax chocolated chewable tablets OTC *laxative* [yellow phenolphthalein]

Ex-Lax Extra Gentle Pills tablets OTC *laxative; stool softener* [docusate sodium; phenolphthalein]
Ex-Lax Gentle Nature tablets OTC *laxative* [sennosides]
Ex-Lax Unflavored tablets OTC *laxative* [yellow phenolphthalein]
Exna tablets ℞ *diuretic; antihypertensive* [benzthiazide]
Exocaine Medicated Rub; Exocaine Plus Rub OTC *counterirritant* [methyl salicylate]
Exocaine Odor Free Creme (discontinued 1993) OTC *topical analgesic* [trolamine salicylate]
Exosurf Neonatal intrathecal suspension, powder for injection ℞ *(orphan: hyaline membrane disease; respiratory distress syndrome)* [colfosceril palmitate]
Exsel lotion/shampoo ℞ *antiseborrheic; antifungal* [selenium sulfide]
exsiccated sodium arsenate [see: sodium arsenate, exsiccated]
Extencaps (trademarked form) *extended-release capsules*
extended insulin zinc [see: insulin zinc, extended]
Extendryl chewable tablets, syrup ℞ *decongestant; antihistamine; anticholinergic* [phenylephrine HCl; chlorpheniramine maleate; methscopolamine nitrate]
Extendryl JR sustained-release capsules ℞ *pediatric decongestant, antihistamine and anticholinergic* [phenylephrine HCl; chlorpheniramine maleate; methscopolamine nitrate]
Extendryl SR sustained-release capsules ℞ *decongestant; antihistamine; anticholinergic* [phenylephrine HCl; chlorpheniramine maleate; methscopolamine nitrate]
Extentabs (trademarked form) *extended-release tablets*
Extenzyme Protein Cleaner tablets (discontinued 1992) OTC *contact lens enzymatic cleaner*

Extra Action Cough syrup OTC *antitussive; expectorant* [dextromethorphan hydrobromide; guaifenesin; alcohol]

Extreme Cold Formula caplets OTC *decongestant; antihistamine; analgesic; antitussive* [phenylpropanolamine HCl; chlorpheniramine maleate; acetaminophen; dextromethorphan hydrobromide]

Eye Wash ophthalmic solution OTC *extraocular irrigating solution* [balanced saline solution]

Eye-Sed Ophthalmic eye drops OTC *ocular astringent* [zinc sulfate]

Eye-Sine ophthalmic solution OTC *artificial tears* [tetrahydrozoline HCl]

Eye-Stream ophthalmic solution OTC *extraocular irrigating solution* [balanced saline solution]

EZ Detect reagent strips OTC *in vitro diagnostic aid for urine occult blood*

EZ Detect Strep-A swab test OTC *in vitro diagnostic aid for streptococci*

EZ Detect test kit OTC *in vitro diagnostic aid for fecal occult blood*

Ezide tablets ℞ *diuretic; antihypertensive* [hydrochlorothiazide]

Ezo cushions OTC *denture cushions*

F

1 + 1-F Creme ℞ *topical corticosteroid; antifungal; antibacterial; anesthetic* [hydrocortisone; clioquinol; pramoxine]

¹⁸**F** [see: fludeoxyglucose F 18]

¹⁸**F** [see: sodium fluoride F 18]

FABRase (*orphan: Fabry's disease*) [alpha-galactosidase A]

FAC (fluorouracil, Adriamycin, cyclophosphamide) *chemotherapy protocol*

FAC-LEV (fluorouracil, Adriamycin, Cytoxin, levamisole) *chemotherapy protocol*

FAC-M (fluorouracil, Adriamycin, cyclophosphamide, methotrexate) *chemotherapy protocol*

Fact Plus home test kit OTC *in vitro diagnostic aid for urine pregnancy test*

factor II (prothrombin)

factor III [see: thromboplastin]

factor VIIa, recombinant, DNA origin (*orphan: hemophilia A and B; von Willebrand's disease*)

factor VIII [see: antihemophilic factor]

factor VIII (rDNA) BAN *blood coagulating factor*

factor VIII, fraction A BAN *blood coagulating factor*

factor IX complex USP *hemostatic; antihemophilic* [also: factor IX fraction]

factor IX fraction BAN *hemostatic* [also: factor IX complex]

factor XIII (placenta-derived) (*orphan: congenital factor XIII deficiency*)

Factrel powder for subcu or IV injection ℞ *gonadotropin releasing hormone* [gonadorelin HCl]

fadrozole INN *antineoplastic; aromatase inhibitor* [also: fadrozole HCl]

fadrozole HCl USAN *antineoplastic; aromatase inhibitor* [also: fadrozole]

falintolol INN

falipamil INN

FAM (fluorouracil, Adriamycin, mitomycin) *chemotherapy protocol*

FAM-CF (fluorouracil, Adriamycin, mitomycin, citrovorum factor) *chemotherapy protocol*

famciclovir INN, BAN

FAME (fluorouracil, Adriamycin, MeCCNU) *chemotherapy protocol*

Family Tabs tablets OTC *vitamin supplement* [multiple vitamins; folic acid]

Familytabs with Calcium, Iron & Zinc tablets OTC *vitamin/mineral supplement* [multiple vitamins; calcium carbonate; ferrous fumarate; zinc oxide]

Familytabs with Iron tablets OTC *vitamin/iron supplement* [multiple vitamins; iron]

famiraprinium chloride INN

FAMMe (fluorouracil, Adriamycin, mitomycin, MeCCNU) *chemotherapy protocol*

famotidine USAN, USP, INN, BAN *treatment of GI ulcers; histamine H_2 antagonist*

famotine INN *antiviral* [also: famotine HCl]

famotine HCl USAN *antiviral* [also: famotine]

famprofazone INN, BAN

FAM-S (fluorouracil, Adriamycin, mitomycin, streptozocin) *chemotherapy protocol*

FAMTX (fluorouracil, Adriamycin, methotrexate) *chemotherapy protocol*

fanetizole INN, BAN *immunoregulator* [also: fanetizole mesylate]

fanetizole mesylate USAN *immunoregulator* [also: fanetizole]

Fansidar tablets ℞ *antimalarial* [sulfadoxine; pyrimethamine]

fanthridone BAN *antidepressant* [also: fantridone HCl; fantridone]

fantridone INN *antidepressant* [also: fantridone HCl; fanthridone]

fantridone HCl USAN *antidepressant* [also: fantridone; fanthridone]

FAP (fluorouracil, Adriamycin, Platinol) *chemotherapy protocol*

Farbee with Vitamin C caplets OTC *vitamin supplement* [multiple B vitamins; vitamin C]

fasiplon INN

Faspak (trademarked form) *flexible plastic bag*

Fastin capsules ℞ *amphetamine-type anorectic* [phentermine HCl]

fat, hard NF *suppository base*

fat emulsion, intravenous *parenteral essential fatty acid replacement*

Father John's Medicine Plus liquid OTC *decongestant; antihistamine; antitussive; expectorant; demulcent* [phenylephrine HCl; chlorpheniramine maleate; dextromethorphan hydrobromide; guaifenesin; ammonium chloride; sodium citrate; citric acid]

fazadinium bromide INN, BAN

fazarabine USAN, INN *antineoplastic*

5-FC (5-fluorocytosine) [see: flucytosine]

FCAP (fluorouracil, cyclophosphamide, Adriamycin, Platinol) *chemotherapy protocol*

FCP (fluorouracil, cyclophosphamide, prednisone) *chemotherapy protocol*

FD&C Red No. 2 (Food, Drug & Cosmetic Act) [see: amaranth]

FD&C Red No. 3 (Food, Drug & Cosmetic Act) [see: erythrosine sodium]

[18]**FDG (fludeoxyglucose)** [see: fludeoxyglucose F 18]

[59]**Fe** [see: ferric chloride Fe 59]

[59]**Fe** [see: ferric citrate (^{59}Fe)]

[59]**Fe** [see: ferrous citrate Fe 59]

[59]**Fe** [see: ferrous sulfate Fe 59]

febantel USAN, INN, BAN *veterinary anthelmintic*

febarbamate INN

Febrol EX sugar-free liquid OTC *analgesic* [acetaminophen]

Febrol sugar-free liquid OTC *analgesic* [acetaminophen]

febuprol INN

febuverine INN

FEC (fluorouracil, epirubicin, cyclophosphamide) *chemotherapy protocol*

feclemine INN

feclobuzone INN

FED (fluorouracil, etoposide, DDP) *chemotherapy protocol*

Fedahist Expectorant syrup, pediatric drops OTC *decongestant; expectorant* [pseudoephedrine HCl; guaifenesin]

Fedahist Timecaps (timed-release capsules), Gyrocaps (extended-release capsules), tablets, syrup ℞ *decongestant; antihistamine* [pseudoephedrine HCl; chlorpheniramine maleate]

fedrilate INN

Feen-A-Mint chocolated chewable tablets OTC *laxative* [yellow phenolphthalein]

Feen-A-Mint Pills tablets OTC *laxative; stool softener* [docusate sodium; phenolphthalein]

Feen-A-Mint tablets, chewable tablets, gum OTC *laxative* [yellow phenolphthalein]

Feiba VH Immuno IV injection or drip ℞ *factor VIII deficiency; correct coagulation deficiency* [anti-inhibitor coagulant complex]

felbamate INN *investigational antiepileptic; (orphan: Lennox-Gastaut syndrome)*

Felbamyl ℞ *(orphan: Lennox-Gastraut syndrome)* [felbamate]

Felbatol ℞ *investigational anticonvulsant* [felbamate]

felbinac USAN, INN, BAN *anti-inflammatory*

Feldene capsules ℞ *nonsteroidal antiinflammatory drug (NSAID); antiarthritic* [piroxicam]

Feldene Melt ℞ *investigational instantaneously dissolving form of Feldene*

felipyrine INN

felodipine USAN, INN, BAN *vasodilator; calcium channel blocker*

felypressin USAN, INN, BAN *vasoconstrictor*

Femazole tablets (discontinued 1992) ℞ *antibiotic; antiprotozoal; amebicide* [metronidazole]

Femcaps tablets OTC *analgesic; muscle relaxant; for menstrual pain and cramps* [atropine sulfate; ephedrine sulfate; caffeine; acetaminophen]

FemCare vaginal cream OTC *antifungal* [clotrimazole]

Femcet capsules ℞ *analgesic; antipyretic; sedative* [acetaminophen; caffeine; butalbital]

Femguard vaginal cream (discontinued 1991) ℞ *bacteriostatic* [sulfathiazole; sulfacetamide; sulfabenzamide; urea]

Femidine Douche solution OTC *antiseptic/germicidal; vaginal cleansing and deodorizing* [povidone-iodine]

Femilax tablets OTC *laxative; stool softener* [docusate sodium; phenolphthalein]

Feminease cream OTC *vaginal moisturizer and lubricant*

Feminique Disposable Douche solution OTC *antiseptic/antifungal; vaginal cleansing and deodorizing; acidity modifier* [sodium benzoate; sorbic acid; lactic acid]

Feminique Disposable Douche solution OTC *vaginal cleansing and deodorizing; acidity modifier* [vinegar (acetic acid)]

Feminone tablets (discontinued 1993) ℞ *estrogen deficiency; inoperable prostatic and breast cancer* [ethinyl estradiol]

Femiron Multi-Vitamins and Iron tablets OTC *vitamin/iron supplement* [multiple vitamins; ferrous fumarate; folic acid]

Femiron tablets OTC *hematinic* [ferrous fumarate]

femoxetine INN

Femstat; Femstat Prefill vaginal cream, prefilled applicator ℞ *antifungal* [butoconazole nitrate]

fenabutene INN

fenacetinol INN
fenaclon INN
fenadiazole INN
fenaftic acid INN
fenalamide USAN, INN *smooth muscle relaxant*
fenalcomine INN
fenamifuril INN
fenamisal INN *antibacterial; tuberculostatic* [also: phenyl aminosalicylate]
fenamole USAN, INN *anti-inflammatory*
fenaperone INN
fenarsone [see: carbarsone]
fenasprate [see: benorilate]
fenbendazole USAN, INN, BAN *anthelmintic*
fenbenicillin INN [also: phenbenicillin]
fenbufen USAN, INN, BAN *anti-inflammatory*
fenbutrazate INN [also: phenbutrazate]
fencamfamin INN, BAN
fencamfamin HCl [see: fencamfamin]
fencarbamide INN *anticholinergic* [also: phencarbamide]
fenchlorphos BAN *systemic insecticide* [also: ronnel; fenclofos]
fencilbutirol USAN, INN *choleretic*
fenclexonium metilsulfate INN
fenclofenac USAN, INN, BAN *anti-inflammatory*
fenclofos INN *systemic insecticide* [also: ronnel; fenchlorphos]
fenclonine USAN, INN *serotonin inhibitor*
fenclorac USAN, INN *anti-inflammatory*
fenclozic acid INN, BAN
fendiline INN
Fendol tablets OTC *decongestant; expectorant; analgesic; antipyretic* [phenylephrine HCl; acetaminophen; salicylamide; caffeine]
fendosal USAN, INN, BAN *anti-inflammatory*
feneritrol INN

Fenesin sustained-release tablet ℞ *expectorant* [guaifenesin]
fenestrel USAN, INN *estrogen*
fenethazine INN
fenethylline BAN *CNS stimulant* [also: fenethylline HCl; fenetylline]
fenethylline HCl USAN *CNS stimulant* [also: fenetylline; fenethylline]
fenetradil INN
fenetylline INN *CNS stimulant* [also: fenethylline HCl; fenethylline]
fenflumizole INN
fenfluramine INN, BAN *anorexiant* [also: fenfluramine HCl]
fenfluramine HCl USAN *anorexiant; CNS stimulant* [also: fenfluramine]
fenfluthrin INN, BAN
fengabine USAN, INN, BAN *mood regulator*
fenharmane INN
fenimide USAN, INN, BAN *antipsychotic*
feniodium chloride INN
fenipentol INN
fenirofibrate INN
fenisorex USAN, INN, BAN *anorexic*
fenmetozole INN *antidepressant; narcotic antagonist* [also: fenmetozole HCl]
fenmetozole HCl USAN *antidepressant; narcotic antagonist* [also: fenmetozole]
fenmetramide USAN, INN, BAN *antidepressant*
fennel oil NF
fenobam USAN, INN *sedative*
fenocinol INN
fenoctimine INN *gastric antisecretory* [also: fenoctimine sulfate]
fenoctimine sulfate USAN *gastric antisecretory* [also: fenoctimine]
fenofibrate INN, BAN
fenoldopam INN, BAN *antihypertensive; dopamine agonist* [also: fenoldopam mesylate]
fenoldopam mesylate USAN *antihypertensive; dopamine agonist* [also: fenoldopam]

fenoprofen USAN, INN, BAN *nonsteroidal anti-inflammatory drug (NSAID); analgesic*
fenoprofen calcium USAN, USP, BAN *antiarthritic; nonsteroidal anti-inflammatory drug (NSAID); analgesic*
fenoterol USAN, INN, BAN *bronchodilator*
fenoterol hydrobromide *bronchodilator*
fenoverine INN
fenoxazol [see: pemoline]
fenoxazoline INN
fenoxazoline HCl [see: fenoxazoline]
fenoxedil INN
fenoxypropazine INN [also: phenoxypropazine]
fenozolone INN
fenpentadiol INN
fenperate INN
fenpipalone USAN, INN *anti-inflammatory*
fenpipramide INN, BAN
fenpiprane INN, BAN
fenpiprane HCl [see: fenpiprane]
fenpiverinium bromide INN
fenprinast INN *bronchodilator; antiallergic* [also: fenprinast HCl]
fenprinast HCl USAN *bronchodilator; antiallergic* [also: fenprinast]
fenproporex INN
fenprostalene USAN, INN, BAN *luteolysin*
fenquizone USAN, INN *diuretic*
fenretinide USAN, INN *antineoplastic*
fenspiride INN *bronchodilator; antiadrenergic (α-receptor)* [also: fenspiride HCl]
fenspiride HCl USAN *bronchodilator; antiadrenergic (α-receptor)* [also: fenspiride]
fentanyl INN, BAN *narcotic analgesic* [also: fentanyl citrate]
fentanyl citrate USAN, USP *narcotic analgesic* [also: fentanyl]
fenthion BAN

fentiazac USAN, INN, BAN *anti-inflammatory*
fenticlor USAN, INN, BAN *topical anti-infective*
fenticonazole INN, BAN *antifungal* [also: fenticonazole nitrate]
fenticonazole nitrate USAN *antifungal* [also: fenticonazole]
fentonium bromide INN
fenyramidol INN *analgesic; skeletal muscle relaxant* [also: phenyramidol HCl]
fenyripol INN *skeletal muscle relaxant* [also: fenyripol HCl]
fenyripol HCl USAN *skeletal muscle relaxant* [also: fenyripol]
Feocyte prolonged-action tablets OTC *hematinic* [ferrous fumarate; ferrous gluconate; ferrous sulfate; desiccated liver; multiple vitamins; folic acid]
Fe-O.D. timed-release tablets OTC *hematinic* [ferrous fumarate; ascorbic acid]
Feosol elixir OTC *hematinic* [ferrous sulfate]
Feosol tablets, timed-release capsules OTC *hematinic* [ferrous sulfate, dried]
Feostat chewable tablets, suspension, drops OTC *hematinic* [ferrous fumarate]
Feostat IM injection (discontinued 1991) ℞ *antianemic* [iron dextran]
fepentolic acid INN
fepitrizol INN
fepradinol INN
feprazone INN, BAN
fepromide INN
feprosidnine INN
Ferancee chewable tablets OTC *hematinic* [ferrous fumarate; vitamin C]
Ferancee-HP film-coated tablets OTC *hematinic* [ferrous fumarate; vitamin C]
Feratab tablets OTC *hematinic* [ferrous sulfate]

Ferate-C tablets (discontinued 1991) OTC *antianemic* [ferrous fumarate; ascorbic acid]

Feratin tablets (discontinued 1991) OTC *antianemic* [ferrous fumarate; desiccated liver; multiple vitamins]

Fergon capsules (discontinued 1991) OTC *antianemic* [ferrous gluconate]

Fergon Iron Plus Calcium timed-release caplets (discontinued 1992) OTC *antianemic; calcium supplement* [ferrous gluconate; calcium; vitamin D]

Fergon Plus caplets ℞ *hematinic* [ferrous gluconate; vitamins B_{12} & C; intrinsic factor concentrate]

Fergon tablets, elixir OTC *hematinic* [ferrous gluconate]

Fer-In-Sol capsules OTC *hematinic* [ferrous sulfate, dried]

Fer-In-Sol drops, syrup OTC *hematinic* [ferrous sulfate]

Fer-Iron drops OTC *hematinic* [ferrous sulfate]

Fermalox tablets (discontinued 1992) OTC *hematinic* [magnesium hydroxide; aluminum hydroxide; ferrous sulfate]

fermium *element (Fm)*

Ferndex tablets (discontinued 1991) ℞ *CNS stimulant; amphetamine* [dextroamphetamine sulfate]

Ferocyl sustained-release tablets OTC *hematinic* [ferrous fumarate; docusate sodium]

Fero-Folic-500 controlled-release Filmtabs (film-coated tablets) ℞ *hematinic* [ferrous sulfate; vitamin C; folic acid]

Fero-Grad-500 controlled-release Filmtabs (film-coated tablets) OTC *hematinic* [ferrous sulfate; sodium ascorbate]

Fero-Gradumet timed-release Filmtabs (film-coated tablets) OTC *hematinic* [ferrous sulfate]

Feronim IM injection (discontinued 1991) ℞ *antianemic* [iron dextran]

Ferospace capsules OTC *hematinic* [ferrous sulfate]

Ferotrinsic capsules ℞ *hematinic* [ferrous fumarate; vitamins B_{12} & C; intrinsic factor concentrate; folic acid]

Ferralet Plus tablets OTC *hematinic* [ferrous gluconate; vitamins B_{12} & C; folic acid]

Ferralet S.R. sustained-release tablets OTC *hematinic* [ferrous gluconate]

Ferralet tablets OTC *hematinic* [ferrous gluconate]

Ferralyn Lanacaps (timed-release capsules) OTC *hematinic* [ferrous sulfate, dried]

Ferra-TD timed-release capsules OTC *hematinic* [ferrous sulfate, dried]

Ferretts tablets OTC *hematinic* [ferrous fumarate]

ferric ammonium citrate NF
ferric ammonium sulfate
ferric cacodylate NF
ferric chloride
ferric chloride Fe 59 USAN *radioactive agent*
ferric citrate (^{59}Fe) INN
ferric citrochloride NF
ferric fructose USAN, INN *hematinic*
ferric glycerophosphate NF
ferric hypophosphite NF
ferric oxide NF *coloring agent*
ferric oxide, red NF
ferric oxide, yellow NF
ferric pyrophosphate, soluble NF
ferric subsulfate NF
ferricholinate [see: ferrocholinate]
ferriclate calcium sodium USAN *hematinic* [also: calcium sodium ferriclate]

Ferro Dok TR timed-release capsules OTC *hematinic* [ferrous fumarate; docusate sodium]

ferrocholate [see: ferrocholinate]
ferrocholinate INN

Ferro-Docusate T.R. timed-release capsules OTC *hematinic* [ferrous fumarate; docusate sodium]

Ferro-DSS S.R. timed-release capsules OTC *hematinic* [ferrous fumarate; docusate sodium]

Ferromar sustained-release caplets OTC *hematinic* [ferrous fumarate; vitamin C]

Ferronex IM injection (discontinued 1991) ℞ *antianemic* [ferrous gluconate; multiple B vitamins; procaine]

ferropolimaler INN

Ferro-Sequels film-coated sustained-release tablets OTC *hematinic* [ferrous fumarate; docusate sodium]

Ferro-Sequels sustained-release capsules (discontinued 1991) OTC *antianemic* [ferrous fumarate; docusate sodium]

ferrotrenine INN

ferrous citrate Fe 59 USAN, USP *radioactive agent*

ferrous fumarate USP *hematinic*

ferrous gluconate USP *hematinic*

ferrous lactate NF

ferrous sulfate USP *hematinic*

ferrous sulfate, dried USP *antianemic*

ferrous sulfate, exsiccated [see: ferrous sulfate, dried]

ferrous sulfate Fe 59 USAN *radioactive agent*

Ferrous-S.Q.L. timed-release capsules (discontinued 1992) OTC *antianemic* [ferrous fumarate; docusate sodium]

fertirelin INN, BAN *veterinary gonadotropin-releasing hormone* [also: fertirelin acetate]

fertirelin acetate USAN *veterinary gonadotropin-releasing hormone* [also: fertirelin]

ferumoxides USAN *diagnostic aid for magnetic imaging*

ferumoxsil USAN *diagnostic aid for magnetic imaging*

Festal II enteric-coated tablets (discontinued 1992) OTC *digestive enzymes* [pancrelipase]

Festalan enteric-coated tablets (discontinued 1992) ℞ *digestive enzymes; antispasmodic; hypermotility reducer* [amylase; protease; lipase; atropine methylnitrate]

Festex Drawing salve (discontinued 1991) OTC *antiseptic; anesthetic; antifungal; anti-infective* [benzalkonium chloride; diperodon HCl; phenol; ichthammol; thymol; camphor; juniper tar]

Fetinic IM injection (discontinued 1991) ℞ *antianemic* [ferrous gluconate; multiple B vitamins]

Fetinic-MW sustained-release capsules (discontinued 1991) ℞ *antianemic* [ferrous fumarate; vitamins B_{12} & C]

fetoxilate INN *smooth muscle relaxant* [also: fetoxylate HCl; fetoxylate]

fetoxylate BAN *smooth muscle relaxant* [also: fetoxylate HCl; fetoxilate]

fetoxylate HCl USAN *smooth muscle relaxant* [also: fetoxilate; fetoxylate]

Feverall, Children's; Infant's Feverall; Junior Feverall suppositories OTC *analgesic; antipyretic* [acetaminophen]

Feverall Sprinkle Caps (powder) OTC *analgesic; antipyretic* [acetaminophen]

fexicaine INN

fexinidazole INN

fezatione INN

fezolamine INN *antidepressant* [also: fezolamine fumarate]

fezolamine fumarate USAN *antidepressant* [also: fezolamine]

fiacitabine (FIAC) USAN, INN *antiviral*

fialuridine (FIAU) *investigational antiviral for AIDS; (orphan: chronic active hepatitis B)*

Fiber Rich timed-release caplets (discontinued 1992) OTC *diet aid* [phenylpropanolamine HCl; grain & citrus fruit fiber]

Fiberall chewable tablets OTC *bulk laxative; antidiarrheal* [calcium polycarbophil]

Fiberall powder, wafers OTC *laxative* [psyllium hydrophilic mucilloid]

FiberCon film-coated tablets OTC *bulk laxative; antidiarrheal* [calcium polycarbophil]

Fiberlan liquid OTC *oral nutritional supplement*

Fiber-Lax tablets OTC *bulk laxative; antidiarrheal* [calcium polycarbophil]

FiberNorm tablets OTC *bulk laxative; antidiarrheal* [calcium polycarbophil]

fibracillin INN

Fibrad powder OTC *oral dietary fiber supplement* [pea, oat and sugar beet fiber]

fibrin INN

fibrinase [see: factor XIII]

fibrinogen (^{125}I) INN [also: fibrinogen I 125]

fibrinogen, human USP

fibrinogen I 125 USAN *vascular patency test; radioactive agent* [also: fibrinogen (^{125}I)]

fibrinoligase [see: factor XIII]

fibrinolysin, human INN [also: plasmin]

fibrinolysin & desoxyribonuclease *topical enzymes for necrotic tissue debridement*

fibrin-stabilizing factor (FSF) [see: factor XIII]

Fibriscint ℞ *investigational imaging aid for deep venous thrombosis* [monoclonal antibodies]

Fibrogammin P *(orphan: congenital factor XIII deficiency)* [factor XIII (placenta-derived)]

fibronectin *(orphan: nonhealing corneal ulcers or epithelial defects)*

filenadol INN

filgrastim USAN, INN, BAN *biological response midifier; bone marrow stimulant; (orphan: severe chronic neutropenia)*

Filibon F.A.; Filibon Forte tablets ℞ *vitamin/calcium/iron supplement* [multiple vitamins; calcium; iron; folic acid]

Filibon tablets OTC *vitamin/calcium/iron supplement* [multiple vitamins; calcium; iron; folic acid]

filipin USAN, INN *antifungal*

Filmix *(orphan: neurosonographic contrast medium, intracranial tumors)* [microbubble contrast agent]

Filmseals (trademarked form) *film-coated tablets*

Filmtab (trademarked form) *film-coated tablets*

FIME (fluorouracil, ICRF-159, MeCCNU) *chemotherapy protocol*

Finac lotion OTC *topical acne treatment* [sulfur; methylbenzethonium chloride; isopropyl alcohol]

finasteride USAN, INN, BAN *antineoplastic; androgen hormone inhibitor*

Fiogesic tablets OTC *decongestant; antihistamine; analgesic* [phenylpropanolamine HCl; pheniramine maleate; pyrilamine maleate; aspirin]

Fiorgen PF tablets ℞ *analgesic; antipyretic; sedative* [acetaminophen; caffeine; butalbital]

Fioricet tablets ℞ *analgesic; antipyretic; sedative* [acetaminophen; caffeine; butalbital]

Fioricet with Codeine capsules ℞ *narcotic analgesic; sedative* [codeine phosphate; acetaminophen; caffeine; butalbital]

Fiorinal tablets, capsules ℞ *analgesic; antipyretic; anti-inflammatory; sedative* [aspirin; caffeine; butalbital]

Fiorinal with Codeine No. 3 capsules ℞ *narcotic analgesic; sedative* [codeine phosphate; aspirin; caffeine; butalbital]

fipexide INN

fire ant venom allergenic extract *(orphan: test for and desensitize fire ant reactions)*

First Choice reagent strips OTC *in vitro diagnostic aid for blood glucose*

First Response home test kit OTC *in vitro diagnostic aid for urine pregnancy test*

First Response Ovulation Predictor test kit OTC *in vitro diagnostic aid to predict ovulation time*

fisalamine [see: mesalamine]

5 Benzagel; 10 Benzagel gel ℞ *keratolytic for acne* [benzoyl peroxide]

566C80 *(orphan: prevent and treat AIDS-related Pneumocystis carinii pneumonia)*

FK-565 *investigational immunomodulator for AIDS*

FLAC (fluorouracil, leucovorin calcium, Adriamycin, cyclophosphamide) *chemotherapy protocol*

Flagyl film-coated tablets ℞ *antibiotic; antiprotozoal; amebicide; (orphan: decubitus ulcers; acne rosacea; perioral dermatitis)* [metronidazole]

Flagyl IV powder for injection ℞ *antibiotic; antiprotozoal; amebicide* [metronidazole HCl]

Flagyl IV RTU (ready-to-use) injection ℞ *antibiotic; antiprotozoal; amebicide* [metronidazole]

flamenol INN

Flanders Buttocks ointment OTC *topical diaper rash treatment* [zinc oxide; balsam Peru]

FLAP (fluorouracil, leucovorin calcium, Adriamycin, Platinol) *chemotherapy protocol*

Flarex eye drop suspension ℞ *ophthalmic topical corticosteroidal anti-inflammatory* [fluorometholone acetate]

Flatulex drops OTC *antiflatulent* [simethicone]

Flatulex tablets OTC *adsorbent; detoxicant; antiflatulent* [activated charcoal; simethicone]

flavamine INN

flavine [see: acriflavine HCl]

flavodic acid INN

flavodilol INN *antihypertensive* [also: flavodilol maleate]

flavodilol maleate USAN *antihypertensive* [also: flavodilol]

flavonoid [see: troxerutin]

Flavons-500 tablets OTC *dietary supplement* [citrus bioflavonoids complex; hesperidin complex]

Flavorcee chewable tablets OTC *vitamin supplement* [ascorbic acid]

flavoxate INN, BAN *smooth muscle relaxant; urinary antispasmodic* [also: flavoxate HCl]

flavoxate HCl USAN *smooth muscle relaxant; urinary antispasmodic* [also: flavoxate]

Flaxedil IV ℞ *neuromuscular blocker* [gallamine triethiodide]

flazalone USAN, INN, BAN *anti-inflammatory*

flecainide INN, BAN *antiarrhythmic* [also: flecainide acetate]

flecainide acetate USAN *antiarrhythmic* [also: flecainide]

Fleet Babylax rectal liquid OTC *hyperosmolar laxative* [glycerin]

Fleet Bagenema rectal liquid OTC *laxative* [Castile soap]

Fleet Bisacodyl Enema; Fleet Bisacodyl Prep rectal liquid OTC *stimulant laxative* [bisacodyl]

Fleet Children's Enema rectal liquid OTC *saline laxative* [monobasic sodium phosphate; dibasic sodium phosphate]

Fleet Enema rectal liquid OTC *saline laxative* [monobasic sodium phosphate; dibasic sodium phosphate]

Fleet Flavored Castor Oil emulsion OTC *stimulant laxative* [castor oil]

Fleet Laxative enteric-coated tablets, suppositories OTC *laxative* [bisacodyl]

Fleet Mineral Oil Enema rectal liquid OTC *lubricant laxative* [mineral oil]

Fleet Phospho-Soda oral solution OTC *buffered saline laxative* [monobasic sodium phosphate; dibasic sodium phosphate]

Fleet Prep Kits No. 1 to No. 6 OTC *pre-procedure bowel evacuant* [other Fleet products in combination kits]

Fleet Relief Anesthetic Hemorrhoidal ointment OTC *topical local anesthetic* [pramoxine HCl]

Fleet Relief anorectal ointment OTC *hemorrhoidal astringent; protectant* [zinc oxide; white petrolatum; mineral oil]

flerobuterol INN

fleroxacin USAN, INN *antibacterial*

flesinoxan INN

flestolol INN *antiadrenergic (β-receptor)* [also: flestolol sulfate]

flestolol sulfate USAN *antiadrenergic (β-receptor)* [also: flestolol]

fletazepam USAN, INN, BAN *skeletal muscle relaxant*

Fletcher's Castoria liquid OTC *laxative* [senna concentrate]

Flex-all 454 gel OTC *topical analgesic; counterirritant; emollient; vulnerary* [menthol; methyl salicylate; trolamine; eucalyptus oil; allantoin; boric acid; aloe]

Flexaphen capsules ℞ *skeletal muscle relaxant; analgesic* [chlorzoxazone; acetaminophen]

Flex-Care solution OTC *contact lens disinfectant*

Flexeril film-coated tablets ℞ *skeletal muscle relaxant* [cyclobenzaprine HCl]

Flexoject IV or IM injection ℞ *skeletal muscle relaxant* [orphenadrine citrate]

Flexon IV or IM injection ℞ *skeletal muscle relaxant* [orphenadrine citrate]

Flint SSD (name changed to SSD cream in 1991)

Flintstones Children's; Flintstones Plus Extra C Children's chewable tablets OTC *vitamin supplement* [multiple vitamins; folic acid]

Flintstones Complete chewable tablets OTC *vitamin/mineral/iron supplement* [multiple vitamins & minerals; iron; folic acid; biotin]

Flintstones Plus Iron chewable tablets OTC *vitamin/iron supplement* [multiple vitamins; iron; folic acid]

Flo-Coat suspension ℞ *GI contrast radiopaque agent* [barium sulfate]

floctafenine USAN, INN, BAN *analgesic*

Flolan *(orphan: primary pulmonary hypertension; heparin replacement for hemodialysis)* [epoprostenol]

flomoxef INN

Flonase ℞ *investigational steroid for asthma*

Flo-Pack (trademarked form) *powder for injection*

flopropione INN

florantyrone INN, BAN

flordipine USAN, INN *antihypertensive*

floredil INN

floretione [see: fluoresone]

florfenicol USAN, INN, BAN *veterinary antibacterial*

Florical capsules, tablets OTC *calcium supplement* [calcium carbonate; sodium fluoride]

florifenine INN

Florinef Acetate tablets ℞ *adrenocortical insufficiency in Addison's disease* [fludrocortisone acetate]

Florone cream, ointment ℞ *topical corticosteroidal anti-inflammatory* [diflorasone diacetate]

Florone E cream ℞ *topical corticosteroidal anti-inflammatory; emollient* [diflorasone diacetate]

floropipamide [now: pipamperone]

floropipeton [see: propyperone]

Floropryl ophthalmic ointment ℞ *antiglaucoma agent; irreversible cholinesterase inhibitor miotic* [isoflurophate]

Florvite; Florvite Half Strength chewable tablets, drops ℞ *pediatric vitamin supplement and dental caries preventative* [multiple vitamins; sodium fluoride; folic acid]

Florvite + Iron chewable tablets, drops ℞ *pediatric vitamin/iron supple-*

ment and dental caries preventative [multiple vitamins & minerals; sodium fluoride; ferrous sulfate; folic acid]

Florvite liquid ℞ *pediatric vitamin deficiency and dental caries prevention* [multiple vitamins; sodium fluoride]

flosequinan USAN, INN, BAN *antihypertensive; vasodilator*

flotrenizine INN

floverine INN

floxacillin USAN *antibacterial* [also: flucloxacillin]

floxacrine INN

Floxin film-coated tablets, IV injection ℞ *broad-spectrum fluoroquinolone-type antibiotic* [ofloxacin]

floxuridine USAN, USP, INN *antiviral; antineoplastic*

Floxyfral ℞ *investigational antidepressant; antipsychotic* [fluvoxamine]

FLT (fluorothymidine) [q.v.]

Flu, Cold & Cough Medicine powder OTC *decongestant; antihistamine; antitussive; analgesic* [pseudoephedrine HCl; chlorpheniramine maleate; dextromethorphan hydrobromide; acetaminophen]

fluacizine INN

flualamide INN

fluanisone INN, BAN

fluazacort USAN, INN *anti-inflammatory*

flubanilate INN *CNS stimulant* [also: flubanilate HCl]

flubanilate HCl USAN *CNS stimulant* [also: flubanilate]

flubendazole USAN, INN, BAN *antiprotozoal*

flubenisolone [see: betamethasone]

flubepride INN

flubuperone [see: melperone]

flucarbril INN

flucetorex INN

flucindole USAN, INN *antipsychotic*

fluciprazine INN

fluclorolone acetonide INN, BAN *glucocorticoid* [also: flucloronide]

flucloronide USAN *glucocorticoid* [also: fluclorolone acetonide]

flucloxacillin INN, BAN *antibacterial* [also: floxacillin]

fluconazole USAN, INN, BAN *broad-spectrum fungistatic*

flucrilate INN *tissue adhesive* [also: flucrylate]

flucrylate USAN *tissue adhesive* [also: flucrilate]

flucytosine USAN, USP, INN, BAN *fungicidal*

fludalanine USAN, INN *antibacterial*

Fludara powder for IV injection ℞ *antineoplastic; (orphan: chronic lymphocytic leukemia; non-Hodgkin's lymphoma)* [fludarabine phosphate]

fludarabine INN *antineoplastic* [also: fludarabine phosphate]

fludarabine phosphate USAN *antineoplastic; (orphan: chronic lymphocytic leukemia; non-Hodgkin's lymphoma)* [also: fludarabine]

fludazonium chloride USAN, INN *topical anti-infective*

fludeoxyglucose (^{18}F) INN *diagnostic aid; radioactive agent* [also: fludeoxyglucose F 18]

fludeoxyglucose F 18 USAN, USP *diagnostic aid; radioactive agent* [also: fludeoxyglucose (^{18}F)]

fludiazepam INN

fludorex USAN, INN *anorexic; antiemetic*

fludoxopone INN

fludrocortisone INN, BAN *salt-regulating adrenocortical steroid; mineralocorticoid* [also: fludrocortisone acetate]

fludrocortisone acetate USP *salt-regulating adrenocortical steroid; mineralocorticoid* [also: fludrocortisone]

fludroxicortide [see: flurandrenolide]

fludroxycortide INN *topical corticosteroid* [also: flurandrenolide; flurandrenolone]

flufenamic acid USAN, INN, BAN *anti-inflammatory*

flufenisal USAN, INN *analgesic*
flufosal INN
flufylline INN
flugestone INN, BAN *progestin* [also: flurogestone acetate]
flugestone acetate [see: flurogestone acetate]
Fluidex tablets (discontinued 1992) OTC *mild diuretic* [buchu; couch grass; corn silk; hydrangea]
Fluidex with Pamabrom capsules (discontinued 1992) OTC *diuretic* [pamabrom]
Flu-Imune IM injection ℞ *flu vaccine* [influenza purified surface antigen]
fluindarol INN
fluindione INN
Flumadine ℞ *investigational antiviral; flu prophylaxis* [rimantadine HCl]
flumazenil USAN, INN, BAN *antagonist to benzodiazepine*
flumazepil [see: flumazenil]
flumecinol INN *(orphan: neonatal hyperbilirubinemia)*
flumedroxone INN, BAN
flumequine USAN, INN, BAN *antibacterial*
flumeridone USAN, INN, BAN *antiemetic*
flumetasone INN *glucocorticoid* [also: flumethasone]
flumethasone USAN, BAN *glucocorticoid* [also: flumetasone]
flumethasone pivalate USAN, USP, BAN *glucocorticoid*
flumethiazide INN, BAN
flumethrin BAN
flumetramide USAN, INN *skeletal muscle relaxant*
flumexadol INN
flumezapine USAN, INN, BAN *antipsychotic; neuroleptic*
fluminorex USAN, INN *anorexic*
flumizole USAN, INN *anti-inflammatory*
flumoxonide USAN, INN *adrenocortical steroid*

Flumucil ℞ *investigational immunomodulator for AIDS* [acetylcysteine]
flunamine INN
flunarizine INN, BAN *vasodilator; (orphan: alternating hemiplegia)* [also: flunarizine HCl]
flunarizine HCl USAN *vasodilator* [also: flunarizine]
flunidazole USAN, INN *antiprotozoal*
flunisolide USAN, USP, INN, BAN *corticosteroid inhalant for asthma; intranasal steroid*
flunisolide acetate USAN *anti-inflammatory*
flunitrazepam USAN, INN, BAN *hypnotic*
flunixin USAN, INN, BAN *anti-inflammatory; analgesic*
flunixin meglumine USAN *anti-inflammatory; analgesic*
flunoprost INN
flunoxaprofen INN
fluocinolide [now: fluocinonide]
fluocinolone BAN *topical corticosteroid* [also: fluocinolone acetonide]
fluocinolone acetonide USAN, USP, INN *topical corticosteroid* [also: fluocinolone]
fluocinonide USAN, USP, INN, BAN *topical corticosteroid*
fluocortin INN *anti-inflammatory* [also: fluocortin butyl]
fluocortin butyl USAN, BAN *anti-inflammatory* [also: fluocortin]
fluocortolone USAN, INN, BAN *glucocorticoid*
fluocortolone caproate USAN *glucocorticoid*
Fluogen IM injection, Steri-Vials, Steri-Dose (disposable syringes) ℞ *flu vaccine* [influenza split-virus vaccine]
Fluonex cream ℞ *topical corticosteroid* [fluocinonide]
Fluonid topical solution ℞ *topical corticosteroid* [fluocinolone acetonide]
fluopromazine BAN *antipsychotic* [also: triflupromazine]

Fluoracaine eye drops ℞ topical ocular anesthetic; disclosing agent [fluorescein sodium; proparacaine HCl]
fluoracizine [see: fluacizine]
fluorescein USP, BAN corneal trauma indicator
fluorescein, soluble [now: fluorescein sodium]
fluorescein sodium USP, BAN corneal trauma indicator
Fluorescite IV injection ℞ corneal disclosing agent [fluorescein sodium]
Fluoresoft solution ℞ ocular topical fluorescent [fluorexon]
fluoresone INN
Fluorets ophthalmic strips OTC corneal disclosing agent [fluorescein sodium]
fluorexon diagnosis and fitting aid for contact lenses
fluorhydrocortisone acetate [see: fludrocortisone acetate]
Fluorigard oral rinse OTC topical dental caries preventative [sodium fluoride]
Fluori-Methane spray ℞ topical vapocoolant anesthetic [trichloromonofluoromethane; dichlorodifluoromethane]
fluorine element (F)
fluorine F 18 fluorodeoxyglucose [see: fludeoxyglucose F 18]
Fluorinse oral rinse ℞ topical dental caries preventative [sodium fluoride]
Fluor-I-Strip; Fluor-I-Strip A.T. ophthalmic strips ℞ corneal disclosing agent [fluorescein sodium]
Fluoritab chewable tablets, drops ℞ dental caries preventative [sodium fluoride]
fluormethylprednisolone [see: dexamethasone]
5-fluorocytosine (5-FC) [see: flucytosine]
fluorodeoxyglucose F 18 [see: fludeoxyglucose F 18]

fluorometholone USP, INN, BAN glucocorticoid; ophthalmic anti-inflammatory
fluorometholone acetate USAN anti-inflammatory
Fluor-Op eye drop suspension ℞ ophthalmic topical corticosteroidal anti-inflammatory [fluorometholone]
Fluoroplex cream, topical solution ℞ antineoplastic for actinic keratoses and basal cell carcinomas [fluorouracil]
fluorosalan USAN disinfectant [also: flusalan]
fluorothymidine (FLT) investigational antiviral for AIDS
fluorouracil USAN, USP, INN, BAN antineoplastic; (orphan: adjuvant to colorectal and esophageal cancer)
fluoruridine deoxyribose [see: floxuridine]
Fluosol emulsion for intracoronary perfusion ℞ myocardial oxygenation during PTCA [intravascular perfluorochemical (PFC) emulsion]
fluostigmine [see: isoflurophate]
Fluothane liquid for vaporization ℞ inhalation general anesthetic [halothane]
fluotracen INN antipsychotic; antidepressant [also: fluotracen HCl]
fluotracen HCl USAN antipsychotic; antidepressant [also: fluotracen]
fluoxetine USAN, INN, BAN antidepressant
fluoxetine HCl USAN antidepressant; used for obsessive-compulsive disorders and bulimia
fluoximesterone [see: fluoxymesterone]
fluoxiprednisolone [see: triamcinolone]
fluoxymesterone USP, INN, BAN oral androgen
fluparoxan INN, BAN antidepressant [also: fluparoxan HCl]
fluparoxan HCl USAN antidepressant [also: fluparoxan]

flupenthixol BAN [also: flupentixol]
flupentixol INN [also: flupenthixol]
fluperamide USAN, INN *antiperistaltic*
fluperlapine INN
fluperolone INN, BAN *glucocorticoid* [also: fluperolone acetate]
fluperolone acetate USAN *glucocorticoid* [also: fluperolone]
fluphenazine INN, BAN *antipsychotic* [also: fluphenazine enanthate]
fluphenazine decanoate *antipsychotic; prolonged parenteral neuroleptic therapy*
fluphenazine enanthate USP *antipsychotic; prolonged parenteral neuroleptic therapy* [also: fluphenazine]
fluphenazine HCl USP, BAN *antipsychotic*
flupimazine INN
flupirtine INN, BAN *analgesic* [also: flupirtine maleate]
flupirtine maleate USAN *analgesic* [also: flupirtine]
flupranone INN
fluprazine INN
fluprednidene INN, BAN
fluprednisolone USAN, NF, INN, BAN *glucocorticoid*
fluprednisolone valerate USAN *glucocorticoid*
fluprofen INN, BAN
fluprofylline INN
fluproquazone USAN, INN, BAN *analgesic*
fluprostenol INN, BAN *prostaglandin* [also: fluprostenol sodium]
fluprostenol sodium USAN *prostaglandin* [also: fluprostenol]
fluquazone USAN, INN *anti-inflammatory*
Flura tablets ℞ *dental caries preventative* [sodium fluoride]
fluracil [see: fluorouracil]
fluradoline INN *analgesic* [also: fluradoline HCl]
fluradoline HCl USAN *analgesic* [also: fluradoline]

Flura-Drops ℞ *dental caries preventative* [sodium fluoride]
Flura-Loz lozenges ℞ *dental caries preventative* [sodium fluoride]
flurandrenolide USAN, USP *topical corticosteroid* [also: fludroxycortide; flurandrenolone]
flurandrenolone BAN *topical corticosteroid* [also: flurandrenolide; fludroxycortide]
flurantel INN
flurazepam INN, BAN *anticonvulsant; hypnotic; muscle relaxant; sedative* [also: flurazepam HCl]
flurazepam HCl USAN, USP *anticonvulsant; hypnotic; muscle relaxant; sedative* [also: flurazepam]
flurbiprofen USAN, USP, INN, BAN *antiarthritic; nonsteroidal anti-inflammatory drug (NSAID); analgesic*
flurbiprofen sodium USP *prostaglandin synthesis inhibitor; antimiotic; ocular nonsteroidal anti-inflammatory drug (NSAID)*
Fluress eye drops ℞ *topical ophthalmic anesthetic; corneal disclosing agent* [benoxinate HCl; fluorescein sodium]
fluretofen USAN, INN *anti-inflammatory; antithrombotic*
flurfamide [now: flurofamide]
flurithromycin INN
flurocitabine USAN, INN *antineoplastic*
Fluro-Ethyl aerosol spray ℞ *topical refrigerant anesthetic* [ethyl chloride; dichlorotetrafluoroethane]
flurofamide USAN, INN *urease enzyme inhibitor*
flurogestone acetate USAN *progestin* [also: flugestone]
Flurosyn ointment, cream ℞ *topical corticosteroid* [fluocinolone acetonide]
flurothyl USAN, USP, BAN *CNS stimulant* [also: flurotyl]

flurotyl INN CNS *stimulant* [also: flurothyl]
fluroxene USAN, NF, INN *inhalation anesthetic*
fluroxyspiramine [see: spiramide]
flusalan INN *disinfectant* [also: fluorosalan]
flusoxolol INN, BAN
fluspiperone USAN, INN *antipsychotic*
fluspirilene USAN, INN, BAN *antipsychotic*
flutamide USAN, INN, BAN *antineoplastic; antiandrogen hormone*
flutazolam INN
flutemazepam INN
Flutex ointment, cream ℞ *topical corticosteroid* [trimacinolone acetonide]
flutiazin USAN, INN *veterinary anti-inflammatory*
fluticasone INN, BAN *topical corticosteroidal anti-inflammatory* [also: fluticasone propionate]
fluticasone propionate USAN *topical corticosteroidal anti-inflammatory* [also: fluticasone]
flutizenol INN
flutomidate INN
flutonidine INN
flutoprazepam INN
flutrimazole INN
flutroline USAN, INN *antipsychotic*
flutropium bromide INN
fluvastatin sodium USAN *antihypercholesterolemic; HMG-CoA reductase inhibitor*
fluvoxamine INN, BAN *investigational antidepressant; antipsychotic; serotonin reuptake inhibitor*
fluzinamide USAN, INN *anticonvulsant*
Fluzone IM injection ℞ *flu vaccine* [influenza split-virus/whole-virus vaccine]
fluzoperine INN
FML Liquifilm; FML Forte eye drop suspension ℞ *ophthalmic topical corticosteroidal anti-inflammatory* [fluorometholone]
FML ophthalmic ointment ℞ *ophthalmic topical corticosteroidal anti-inflammatory* [fluorometholone]
FML-S eye drop suspension ℞ *ophthalmic topical corticosteroidal anti-inflammatory; bacteriostatic antibiotic* [fluorometholone; sulfacetamide sodium]
FNM (fluorouracil, Novantrone, methotrexate) *chemotherapy protocol*
FOAM (fluorouracil, Oncovin, Adriamycin, mitomycin) *chemotherapy protocol*
Foamicon Antacid chewable tablets OTC *antacid* [aluminum hydroxide; magnesium trisilicate]
Focalpak kit ℞ *fluorescein angiography* [fluorescein]
focofilcon A USAN *hydrophilic contact lens material*
Foille Medicated First Aid lotion (discontinued 1991) OTC *topical local anesthetic* [benzocaine; chloroxylenol]
Foille Medicated First Aid ointment, aerosol spray OTC *topical antiseptic, analgesic, and anesthetic* [benzocaine; chloroxylenol]
Foille Plus aerosol spray OTC *topical antiseptic, analgesic, and anesthetic* [benzocaine; chloroxylenol]
Foille spray OTC *topical antiseptic, analgesic, and anesthetic* [benzocaine; chloroxylenol]
FoilleCort cream OTC *topical corticosteroid* [hydrocortisone acetate]
Folabee IM ℞ *antianemic; vitamin supplement* [liver extracts; vitamin B_{12}; folic acid]
folacin [see: folic acid]
folate [see: folic acid]
folate sodium USP
folescutol INN
Folex PFS powder for IV or IM injection ℞ *antineoplastic for leukemia;*

systemic antipsoriatic; antirheumatic [methotrexate sodium]

Folex powder for IV or IM injection (discontinued 1992) ℞ *antineoplastic for leukemia; systemic antipsoriatic; antirheumatic* [methotrexate sodium]

folic acid USP, INN, BAN *vitamin B_c; vitamin M; hematopoietic*

folinate-SF calcium [see: leucovorin calcium]

folinic acid [see: leucovorin calcium]

follicle-stimulating hormone (FSH) BAN [also: menotropins]

follidrin [see: estradiol benzoate]

follotropin [see: menotropins]

Follow-Up [see: Carnation Follow-Up]

Follutein powder for injection ℞ *hormone for prepubertal cryptorchidism and hypogonadism* [chorionic gonadotropin]

Foltrin capsules ℞ *hematinic* [liver-stomach concentrate; multiple vitamins; ferrous fumarate]

Folvite tablets, IM injection ℞ *antianemic* [folic acid]

fomepizole USAN *antidote; alcohol dehydrogenase inhibitor; (orphan: methanol or ethylene glycol poisoning)*

FOMI; FOMi (fluorouracil, Oncovin, mitomycin) *chemotherapy protocol*

fomidacillin INN, BAN

fominoben INN

fomocaine INN, BAN

fonatol [see: diethylstilbestrol]

fonazine mesylate USAN *serotonin inhibitor* [also: dimetotiazine; dimethothiazine]

fontarsol [see: dichlorophenarsine HCl]

Footwork aerosol powder (discontinued 1991) OTC *topical antifungal* [tolnaftate]

fopirtoline INN

Forane liquid for vaporization ℞ *inhalation general anesthetic* [isoflurane]

forfenimex INN

formaldehyde solution USP *disinfectant*

Formalyde-10 spray ℞ *for hyperhidrosis and bromhidrosis* [formaldehyde]

formebolone INN, BAN

formetamide [see: formetorex]

formetorex INN

formidacillin [see: fomidacillin]

forminitrazole INN, BAN

formocortal USAN, INN, BAN *glucocorticoid*

formoterol INN

Formula 44 Cough Control Disks; Formula 44 Cough Silencers lozenges OTC *antitussive; topical local anesthetic* [dextromethorphan hydrobromide; benzocaine]

Formula 44 Cough Medicine liquid (discontinued 1992) OTC *antihistamine; antitussive* [chlorpheniramine maleate; dextromethorphan hydrobromide; alcohol]

Formula 44; Formula 44 Pediatric Formula syrup OTC *antitussive* [dextromethorphan hydrobromide]

Formula 44D liquid OTC *decongestant; antitussive* [pseudoephedrine HCl; dextromethorphan hydrobromide; alcohol]

Formula 44e, Pediatric liquid OTC *antitussive; expectorant* [dextromethorphan hydrobromide; guaifenesin]

Formula 44M Cough and Cold liquid OTC *decongestant; antihistamine; antitussive; analgesic* [pseudoephedrine HCl; chlorpheniramine maleate; dextromethorphan hydrobromide; acetaminophen; alcohol]

Formula B Plus tablets ℞ *vitamin/mineral/iron supplement* [multiple vitamins & minerals; ferrous fumarate; folic acid; biotin]

Formula B tablets ℞ *vitamin supplement* [multiple B vitamins; vitamin C; folic acid]

Formula E 400; Formula E 1000
perles OTC *vitamin supplement* [vitamin E]
Formula N sustained-release tablets OTC *vitamin supplement* [niacin]
Formula N-AM sustained-release tablets OTC *vitamin supplement* [niacinamide]
Formula Q capsules OTC *prevention and treatment of nocturnal leg cramps* [quinine sulfate]
Formula VM-2000 tablets OTC *dietary supplement* [multiple vitamins, minerals & amino acids; folic acid; biotin]
4′-formylacetanilide thiosemicarbazone [see: amithiozone]
forskolin [see: colforsin]
Forta Drink; Forta Shake powder OTC *oral nutritional supplement*
Fortaz powder for IV or IM injection ℞ *cephalosporin-type antibiotic* [ceftazidime]
Forte L.I.V. IM injection ℞ *antianemic* [ferrous gluconate; multiple B vitamins; procaine]
Fortel Home Ovulation Test kit OTC *in vitro diagnostic aid to predict ovulation time*
fortimicin A [now: astromicin sulfate]
Fosamax ℞ *investigational osteoporosis treatment* [alendronate]
fosarilate USAN, INN *antiviral*
fosazepam USAN, INN, BAN *hypnotic*
foscarnet sodium USAN, INN, BAN *antiviral*
Foscavir IV injection ℞ *antiviral for cytomegalovirus retinitis in AIDS* [foscarnet sodium]
foscolic acid INN
fosenazide INN
fosenopril sodium [see: fosinopril sodium]
fosfestrol INN, BAN *antineoplastic; estrogen* [also: diethylstilbestrol diphosphate]
fosfocreatinine INN

fosfomycin USAN, INN, BAN *antibacterial*
fosfomycin tromethamine USAN *antibacterial*
fosfonet sodium USAN, INN *antiviral*
fosfosal INN
Fosfree tablets OTC *vitamin/calcium/iron supplement* [multiple vitamins; calcium; iron]
fosinopril INN, BAN *antihypertensive; angiotensin-converting enzyme (ACE) inhibitor* [also: fosinopril sodium]
fosinopril sodium USAN *antihypertensive; angiotensin-converting enzyme (ACE) inhibitor* [also: fosinopril]
fosinoprilat USAN, INN *antihypertensive*
fosmenic acid INN
fosmidomycin INN
fosphenytoin INN *(orphan: grand mal status epilepticus)*
fospirate USAN, INN *veterinary anthelmintic*
fosquidone USAN, INN, BAN *antineoplastic*
fostedil USAN, INN *vasodilator; calcium channel blocker*
Fostex 10% BPO wash (liquid), bar, gel, tinted cream OTC *topical keratolytic for acne* [benzoyl peroxide]
Fostex 5% BPO gel OTC *topical keratolytic for acne* [benzoyl peroxide]
Fostex Medicated Cleansing Bar OTC *acne cleansing bar* [sulfur; salicylic acid; boric acid; docusate sodium; urea]
Fostex Medicated Cleansing Shampoo OTC *antiseborrheic; keratolytic* [sulfur; salicylic acid]
Fostex Medicated Cover-Up cream OTC *antibacterial; exfoliant* [sulfur]
fostriecin INN *antineoplastic* [also: fostriecin sodium]
fostriecin sodium USAN *antineoplastic* [also: fostriecin]
Fostril lotion OTC *topical acne treatment* [sulfur; zinc oxide]

fotemustine INN, BAN
Fototar cream OTC *topical antipsoriatic; antiseborrheic* [coal tar]
Fototar stick (discontinued 1991) OTC *topical antipsoriatic; antiseborrheic* [coal tar]
fotretamine INN
Fouchet's reagent (solution)
4-Way Cold tablets OTC *decongestant; antihistamine; analgesic* [phenylpropanolamine HCl; chlorpheniramine maleate; acetaminophen]
4-Way Fast Acting nasal spray OTC *nasal decongestant; antihistamine* [phenylephrine HCl; naphazoline HCl; pyrilamine maleate]
4-Way Long Lasting nasal spray OTC *nasal decongestant* [oxymetazoline HCl]
Fourneau 309 (available only from the Centers for Disease Control) ℞ *investigational anti-infective for trypanosomiasis and onchocerciasis* [suramin sodium]
frabuprofen INN
Fractar (trademarked ingredient) OTC *antipsoriatic; antiseborrheic* [crude coal tar]
Fragmin ℞ *investigational anticoagulant*
framycetin INN, BAN
francium *element (Fr)*
FreAmine III 3% (8.5%) with Electrolytes IV infusion ℞ *total parenteral nutrition (8.5% only); peripheral parenteral nutrition (both)* [multiple essential & nonessential amino acids & electrolytes]
FreAmine III 3% IV infusion (discontinued 1992) ℞ *peripheral parenteral nutrition* [multiple essential & nonessential amino acids]
FreAmine III 8.5%; FreAmine III 10% IV infusion ℞ *total parenteral nutrition; peripheral parenteral nutrition* [multiple essential & nonessential amino acids]
FreAmine HBC 6.9% IV infusion ℞ *nutritional therapy for high metabolic stress* [multiple branched-chain essential & nonessential amino acids; electrolytes]
Freedavite tablets OTC *vitamin/mineral/iron supplement* [multiple vitamins & minerals; ferrous fumarate]
Freedox ℞ *investigational lazaroid for subarachnoid hemorrhage, ischemic stroke, spinal cord and head injury*
Freezone liquid OTC *topical keratolytic* [salicylic acid]
frentizole USAN, INN, BAN *immunoregulator*
Frepp scrub applicators (discontinued 1991) OTC *broad-spectrum antimicrobial* [povidone-iodine]
Frepp/Sepp kit (discontinued 1991) OTC *broad-spectrum antimicrobial* [povidone-iodine]
Frisium ℞ *investigational benzodiazepine-type tranquilizer; anxiolytic* [clobazam]
fronepidil INN
froxiprost INN
fructose (D-fructose) USP *nutrient; caloric replacement* [also: levulose]
Fruity Chews chewable tablets OTC *vitamin supplement* [multiple vitamins; folic acid]
Fruity Chews with Iron chewable tablets OTC *vitamin/mineral/iron supplement* [multiple vitamins & minerals; iron; folic acid]
frusemide BAN *diuretic* [also: furosemide]
FS Shampoo ℞ *topical corticosteroid; antiseborrheic* [fluocinolone acetonide]
FSF (fibrin-stabilizing factor) [see: factor XIII]
FSH (follicle-stimulating hormone) [see: menotropins]
ftalofyne INN *veterinary anthelmintic* [also: phthalofyne]
ftaxilide INN
ftivazide INN
ftormetazine INN
ftorpropazine INN

5-FU (5-fluorouracil) [see: fluorouracil]
fubrogonium iodide INN
fuchsin, basic USP *topical antibacterial/antifungal*
FUDR; FUdR (5-fluorouracil deoxyribonucleoside) [see: floxuridine]
FUDR powder for IV injection ℞ *antineoplastic for GI adenocarcinoma metastatic to liver* [floxuridine]
Ful-Glo ophthalmic strips ℞ *corneal disclosing agent* [fluorescein sodium]
fulmicoton [see: pyroxylin]
Fulvicin P/G tablets ℞ *systemic antifungal* [griseofulvin (ultramicrosize)]
Fulvicin U/F tablets ℞ *systemic antifungal* [griseofulvin (microsize)]
FUM (fluorouracil, methotrexate) *chemotherapy protocol*
fumagillin INN, BAN
Fumaral Spancaps (timed-release capsules) OTC *antianemic* [ferrous fumarate; ascorbic acid]
fumaric acid NF *acidifier*
Fumasorb tablets OTC *hematinic* [ferrous fumarate]
Fumatinic sustained-release capsules ℞ *hematinic* [ferrous fumarate; vitamins B_{12} & C; folic acid]
Fumatrin Forte tablets (discontinued 1991) ℞ *antianemic* [ferrous fumarate; desiccated liver; multiple vitamins]
Fumerin sugar-coated tablets OTC *hematinic* [ferrous fumarate]
Fumide tablets ℞ *loop diuretic* [furosemide]
fumoxicillin USAN, INN *antibacterial*
Funduscein-10; Funduscein-25 IV injection ℞ *corneal disclosing agent* [fluorescein sodium]
Fungacetin ointment (discontinued 1991) OTC *topical antifungal* [triacetin]
Fungatin cream OTC *topical antifungal* [tolnaftate]
fungimycin USAN *antifungal*

Fungi-Nail liquid OTC *topical antifungal; keratolytic; anesthetic* [resorcinol; salicylic acid; chloroxylenol; benzocaine; alcohol]
Fungizone cream, lotion, ointment ℞ *topical antifungal* [amphotericin B]
Fungizone IV infusion ℞ *systemic antifungal* [amphotericin B]
Fungoid cream, solution, tincture ℞ *topical antifungal* [triacetin; cetylpyridinium chloride; chloroxylenol]
Fungoid-HC cream ℞ *topical corticosteroid; antipruritic; antifungal; antibacterial* [hydrocortisone; triacetin; cetylpyridinium chloride; chloroxylenol]
fuprazole INN
furacilin [see: nitrofurazone]
Furacin soluble dressing (ointment), cream ℞ *broad-spectrum antibacterial for adjunctive burn therapy* [nitrofurazone]
furacrinic acid INN, BAN
Furadantin tablets, oral suspension ℞ *urinary antibacterial* [nitrofurantoin]
furafylline INN
Furalan tablets ℞ *urinary antibacterial* [nitrofurantoin]
furalazine INN
furaltadone INN, BAN
Furamide (available only from the Centers for Disease Control) ℞ *investigational anti-infective for amebiasis* [diloxanide furoate]
Furan tablets (discontinued 1992) ℞ *urinary antibacterial* [nitrofurantoin]
Furanite tablets ℞ *urinary antibacterial* [nitrofurantoin]
furaprofen USAN, INN *anti-inflammatory*
furazabol INN
furazolidone USP, INN, BAN *bactericidal; antiprotozoal (Trichomonas); antidiarrheal*
furazolium chloride USAN, INN *antibacterial*
furazolium tartrate USAN *antibacterial*

furbucillin INN
furcloprofen INN
furegrelate INN *thromboxane synthetase inhibitor* [also: furegrelate sodium]
furegrelate sodium USAN *thromboxane synthetase inhibitor* [also: furegrelate]
furethidine INN, BAN
furfenorex INN
furfuryltrimethylammonium iodide [see: furtrethonium iodide]
furidarone INN
furmethoxadone INN
furobufen USAN, INN *anti-inflammatory*
furodazole USAN, INN *anthelmintic*
furofenac INN
furomazine INN
Furomide M.D. injection ℞ *loop diuretic* [furosemide]
Furonatal F.A. tablets ℞ *antianemic* [multiple vitamins & minerals]
furosemide USAN, USP, INN *loop diuretic; antihypertensive* [also: frusemide]
furostilbestrol INN
furoxicillin [see: fumoxicillin]
Furoxone tablets, liquid ℞ *antibacterial* [furazolidone]
fursalan USAN, INN *disinfectant*
fursultiamine INN
furterene INN
furtrethonium iodide INN
furtrimethonium iodide [see: furtrethonium iodide]
fusafungine INN, BAN
fusidate sodium USAN *antibacterial*
fusidic acid USAN, INN, BAN *antibacterial*
fusidic acid, sodium salt [see: fusidate sodium]
FUVAC (5-FU, vinblastine, Adriamycin, cyclophosphamide) *chemotherapy protocol*
fuzlocillin INN, BAN
fytic acid INN

G

G-1 capsules (name changed to Tencet in 1991)
G-201 ℞ *investigational topical nonsteroidal anti-inflammatory drug (NSAID) for skin disorders*
G-203 wipe ℞ *investigational topical corticosteroid for eczema and atopic dermatitis* [fluocinonide]
67Ga [see: gallium citrate Ga 67]
gabapentin USAN, INN *anticonvulsant*
gabexate INN
gaboxadol INN
gadodiamide USAN, INN *diagnostic aid for magnetic imaging*
gadolinium *element (Gd)*
gadopenamide INN
gadopentetate dimeglumine USAN *radiopaque medium* [also: gadopentetic acid]
gadopentetic acid INN, BAN *diagnostic aid* [also: gadopentetate dimeglumine]
gadoteric acid INN
gadoteridol USAN, INN, BAN *diagnostic aid for magnetic imaging*
gaiactamine [see: guaiactamine]
gaietamine [see: guaiactamine]
galamustine INN
galantamine INN
galantamine hydrobromide
galanthamine [see: galantamine]
Galardin ℞ *investigational treatment for corneal ulcers*

gallamine BAN *neuromuscular blocker* [also: gallamine triethiodide]
gallamine triethiodide USP, INN *neuromuscular blocker; muscle relaxant* [also: gallamine]
gallamone triethiodide [see: gallamine triethiodide]
gallic acid NF
gallic acid, bismuth basic salt [see: bismuth subgallate]
gallium *element (Ga)*
gallium (^{67}Ga) citrate INN *radiopaque medium; radioactive agent* [also: gallium citrate Ga 67]
gallium citrate Ga 67 USAN, USP *radiopaque medium; radioactive agent* [also: gallium (^{67}Ga) citrate]
gallium nitrate USAN *calcium regulator; (orphan: hypercalcemia of malignancy)*
gallium nitrate nonahydrate [see: gallium nitrate]
gallopamil INN, BAN
gallotannic acid [see: tannic acid]
galosemide INN
galtifenin INN
Gamastan IM injection ℞ *passive immunizing agent* [immune globulin]
gamfexine USAN, INN *antidepressant*
Gamimune N IV infusion ℞ *passive immunizing agent; investigational immunomodulator for AIDS* [immune globulin]
gamma benzene hexachloride [now: lindane]
gamma globulin [see: globulin, immune]
Gammagard powder for IV infusion ℞ *passive immunizing agent* [immune globulin]
gamma-hydroxybutyrate sodium [see: hydroxybutyrate sodium, gamma]
gamma-linolenic acid (GLA)
gammaphos [now: ethiofos]
Gammar IM injection ℞ *immunizing agent* [immune globulin]

Gammar-IV powder for IV infusion ℞ *immunizing agent* [immune globulin]
gamma-vinyl GABA (gamma-aminobutyric acid) [see: vigabatrin]
gamolenic acid INN, BAN
Gamulin Rh IM injection ℞ *obstetric Rh factor immunity suppressant* [Rh$_0$(D) immune globulin]
ganciclovir USAN, INN, BAN *antiviral* [also: ganciclovir sodium]
ganciclovir sodium USAN *antiviral; (orphan: cytomegalovirus retinitis in AIDS)* [also: ganciclovir]
ganglefene INN
gangliosides, sodium salts *(orphan: retinitis pigmentosa)*
ganirelix INN *gonad-stimulating principle* [also: ganirelix acetate]
ganirelix acetate USAN *gonad-stimulating principle* [also: ganirelix]
Ganite IV infusion ℞ *calcium resorption inhibitor; (orphan: hypercalcemia of malignancy)* [gallium nitrate]
Gantanol tablets, oral suspension ℞ *broad-spectrum bacteriostatic* [sulfamethoxazole]
Gantrisin eye drops ℞ *ophthalmic bacteriostatic* [sulfisoxazole diolamine]
Gantrisin ophthalmic ointment (discontinued 1992) ℞ *ophthalmic bacteriostatic* [sulfisoxazole diolamine]
Gantrisin syrup, pediatric suspension ℞ *broad-spectrum bacteriostatic* [sulfisoxazole acetyl]
Gantrisin tablets ℞ *broad-spectrum bacteriostatic* [sulfisoxazole]
gapicomine INN
gapromidine INN
Garamicina (Mexican name for U.S. product Garamycin)
Garamycin cream, ointment ℞ *topical antibiotic* [gentamicin sulfate]
Garamycin IV, IM or intrathecal injection, IV piggyback ℞ *aminoglycoside-type antibiotic* [gentamicin sulfate]

Garamycin Ophthalmic ointment, eye drops ℞ *ophthalmic antibiotic* [gentamicin sulfate]

Garamycin Pediatric IV or IM injection ℞ *aminoglycoside-type antibiotic* [gentamicin sulfate]

Garden Fresh bar soap OTC *cleansing* [vegetable-based]

gas gangrene antitoxin, pentavalent

gas gangrene antitoxin, polyvalent [see: gas gangrene antitoxin, pentavalent]

Gas Permeable Daily Cleaner solution OTC *contact lens cleaning solution*

Gas Permeable Wetting and Soaking solution OTC *contact lens wetting/soaking solution*

Gas Relief chewable tablets, drops OTC *antiflatulent* [simethicone]

gastric mucin BAN

Gastroccult test kit OTC *in vitro diagnostic aid for gastric occult blood*

Gastrocrom capsules ℞ *bronchodilator for bronchial asthma; (orphan: mastocytosis)* [cromolyn sodium]

Gastrografin solution ℞ *GI contrast radiopaque agent* [diatrizoate meglumine; diatrizoate sodium]

Gastrolyte oral concentrate (discontinued 1991) OTC *electrolyte replacement* [sodium, potassium, and chloride electrolytes]

Gastrosed drops, tablets ℞ *anticholinergic* [hyoscyamine sulfate]

Gastro-Test OTC *in vitro diagnostic aid for determining stomach pH and gastric bleeding*

Gastrozepine ℞ *investigational antiulcerative* [pirenzepine HCl]

Gas-X chewable tablets OTC *antiflatulent* [simethicone]

gaultheria oil [see: methyl salicylate]

gauze, absorbent USP *surgical aid*

gauze, petrolatum USP *surgical aid*

gauze bandage [see: bandage, gauze]

Gaviscon ESR liquid, chewable tablets OTC *antacid* [aluminum hydroxide; magnesium carbonate; sodium bicarbonate]

Gaviscon; Gaviscon-2 chewable tablets OTC *antacid* [aluminum hydroxide; magnesium trisilicate; sodium bicarbonate]

Gaviscon liquid OTC *antacid* [aluminum hydroxide; magnesium carbonate]

G.B.S. tablets (discontinued 1992) ℞ *laxative; hydrocholeretic; sedative* [dehydrocholic acid; homatropine methylbromide; phenobarbital]

G-CSF (granulocyte colony-stimulating factor) [see: filgrastim]

gedocarnil INN

Gee-Gee tablets OTC *expectorant* [guaifenesin]

gefarnate INN, BAN

Gel Clean (discontinued 1992) OTC *contact lens cleaning gel*

Gel II gel (discontinued 1991) ℞ *topical dental caries preventative* [sodium fluoride; acidulated phosphate fluoride]

Gelamal suspension OTC *antacid*

gelatin NF *encapsulating, suspending, binding and coating agent*

gelatin film, absorbable USP *topical hemostatic*

gelatin powder, absorbable *topical hemostatic*

gelatin solution, special intravenous [see: polygeline]

gelatin sponge, absorbable USP *local hemostatic*

Gelfilm; Gelfilm Ophthalmic gelatin film ℞ *topical hemostatic aid in surgical hemostasis* [absorbable gelatin film]

Gelfoam sponge, packs, prostatectomy cones, powder ℞ *topical hemostatic aid in surgical hemostasis* [absorbable gelatin sponge]

Gel-Kam gel ℞ *topical dental caries preventative* [stannous fluoride]

Gelpirin tablets OTC *analgesic; antipyretic; anti-inflammatory* [acetaminophen; buffered aspirin; caffeine]

Gelpirin-CCF tablets OTC *antipyretic; analgesic; expectorant; decongestant; antihistamine* [acetaminophen; guaifenesin; phenylpropanolamine HCl; chlorpheniramine maleate]

Gelseals (trademarked form) *filled elastic capsules*

Gel-Tin gel OTC *topical dental caries preventative* [stannous fluoride]

Gelusil; Gelusil-II chewable tablets, liquid OTC *antacid; antiflatulent* [aluminum hydroxide; magnesium hydroxide; simethicone]

Gelusil-M liquid, chewable tablets (discontinued 1991) OTC *antacid; antiflatulent* [aluminum hydroxide; magnesium hydroxide; simethicone]

gemazocine INN

gemcadiol USAN, INN *antihyperlipoproteinemic*

gemcitabine USAN *antineoplastic*

gemcitabine HCl USAN *antineoplastic*

gemeprost USAN, INN, BAN *prostaglandin*

gemfibrozil USAN, USP, INN, BAN *antihyperlipoproteinemic*

Gemnisyn tablets OTC *analgesic; antipyretic; anti-inflammatory* [acetaminophen; aspirin]

Gemonil tablets (discontinued 1991) ℞ *anticonvulsant* [metharbital]

Genabid timed-release capsules ℞ *peripheral vasodilator* [papaverine HCl]

Genac tablets OTC *decongestant; antihistamine* [pseudoephedrine HCl; triprolidine HCl]

Genacol tablets OTC *decongestant; antihistamine; antitussive; analgesic* [phenylpropanolamine HCl; chlorpheniramine maleate; dextromethorphan hydrobromide; acetaminophen]

Genagesic tablets ℞ *narcotic analgesic* [propoxyphene HCl; acetaminophen]

Genahist capsules, tablets, elixir ℞ *antihistamine; motion sickness preventative; sleep aid; antiparkinsonian* [diphenhydramine HCl]

Genalac chewable tablets OTC *antacid* [calcium carbonate; glycine]

Genamin Cold syrup OTC *antihistamine; decongestant* [phenylpropanolamine HCl; chlorpheniramine maleate]

Genapap, Children's chewable tablets, elixir OTC *analgesic; antipyretic* [acetaminophen]

Genapap, Infants' drops OTC *analgesic; antipyretic* [acetaminophen]

Genapap tablets OTC *analgesic; antipyretic* [acetaminophen]

Genapax medicated tampons ℞ *antifungal* [gentian violet]

Genaphed tablets OTC *nasal decongestant* [pseudoephedrine HCl]

Genasal nasal spray OTC *nasal decongestant* [oxymetazoline HCl]

Genasoft Plus softgels OTC *laxative; stool softener* [docusate sodium; casanthranol]

Genaspor cream OTC *topical antifungal* [tolnaftate]

Genatap elixir OTC *decongestant; antihistamine* [phenylpropanolamine HCl; brompheniramine maleate]

Genaton chewable tablets OTC *antacid* [aluminum hydroxide; magnesium trisilicate]

Genatuss DM syrup OTC *antitussive; expectorant* [dextromethorphan hydrobromide; guaifenesin; alcohol]

Genatuss syrup OTC *expectorant* [guaifenesin; alcohol]

Gen-bee with C caplets OTC *vitamin supplement* [multiple B vitamins; vitamin C]

Gencalc 600 film-coated tablets OTC *calcium supplement* [calcium carbonate]

GenCept tablets ℞ *oral contraceptive* [norethindrone; ethinyl estradiol]

Gencold sustained-release capsules OTC *decongestant; antihistamine* [phenylpropanolamine HCl; chlorpheniramine maleate]

Gendecon tablets OTC *decongestant; antihistamine; analgesic* [phenylephrine HCl; chlorpheniramine maleate; acetaminophen]

Gen-D-phen syrup OTC *antihistamine; antitussive* [diphenhydramine HCl]

Genebs tablets OTC *analgesic; antipyretic* [acetaminophen]

Generet-500 timed-release tablets OTC *hematinic* [ferrous sulfate; multiple B vitamins; sodium ascorbate]

Generix-T tablets OTC *vitamin/mineral/iron supplement* [multiple vitamins & minerals; iron]

Genex capsules OTC *decongestant; analgesic* [phenylpropanolamine HCl; acetaminophen]

Genite liquid OTC *decongestant; antihistamine; antitussive; analgesic* [pseudoephedrine HCl; doxylamine succinate; dextromethorphan hydrobromide; acetaminophen; alcohol]

Gen-K powder packets ℞ *potassium supplement* [potassium chloride]

genophyllin [see: aminophylline]

Genoptic Ophthalmic Liquifilm eye drops ℞ *ophthalmic antibiotic* [gentamicin]

Genoptic S.O.P. Ophthalmic ointment ℞ *ophthalmic antibiotic* [gentamicin sulfate]

Genora 1/35; 0.5/35 tablets ℞ *oral contraceptive* [ethinyl estradiol; norethindrone]

Genora 1/50 tablets ℞ *oral contraceptive* [mestranol; norethindrone]

Genpril tablets, caplets OTC *nonsteroidal anti-inflammatory drug (NSAID); antiarthritic; analgesic* [ibuprofen]

Genprin tablets OTC *analgesic; antipyretic; anti-inflammatory; antirheumatic* [aspirin]

Gensan tablets OTC *analgesic; antipyretic; anti-inflammatory* [aspirin; caffeine]

Gentab-LA long-acting tablets ℞ *decongestant; expectorant* [phenylpropanolamine HCl; guaifenesin]

Gentacidin eye drops, ophthalmic ointment ℞ *ophthalmic antibiotic* [gentamicin]

Gent-AK eye drops, ophthalmic ointment ℞ *ophthalmic antibiotic* [gentamicin sulfate]

gentamicin BAN *aminoglycoside bactericidal antibiotic* [also: gentamicin sulfate]

gentamicin liposome (*orphan:* disseminated Mycobacterium avium-intracellulare)

gentamicin sulfate USAN, USP *aminoglycoside bactericidal antibiotic* [also: gentamicin]

gentamicin-impregnated PMMA beads (*orphan:* osteomyelitis)

gentian violet USP *topical anti-infective/antifungal* [also: methylrosanilinium chloride]

gentisic acid ethanolamide NF *complexing agent*

Gentlax granules OTC *laxative* [senna concentrate]

Gentlax S tablets OTC *laxative; stool softener* [docusate sodium; sennosides]

Gentran 40 IV injection ℞ *plasma volume expander; shock due to hemorrhage, burns, surgery* [dextran 40]

Gentran 70; Gentran 75 IV infusion ℞ *plasma volume expander; shock due to hemorrhage, burns, surgery* [dextran 70]

Gentrasul eye drops, ophthalmic ointment ℞ *ophthalmic antibiotic* [gentamicin]

Gentz anorectal wipes OTC *antipruritic; astringent* [pramoxine HCl; alcloxa; hamamelis water]

Genvite tablets OTC *antianemic* [ferrous fumarate; multiple vitamins]

Gen-Xene tablets ℞ *anxiolytic; minor tranquilizer; anticonvulsant adjunct* [chlorazepate dipotassium]

Geocillin film-coated tablets ℞ *extended-spectrum penicillin-type antibiotic* [carbenicillin indanyl sodium]

gepefrine INN

gepirone INN *tranquilizer; anxiolytic; antidepressant* [also: gepirone HCl]

gepirone HCl USAN *tranquilizer; anxiolytic; antidepressant* [also: gepirone]

2-geranylhydroquinone [see: geroquinol]

Geravim elixir OTC *vitamin/mineral supplement* [multiple B vitamins & minerals]

Geravite elixir OTC *geriatric dietary supplement* [multiple B vitamins; lysine]

Geref powder for IV injection ℞ *pituitary diagnostic aid; (orphan: growth hormone deficiency; anovulation; AIDS-related weight loss)* [sermorelin acetate]

Geriamic tablets OTC *antianemic* [ferrous sulfate; multiple B vitamins; vitamin C]

Geridium tablets ℞ *urinary analgesic* [phenazopyridine HCl]

Gerilets Filmtabs (film-coated tablets) (discontinued 1991) OTC *antianemic* [ferrous sulfate; multiple vitamins]

Gerimal sublingual tablets, tablets ℞ *for age-related mental capacity decline* [ergoloid mesylates]

Gerimed film-coated tablets OTC *geriatric vitamin/mineral supplement* [multiple vitamins & minerals]

Geriot film-coated tablets OTC *vitamin/mineral/iron supplement* [multiple vitamins & minerals; ferrous fumarate; folic acid; biotin]

Geriplex-FS Kapseals (capsules) OTC *geriatric dietary supplement* [multiple vitamins & minerals; choline; sodium bisulfite; aspergillus oryzea enzymes]

Geriplex-FS liquid (discontinued 1991) OTC *vitamin/iron supplement* [multiple B vitamins; iron]

Geritol Complete tablets OTC *vitamin/mineral/iron supplement* [multiple vitamins & minerals; ferrous fumarate; folic acid; biotin]

Geritol Extend caplets OTC *vitamin/mineral/iron supplement* [multiple vitamins & minerals; ferrous fumarate; folic acid]

Geritol Tonic liquid OTC *hematinic* [ferric ammonium citrate; multiple B vitamins; alcohol]

Geritonic liquid OTC *hematinic* [ferric ammonium citrate; liver fraction 1; multiple B vitamins; alcohol]

Gerivite liquid OTC *geriatric vitamin/mineral supplement* [multiple B vitamins & minerals; alcohol]

Gerivites tablets OTC *hematinic* [ferrous sulfate; multiple B vitamins; vitamin C]

Gerix (discontinued 1991) *vitamin/iron supplement* [multiple vitamins; ferrous sulfate]

Germanin (available only from the Centers for Disease Control) ℞ *investigational anti-infective for trypanosomiasis and onchocerciasis* [suramin sodium]

germanium *element* (Ge)

Germicin solution OTC *topical antiseptic* [benzalkonium chloride]

Ger-O-Foam aerosol (discontinued 1992) OTC *counterirritant; topical anesthetic* [methyl salicylate; benzocaine]

geroquinol INN

gesarol [see: chlorophenothane]

gestaclone USAN, INN *progestin*

gestadienol INN
gestanin [see: allyloestrenol]
Gesterol 50 IM injection ℞ *progestin; amenorrhea; functional uterine bleeding* [progesterone]
Gesterol L.A. 250 IM injection ℞ *progestin; amenorrhea; functional uterine bleeding* [hydroxyprogesterone caproate]
gestodene USAN, INN, BAN *progestin*
gestonorone caproate USAN, INN *progestin* [also: gestronol]
gestrinone USAN, INN *progestin*
gestronol BAN *progestin* [also: gestonorone caproate]
Gets-It liquid OTC *topical keratolytic* [salicylic acid; zinc chloride]
gevotroline INN *antipsychotic* [also: gevotroline HCl]
gevotroline HCl USAN *antipsychotic* [also: gevotroline]
Gevrabon liquid OTC *vitamin/mineral supplement* [multiple B vitamins & minerals; alcohol]
Gevral Protein powder OTC *oral protein supplement* [calcium caseinate; sucrose]
Gevral T film-coated tablets OTC *vitamin/mineral/iron supplement* [multiple vitamins & minerals; ferrous fumarate; folic acid]
Gevral tablets OTC *vitamin/mineral/iron supplement* [multiple vitamins & minerals; ferrous fumarate; folic acid]
GG-Cen capsules OTC *expectorant* [guaifenesin]
GHRF; GH-RF (growth hormone-releasing factor) [q.v.]
giparmen INN
giractide INN
gitalin NF [also: gitalin amorphous]
gitalin amorphous INN [also: gitalin]
gitaloxin INN
gitoformate INN
gitoxin 16-formate [see: gitaloxin]

gitoxin pentaacetate [see: pengitoxin]
GLA (gamma-linolenic acid)
glacial acetic acid [see: acetic acid, glacial]
glafenine INN
glaphenine [see: glafenine]
Glauber salt [see: sodium sulfate]
glaucarubin
Glaucon Drop-Tainers (eye drops) ℞ *antiglaucoma agent* [epinephrine HCl]
glaze, pharmaceutical NF *tablet-coating agent*
glaziovine INN
gleptoferron USAN, INN, BAN *veterinary hematinic*
gliamilide USAN, INN *antidiabetic*
glibenclamide INN, BAN *sulfonylurea-type antidiabetic* [also: glyburide]
glibornuride USAN, INN, BAN *antidiabetic*
glibutimine INN
glicaramide INN
glicetanile INN *antidiabetic* [also: glicetanile sodium]
glicetanile sodium USAN *antidiabetic* [also: glicetanile]
gliclazide INN, BAN
glicondamide INN
glidazamide INN
gliflumide USAN, INN *antidiabetic*
glimepiride INN, BAN *antihypoglycemic; blood glucose regulator*
glipentide [see: glisentide]
glipizide USAN, INN, BAN *sulfonylurea-type antidiabetic*
gliquidone INN, BAN
glisamuride INN
glisentide INN
glisindamide INN
glisolamide INN
glisoxepide INN, BAN
globin zinc insulin INN [also: insulin, globin zinc]
globulin, aerosolized pooled immune (orphan: *respiratory syncytial virus*)

globulin, immune USP *passive immunizing agent; investigational immunomodulator for AIDS*

globulin, immune human serum [now: globulin, immune]

Glossets (trademarked form) *sublingual or rectal administration*

gloxazone USAN, INN, BAN *veterinary anaplasmodastat*

gloximonam USAN, INN *antibacterial*

GLQ223 ℞ *investigational antiviral for AIDS* [trichosanthin]

glucagon USP, INN, BAN *antidiabetic; glucose elevating agent*

Glucagon Emergency Kit Hyporets (prefilled disposable syringes) ℞ *emergency treatment for hypoglycemic crisis* [glucagon; lactose]

glucalox INN [also: glycalox]

glucametacin INN

D-glucaric acid, calcium salt tetrahydrate [see: calcium saccharate]

gluceptate sodium USAN *pharmaceutic aid*

Glucerna liquid OTC *oral nutritional supplement for abnormal glucose tolerance*

D-glucitol [see: sorbitol]

D-glucitol hexanicotinate [see: sorbinicate]

glucocerebrosidase-β-glucosidase [see: alglucerase]

glucoheptonic acid, calcium salt [see: calcium gluceptate]

D-gluconic acid, calcium salt [see: calcium gluconate]

D-gluconic acid, magnesium salt [see: magnesium gluconate]

D-gluconic acid, monopotassium salt [see: potassium gluconate]

D-gluconic acid, monosodium salt [see: sodium gluconate]

β-D-glucopyranuronamide [see: glucuronamide]

glucosamine USAN, INN *pharmaceutic aid*

D-glucose [see: dextrose]

glucose, liquid NF *tablet binder and coating agent; antihypoglycemic*

Glucose & Ketone Urine Test reagent strips OTC *in vitro diagnostic aid for multiple urine products*

D-glucose monohydrate [see: dextrose]

glucose oxidase

glucose polymers *caloric replacement*

Glucose-40 Ophthalmic ointment ℞ *topical osmotherapeutic agent for reducing corneal edema* [glucose]

Glucostix reagent strips OTC *in vitro diagnostic aid for blood glucose*

glucosulfamide INN

glucosulfone INN

Glucotrol tablets ℞ *antidiabetic* [glipizide]

glucurolactone INN

glucuronamide INN, BAN

Glukor powder for injection ℞ *hormone for prepubertal cryptorchidism and hypogonadism* [chorionic gonadotropin]

glunicate INN

gluside [see: saccharin]

gluside, soluble [see: saccharin sodium]

glusoferron INN

glutamic acid (L-glutamic acid) USAN, INN *nonessential amino acid; symbols: Glu, E*

glutamic acid HCl *gastric acidifier*

glutamine (L-glutamine) *nonessential amino acid; symbols: Gln, Q* [see: levoglutamide]

glutaral USAN, USP, INN *disinfectant*

glutaraldehyde [see: glutaral]

glutasin [see: glutamic acid HCl]

glutaurine INN

glutethimide USP, INN, BAN *sedative*

Glutofac tablets OTC *vitamin/mineral supplement* [multiple vitamins & minerals]

Glutose gel OTC *glucose elevating agent* [glucose]

Glyate syrup OTC *expectorant* [guaifenesin; alcohol]
glyburide USAN *sulfonylurea-type antidiabetic* [also: glibenclamide]
glybutamide [see: carbutamide]
glybuthiazol INN
glybuthizol [see: glybuthiazol]
glybuzole INN
glycalox BAN [also: glucalox]
Glycate chewable tablets (discontinued 1992) OTC *antacid* [calcium carbonate; glycine]
glycerides oleiques polyoxyethylenes [see: peglicol 5 oleate]
glycerin USP *humectant; solvent; osmotic diuretic; laxative; emollient/protectant* [also: glycerol]
glycerol INN *humectant; solvent; osmotic diuretic; laxative; emollient/protectant; monoctanoin component D* [also: glycerin]
glycerol, iodinated USAN, BAN *(disapproved for use as an expectorant in 1991)*
glycerol 1-decanoate *monoctanoin component B* [see: monoctanoin]
glycerol 1,2-dioctanoate *monoctanoin component C* [see: monoctanoin]
glycerol 1-octanoate *monoctanoin component A* [see: monoctanoin]
glycerol phosphate, manganese salt [see: manganese glycerophosphate]
glyceryl behenate NF *tablet and capsule lubricant*
glyceryl borate [see: boroglycerin]
glyceryl guaiacolate [now: guaifenesin]
glyceryl monostearate NF *emulsifying agent*
glyceryl triacetate [now: triacetin]
glyceryl trinitrate BAN *coronary vasodilator* [also: nitroglycerin]
glycerylaminophenaquine [see: glafenine]
Glyceryl-T capsules, liquid ℞ *antiasthmatic; bronchodilator; expectorant* [theophylline; guaifenesin]

glycinato dihydroxyaluminum hydrate [see: dihydroxyaluminum aminoacetate]
glycine USP, INN *nonessential amino acid; urologic irrigant; symbols: Gly, G*
glycine aluminum-zirconium complex [see: aluminum zirconium trichlorohydrex gly]
glyclopyramide INN
glycobiarsol USP, INN [also: bismuth glycollylarsanilate]
glycocholate sodium [see: sodium glycocholate]
glycocoll [see: glycine]
Glycofed tablets OTC *decongestant; expectorant* [pseudoephedrine HCl; guaifenesin]
glycol distearate USAN *thickening agent*
p-**glycolophenetidide** [see: fenacetinol]
glycophenylate [see: mepenzolate bromide]
glycopyrrolate USAN, USP *peptic ulcer adjunct* [also: glycopyrronium bromide]
glycopyrrone bromide [see: glycopyrrolate]
glycopyrronium bromide INN, BAN *anticholinergic* [also: glycopyrrolate]
Glycotuss tablets OTC *expectorant* [guaifenesin]
Glycotuss-DM tablets OTC *antitussive; expectorant* [dextromethorphan hydrobromide; guaifenesin]
glycyclamide INN, BAN
glycyrrhetinic acid [see: enoxolone]
glycyrrhiza NF
glydanile sodium [now: glicetanile sodium]
glyhexamide USAN, INN *antidiabetic*
glyhexylamide [see: metahexamide]
glymidine BAN *antidiabetic* [also: glymidine sodium]
glymidine sodium USAN, INN *antidiabetic* [also: glymidine]

glymol [see: mineral oil]

Glynase PresTabs (tablets) ℞ *antidiabetic* [glyburide]

glyoctamide USAN, INN *antidiabetic*

Gly-Oxide oral solution OTC *oral anti-inflammatory/anti-infective* [carbamide peroxide]

glyparamide USAN *antidiabetic*

glyphylline [see: dyphylline]

glypinamide INN

Glypressin *(orphan: bleeding esophageal ulcers)* [terlipressin]

glyprothiazol INN

glyprothizol [see: glyprothiazol]

Glyrol solution (discontinued 1991) ℞ *osmotic diuretic* [glycerin]

glysobuzole INN [also: isobuzole]

Glytuss film-coated tablets OTC *expectorant* [guaifenesin]

GM 6001 *(orphan: corneal ulcers)*

GM-CSF (granulocyte macrophage colony-stimulating factor) [see: sargramostim; molgramostim]

G-myticin cream, ointment ℞ *topical antibiotic* [gentamicin sulfate]

Go-Evac powder for oral solution ℞ *pre-procedure bowel evacuant* [polyethylene glycol-electrolyte solution]

gold *element (Au)*

gold Au 198 USAN, USP *antineoplastic; liver imaging aid; radioactive agent*

gold sodium thiomalate USP *antirheumatic (50% gold)* [also: sodium aurothiomalate]

gold sodium thiosulfate NF [also: sodium aurotiosulfate]

gold thioglucose [see: aurothioglucose]

GoLYTELY powder for oral solution ℞ *pre-procedure bowel evacuant* [polyethylene glycol-electrolyte solution]

gonacrine [see: acriflavine]

gonadorelin INN, BAN *gonad-stimulating principle* [also: gonadorelin acetate]

gonadorelin acetate USAN *gonad-stimulating principle; (orphan: hypothalamic amenorrhea)* [also: gonadorelin]

gonadorelin HCl USAN *gonad-stimulating principle*

gonadotrophin, chorionic INN, BAN *gonad-stimulating principle* [also: gonadotropin, chorionic]

gonadotrophin, serum INN

gonadotropin, chorionic USP *gonad-stimulating principle* [also: gonadotrophin, chorionic]

gonadotropin, serum [see: gonadotrophin, serum]

Gonak ophthalmic solution OTC *ophthalmic surgical aid; gonioscopic examination aid* [hydroxypropyl methylcellulose]

Gonal-F ℞ *investigational fertility stimulant* [recombinant human follicle-stimulating hormone]

Gonic powder for injection ℞ *hormone for prepubertal cryptorchidism and hypogonadism* [chorionic gonadotropin]

Gonioscopic Prism Solution OTC *agent for bonding gonioscopic prisms to eye* [hydroxyethylcellulose]

Goniosol ophthalmic solution ℞ *ophthalmic surgical aid; gonioscopic examination aid* [hydroxypropyl methylcellulose]

Gonodecten tube test OTC *in vitro diagnostic aid for gonorrhea in males*

Gonozyme Diagnostic Kit swab test OTC *in vitro diagnostic aid for gonorrhea*

GoodStart [see: Carnation GoodStart]

Goody's Headache powder OTC *analgesic; antipyretic; anti-inflammatory* [acetaminophen; aspirin; caffeine]

Gordobalm OTC *counterirritant; topical antiseptic* [methyl salicylate; menthol; camphor; alcohol]

Gordochom solution ℞ *topical antifungal; antiseptic* [undecylenic acid; chloroxylenol]

Gordofilm liquid ℞ *topical keratolytic* [salicylic acid; lactic acid]

Gordogesic Creme OTC *counterirritant* [methyl salicylate]

Gordon's Urea 40% cream ℞ *for removal of dystrophic nails* [urea]
Gordo-Vite E cream (discontinued 1992) OTC *emollient* [vitamin E]
Gormel Creme OTC *moisturizer; emollient; keratolytic* [urea]
goserelin USAN, INN, BAN *luteinizing hormone-releasing hormone (LHRH) agonist*
goserelin acetate *antineoplastic; gonadotropin-releasing hormone*
gossypol (*orphan: adrenal cortex cancer*)
govafilcon A USAN *hydrophilic contact lens material*
Gp120 ℞ *investigational vaccine for AIDS*
GP-500 tablets ℞ *decongestant; expectorant* [pseudoephedrine HCl; guaifenesin]
Gradumet (trademarked form) *sustained-release tablets*
gramicidin USP, INN *antibacterial antibiotic*
gramicidin S INN
granisetron USAN, INN, BAN *antiemetic*
granisetron HCl USAN *antiemetic*
Granulderm aerosol spray ℞ *topical enzyme for wound debridement* [trypsin; balsam Peru]
Granulex aerosol spray ℞ *topical enzyme for wound debridement* [trypsin; balsam Peru]
granulocyte macrophage-colony stimulating factor (GM-CSF) [see: sargramostim]
granulocyte-colony stimulating factor (G-CSF), recombinant [see: filgrastim]
GranuMed aerosol spray ℞ *topical enzyme for wound debridement* [trypsin; balsam Peru]
Grapefruit Diet Plan with Diadax sustained-release capsules, chewable tablets (discontinued 1992) OTC *diet aid* [phenylpropanolamine HCl; grapefruit extract]

green soap [see: soap, green]
Grifulvin V tablets, oral suspension ℞ *systemic antifungal* [griseofulvin (microsize)]
Grisactin 500 tablets ℞ *systemic antifungal* [griseofulvin (microsize)]
Grisactin capsules ℞ *systemic antifungal* [griseofulvin (microsize)]
Grisactin Ultra tablets ℞ *systemic antifungal* [griseofulvin (ultramicrosize)]
griseofulvin USP, INN, BAN *fungistatic*
Gris-PEG film-coated tablets ℞ *systemic antifungal* [griseofulvin (ultramicrosize)]
growth hormone, human [see: somatropin]
growth hormone-releasing factor (GHRF; GH-RF) (*orphan: inadequate endogenous growth hormone*)
GS 393 *investigational anti-HIV drug*
G-strophanthin [see: ouabain]
guabenxan INN
guacetisal INN
guafecainol INN
guaiac
guaiacol NF
guaiacol carbonate NF
guaiacol glyceryl ether [see: guaifenesin]
guaiactamine INN
guaiapate USAN, INN *antitussive*
guaiazulene soluble [see: sodium gualenate]
guaietolin INN
Guaifed; Guaifed-PD timed-release capsules ℞ *decongestant; expectorant* [pseudoephedrine HCl; guaifenesin]
Guaifed syrup OTC *decongestant; expectorant* [pseudoephedrine HCl; guaifenesin]
guaifenesin USAN, USP, INN *expectorant* [also: guaiphenesin]
guaifylline INN *bronchodilator; expectorant* [also: guaithylline]

GuaiMAX-D extended-release tablets OTC *decongestant; expectorant* [pseudoephedrine HCl; guaifenesin]

guaimesal INN

Guaipax sustained-release tablets ℞ *decongestant; expectorant* [phenylpropanolamine HCl; guaifenesin]

guaiphenesin BAN *expectorant* [also: guaifenesin]

guaisteine INN

Guaitab tablets OTC *decongestant; expectorant* [pseudoephedrine HCl; guaifenesin]

guaithylline USAN *bronchodilator; expectorant* [also: guaifylline]

guamecycline INN, BAN

guanabenz USAN, INN *antihypertensive*

guanabenz acetate USAN, USP *antihypertensive*

guanacline INN, BAN *antihypertensive* [also: guanacline sulfate]

guanacline sulfate USAN *antihypertensive* [also: guanacline]

guanadrel INN *antihypertensive* [also: guanadrel sulfate]

guanadrel sulfate USAN, USP *antihypertensive* [also: guanadrel]

guanatol HCl [see: chloroguanide HCl]

guanazodine INN

guancidine INN *antihypertensive* [also: guancydine]

guancydine USAN *antihypertensive* [also: guancidine]

guanethidine INN, BAN *antihypertensive* [also: guanethidine monosulfate]

guanethidine monosulfate USAN, USP *antihypertensive; (orphan: reflex sympathetic dystrophy and causalgia)* [also: guanethidine]

guanethidine sulfate USAN, USP *antihypertensive*

guanfacine INN, BAN *antihypertensive* [also: guanfacine HCl]

guanfacine HCl USAN *antihypertensive* [also: guanfacine]

guanidine HCl *cholinergic muscle stimulant*

guanisoquin sulfate USAN *antihypertensive* [also: guanisoquine]

guanisoquine INN *antihypertensive* [also: guanisoquin sulfate]

guanoclor INN, BAN *antihypertensive* [also: guanoclor sulfate]

guanoclor sulfate USAN *antihypertensive* [also: guanoclor]

guanoctine INN *antihypertensive* [also: guanoctine HCl]

guanoctine HCl USAN *antihypertensive* [also: guanoctine]

guanoxabenz USAN, INN *antihypertensive*

guanoxan INN, BAN *antihypertensive* [also: guanoxan sulfate]

guanoxan sulfate USAN *antihypertensive* [also: guanoxan]

guanoxyfen INN *antihypertensive; antidepressant* [also: guanoxyfen sulfate]

guanoxyfen sulfate USAN *antihypertensive; antidepressant* [also: guanoxyfen]

guar gum NF *tablet binder and disintegrant*

guaranine [see: caffeine]

GuiaCough CF syrup OTC *expectorant; decongestant; antitussive* [guaifenesin; phenylpropanolamine HCl; dextromethorphan hydrobromide]

GuiaCough DM syrup OTC *expectorant; antitussive* [guaifenesin; dextromethorphan hydrobromide]

GuiaCough PE syrup OTC *expectorant; decongestant* [guaifenesin; pseudoephedrine HCl]

GuiaCough syrup OTC *expectorant* [guaifenesin]

Guiafenesin-DAC syrup ℞ *decongestant; antitussive; expectorant* [pseudoephedrine HCl; codeine phosphate; guaifenesin; alcohol]

Guiaphed elixir OTC *antiasthmatic; bronchodilator; decongestant; expectorant; sedative* [theophylline; ephed-

rine sulfate; guaifenesin; phenobarbital]
Guiatuss AC syrup ℞ *antitussive; expectorant* [guaifenesin; codeine phosphate; alcohol]
Guiatuss CF liquid OTC *expectorant; decongestant; antitussive* [guaifenesin; phenylpropanolamine HCl; dextromethorphan hydrobromide; alcohol]
Guiatuss DAC syrup ℞ *expectorant; decongestant; antitussive* [guaifenesin; pseudoephedrine HCl; codeine phosphate; alcohol]
Guiatuss DM liquid OTC *antitussive; expectorant* [guaifenesin; dextromethorphan hydrobromide]
Guiatuss PE liquid OTC *antitussive; expectorant* [guaifenesin; pseudoephedrine HCl; alcohol]
Guiatuss syrup OTC *expectorant* [guaifenesin]
Guiatuss-DM liquid OTC *antitussive; expectorant* [dextromethorphan hydrobromide; guaifenesin]
Guiatussin DAC syrup ℞ *decongestant; antitussive; expectorant* [pseudoephedrine HCl; codeine phosphate; guaifenesin; alcohol]
Guiatussin with Codeine Expectorant liquid ℞ *antitussive; expectorant* [codeine phosphate; guaifenesin; alcohol]
Guiatussin with Dextromethorphan liquid OTC *antitussive; expectorant* [dextromethorphan hydrobromide; guaifenesin; alcohol]
Guipax tablets ℞ *decongestant; expectorant* [phenylpropanolamine HCl; guaifenesin]
gum arabic [see: acacia]
gum senegal [see: acacia]
guncotton, soluble [see: pyroxylin]
Gustase Plus tablets ℞ *digestive enzymes; sedative* [amylase; protease;

cellulase; homatropine methylbromide; phenobarbital]
Gustase tablets OTC *digestive enzymes* [amylase; protease; cellulase]
gutta percha USP *dental restoration agent*
G-Well lotion, shampoo ℞ *scabicide; pediculicide* [lindane]
Gynecort 5; Gynecort 10 cream OTC *topical corticosteroid* [hydrocortisone acetate]
Gyne-Lotrimin vaginal cream, vaginal tablets (100 mg) OTC *antifungal* [clotrimazole]
Gyne-Lotrimin vaginal tablets (500 mg) ℞ *antifungal* [clotrimazole]
Gyne-Moistrin gel OTC *vaginal lubricant*
gynergon [see: estradiol]
Gyne-Sulf vaginal cream ℞ *bacteriostatic* [sulfathiazole; sulfacetamide; sulfabenzamide; urea]
gynoestryl [see: estradiol]
Gynogen IM injection (discontinued 1992) ℞ *estrogen replacement therapy; antineoplastic for prostatic and breast cancer* [estrone]
Gynogen L.A. "10" IM injection (discontinued 1992) ℞ *estrogen replacement therapy; antineoplastic for prostatic cancer* [estradiol valerate in oil]
Gynogen L.A. "20"; Gynogen L.A. "40" IM injection ℞ *estrogen replacement therapy; antineoplastic for prostatic cancer* [estradiol valerate in oil]
Gynol II Contraceptive vaginal jelly OTC *spermicidal contraceptive* [nonoxynol 9]
Gynovite Plus tablets OTC *vitamin/mineral/calcium/iron supplement* [multiple vitamins & minerals; calcium; iron; folic acid; biotin]
Gyrocaps (trademarked form) *extended-release capsules*

H

²H (deuterium) [see: deuterium oxide]

³H (tritium) [see: tritiated water]

HA-1A ℞ *investigational monoclonal antibody for gram-negative bacteremia and septic shock*

Habitrol transdermal patch ℞ *smoking deterrent; nicotine withdrawal aid* [nicotine]

hachimycin INN, BAN

HAD (hexamethylmelamine, Adriamycin, DDP) *chemotherapy protocol*

hafnium *element (Hf)*

Hair Booster Vitamin tablets OTC *vitamin/mineral/iron supplement* [multiple B vitamins & minerals; iron; folic acid]

halarsol [see: dichlorophenarsine HCl]

halazepam USAN, USP, INN, BAN *anxiolytic; sedative*

halazone USP, INN *disinfectant; water purifier*

halcinonide USAN, USP, INN, BAN *topical corticosteroidal anti-inflammatory*

Halcion tablets ℞ *sedative; hypnotic* [triazolam]

Haldol Decanoate 50; Haldol Decanoate 100 long-acting IM injection ℞ *antipsychotic* [haloperidol decanoate]

Haldol oral concentrate, IM injection ℞ *antipsychotic; control manifestations of Tourette syndrome* [haloperidol lactate]

Haldol tablets ℞ *antipsychotic; control manifestations of Tourette syndrome* [haloperidol]

Halenol Children's liquid OTC *analgesic; antipyretic* [acetaminophen]

Halenol tablets (discontinued 1992) OTC *analgesic; antipyretic* [acetaminophen]

Halercol capsules OTC *vitamin supplement* [multiple vitamins]

haletazole INN [also: halethazole]

halethazole BAN [also: haletazole]

Haley's M-O liquid OTC *laxative* [magnesium hydroxide; mineral oil]

Halfan ℞ *(orphan: acute multi-drug resistant malaria)* [halofantrine HCl]

Halfprin enteric-coated tablets OTC *analgesic; antipyretic; anti-inflammatory; antirheumatic* [aspirin]

Hall's Mentho-Lyptus lozenges OTC *antipruritic/counterirritant; mild local anesthetic; antiseptic* [menthol; eucalyptus oil]

halobetasol propionate USAN *topical corticosteroidal anti-inflammatory* [also: ulobetasol]

halocarban INN *disinfectant* [also: cloflucarban]

halocortolone INN

halocrinic acid [see: brocrinat]

Halodrin tablets ℞ *estrogen/androgen for menopausal vasomotor symptoms* [ethinyl estradiol; fluoxymesterone]

halofantrine INN, BAN *antimalarial; (orphan: acute malaria)* [also: halofantrine HCl]

halofantrine HCl USAN *antimalarial* [also: halofantrine]

Halofed syrup (discontinued 1993) OTC *nasal decongestant* [pseudoephedrine HCl]

Halofed tablets OTC *nasal decongestant* [pseudoephedrine HCl]

halofenate USAN, INN, BAN *antihyperlipoproteinemic; uricosuric*

halofuginone INN, BAN *antiprotozoal* [also: halofuginone hydrobromide]

halofuginone hydrobromide USAN *antiprotozoal* [also: halofuginone]

Halog ointment, cream, solution ℞ *topical corticosteroidal anti-inflammatory* [halcinonide]

Halog-E cream ℞ *topical corticosteroidal anti-inflammatory; emollient* [halcinonide]

Halogen Ear Drops (discontinued 1991) OTC *antibacterial/antifungal* [chloroxylenol; acetic acid; benzalkonium chloride]
halometasone INN
halonamine INN
halopemide USAN, INN *antipsychotic*
halopenium chloride INN, BAN
haloperidol USAN, USP, INN, BAN *antidyskinetic for Tourette's disease; antipsychotic*
haloperidol decanoate USAN, BAN *antipsychotic*
haloperidol lactate *antidyskinetic for Tourette's disease; antipsychotic*
halopone chloride [see: halopenium chloride]
halopredone INN *topical anti-inflammatory* [also: halopredone acetate]
halopredone acetate USAN *topical anti-inflammatory* [also: halopredone]
haloprogesterone USAN, INN *progestin*
haloprogin USAN, USP, INN *antibacterial; antifungal*
halopyramine BAN [also: chloropyramine]
Halotestin tablets ℞ *androgenic hormone for male hypogonadism and breast cancer* [fluoxymesterone]
Halotex cream, solution ℞ *topical antifungal* [haloprogin]
halothane USP, INN, BAN *inhalation general anesthetic*
Halotussin AC liquid ℞ *expectorant; antitussive* [guaifenesin; codeine phosphate]
Halotussin PE liquid OTC *expectorant; decongestant* [guaifenesin; pseudoephedrine HCl]
Halotussin syrup OTC *expectorant* [guaifenesin; alcohol]
Halotussin-DAC liquid ℞ *expectorant; antitussive; decongestant* [guaifenesin; pseudoephedrine HCl; codeine]
Halotussin-DM syrup, sugar-free liquid OTC *expectorant; antitussive* [guaifenesin; dextromethorphan hydrobromide]
haloxazolam INN
haloxon INN, BAN
halquinol BAN *topical anti-infective* [also: halquinols]
halquinols USAN *topical anti-infective* [also: halquinol]
Haltran tablets OTC *nonsteroidal anti-inflammatory drug (NSAID); antiarthritic; analgesic* [ibuprofen]
HAM (hexamethylmelamine, Adriamycin, melphalan) *chemotherapy protocol*
HAM (hexamethylmelamine, Adriamycin, methotrexate) *chemotherapy protocol*
hamamelis water *astringent*
hamycin USAN, INN *antifungal*
hard fat [see: fat, hard]
Harmonyl tablets (discontinued 1991) ℞ *antihypertensive* [deserpidine]
Havrix ℞ *investigational vaccine for hepatitis A*
Hayfebrol liquid OTC *decongestant; antihistamine* [pseudoephedrine HCl; chlorpheniramine maleate]
HBIG (hepatitis B immune globulin) [q.v.]
H-BIG IM injection ℞ *hepatitis B immunizing agent* [hepatitis B immune globulin]
HC (hydrocortisone) [q.v.]
4-HC (4-hydroperoxycyclophosphamide) [q.v.]
HC Derma-Pax liquid OTC *topical corticosteroid; antihistamine; antiseptic* [hydrocortisone; pyrilamine maleate; chlorpheniramine maleate; alcohol; chlorobutanol]
1% HC ointment ℞ *topical corticosteroid* [hydrocortisone]
HCA (hydrocortisone acetate) [q.v.]
H-CAP (hexamethylmelamine, cyclophosphamide, Adriamycin, Platinol) *chemotherapy protocol*

hCG (human chorionic gonadotropin) [see: gonadotropin, chorionic]
HCG-nostick test kit ℞ *in vitro diagnostic aid for urine pregnancy test*
HCT (hydrochlorothiazide) [q.v.]
HCTZ (hydrochlorothiazide) [q.v.]
HD 200 Plus powder for suspension ℞ *GI contrast radiopaque agent* [barium sulfate]
HD 85 suspension ℞ *GI contrast radiopaque agent* [barium sulfate]
HDCV (human diploid cell vaccine) [see: rabies vaccine]
HDMTX-CF (high-dose methotrexate, citrovorum factor) *chemotherapy protocol*
HDMTX/LV (high-dose methotrexate, leucovorin) *chemotherapy protocol*
HDPEB (high-dose PEB protocol) *chemotherapy protocol* [see: PEB]
HD-VAC (high-dose [methotrexate], vinblastine, Adriamycin, cisplatin) *chemotherapy protocol*
Head & Shoulders cream shampoo, lotion shampoo OTC *antiseborrheic; antibacterial; antifungal* [pyrithione zinc]
Head & Shoulders Dry Scalp shampoo OTC *antiseborrheic; antibacterial; antifungal* [pyrithione zinc]
Head & Shoulders Intensive Treatment Dandruff Shampoo OTC *antiseborrheic* [selenium sulfide]
Healon intraocular injection ℞ *viscoelastic agent for ophthalmic surgery* [sodium hyaluronate]
Healon-GV ℞ *investigational viscoelastic agent for ophthalmic surgery* [sodium hyaluronate]
Heatrol tablets OTC *salt replacement; electrolyte replacement* [sodium chloride; potassium chloride; calcium phosphate; magnesium carbonate]
heavy liquid petrolatum [see: mineral oil]
heavy water (D_2O) [see: deuterium oxide]

Heb Cream Base OTC *cream base*
hedaquinium chloride INN, BAN
Heet Liniment OTC *counterirritant; topical antiseptic* [methyl salicylate; camphor; capsicum oleoresin; alcohol]
Heet Spray OTC *counterirritant; topical antiseptic* [methyl salicylate; camphor; menthol; methyl nicotinate; alcohol]
hefilcon A USAN *hydrophilic contact lens material*
hefilcon B USAN *hydrophilic contact lens material*
helenien [see: xantofyl palmitate]
helicon [see: aspirin]
heliomycin INN
Helistat sponge ℞ *hemostasis adjunct during surgery* [absorbable collagen hemostatic sponge]
helium USP *diluent for gases; element (He)*
Hemabate IM injection ℞ *abortifacient; for postpartum uterine bleeding* [carboprost tromethamine]
Hema-Check test slides OTC *in vitro diagnostic aid for fecal occult blood*
Hema-Combistix reagent strips OTC *in vitro diagnostic aid for multiple urine products*
Hemaspan timed-release tablets OTC *hematinic* [ferrous fumarate; vitamin C]
Hemastix reagent strips OTC *in vitro diagnostic aid for urine occult blood*
Hematest tablets OTC *in vitro diagnostic aid for fecal occult blood*
Hematran IV, IM injection (discontinued 1991) ℞ *antianemic* [iron dextran]
heme arginate *(orphan: acute symptomatic porphyria)*
HemeSelect OTC *in vitro diagnostic aid for fecal occult blood*
Hemet Hemorrhoidal suppositories (discontinued 1991) OTC *topical anesthetic; astringent* [benzocaine;

zinc oxide; bismuth subgallate; balsam Peru]

Hemet Rectal ointment OTC *topical anesthetic; vasoconstrictor; astringent* [diperodon HCl; pyrilamine maleate; phenylephrine HCl; bismuth subcarbonate; zinc oxide]

hemiacidrin [see: citric acid, glucono-delta-lactone & magnesium carbonate]

hemin (*orphan: acute intermittent porphyria; hereditary coproporphyria*)

Hemocaine anorectal ointment OTC *topical anesthetic; vasoconstrictor; astringent* [diperodon HCl; pyrilamine maleate; phenylephrine HCl; bismuth subcarbonate; zinc oxide]

Hemoccult II test kit OTC *in vitro diagnostic aid for fecal occult blood*

Hemoccult SENSA OTC *in vitro diagnostic aid for fecal occult blood*

Hemoccult test slides OTC *in vitro diagnostic aid for fecal occult blood*

Hemocyte IM injection ℞ *hematinic* [ferrous gluconate; multiple B vitamins; procaine HCl]

Hemocyte Plus tablets ℞ *hematinic* [ferrous fumarate; multiple B vitamins; sodium ascorbate; folic acid]

Hemocyte tablets OTC *hematinic* [ferrous fumarate]

Hemocyte-F tablets ℞ *hematinic* [ferrous fumarate; folic acid]

Hemocyte-V IM injection ℞ *hematinic* [ferrous gluconate; multiple B vitamins]

Hemofil M IV ℞ *antihemophilic; correct coagulation deficiency* [antihemophilic factor]

Hemophilus b conjugate vaccine active bacterin for *Haemophilus influenzae* type b

Hemorrhoidal HC rectal suppositories ℞ *topical corticosteroidal anti-inflammatory; antipruritic* [hydrocortisone acetate; zinc oxide; bismuth salts]

Hemorrhoidal Uniserts (name changed to Hemril Uniserts in 1990)

Hemotene ℞ *topical hemostatic aid in surgery* [microfibrillar collagen hemostat]

Hemo-Vite liquid ℞ *antianemic* [ferric pyrophosphate; multiple B vitamins; folic acid]

Hemo-Vite tablets ℞ *antianemic* [ferrous fumarate; intrinsic factor; vitamin C; multiple B vitamins; folic acid]

Hem-Prep rectal suppositories OTC *topical antiseptic; astringent; anesthetic; emollient* [phenylmercuric nitrate; bismuth subgallate; zinc oxide; benzocaine]

Hemril Uniserts (suppositories) OTC *astringent; emollient/protectant* [bismuth subgallate; bismuth resorcin compound; benzyl benzoate; zinc oxide; balsam Peru]

Hemril-HC Uniserts (suppositories) ℞ *topical corticosteroidal anti-inflammatory; antipruritic* [hydrocortisone acetate]

heneicosafluorotripropylamine [see: perfluamine]

HEOD (hexachloro-epoxy-octahydro-dimethanonaphthalene) [see: dieldrin]

heparin BAN *anticoagulant* [also: heparin calcium]

heparin calcium USP *anticoagulant* [also: heparin]

heparin sodium USP, INN, BAN *anticoagulant*

HepatAmine IV infusion ℞ *nutritional therapy for hepatic failure and hepatic encephalopathy* [multiple branched-chain essential & nonessential amino acids; electrolytes]

Hepatic-Aid II Instant Drink powder OTC *oral nutritional supplement for liver disease*

hepatitis B immune globulin (HBIG) USP *passive immunizing agent*

hepatitis B surface antigen [see: hepatitis B virus vaccine, inactivated]

hepatitis B virus vaccine, inactivated USP *active immunizing agent*

Hep-B-Gammagee IM injection ℞ *hepatitis B immunizing agent* [hepatitis B immune globulin]

Hepfomin-R IM ℞ *antianemic; vitamin supplement* [liver extracts; vitamin B$_{12}$; folic acid]

Hep-Forte capsules OTC *geriatric dietary supplement* [multiple B vitamins & minerals; folic acid; biotin; liver fraction; desiccated liver]

Hepicebrin tablets (discontinued 1991) OTC *vitamin supplement* [multiple vitamins; sodium bisulfite]

Hep-Lock; Hep-Lock U/P solution ℞ *IV flush for catheter patency (not therapeutic)* [heparin sodium]

Hep-Lock PF solution (discontinued 1992) ℞ *IV flush for catheter patency (not therapeutic)* [heparin sodium]

HEPP (H-chain ε [IgE] pentapeptide) [see: pentigetide]

hepronicate INN

heptabarb INN [also: heptabarbitone]

heptabarbital [see: heptabarb; heptabarbitone]

heptabarbitone BAN [also: heptabarb]

heptaminol INN, BAN

heptaminol HCl [see: heptaminol]

2-heptanamine [see: tuaminoheptane]

2-heptanamine sulfate [see: tuaminoheptane sulfate]

Heptavax-B IM injection (discontinued 1991) ℞ *hepatitis B vaccine* [hepatitis B virus vaccine, inactivated]

heptaverine INN

heptolamide INN

Heptuna Plus capsules ℞ *hematinic* [ferrous sulfate; multiple B vitamins; multiple minerals; vitamin C; intrinsic factor concentrate]

hepzidine INN

HER2 ℞ *investigational antineoplastic for breast and ovarian cancer* [monoclonal antibodies]

Herbal Cellulex tablets (discontinued 1992) OTC *dietary supplement* [vitamin C; multiple minerals]

Herbal Laxative tablets OTC *laxative* [senna leaves; cascara sagrada bark]

heroin *(banned in USA)*

heroin HCl *(banned in USA)* [see: diacetylmorphine HCl]

Herpecin-L lip balm OTC *topical protectant; sunblock; vulnerary* [pyridoxine HCl; allantoin; padimate O; titanium dioxide]

Herpetrol tablets OTC *dietary supplement; claimed to prevent and treat herpes simplex infections* [L-lysine; multiple vitamins; zinc]

Herplex Liquifilm eye drops ℞ *ophthalmic antiviral* [idoxuridine]

HES (hydroxyethyl starch) [see: hetastarch]

Hespan IV infusion ℞ *plasma volume expander in shock due to hemorrhage, burns, surgery* [hetastarch]

hesperidin

hesperidin methyl chalcone [see: bioflavonoids]

hetacillin USAN, USP, INN, BAN *antibacterial*

hetacillin potassium USAN, USP *antibacterial*

hetaflur USAN, INN, BAN *dental caries prophylactic*

hetastarch USAN, BAN *plasma volume extender*

heteronium bromide USAN, INN, BAN *anticholinergic*

Hetrazan tablets (discontinued 1991) ℞ *anthelmintic* [diethylcarbamazine citrate]

hexaammonium molybdate tetrahydrate [see: ammonium molybdate]

Hexabrix injection ℞ *parenteral radiopaque agent* [ioxaglate meglumine; ioxaglate sodium]
HexaCAF; Hexa-CAF (hexamethylmelamine, cyclophosphamide, amethopterin, fluorouracil) *chemotherapy protocol*
hexacarbacholine bromide INN [also: carbolonium bromide]
hexachlorane [see: lindane]
hexachlorocyclohexane [see: lindane]
hexachlorophane BAN *topical anti-infective; detergent* [also: hexachlorophene]
hexachlorophene USP, INN *topical anti-infective; detergent* [also: hexachlorophane]
hexacyclonate sodium INN
hexacyprone INN
hexadecanoic acid, methylethyl ester [see: isopropyl palmitate]
hexadecanol [see: cetyl alcohol]
hexadecylamine hydrofluoride [see: hetaflur]
hexadecylpyridinium chloride [see: cetylpyridinium chloride]
hexadecyltrimethylammonium bromide [see: cetrimonium bromide]
hexadecyltrimethylammonium chloride [see: cetrimonium chloride]
2,4-hexadienoic acid, potassium salt [see: potassium sorbate]
hexadiline INN
hexadimethrine bromide INN, BAN
hexadiphane [see: prozapine]
Hexadrol Phosphate intra-articular, intralesional, soft tissue, or IM injection ℞ *glucocorticoids* [dexamethasone sodium phosphate]
Hexadrol tablets, elixir ℞ *glucocorticoids* [dexamethasone]
hexadylamine [see: hexadiline]
hexafluorenium bromide USAN, USP *skeletal muscle relaxant; succinylcholine synergist* [also: hexafluronium bromide]
hexafluorodiethyl ether [see: flurothyl]
hexaflurone bromide [see: hexafluorenium bromide]
hexafluronium bromide INN *skeletal muscle relaxant; succinylcholine synergist* [also: hexafluorenium bromide]
Hexalen capsules ℞ *antineoplastic for ovarian adenocarcinoma (orphan)* [altretamine]
Hexalol tablets ℞ *urinary anti-infective; analgesic; antispasmodic; acidifier* [atropine sulfate; hyoscyamine; methylene blue; phenyl salicylate; benzoic acid]
hexamarium bromide [see: distigmine bromide]
hexametazime BAN
hexamethone bromide [see: hexamethonium bromide]
hexamethonium bromide INN, BAN
hexamethylenamine [now: methenamine]
hexamethylenamine mandelate [see: methenamine mandelate]
hexamethylenetetramine [see: methenamine]
hexamethylmelamine (HMM; HXM) [see: altretamine]
hexamidine INN
hexamine hippurate BAN *urinary antibacterial* [also: methenamine hippurate]
hexamine mandelate [see: methenamine mandelate]
hexapradol INN
hexaprofen INN, BAN
hexapropymate INN, BAN
hexasonium iodide INN
Hexastat *(orphan: advanced ovarian adenocarcinoma)* [hexamethylmelamine]
hexavitamin USP
Hexavitamin tablets OTC *vitamin supplement* [multiple vitamins]

hexcarbacholine bromide INN [also: carbolonium bromide]
hexedine USAN, INN *antibacterial*
hexemal [see: cyclobarbital]
hexestrol NF, INN
hexetidine BAN
hexicide [see: lindane]
hexinol [see: cyclomenol]
hexobarbital USP, INN
hexobarbital sodium NF
hexobendine USAN, INN, BAN *vasodilator*
hexocyclium methylsulfate *peptic ulcer adjunct* [also: hexocyclium metilsulfate; hexocyclium methylsulphate]
hexocyclium methylsulphate BAN [also: hexocyclium methylsulfate; hexocyclium metilsulfate]
hexocyclium metilsulfate INN [also: hexocyclium methylsulfate; hexocyclium methylsulphate]
hexoprenaline INN, BAN
hexoprenaline sulfate *investigational tocolytic agent*
hexopyrimidine [see: hexetidine]
hexopyrrolate [see: hexopyrronium bromide]
hexopyrronium bromide INN
hexydaline [see: methenamine mandelate]
hexylcaine INN *local anesthetic* [also: hexylcaine HCl]
hexylcaine HCl USP *local anesthetic* [also: hexylcaine]
hexylene glycol NF *humectant; solvent*
hexylresorcinol USP *anthelmintic; topical antiseptic*
1-hexyltheobromine [see: pentifylline]
H-F Gel (*orphan: hydrofluoric acid burns*) [calcium gluconate]
hFSH (human follicle-stimulating hormone) [now: menotropins]
HFZ (homofenazine) [q.v.]
^{197}**Hg** [see: chlormerodrin Hg 197]
^{197}**Hg** [see: merisoprol acetate Hg 197]
^{197}**Hg** [see: merisoprol Hg 197]
^{203}**Hg** [see: chlormerodrin Hg 203]
^{203}**Hg** [see: merisoprol acetate Hg 203]
H-H-R tablets (discontinued 1993) ℞ *antihypertensive* [hydralazine HCl; hydrochlorothiazide; reserpine]
Hibiclens Antiseptic/AntiMicrobial Skin Cleanser liquid OTC *broad-spectrum antimicrobial; germicidal* [chlorhexidine gluconate; alcohol]
Hibiclens sponge/brush OTC *broad-spectrum antimicrobial; germicidal* [chlorhexidine gluconate; alcohol]
Hibistat Germicidal Hand Rinse liquid OTC *broad-spectrum antimicrobial; germicidal* [chlorhexidine gluconate; alcohol]
Hibistat Towelette wipes OTC *broad-spectrum antimicrobial; germicidal* [chlorhexidine gluconate; alcohol]
HibTITER IM injection ℞ *Haemophilus influenzae type b (HIB) vaccine* [Hemophilus b conjugate vaccine]
Hi-Cor 1.0; Hi-Cor 2.5 cream ℞ *topical corticosteroid* [hydrocortisone]
HIDA (hepatoiminodiacetic acid) [see: lidofenin]
high molecular weight dextran [see: dextran 70]
High Potency N-Vites tablets OTC *vitamin supplement* [multiple B vitamins; vitamin C]
Hipotest tablets OTC *dietary supplement* [multiple vitamins, minerals & food products; calcium; iron; folic acid; biotin]
Hi-Po-Vites tablets OTC *dietary supplement* [multiple vitamins, minerals & food products; iron; folic acid; biotin]
Hiprex tablets ℞ *urinary antibacterial* [methenamine hippurate]
Hirulog ℞ *investigational agent for deep venous thrombosis and unstable angina*
Hismanal tablets ℞ *antihistamine* [astemizole]
Hismanal-D ℞ *investigational antihistamine/decongestant combination*

Hispril Spansules (sustained-release capsules) (discontinued 1991) ℞ *antihistamine* [diphenylpyraline HCl]

Histabid Duracaps (sustained-release capsules) (discontinued 1991) ℞ *decongestant; antihistamine* [phenylpropanolamine HCl; chlorpheniramine maleate]

Histagesic Modified tablets OTC *decongestant; antihistamine; analgesic* [phenylephrine HCl; chlorpheniramine maleate; acetaminophen]

Histaject subcu or IM injection ℞ *antihistamine; anaphylaxis* [brompheniramine maleate]

Histalet Forte tablets ℞ *decongestant; antihistamine* [phenylpropanolamine HCl; phenylephrine HCl; chlorpheniramine maleate; pyrilamine maleate]

Histalet syrup ℞ *decongestant; antihistamine* [pseudoephedrine HCl; chlorpheniramine maleate]

Histalet X tablets, syrup ℞ *decongestant; expectorant* [pseudoephedrine HCl; guaifenesin]

Histamic sustained-release capsules ℞ *decongestant; antihistamine* [phenylpropanolamine HCl; phenylephrine HCl; chlorpheniramine maleate; phenyltoloxamine citrate]

histamine dihydrochloride USAN

histamine phosphate USP *gastric secretory stimulant; diagnostic aid for pheochromocytoma*

histantin [see: chlorcyclizine HCl]

histapyrrodine INN

Histatab Plus tablets OTC *decongestant; antihistamine* [phenylephrine HCl; chlorpheniramine maleate]

Histatan Pediatric suspension ℞ *decongestant; antihistamine* [phenylephrine tannate; chlorpheniramine tannate; pyrilamine tannate]

Histatime Forte tablets ℞ *decongestant; antihistamine* [phenylpropanolamine HCl; phenylephrine HCl; chlorpheniramine maleate; pyrilamine maleate]

Histatrol intracutaneous injection, topical solution ℞ *intradermal or prick, puncture and scratch allergenic skin test* [histamine phosphate]

Hista-Vadrin Decongestant tablets ℞ *decongestant; antihistamine* [phenylpropanolamine HCl; phenylephrine HCl; chlorpheniramine maleate]

Histerone 50; Histerone 100 IM injection ℞ *androgen replacement for delayed puberty or breast cancer* [testosterone]

histidine (L-histidine) USAN, USP, INN *amino acid (essential in infants and in renal failure, nonessential otherwise); symbols:* His, H

histidine monohydrochloride NF

Histodrix sustained-release tablets OTC *decongestant; antihistamine* [pseudoephedrine sulfate; dexbrompheniramine maleate]

Histolyn-CYL intradermal injection ℞ *diagnostic aid for histoplasmosis* [histoplasmin]

histoplasmin USP *dermal histoplasmosis test*

Histor-D syrup ℞ *decongestant; antihistamine* [phenylephrine HCl; chlorpheniramine maleate; alcohol]

Histor-D Timecelles (sustained-release capsules) ℞ *decongestant; antihistamine; anticholinergic* [phenylephrine HCl; chlorpheniramine maleate; methscopolamine nitrate]

Histosal tablets OTC *decongestant; antihistamine; analgesic* [phenylpropanolamine HCl; pyrilamine maleate; acetaminophen; caffeine]

histrelin USAN, INN *LHRH agonist; (orphan: acute intermittent porphyria; central precocious puberty)*

histrelin acetate *LHRH agonist; (orphan: acute intermittent porphyria; central precocious puberty)*

Histussin HC syrup ℞ *decongestant; antihistamine; antitussive* [phenylephrine HCl; chlorpheniramine maleate; hydrocodone bitartrate]

HIV immune globulin [see: human immunodeficiency virus immune globulin]

HIV immunotherapeutic *investigational immunomodulator for AIDS*

HIV neutralizing antibodies *(orphan: AIDS)*

HIV vaccine *investigational antiviral for AIDS* [also: RG 83894]

HIVAB HIV-1/HIV-2 (rDNA) EIA test kit OTC *in vitro diagnostic aid for HIV-1 and HIV-2 antibody*

Hi-Value III; Hi-Value V *investigational in vitro diagnostic aid for glucose levels*

Hi-Vegi-Lip tablets OTC *digestive enzymes* [pancreatin]

Hivid film-coated tablets ℞ *antiviral for advanced HIV infection; (orphan: AIDS)* [zalcitabine]

HMB (homatropine methylbromide) [q.v.]

HMDP (hydroxymethylene diphosphonate) [see: oxidronic acid]

hMG (human menopausal gonadotropin) [see: menotropins]

HMM (hexamethylmelamine) [see: altretamine]

HMS Liquifilm eye drop suspension ℞ *ophthalmic topical corticosteroidal anti-inflammatory* [medrysone]

HN₂ (nitrogen mustard) [see: mechlorethamine HCl]

HOAP-BLEO (hydroxydaunomycin, Oncovin, ara-C, prednisone, bleomycin) *chemotherapy protocol*

Hold DM; Children's Hold lozenges OTC *antitussive* [dextromethorphan hydrobromide]

holmium *element (Ho)*

homarylamine INN

Homatrine eye drops (discontinued 1991) ℞ *cycloplegic; mydriatic* [homatropine hydrobromide]

homatropine BAN *ophthalmic anticholinergic* [also: homatropine hydrobromide]

homatropine hydrobromide USP *ophthalmic anticholinergic; cycloplegic; mydriatic* [also: homatropine]

homatropine methylbromide USP, INN, BAN *GI anticholinergic/antispasmodic*

Home Treatment Fluoride Gelution gel ℞ *topical dental caries preventative* [acidulated phosphate fluoride]

Homicebrin liquid (discontinued 1992) OTC *vitamin supplement* [multiple vitamins]

homidium bromide INN, BAN

homochlorcyclizine INN, BAN

homofenazine (HFZ) INN

homomenthyl salicylate [now: homosalate]

homopipramol INN

homosalate USAN, INN *ultraviolet screen*

4-homosulfanilamide [see: mafenide]

homprenorphine INN, BAN

HOP (hydroxydaunomycin, Oncovin, prednisone) *chemotherapy protocol*

hopantenic acid INN

hoquizil INN *bronchodilator* [also: hoquizil HCl]

hoquizil HCl USAN *bronchodilator* [also: hoquizil]

H.P. Acthar IM or subcu injectable gel ℞ *steroid* [repository corticotropin]

HPA-23 *(orphan: AIDS)*

HRT ℞ *investigational osteoporosis treatment* [norethindrone acetate; ethinyl estradiol]

HT (human thrombin) [see: thrombin]

HT; 3-HT (3-hydroxytyramine) [see: dopamine]

Hulk Hogan Complete Multi-Vitamins chewable tablets OTC *vitamin/*

mineral supplement [multiple vitamins & minerals; folic acid; biotin]
Hulk Hogan Multi-Vitamins Plus Extra C chewable tablets OTC *vitamin supplement* [multiple vitamins; folic acid]
Hulk Hogan Multi-Vitamins Plus Iron chewable tablets OTC *vitamin/iron supplement* [multiple vitamins; iron; folic acid]
human albumin [see: albumin, human]
human amniotic fluid-derived surfactant [see: surfactant, human amniotic fluid derived]
human antihemophilic factor [see: antihemophilic factor]
human chorionic gonadotropin (hCG) [see: gonadotropin, chorionic]
human cytomegalovirus immune globulin [see: cytomegalovirus immune globulin, human]
human diploid cell vaccine (HDCV) [see: rabies vaccine]
human epidermal growth factor [see: epidermal growth factor, human]
human fibrinogen [see: fibrinogen, human]
human fibrinolysin [see: fibrinolysin, human]
human follicle-stimulating hormone (hFSH) [now: menotropins]
human growth hormone, recombinant *(orphan status withdrawn 1993)*
human growth hormone releasing factor [see: growth hormone-releasing factor]
human IgM monoclonal antibody (C-58) to cytomegalovirus (CMV) *(orphan: prophylaxis and treatment of CMV in bone marrow transplants)*
human immunodeficiency virus (HIV-1) immune globulin *(orphan: AIDS; HIV-infected pregnant women and infants of HIV-infected mothers)*
human insulin [see: insulin, human]
human menopausal gonadotropin (hMG) [see: menotropins]
human respiratory syncytial virus immune globulin [see: respiratory syncytial virus immune globulin, human]
human superoxide dismutase (SOD) [see: superoxide dismutase, human]
Human Surf *(orphan: neonatal respiratory distress syndrome)* [surfactant, human amniotic fluid derived]
human T-cell inhibitor [see: muromonab-CD3]
human T-lymphotrophic virus type III (HTLV-III) gp-160 antigens *(orphan: AIDS)*
Humate-P IV injection ℞ *antihemophilic* [antihemophilic factor]
Humatin capsules ℞ *aminoglycoside-type antibiotic; amebicide* [paromomycin sulfate]
Humatrope powder for injection ℞ *growth hormone; (orphan: growth failure; Turner syndrome; anovulation; severe burns)* [somatropin]
Humibid DM sustained-release tablets ℞ *expectorant; antitussive* [guaifenesin; dextromethorphan hydrobromide]
Humibid L.A. sustained-release tablets ℞ *expectorant* [guaifenesin]
Humibid Sprinkle sustained-release capsules ℞ *expectorant* [guaifenesin]
HuMist nasal mist OTC *nasal moisturizer* [sodium chloride (saline)]
Humorphan H.P. *(orphan: narcotic-tolerant pain)* [oxymorphone HCl]
Humorsol Ocumeter (eye drops) ℞ *antiglaucoma agent; reversible cholinesterase inhibitor miotic* [demecarium bromide]
Humulin 50/50 subcu injection OTC *antidiabetic* [isophane insulin; human insulin]

Humulin 70/30 subcu injection OTC *antidiabetic* [isophane insulin; insulin]
Humulin BR subcu injection OTC *antidiabetic* [insulin]
Humulin L subcu injection OTC *antidiabetic* [insulin zinc]
Humulin N subcu injection OTC *antidiabetic* [isophane insulin]
Humulin R subcu injection OTC *antidiabetic* [insulin]
Humulin U Ultralente subcu injection OTC *antidiabetic* [insulin zinc]
Hurricaine spray, liquid, gel OTC *topical oral anesthetic* [benzocaine]
HVS 1 + 2 solution OTC *oral antibacterial* [benzalkonium chloride]
HXM (hexamethylmelamine) [see: altretamine]
Hyalex tablets OTC *vitamin/mineral supplement* [multiple vitamins; magnesium salicylate; magnesium PABA; zinc]
hyalosidase INN, BAN
hyaluronate sodium USAN, BAN *veterinary synovitis agent; ophthalmic surgical aid*
hyaluronidase USP, INN, BAN *dispersion aid*
hyaluronoglucosaminidase [see: hyalosidase]
hyamate [see: buramate]
Hybalamin IM injection (discontinued 1991) ℞ *antianemic; vitamin supplement* [hydroxocobalamin]
Hybolin Decanoate-50; Hybolin Decanoate-100 IM injection ℞ *anabolic steroid for anemia of renal insufficiency* [nandrolone decanoate]
Hybolin Improved IM injection ℞ *anabolic steroid for metastatic breast cancer in women* [nandrolone phenpropionate]
Hybri-CEAker (*orphan: diagnostic aid in colorectal carcinoma*) [indium In 111 altumomab pentetate]
hycanthone USAN, INN *antischistosomal*

hycanthone mesylate
Hycodan tablets, syrup ℞ *antitussive; anticholinergic* [hydrocodone bitartrate; homatropine methylbromide]
Hycomine Compound tablets ℞ *decongestant; antihistamine; antitussive; analgesic* [phenylephrine HCl; chlorpheniramine maleate; hydrocodone bitartrate; acetaminophen; caffeine]
Hycomine syrup, pediatric syrup ℞ *decongestant; antitussive* [phenylpropanolamine HCl; hydrocodone bitartrate]
Hycort cream, ointment ℞ *topical corticosteroid* [hydrocortisone]
Hycotuss Expectorant syrup ℞ *antitussive; expectorant* [hydrocodone bitartrate; guaifenesin; alcohol]
Hydeltrasol IV, IM injection ℞ *glucocorticoids* [prednisolone sodium phosphate]
Hydeltra-T.B.A. intra-articular, intralesional, or soft tissue injection ℞ *glucocorticoids* [prednisolone tebutate]
Hydergine LC liquid capsules ℞ *for age-related mental capacity decline* [ergoloid mesylates]
Hydergine sublingual tablets, tablets, liquid ℞ *for age-related mental capacity decline* [ergoloid mesylates]
Hydextran IV, IM injection (discontinued 1991) ℞ *antianemic* [iron dextran]
hydracarbazine INN
hydralazine INN, BAN *antihypertensive* [also: hydralazine HCl]
hydralazine HCl USP *antihypertensive; peripheral vasodilator* [also: hydralazine]
hydralazine polistirex USAN *antihypertensive*
Hydramine syrup, elixir ℞ *antitussive* [diphenhydramine HCl]
Hydramyn syrup ℞ *antihistamine; antitussive* [diphenhydramine HCl]

Hydrap-ES tablets ℞ *antihypertensive* [hydrochlorothiazide; reserpine; hydralazine HCl]
hydrargaphen INN, BAN
hydrastine USP
hydrastine HCl USP
hydrastinine HCl NF
Hydrate IV or IM injection ℞ *antinauseant; antiemetic; antivertigo; motion sickness preventative* [dimenhydrinate]
Hydrazide 25/25; Hydrazide 50/50 capsules ℞ *antihypertensive* [hydrochlorothiazide; hydralazine HCl]
Hydra-Zide capsules ℞ *antihypertensive* [hydrochlorothiazide; hydralazine HCl]
hydrazinoxane [see: domoxin]
Hydrea capsules ℞ *antineoplastic for melanoma, ovarian carcinoma and myelocytic leukemia; (orphan: sickle cell anemia)* [hydroxyurea]
Hydrex tablets ℞ *diuretic; antihypertensive* [benzthiazide]
Hydrisalic gel ℞ *topical keratolytic* [salicylic acid]
Hydrisea lotion OTC *moisturizer; emollient* [Dead Sea salts]
Hydrisinol cream, lotion OTC *moisturizer; emollient*
hydrobentizide INN
Hydrobexan IM injection ℞ *antianemic; vitamin supplement* [hydroxocobalamin]
hydrobutamine [see: butidrine]
Hydrocare solution OTC *contact lens aid*
Hydrocet capsules ℞ *narcotic analgesic* [hydrocodone bitartrate; acetaminophen]
Hydro-Chlor tablets ℞ *diuretic; antihypertensive* [hydrochlorothiazide]
hydrochloric acid NF *acidifying agent*
hydrochloric acid, diluted NF *acidifying agent*
hydrochlorothiazide (HCT; HCTZ) USP, INN, BAN *diuretic; antihypertensive*

Hydrocil Instant powder OTC *bulk laxative* [psyllium hydrophilic mucilloid]
hydrocodone INN, BAN *antitussive* [also: hydrocodone bitartrate]
hydrocodone bitartrate USAN, USP *antitussive* [also: hydrocodone]
hydrocodone polistirex USAN *antitussive*
hydrocolloid gel *dressings for wet wounds*
Hydrocort cream ℞ *topical corticosteroid* [hydrocortisone]
hydrocortamate INN
hydrocortamate HCl [see: hydrocortamate]
hydrocortisone (HC) USP, INN, BAN *topical/ophthalmic corticosteroid*
hydrocortisone aceponate INN
hydrocortisone acetate (HCA) USP, BAN *topical/ophthalmic corticosteroid*
hydrocortisone buteprate USAN *glucocorticoid*
hydrocortisone butyrate USAN, USP, BAN *topical corticosteroid*
hydrocortisone cyclopentylpropionate [see: hydrocortisone cypionate]
hydrocortisone cypionate USP *glucocorticoid*
hydrocortisone hemisuccinate USP *adrenocortical steroid*
hydrocortisone sodium phosphate USP, BAN *glucocorticoid*
hydrocortisone sodium succinate USP, BAN *glucocorticoid*
hydrocortisone valerate USAN, USP *topical corticosteroid*
Hydrocortone Acetate intralesional, intra-articular, or soft tissue injection ℞ *glucocorticoids* [hydrocortisone acetate]
Hydrocortone Phosphate IV, subcu, or IM injection ℞ *glucocorticoids* [hydrocortisone sodium phosphate]
Hydrocortone tablets ℞ *glucocorticoids* [hydrocortisone]

Hydrocream Base OTC *cream base*

Hydro-Crysti 12 IM injection ℞ *antianemic; vitamin supplement* [hydroxocobalamin]

HydroDIURIL tablets ℞ *diuretic; antihypertensive* [hydrochlorothiazide]

Hydro-Ergoloid oral tablets, sublingual tablets ℞ *cognition adjuvant* [ergoloid mesylates]

hydrofilcon A USAN *hydrophilic contact lens material*

hydroflumethiazide USP, INN, BAN *antihypertensive; diuretic*

hydrofluoric acid *dental caries prophylactic*

Hydro-Fluserpine #2 tablets ℞ *antihypertensive* [hydroflumethiazide; reserpine]

hydrogen *element (H)*

hydrogen peroxide USP *topical antiinfective*

hydrogen tetrabromoaurate [see: bromauric acid]

hydrogenated ergot alkaloids [now: ergoloid mesylates]

hydrogenated vegetable oil [see: vegetable oil, hydrogenated]

Hydrogesic capsules ℞ *narcotic analgesic* [hydrocodone bitartrate; acetaminophen]

hydromadinone INN

Hydromal tablets ℞ *diuretic; antihypertensive* [hydrochlorothiazide]

Hydromet syrup ℞ *antitussive; GI antispasmodic* [hydrocodone bitartrate; homatropine methylbromide]

hydromorphinol INN, BAN

hydromorphone INN, BAN *narcotic analgesic* [also: hydromorphone HCl]

hydromorphone HCl USP *narcotic analgesic* [also: hydromorphone]

hydromorphone sulfate

Hydromox R tablets (discontinued 1992) ℞ *antihypertensive* [quinethazone; reserpine]

Hydromox tablets ℞ *diuretic; antihypertensive* [quinethazone]

Hydromycin ophthalmic suspension, otic suspension ℞ *topical antibiotic* [neomycin sulfate; polymyxin B sulfate; hydrocortisone]

Hydropane syrup ℞ *antitussive; GI antispasmodic* [hydrocodone bitartrate; homatropine hydrobromide]

Hydropel ointment OTC *skin protectant* [silicone; hydrophobic starch derivative; petrolatum]

4-hydroperoxycyclophosphamide (4-HC) *(orphan: ex vivo treatment of autologous bone marrow for acute myelogenous leukemia)*

Hydrophed tablets ℞ *antiasthmatic; bronchodilator; decongestant; anxiolytic* [theophylline; ephedrine sulfate; hydroxyzine HCl]

Hydrophen Pediatric liquid (discontinued 1992) ℞ *decongestant; antitussive* [phenylpropanolamine HCl; hydrocodone bitartrate]

Hydrophilic OTC *ointment base*

hydrophilic ointment [see: ointment, hydrophilic]

hydrophilic petrolatum [see: petrolatum, hydrophilic]

Hydropine; Hydropine H.P. tablets (discontinued 1993) ℞ *antihypertensive* [hydroflumethiazide; reserpine]

Hydropres 25; Hydropres 50 tablets ℞ *antihypertensive* [hydrochlorothiazide; reserpine]

Hydro-Propanolamine syrup ℞ *decongestant; antitussive* [hydrocodone bitartrate; phenylpropanolamine HCl]

hydroquinone USP *hyperpigmentation bleaching agent*

Hydro-Serp tablets ℞ *antihypertensive* [hydrochlorothiazide; reserpine]

Hydroserpine #1; Hydroserpine #2 tablets ℞ *antihypertensive* [hydrochlorothiazide; reserpine]

Hydrosine 25, Hydrosine 50 tablets ℞ *antihypertensive* [hydrochlorothiazide; reserpine]

Hydro-T tablets ℞ *diuretic; antihypertensive* [hydrochlorothiazide]
hydrotalcite INN, BAN
HydroTex cream ℞ *topical corticosteroid* [hydrocortisone]
HydroTex ointment (discontinued 1993) ℞ *topical corticosteroid* [hydrocortisone]
Hydroxacen injection ℞ *anxiolytic; antihistamine* [hydroxyzine HCl]
hydroxamethocaine BAN [also: hydroxytetracaine]
hydroxidione sodium succinate [see: hydroxydione sodium succinate]
hydroxindasate INN
hydroxindasol INN
hydroxizine chloride [see: hydroxyzine HCl]
Hydroxo-12 IM injection ℞ *antianemic; vitamin supplement* [hydroxocobalamin]
hydroxocobalamin USAN, USP, INN, BAN *vitamin; hematopoietic*
hydroxocobemine [see: hydroxocobalamin]
4'-hydroxyacetanilide [see: acetaminophen]
4'-hydroxyacetanilide salicylate [see: acetaminosalol]
hydroxyamfetamine INN *ophthalmic adrenergic; mydriatic* [also: hydroxyamphetamine hydrobromide; hydroxyamphetamine]
hydroxyamphetamine BAN *ophthalmic adrenergic; mydriatic* [also: hydroxyamphetamine hydrobromide; hydroxyamfetamine]
hydroxyamphetamine hydrobromide USP *ophthalmic adrenergic; mydriatic* [also: hydroxyamfetamine; hydroxyamphetamine]
hydroxyapatite BAN *prosthetic aid* [also: durapatite; calcium phosphate, tribasic]
2-hydroxybenzamide [see: salicylamide]
2-hydroxybenzoic acid [see: salicylic acid]
o-hydroxybenzyl alcohol [see: salicyl alcohol]
hydroxybutanedioic acid [see: malic acid]
hydroxybutyrate sodium, gamma *(orphan: narcolepsy; cataplexy; sleep paralysis; hypnagogic hallucinations)*
hydroxycarbamide INN *antineoplastic* [also: hydroxyurea]
hydroxychloroquine INN, BAN *antimalarial; lupus erythematosus suppressant* [also: hydroxychloroquine sulfate]
hydroxychloroquine sulfate USP *antimalarial; antirheumatic; lupus erythematosus suppressant* [also: hydroxychloroquine]
25-hydroxycholecalciferol [see: calcifediol]
hydroxycincophene [see: oxycinchophen]
hydroxycobalamin & sodium thiosulfate *(orphan: severe acute cyanide poisoning)*
hydroxydaunomycin [see: doxorubicin]
14-hydroxydihydromorphine [see: hydromorphinol]
hydroxydione sodium succinate INN, BAN
hydroxyethyl cellulose NF *suspending and viscosity-increasing agent; ophthalmic aid*
hydroxyethyl starch (HES) [see: hetastarch]
hydroxyhexamide
hydroxylapatite [see: durapatite; calcium phosphate, tribasic]
hydroxymagnesium aluminate [see: magaldrate]
hydroxymesterone [see: medrysone]
hydroxymethylene diphosphonate (HMDP) [see: oxidronic acid]
hydroxymethylgramicidin [see: methocidin]

N-hydroxynaphthalimide diethyl phosphate [see: naftalofos]
hydroxypethidine INN, BAN
hydroxyphenamate USAN *minor tranquilizer* [also: oxyfenamate]
hydroxyprocaine INN, BAN
hydroxyprogesterone INN, BAN *progestin* [also: hydroxyprogesterone caproate]
hydroxyprogesterone caproate USP, INN *progestin* [also: hydroxyprogesterone]
hydroxypropyl cellulose NF *topical protectant; emulsifying and coating agent*
hydroxypropyl methylcellulose USP *suspending and viscosity-increasing agent; ophthalmic surgical aid* [also: hypromellose]
hydroxypropyl methylcellulose 1828 USP
hydroxypropyl methylcellulose phthalate NF *tablet-coating agent*
hydroxypropyl methylcellulose phthalate 200731 NF *tablet-coating agent*
hydroxypropyl methylcellulose phthalate 220824 NF *tablet-coating agent*
hydroxypyridine tartrate INN
hydroxyquinoline *topical antiseptic*
4′-hydroxysalicylanilide [see: osalmid]
hydroxystearin sulfate NF
hydroxystenozole INN
hydroxystilbamidine INN, BAN *antileishmanial* [also: hydroxystilbamidine isethionate]
hydroxystilbamidine isethionate USP *antileishmanial* [also: hydroxystilbamidine]
hydroxysuccinic acid [see: malic acid]
hydroxytetracaine INN [also: hydroxamethocaine]
hydroxytoluic acid INN, BAN
hydroxytryptophan [see: L-5 hydroxytryptophan]

3-hydroxytyramine (HT; 3-HT) [see: dopamine]
hydroxyurea USAN, USP, BAN *antineoplastic; (orphan: sickle cell anemia)* [also: hydroxycarbamide]
hydroxyzine INN, BAN *anxiolytic; minor tranquilizer; antihistamine; antipruritic* [also: hydroxyzine HCl]
hydroxyzine HCl USP *anxiolytic; minor tranquilizer; antihistamine; antipruritic* [also: hydroxyzine]
hydroxyzine pamoate USP *minor tranquilizer*
Hydro-Z-50 tablets (discontinued 1992) ℞ *diuretic; antihypertensive* [hydrochlorothiazide]
Hydrozide-50 tablets ℞ *diuretic; antihypertensive* [hydrochlorothiazide]
hy-Flow solution OTC *contact lens wetting solution*
Hygroton tablets ℞ *antihypertensive; diuretic* [chlorthalidone]
Hylidone tablets ℞ *antihypertensive* [chlorthalidone]
Hyliver Plus IM injection ℞ *antianemic; vitamin supplement* [liver extracts; vitamin B_{12}; folic acid]
Hylorel tablets ℞ *antihypertensive* [guanadrel sulfate]
Hylutin IM injection ℞ *progestin; amenorrhea; functional uterine bleeding* [hydroxyprogesterone caproate]
hymecromone USAN, INN *choleretic*
hyoscine hydrobromide BAN *GI antispasmodic; prevent motion sickness; cycloplegic; mydriatic* [also: scopolamine hydrobromide]
hyoscine methobromide BAN *anticholinergic* [also: methscopolamine bromide]
hyoscyamine (L-hyoscyamine) USP, BAN *anticholinergic*
hyoscyamine hydrobromide USP *anticholinergic*
hyoscyamine sulfate USP *GI anticholinergic/antispasmodic* [also: hyoscyamine sulphate]

hyoscyamine sulphate BAN GI *anticholinergic/antispasmodic* [also: hyoscyamine sulfate]
Hyosophen tablets, elixir ℞ *anticholinergic; sedative* [atropine sulfate; scopolamine hydrobromide; hyoscyamine hydrobromide; phenobarbital]
Hypaque Meglumine injection ℞ *parenteral radiopaque agent* [diatrizoate meglumine]
Hypaque Sodium solution, powder, injection ℞ *GI contrast radiopaque agent* [diatrizoate sodium]
Hypaque-Cysto intracavitary instillation ℞ *cholecystographic radiopaque agent* [diatrizoate meglumine]
Hypaque-M; Hypaque-76 injection ℞ *parenteral radiopaque agent* [diatrizoate meglumine; diatrizoate sodium]
Hyperab IM injection ℞ *rabies prophylaxis* [rabies immune globulin]
HyperHep IM injection ℞ *hepatitis B immunizing agent* [hepatitis B immune globulin]
hypericin *investigational antiviral for AIDS*
Hyperlyte; Hyperlyte CR; Hyperlyte R IV admixture ℞ *intravenous electrolyte therapy* [combined electrolyte solution]
Hypermune RSV (*orphan: prophylaxis and treatment of respiratory syncytial virus*) [respiratory syncytial virus immune globulin, human]
Hyperstat IV injection ℞ *antihypertensive for hypertensive emergencies* [diazoxide]
Hyper-Tet IM injection ℞ *tetanus immunizing agent* [tetanus immune globulin]
Hy-Phen tablets ℞ *narcotic analgesic* [hydrocodone bitartrate; acetaminophen]
hyphylline [see: dyphylline]
hypnogene [see: barbital]
hypochlorous acid, sodium salt [see: sodium hypochlorite]

Hypo-Clear solution (discontinued 1992) OTC *contact lens rinsing and storage solution* [saline solution]
α-hypophamine [see: oxytocin]
β-hypophamine [see: vasopressin]
hypophosphorous acid NF *antioxidant*
Hyporet (trademarked form) *prefilled disposable syringe*
Hypotears; Hypotears PF eye drops, ophthalmic ointment OTC *ocular moisturizer/lubricant*
HypRho-D; HypRho-D Mini Dose IM injection ℞ *obstetric Rh factor immunity suppressant* [Rh$_0$(D) immune globulin]
Hyprogest 250 IM injection ℞ *progestin; amenorrhea; functional uterine bleeding* [hydroxyprogesterone caproate]
hyprolose [see: hydroxypropyl cellulose]
hypromellose INN, BAN *suspending and viscosity-increasing agent* [also: hydroxypropyl methylcellulose]
Hyrexin-50 injection ℞ *antihistamine; motion sickness preventative; sleep aid; antiparkinsonian* [diphenhydramine HCl]
Hyskon uterine infusion ℞ *hysteroscopy aid* [dextran 70; dextrose]
Hysone cream (discontinued 1992) ℞ *topical corticosteroid; antifungal; antibacterial* [hydrocortisone; clioquinol]
Hytakerol capsules, oral solution ℞ *vitamin deficiency therapy* [dihydrotachysterol]
Hytinic capsules OTC *hematinic* [polysaccharide-iron complex]
Hytinic elixir (discontinued 1991) OTC *hematinic* [polysaccharide-iron complex]
Hytinic IM injection ℞ *hematinic* [ferrous gluconate; multiple B vitamins; procaine HCl]
Hytone cream, lotion, ointment ℞ *topical corticosteroid* [hydrocortisone]

Hytrin tablets ℞ *antihypertensive* [terazosin HCl]
Hytuss 2X capsules OTC *expectorant* [guaifenesin]
Hytuss tablets OTC *expectorant* [guaifenesin]
Hyzine-50 IM injection ℞ *anxiolytic* [hydroxyzine HCl]

I

I Rinse ophthalmic solution (discontinued 1991) OTC *extraocular irrigating solution* [balanced saline solution]
^{123}**I** [see: iodohippurate sodium I 123]
^{123}**I** [see: sodium iodide I 123]
^{125}**I** [see: albumin, iodinated I 125 serum]
^{125}**I** [see: diatrizoate sodium I 125]
^{125}**I** [see: diohippuric acid I 125]
^{125}**I** [see: diotyrosine I 125]
^{125}**I** [see: fibrinogen I 125]
^{125}**I** [see: insulin I 125]
^{125}**I** [see: iodohippurate sodium I 125]
^{125}**I** [see: iodopyracet I 125]
^{125}**I** [see: iomethin I 125]
^{125}**I** [see: iothalamate sodium I 125]
^{125}**I** [see: liothyronine I 125]
^{125}**I** [see: oleic acid I 125]
^{125}**I** [see: povidone I 125]
^{125}**I** [see: rose bengal sodium I 125]
^{125}**I** [see: sodium iodide I 125]
^{125}**I** [see: thyroxine I 125]
^{125}**I** [see: triolein I 125]
^{131}**I** [see: albumin, aggregated iodinated I 131 serum]
^{131}**I** [see: albumin, iodinated I 131 serum]
^{131}**I** [see: diatrizoate sodium I 131]
^{131}**I** [see: diohippuric acid I 131]
^{131}**I** [see: diotyrosine I 131]
^{131}**I** [see: ethiodized oil I 131]
^{131}**I** [see: insulin I 131]
^{131}**I** [see: iodipamide sodium I 131]
^{131}**I** [see: iodoantipyrine I 131]
^{131}**I** [see: iodocholesterol I 131]
^{131}**I** [see: iodohippurate sodium I 131]
^{131}**I** [see: iodopyracet I 131]
^{131}**I** [see: iomethin I 131]
^{131}**I** [see: iothalamate sodium I 131]
^{131}**I** [see: iotyrosine I 131]
^{131}**I** [see: liothyronine I 131]
^{131}**I** [see: macrosalb (^{131}I)]
^{131}**I** [see: oleic acid I 131]
^{131}**I** [see: povidone I 131]
^{131}**I** [see: rose bengal sodium I 131]
^{131}**I** [see: sodium iodide I 131]
^{131}**I** [see: thyroxine I 131]
^{131}**I** [see: tolpovidone I 131]
^{131}**I** [see: triolein I 131]
ibacitabine INN
ibafloxacin USAN, INN, BAN *antibacterial*
ibazocine INN
IBC (isobutyl cyanoacrylate) [see: bucrylate]
Iberet; Iberet-500 liquid, controlled-release Filmtabs (film-coated tablets) OTC *hematinic* [ferrous sulfate; multiple B vitamins; sodium ascorbate]
Iberet-Folic-500 controlled-release Filmtabs (film-coated tablets) ℞ *hematinic* [ferrous sulfate; multiple B vitamins; folic acid; sodium ascorbate]
Iberol Filmtabs (film-coated tablets) (discontinued 1991) OTC *antianemic* [ferrous sulfate; multiple B vitamins; sodium ascorbate]
Iberol-F Filmtabs (discontinued 1991) OTC *vitamin/iron supplement* [ferrous sulfate; vitamin C; multiple B vitamins; folic acid]
ibopamine USAN, INN, BAN *peripheral dopaminergic agent*
ibrotal [see: ibrotamide]

ibrotamide INN
ibudilast INN
ibufenac USAN, INN, BAN *analgesic; anti-inflammatory*
Ibuprin tablets OTC *nonsteroidal anti-inflammatory drug (NSAID); antiarthritic; analgesic* [ibuprofen]
ibuprofen USAN, USP, INN, BAN *antiarthritic; nonsteroidal anti-inflammatory drug (NSAID); analgesic*
ibuprofen aluminum USAN *anti-inflammatory*
ibuprofen piconol USAN *topical anti-inflammatory*
Ibuprohm caplets OTC *nonsteroidal anti-inflammatory drug (NSAID); antiarthritic; analgesic* [ibuprofen]
Ibuprohm tablets ℞/OTC *nonsteroidal anti-inflammatory drug (NSAID); antiarthritic; analgesic* [ibuprofen]
ibuproxam INN
Ibu-Tab film-coated tablets ℞/OTC *nonsteroidal anti-inflammatory drug (NSAID); antiarthritic; analgesic* [ibuprofen]
ibuterol INN
ibutilide INN *antiarrhythmic* [also: ibutilide fumarate]
ibutilide fumarate USAN *antiarrhythmic* [also: ibutilide]
ibuverine INN
ibylcaine chloride [see: butethamine HCl]
ICE (ifosfamide, carboplatin, etoposide) *chemotherapy protocol*
ichthammol USP, BAN *topical anti-infective*
ICI 139603 (tetronasin) [see: tetronasin 5930]
iclazepam INN
icosapent INN [also: doconexent; omega-3 marine triglycerides]
icospiramide INN
icotidine USAN *antagonist to histamine H_1 and H_2 receptors*
ictasol USAN *disinfectant*
Ictotest tablets OTC *in vitro diagnostic aid for bilirubin in the urine*

Icy Hot balm, cream, stick OTC *counterirritant* [methyl salicylate; menthol]
Idamycin powder for IV injection ℞ *antineoplastic antibiotic; (orphan: leukemia)* [idarubicin HCl]
Idarac ℞ *investigational nonsteroidal anti-inflammatory drug (NSAID); analgesic*
idarubicin INN, BAN *antineoplastic* [also: idarubicin HCl]
idarubicin HCl USAN, INN *antineoplastic; (orphan: leukemia)* [also: idarubicin]
idaverine INN
idazoxan INN, BAN
idebenone INN
idenast INN
Identi-Dose (trademarked form) *unit dose package*
idoxuridine (IDU) USAN, USP, INN, BAN *ophthalmic antiviral*
idralfidine INN
idrobutamine [see: butidrine]
idrocilamide INN
idropranolol INN
IDU (idoxuridine) [q.v.]
ifenprodil INN
Ifex powder for IV injection ℞ *antineoplastic; (orphan: testicular cancer; bone and soft tissue sarcomas)* [ifosfamide]
IFN (interferon) [q.v.]
IFN-alpha 2 (interferon alfa-2) [see: interferon alfa-2b, recombinant]
ifosfamide USAN, USP, INN, BAN *antineoplastic; (orphan: testicular cancer; bone and soft tissue sarcomas)*
ifoxetine INN
IG (immune globulin) [see: globulin, immune]
IgE pentapeptide [see: pentigetide]
IGIV (immune globulin intravenous) [see: globulin, immune]
IL-2 (interleukin-2) [see: aldesleukin; teceleukin; celmoleukin]

Iletin *insulin* [see under: Regular, NPH, Protamine, Lente, Semilente & Ultralente]
I-Liqui Tears eye drops (discontinued 1991) OTC *ocular moisturizer/lubricant*
ilmofosine USAN, INN *antineoplastic*
Ilopan IM injection, IV infusion ℞ *postoperative ileus prophylactic* [dexpanthenol]
Ilopan-Choline tablets ℞ *antiflatulent for splenic flexure syndrome* [dexpanthenol; choline bitartrate]
iloprost INN, BAN *(orphan: Raynaud's phenomenon; thrombocytopenia)*
Ilosone drops, chewable tablets (discontinued 1991) ℞ *macrolide antibiotic* [erythromycin estolate]
Ilosone tablets, Pulvules (capsules), oral suspension ℞ *macrolide antibiotic* [erythromycin estolate]
Ilotycin Gluceptate injection ℞ *macrolide antibiotic* [erythromycin gluceptate]
Ilotycin ophthalmic ointment ℞ *ophthalmic antibiotic* [erythromycin]
Ilozyme tablets ℞ *digestive enzymes* [pancrelipase]
I-L-X B$_{12}$ elixir OTC *hematinic* [ferric ammonium citrate; liver fraction 1; multiple B vitamins]
I-L-X B$_{12}$ tablets OTC *hematinic* [ferrous gluconate; desiccated liver; multiple vitamins]
I-L-X elixir OTC *hematinic* [ferrous gluconate; liver concentrate 1:20; multiple B vitamins]
imafen INN *antidepressant* [also: imafen HCl]
imafen HCl USAN *antidepressant* [also: imafen]
Imagent GI ℞ *investigational oral GI contrast agent for MRI and x-ray imaging*
imanixil INN
imazodan INN *cardiotonic* [also: imazodan HCl]

imazodan HCl USAN *cardiotonic* [also: imazodan]
imcarbofos USAN, INN *veterinary anthelmintic*
Imdur ℞ *investigational coronary vasodilator for angina*
I-Methasone eye drops (discontinued 1991) ℞ *ophthalmic topical corticosteroidal anti-inflammatory* [dexamethasone sodium phosphate]
imexon INN
Imfergen IM (discontinued 1991) ℞ *antianemic* [iron dextran]
Imferon IM injection (discontinued 1992) ℞ *antianemic* [iron dextran]
imiclopazine INN
imidapril INN, BAN
imidazole carboxamide [see: dacarbazine]
imidazole salicylate INN
imidecyl iodine USAN *topical anti-infective*
imidocarb INN, BAN *antiprotozoal (Babesia)* [also: imidocarb HCl]
imidocarb HCl USAN *antiprotozoal (Babesia)* [also: imidocarb]
imidoline INN *antipsychotic* [also: imidoline HCl]
imidoline HCl USAN *antipsychotic* [also: imidoline]
imidurea NF *antimicrobial*
Imigran (foreign name for U.S. product Imitrex)
imiloxan INN *antidepressant* [also: imiloxan HCl]
imiloxan HCl USAN *antidepressant* [also: imiloxan]
iminophenimide INN
iminostilbene [see: carbamazepine]
imipemide [now: imipenem]
imipenem USAN, INN, BAN *bactericidal antibiotic*
imipramine INN, BAN *antidepressant* [also: imipramine HCl]
imipramine HCl USP *tricyclic antidepressant; treatment of childhood enuresis* [also: imipramine]

imipramine pamoate *tricyclic antidepressant*
imipraminoxide INN
imiquimod USAN *immunomodulator*
imirestat INN
Imitrex subcu injection in vials, prefilled syringes, or SELFdose kits (two prefilled syringes) ℞ *serotonin agonist to relieve migraine attacks* [sumatriptan succinate]
Immther *(orphan: pulmonary and hepatic metastases of colorectal adenocarcinoma)* [disaccharide tripeptide glycerol dipalmitoyl]
immune globulin (IG) [see: globulin, immune]
immune globulin intramuscular [see: globulin, immune]
immune globulin intravenous (IGIV) [see: globulin, immune]
immune serum globulin (ISG) [see: globulin, immune]
Immunex CRP test kit ℞ *in vitro diagnostic aid for C-reactive protein to diagnose inflammatory conditions*
Immuno C1-Inhibitor (Human) Vapor Heated *(orphan: prevent angioedema)* [C1-inhibitor]
ImmuRAID-AFP *(orphan: diagnostic aid for hepatic cancer in AFP-producing tumors)* [technetium Tc 99m murine monoclonal antibody to human alpha-fetoprotein (AFP)]
ImmuRAID-CEA ℞ *investigational monoclonal antibody-based diagnostic aid for colorectal cancer*
ImmuRAID-hCG *(orphan: diagnostic aid for hCG-producing tumors)* [technetium Tc 99m murine monoclonal antibody to human chorionic gonadotropin (hCG)]
ImmuRAID-LL2 ℞ *investigational monoclonal antibody-based diagnostic aid for non-Hodgkin's B-cell lymphoma*
ImmuRAID-MN3 ℞ *investigational monoclonal antibody-based diagnostic aid for infectious diseases*

ImmuRAIT-LL2 ℞ *(orphan: B-cell leukemia and lymphoma therapy)* [iodine I 131 murine monoclonal antibody IgG2a to B cell]
IM-Nutrients soft capsules OTC *vitamin/mineral supplement* [vitamins A & E; buffered vitamin C; selenium methionine; zinc citrate]
Imodium A-D caplets, liquid ℞ *antidiarrheal* [loperamide HCl]
Imodium capsules ℞ *antidiarrheal* [loperamide HCl]
Imogam IM injection ℞ *rabies prophylaxis* [rabies immune globulin]
imolamine INN, BAN
Imovax intradermal or IM injection ℞ *rabies prophylaxis* [rabies vaccine (HDCV)]
imoxiterol INN
impacarzine INN
Impact liquid OTC *oral nutritional supplement*
IMPE [see: etipirium iodide]
impromidine INN, BAN *gastric secretion indicator* [also: impromidine HCl]
impromidine HCl USAN *gastric secretion indicator* [also: impromidine]
improsulfan INN
Improved Analgesic ointment OTC *counterirritant* [methyl salicylate; menthol]
Imreg-1; Imreg-2 ℞ *investigational immunomodulator for AIDS*
imuracetam INN
Imuran tablets, IV injection ℞ *immunosuppressant for organ transplantation* [azathioprine]
Imuthiol ℞ *investigational immunomodulator; (orphan: AIDS)* [diethyldithiocarbamate]
Imuvert *(orphan: primary brain malignancies)* [*Serratia marcescens* extract (polyribosomes)]
¹¹¹In [see: indium In 111 pentetate]
¹¹¹In [see: pentetate indium disodium In 111]
¹¹³ᵐIn [see: indium chlorides In 113m]

inactivated mumps vaccine [see: mumps virus vaccine, inactivated]
inactivated poliomyelitis vaccine (IPV) [see: poliovirus vaccine inactivated]
inactivated poliovirus vaccine (IPV) [see: poliovirus vaccine, inactivated]
inaperisone INN
I-Naphline eye drops (discontinued 1991) ℞ *topical ocular vasoconstrictor* [naphazoline HCl]
Inapsine IV or IM injection ℞ *general anesthetic* [droperidol]
Incremin with Iron syrup OTC *hematinic* [ferric pyrophosphate; multiple B vitamins; lysine; alcohol]
indacrinic acid [see: indacrinone]
indacrinone USAN, INN *antihypertensive; diuretic*
indalpine INN, BAN
Indameth capsules, sustained-release capsules (discontinued 1991) ℞ *nonsteroidal anti-inflammatory drug (NSAID); antiarthritic; analgesic* [indomethacin]
indanazoline INN
indandione *anticoagulant*
indanidine INN
indanorex INN
indapamide USAN, INN, BAN *antihypertensive; diuretic*
indatraline INN
indecainide INN *antiarrhythmic* [also: indecainide HCl]
indecainide HCl USAN *antiarrhythmic* [also: indecainide]
indeloxazine INN *antidepressant* [also: indeloxazine HCl]
indeloxazine HCl USAN *antidepressant* [also: indeloxazine]
indenolol INN, BAN
Inderal LA long-acting capsules ℞ *antianginal; antihypertensive; migraine preventative* [propranolol HCl]
Inderal tablets, IV injection ℞ *antianginal; antihypertensive; migraine preventative* [propranolol HCl]

Inderide 40/25; Inderide 80/25 tablets ℞ *antihypertensive* [propranolol HCl; hydrochlorothiazide]
Inderide LA 80/50; Inderide LA 120/50; Inderide LA 160/50 long-acting capsules ℞ *antihypertensive* [propranolol HCl; hydrochlorothiazide]
indigo carmine BAN *cystoscopy aid* [also: indigotindisulfonate sodium]
indigotindisulfonate sodium USP *cystoscopy aid* [also: indigo carmine]
indium *element (In)*
indium chlorides In 113m USAN, USP *radioactive agent*
indium In 111 altumomab pentetate (orphan: *diagnostic aid for colorectal carcinoma*)
indium In 111 antimelanoma antibody XMMME-0001-DTPA [see: antimelanoma antibody]
indium In 111 murine anti-CEA monoclonal antibody type ZCE 025 (orphan: *diagnostic aid in colorectal carcinoma*)
indium In 111 murine monoclonal antibody B72.3 (orphan: *diagnostic aid in ovarian carcinoma*)
indium In 111 murine monoclonal antibody Fab to myosin (orphan: *diagnostic aid for cardiac necrosis and myocarditis*)
indium In 111 oxyquinoline USAN, USP *radioactive agent; diagnostic aid*
indium In 111 pentetate USP *radionuclide cisternography aid; radioactive agent*
indobufen INN
indocate INN
Indocin capsules, oral suspension, suppositories ℞ *nonsteroidal anti-inflammatory drug (NSAID); antiarthritic; analgesic* [indomethacin]
Indocin I.V. powder for IV injection ℞ *prostaglandin synthesis inhibitor for patent ductus arteriosus* [indomethacin sodium trihydrate]

Indocin SR sustained-release capsules ℞ *nonsteroidal anti-inflammatory drug (NSAID); antiarthritic; analgesic* [indomethacin]

indocyanine green USP *cardiac output test; hepatic function test*

indolapril INN *antihypertensive* [also: indolapril HCl]

indolapril HCl USAN *antihypertensive* [also: indolapril]

Indo-Lemmon capsules (discontinued 1991) ℞ *nonsteroidal anti-inflammatory drug (NSAID); antiarthritic; analgesic* [indomethacin]

indolidan USAN, INN, BAN *cardiotonic*

indometacin INN *nonsteroidal anti-inflammatory drug (NSAID); antiarthritic; analgesic* [also: indomethacin]

indomethacin USAN, USP, BAN *nonsteroidal anti-inflammatory drug (NSAID); antiarthritic; analgesic* [also: indometacin]

indomethacin sodium USAN *anti-inflammatory*

indomethacin sodium trihydrate *neonatal closure of patent ductus arteriosus*

indopanolol INN

indopine INN

indoprofen USAN, INN, BAN *analgesic; anti-inflammatory*

indoramin USAN, INN, BAN *antihypertensive*

indoramin HCl USAN, BAN *antihypertensive*

indorenate INN *antihypertensive* [also: indorenate HCl]

indorenate HCl USAN *antihypertensive* [also: indorenate]

indoxole USAN, INN *antipyretic; anti-inflammatory*

indriline INN *CNS stimulant* [also: indriline HCl]

indriline HCl USAN *CNS stimulant* [also: indriline]

inductin [see: diphoxazide]

Infalyte powder (discontinued 1991) OTC *electrolyte replacement* [sodium, potassium, and chloride electrolytes]

Infasurf *(orphan: respiratory failure in premature infants)* [surface active extract of saline lavage of bovine lungs]

Infatabs (trademarked form) *chewable tablets*

Infectrol eye drop suspension, ophthalmic ointment ℞ *topical ophthalmic corticosteroidal anti-inflammatory; antibiotic* [dexamethasone; neomycin sulfate; polymyxin B sulfate]

InFeD IV injection ℞ *hematinic* [iron dextran]

Inflamase Mild Ophthalmic; Inflamase Forte Ophthalmic eye drops ℞ *ophthalmic topical corticosteroidal anti-inflammatory* [prednisolone sodium phosphate]

influenza virus vaccine USP *active immunizing agent for influenza*

infraRUB cream OTC *counterirritant* [methyl salicylate; menthol]

Infumorph 200; Infumorph 500 concentrate for continuous microinfusion ℞ *(orphan: intraspinal microinfusion for intractable pain)* [morphine sulfate]

INH (isonicotinic acid hydrazide) [see: isoniazid]

Inhal-Aid (trademarked form) *portable inhalation device*

Inhibace ℞ *investigational antihypertensive; ACE inhibitor* [cilazapril]

inicarone INN

Inlay-Tabs (trademarked form) *tablets with contrasting inlay*

Inner Rinse Concentrate Douche powder (discontinued 1991) OTC *antiseptic/germicidal; vaginal cleansing and deodorizing; acidity modifier* [sodium borate; citric acid]

Innovar injection ℞ *narcotic analgesic; major tranquilizer* [fentanyl citrate; droperidol]

Inocor IV injection ℞ *vasodilator for congestive heart failure* [amrinone lactate]

inocoterone INN *anti-acne* [also: inocoterone acetate]

inocoterone acetate USAN *anti-acne* [also: inocoterone]

inosine INN

inosine pranobex BAN *immunomodulating agent; (orphan: subacute sclerosing panencephalitis)*

inosiplex [now: inosine pranobex]

inositol NF *dietary lipotropic supplement*

inositol niacinate USAN *peripheral vasodilator* [also: inositol nicotinate]

inositol nicotinate INN, BAN *peripheral vasodilator* [also: inositol niacinate]

Inpersol; Inpersol-LM solution ℞ *peritoneal dialysis solution* [dextrose; multiple electrolytes]

inprochone [see: inproquone]

inproquone INN, BAN

Insect Antigens subcu or IM injection (discontinued 1991) ℞ *venom sensitivity testing; allergenic hyposensitization therapy* [antigen extracts available: bee, wasp, hornet, yellow jacket & fire ant]

INSH (isonicotinoyl-salicylidenehydrazine) [see: salinazid]

InspirEase (trademarked form) *portable inhalation device*

Insta-Glucose gel OTC *glucose elevating agent* [glucose]

Insulatard NPH Human suspension for injection OTC *antidiabetic* [isophane insulin (human)]

Insulatard NPH suspension for injection OTC *antidiabetic* [isophane insulin (pork)]

insulin USP *antidiabetic*

insulin, biphasic INN, BAN

insulin, dalanated USAN, INN *antidiabetic*

insulin, globin zinc USP [also: globin zinc insulin]

insulin, human USAN, USP, INN, BAN *antidiabetic*

insulin, isophane USP, INN *antidiabetic* [also: isophane insulin]

insulin, neutral USAN *antidiabetic* [also: neutral insulin]

insulin, NPH (neutral protamine Hagedorn) [see: insulin, isophane]

insulin, protamine zinc USP *antidiabetic* [also: protamine zinc insulin]

insulin argine INN

insulin defalan INN

insulin I 125 USAN *radioactive agent*

insulin I 131 USAN *radioactive agent*

Insulin Reaction gel OTC *glucose elevating agent* [glucose]

insulin zinc USP, BAN *antidiabetic* [also: compound insulin zinc suspension]

insulin zinc, extended USP *antidiabetic* [also: insulin zinc suspension (crystalline)]

insulin zinc, prompt USP *antidiabetic* [also: insulin zinc suspension (amorphous)]

insulin zinc suspension (amorphous) INN, BAN *antidiabetic* [also: insulin zinc, prompt]

insulin zinc suspension (crystalline) INN, BAN *antidiabetic* [also: insulin zinc, extended]

insulin-like growth factor-1 *investigational agent for peripheral neuropathy; (orphan: amyotrophic lateral sclerosis)*

insulinotropin *investigational blood glucose regulating agent*

Intal capsules for inhalation, solution for nebulization, aerosol spray ℞ *bronchodilator for bronchial asthma and bronchospasm* [cromolyn sodium]

Intensol (trademarked form) *concentrated oral solution*

Intercept Contraceptive Inserts vaginal suppositories (discontinued 1992) OTC *spermicidal contraceptive* [nonoxynol 9]

α-2-interferon [see: interferon alfa-2b, recombinant]

interferon (recombinant human, beta) *(orphan: AIDS; multiple sclerosis)*

interferon αA [see: interferon alfa-2a, recombinant]

interferon alfa-2a, recombinant (rIFN-A) USAN, INN, BAN *antineoplastic; antiviral; investigational cytokine for AIDS; (orphan: various cancers)*

interferon alfa-2b, recombinant (rIFN-2) USAN, INN, BAN *antineoplastic; antiviral; (orphan: various cancers; hepatitis B)*

interferon alfa-n1 USAN, INN, BAN *antineoplastic; antiviral; (orphan: Kaposi sarcoma; human papillomavirus)*

interferon alfa-n3 USAN *antiviral; antineoplastic*

interferon beta, recombinant (rIFN-beta) *(orphan: metastatic renal cell carcinoma; malignant melanoma; Kaposi sarcoma; multiple sclerosis)*

interferon beta, recombinant human *(orphan: non-A, non-B hepatitis; AIDS; multiple sclerosis)*

interferon gamma-1b USAN, INN, BAN *antineoplastic; antiviral; immunoregulator; (orphan: chronic granulomatous disease)* [also: interferon gamma-2a]

interferon gamma-2a [see: interferon gamma-1b]

α-interferons [see: interferon alfa-n1 & -n3]

interleukin-1 alpha, recombinant human *(orphan: bone marrow transplants; aplastic anemia)*

interleukin-1 receptor antagonist, recombinant human *(orphan: juvenile rheumatoid arthritis)*

interleukin-2, liposome-encapsulated recombinant *(orphan: brain and central nervous system tumors)*

interleukin-2, recombinant (IL-2) [see: aldesleukin; teceleukin; celmoleukin]

interleukin-2 PEG [see: PEG-interleukin-2]

interleukin-3, recombinant human *investigational AIDS drug; (orphan: diamond-blackfan anemia)*

interleukin-6 *investigational bone marrow stimulant following chemotherapy*

intermedine INN

Intralipid 10%; Intralipid 20% IV infusion ℞ *nutritional therapy* [intravenous fat emulsion]

IntraSite gel OTC *wound dressing* [graft T starch copolymer]

intravascular perfluorochemical emulsion *synthetic blood oxygen carrier for PTCA*

intravenous fat emulsion [see: fat emulsion, intravenous]

intrazole USAN, INN *anti-inflammatory*

Intrinsitinic capsules ℞ *dietary supplement* [liver-stomach concentrate; multiple vitamins; ferrous fumarate]

intriptyline INN *antidepressant* [also: intriptyline HCl]

intriptyline HCl USAN *antidepressant* [also: intriptyline]

Introlan liquid OTC *oral nutritional supplement*

Introlite liquid in prefilled enteral feeding containers OTC *oral nutritional supplement*

Intron A subcu or IM injection ℞ *antineoplastic for hairy cell leukemia and Kaposi sarcoma; antiviral for chronic hepatitis (orphan)* [interferon alfa-2b]

Intropin IV injection ℞ *vasopressor used in shock* [dopamine HCl]

inulin USP *renal function test*

invenol [see: carbutamide]

Inversine tablets ℞ *antihypertensive* [mecamylamine HCl]

invert sugar [see: sugar, invert]

iobenguane (^{131}I) INN

iobenzamic acid USAN, INN, BAN *cholecystographic radiopaque medium*

iobutoic acid INN

Iocare solution OTC *irrigating solution for EENT surgery* [balanced saline solution]

iocarmate meglumine USAN *radiopaque medium* [also: meglumine iocarmate]

iocarmic acid USAN, INN, BAN *radiopaque medium*

iocetamic acid USAN, USP, INN, BAN *cholecystographic radiopaque medium*

Iocon shampoo OTC *antiseborrheic; antipsoriatic; antipruritic; antibacterial* [coal tar; alcohol]

iodamide USAN, INN, BAN *radiopaque medium*

iodamide meglumine USAN *radiopaque medium*

iodecimol INN

iodecol [see: iodecimol]

iodetryl INN

Iodex; Iodex-P ointment OTC *broad-spectrum antimicrobial* [povidone-iodine]

Iodex M/S (name changed to Iodex with Methyl Salicylate in 1992)

Iodex with Methyl Salicylate salve OTC *counterirritant; topical anti-infective* [methyl salicylate; iodine; oil of wintergreen]

iodinated (^{125}I) human serum albumin INN *blood volume test* [also: albumin, iodinated I 125 serum]

iodinated (^{131}I) human serum albumin INN *blood volume test* [also: albumin, iodinated I 131 serum]

iodinated glycerol [see: glycerol, iodinated]

Iodinated Glycerol DM liquid ℞ *antitussive; expectorant* [iodinated glycerol; dextromethorphan hydrobromide]

iodinated I 125 albumin [see: albumin, iodinated I 125]

iodinated I 131 aggregated albumin [see: albumin, iodinated I 131 aggregated]

iodinated I 131 albumin [see: albumin, iodinated I 131]

iodine USP *broad-spectrum topical anti-infective; element (I)*

iodine I 123 murine monoclonal antibody to alpha-fetoprotein (AFP) (*orphan: diagnostic aid in AFP-producing tumors and hepatic cancer*)

iodine I 123 murine monoclonal antibody to human chorionic gonadotropin (hCG) (*orphan: diagnostic aid in hCG-producing tumors*)

iodine I 131 6B-iodomethyl-19-norcholesterol (*orphan: adrenal cortical imaging*)

iodine I 131 Lym-1 monoclonal antibody (*orphan: B-cell lymphoma*)

iodine I 131 meta-iodobenzylguanidine sulfate (*orphan: diagnostic aid in pheochromocytoma*)

iodine I 131 murine monoclonal antibody IgG$_2$a to B cell (*orphan: B-cell leukemia and lymphoma*)

iodine I 131 murine monoclonal antibody to alpha-fetoprotein (AFP) (*orphan: AFP-producing tumors; hepatocellular carcinoma; hepatoblastoma*)

iodine I 131 murine monoclonal antibody to human chorionic gonadotropin (hCG) (*orphan status withdrawn 1993*)

iodipamide USP, BAN [also: adipiodone]

iodipamide meglumine USP, BAN *radiopaque medium*

iodipamide methylglucamine [see: iodipamide meglumine]

iodipamide sodium USP

iodipamide sodium I 131 USAN *radioactive agent*

iodisan [see: prolonium iodide]

iodixanol USAN, INN, BAN *radiopaque medium*

iodized oil NF
iodoalphionic acid NF [also: pheniodol sodium]
iodoantipyrine I 131 USAN *radioactive agent*
iodobehenate calcium NF
iodocetylic acid (^{123}I) INN *diagnostic aid* [also: iodocetylic acid I 123]
iodocetylic acid I 123 USAN *diagnostic aid* [also: iodocetylic acid (^{123}I)]
iodochlorhydroxyquin [now: clioquinol]
iodocholesterol (^{131}I) INN *radioactive agent* [also: iodocholesterol I 131]
iodocholesterol I 131 USAN *radioactive agent* [also: iodocholesterol (^{131}I)]
iodoform NF
iodohippurate sodium I 123 USAN, USP *renal function test; radioactive agent*
iodohippurate sodium I 125 USAN *radioactive agent*
iodohippurate sodium I 131 USAN, USP *renal function test; radioactive agent* [also: sodium iodohippurate (^{131}I)]
iodohydroxyquin [see: clioquinol]
iodol USP
iodomethamate sodium NF
Iodo-Niacin controlled-action tablets ℞ *expectorant* [potassium iodide; niacinamide hydroiodide]
Iodo-Pak IV injection ℞ *intravenous nutritional therapy* [sodium iodide]
iodopanoic acid [see: iopanoic acid]
Iodopen IV injection ℞ *intravenous nutritional therapy* [sodium iodide]
iodophthalein, soluble [now: iodophthalein sodium]
iodophthalein sodium NF, INN
iodopyracet NF [also: diodone]
iodopyracet I 125 USAN *radioactive agent*
iodopyracet I 131 USAN *radioactive agent*

iodoquinol USAN, USP *amebicide; antimicrobial* [also: diiodohydroxyquinoline]
iodothiouracil INN, BAN
iodothymol [see: thymol iodide]
Iodotope capsules, oral solution ℞ *radioactive agent for thyroid carcinoma* [sodium iodide I 131]
iodoxamate meglumine USAN, BAN *radiopaque medium*
iodoxamic acid USAN, INN, BAN *radiopaque medium*
iodoxyl [see: iodomethamate sodium]
iofendylate INN *radiopaque medium* [also: iophendylate]
iofetamine (^{123}I) INN *diagnostic aid; radioactive agent* [also: iofetamine HCl I 123]
iofetamine HCl I 123 USAN *diagnostic aid; radioactive agent* [also: iofetamine (^{123}I)]
Iofoam (trademarked form) *foaming skin cleanser*
ioglicic acid USAN, INN, BAN *radiopaque medium*
ioglucol USAN, INN *radiopaque medium*
ioglucomide USAN, INN *radiopaque medium*
ioglunide INN
ioglycamic acid USAN, INN, BAN *cholecystographic radiopaque medium*
iogulamide USAN *radiopaque medium*
iohexol USAN, INN, BAN *radiopaque medium*
iolidonic acid INN
iolixanic acid INN
iomeglamic acid INN
iomeprol USAN, INN, BAN *radiopaque medium*
iomethin I 125 USAN *neoplasm test; radioactive agent* [also: iometin (^{125}I)]
iomethin I 131 USAN *neoplasm test; radioactive agent* [also: iometin (^{131}I)]
iometin (^{125}I) INN *neoplasm test; radioactive agent* [also: iomethin I 125]
iometin (^{131}I) INN *neoplasm test; radioactive agent* [also: iomethin I 131]

iomorinic acid INN
Ionamin capsules ℞ *anorexiant* [phentermine HCl]
Ionax Astringent Skin Cleanser liquid OTC *topical acne cleanser* [salicylic acid; allantoin; acetone; isopropyl alcohol]
Ionax foam OTC *topical acne cleanser* [benzalkonium chloride]
Ionax Scrub OTC *abrasive cleanser for acne* [polyethylene granules; benzalkonium chloride; alcohol]
Ionil Plus shampoo OTC *antiseborrheic; keratolytic* [salicylic acid]
Ionil shampoo OTC *antiseborrheic; keratolytic; antiseptic* [salicylic acid; benzalkonium chloride]
Ionil-T Plus shampoo OTC *antiseborrheic; antipsoriatic; antipruritic; antibacterial* [coal tar]
Ionil T shampoo OTC *antiseborrheic; antipsoriatic; keratolytic; antiseptic* [coal tar; salicylic acid; benzalkonium chloride]
Ionosil B (D; G) and 10% Invert Sugar IV infusion (discontinued 1991) ℞ *intravenous nutritional/electrolyte therapy* [combined electrolyte solution; invert sugar (50% dextrose + 50% fructose)]
Ionosol B (MB; T) and 5% Dextrose; Ionosol MB and 10% Dextrose IV infusion (discontinued 1991) ℞ *intravenous nutritional/electrolyte therapy* [combined electrolyte solution; dextrose]
ionphylline [see: aminophylline]
iopamidol USAN, USP, INN, BAN *radiopaque medium*
iopanoic acid USP, INN, BAN *cholecystographic radiopaque medium*
iopentol USAN, INN, BAN *radiopaque medium*
Iophen tablets, elixir, solution ℞ *expectorant* [iodinated glycerol]
Iophen-C liquid ℞ *antitussive; expectorant* [iodinated glycerol; codeine phosphate]

Iophen-DM liquid ℞ *antitussive; expectorant* [iodinated glycerol; dextromethorphan hydrobromide]
iophendylate USP, BAN *radiopaque medium* [also: iofendylate]
iophenoic acid INN [also: iophenoxic acid]
iophenoxic acid USP [also: iophenoic acid]
Iophylline elixir ℞ *antiasthmatic; bronchodilator; expectorant* [theophylline; iodinated glycerol]
Iopidine eye drops ℞ *antiglaucoma agent* [apraclonidine HCl]
ioprocemic acid USAN, INN *radiopaque medium*
iopromide INN, BAN
iopronic acid USAN, INN, BAN *cholecystographic radiopaque medium*
iopydol USAN, INN, BAN *bronchographic radiopaque medium*
iopydone USAN, INN, BAN *bronchographic radiopaque medium*
iosarcol INN
iosefamic acid USAN, INN *radiopaque medium*
ioseric acid USAN, INN *radiopaque medium*
iosimide INN
iosulamide INN *radiopaque medium* [also: iosulamide meglumine]
iosulamide meglumine USAN *radiopaque medium* [also: iosulamide]
iosulfan blue *lymphography radiopaque medium*
iosumetic acid USAN, INN *radiopaque medium*
iotalamic acid INN *radiopaque medium* [also: iothalamic acid]
iotasul USAN, INN *radiopaque medium*
iotetric acid USAN, INN *radiopaque medium*
iothalamate meglumine USP *radiopaque medium* [also: meglumine iothalamate]
iothalamate sodium USP *radiopaque medium* [also: sodium iothalamate]

iothalamate sodium I 125 USAN *radioactive agent* [also: sodium iotalamate (^{125}I)]
iothalamate sodium I 131 USAN *radioactive agent* [also: sodium iotalamate (^{131}I)]
iothalamic acid USP, BAN *radiopaque medium* [also: iotalamic acid]
iothiouracil sodium
iotranic acid INN
iotriside INN
iotrizoic acid INN
iotrol [now: iotrolan]
iotrolan USAN, INN, BAN *radiopaque medium*
iotroxic acid USAN, INN, BAN *radiopaque medium*
IoTuss liquid ℞ *antitussive; expectorant* [codeine phosphate; iodinated glycerol]
IoTuss-DM liquid ℞ *antitussive; expectorant* [dextromethorphan hydrobromide; iodinated glycerol]
iotyrosine I 131 USAN *radioactive agent*
ioversol USAN, INN, BAN *radiopaque medium*
ioxabrolic acid INN
ioxaglate meglumine USAN *radiopaque medium* [also: meglumine ioxaglate]
ioxaglate sodium USAN *radiopaque medium* [also: sodium ioxaglate]
ioxaglic acid USAN, INN, BAN *radiopaque medium*
ioxilan USAN, INN *diagnostic aid*
ioxitalamic acid INN
ioxotrizoic acid USAN, INN *radiopaque medium*
iozomic acid INN
I-Paracaine eye drops (discontinued 1991) ℞ *topical ophthalmic anesthetic* [proparacaine HCl]
I-Parescein eye drops (discontinued 1991) ℞ *topical ophthalmic anesthetic; corneal diclosing agent* [proparacaine HCl; fluorescein sodium]

ipazilide fumarate USAN *antiarrhythmic*
ipecac USP *emetic*
ipecac, powdered USP
I-Pentolate eye drops (discontinued 1991) ℞ *cycloplegic; mydriatic* [cyclopentolate HCl]
ipexidine INN *dental caries prophylactic* [also: ipexidine mesylate]
ipexidine mesylate USAN, INN *dental caries prophylactic* [also: ipexidine]
I-Phrine 2.5%; I-Phrine 10% eye drops (discontinued 1991) ℞ *ophthalmic decongestant/vasoconstrictor; mydriatic* [phenylephrine HCl]
I-Picamide eye drops (discontinued 1991) ℞ *cycloplegic; mydriatic* [tropicamide]
I-Pilopine eye drops (discontinued 1992) ℞ *antiglaucoma agent; miotic* [pilocarpine HCl]
ipodate calcium USP *cholecystographic radiopaque medium*
ipodate sodium USAN, USP *cholecystographic radiopaque medium* [also: sodium iopodate]
IPOL subcu injection ℞ *poliomyelitis vaccine* [poliovirus vaccine, inactivated]
ipragratine INN
ipramidil INN
Ipran tablets ℞ *antianginal; antihypertensive; antimigrainal* [propranolol HCl]
ipratropium bromide USAN, INN, BAN *bronchodilator; anticholinergic*
iprazochrome INN
iprazone [see: isoprazone]
ipriflavone INN
iprindole USAN, INN, BAN *antidepressant*
iprocinodine HCl USAN, BAN *veterinary antibacterial*
iproclozide INN, BAN
iprocrolol INN
iprofenin USAN *hepatic function test*
iproheptine INN
iproniazid INN, BAN

ipronidazole USAN, INN, BAN *antiprotozoal (Histomonas)*
ipropethidine [see: properidine]
iproplatin USAN, INN, BAN *antineoplastic*
iprotiazem INN
iproxamine INN *vasodilator* [also: iproxamine HCl]
iproxamine HCl USAN *vasodilator* [also: iproxamine]
iprozilamine INN
ipsalazide INN, BAN
ipsapirone INN, BAN *anxiolytic* [also: ipsapirone HCl]
ipsapirone HCl USAN *anxiolytic* [also: ipsapirone]
Ipsatol Cough Formula for Children syrup OTC *pediatric decongestant, antitussive and expectorant* [phenylpropanolamine HCl; dextromethorphan hydrobromide; guaifenesin]
Ipsatol Cough Formula liquid OTC *decongestant; antitussive; expectorant* [phenylpropanolamine HCl; dextromethorphan hydrobromide; guaifenesin]
IPTD (isopropyl-thiadiazol) [see: glyprothiazol]
IPV (inactivated poliomyelitis vaccine) [see: poliovirus vaccine, inactivated]
IPV (inactivated poliovaccine) [see: poliovirus vaccine, inactivated]
iquindamine INN
¹⁹²Ir [see: iridium Ir 192]
Ircon tablets OTC *hematinic* [ferrous fumarate]
Ircon-FA tablets OTC *hematinic* [ferrous fumarate; folic acid]
I-Rescein IV injection (discontinued 1991) ℞ *corneal disclosing agent* [fluorescein sodium]
irgasan [see: triclosan]
iridium *element (Ir)*
iridium Ir 192 USAN *radioactive agent*
irindalone INN

irloxacin INN
Irodex IV, IM injection (discontinued 1992) ℞ *antianemic* [iron dextran]
irolapride INN
Iromide IM injection (discontinued 1991) ℞ *antianemic* [ferrous gluconate; multiple B vitamins]
Iromin-G tablets OTC *vitamin/iron supplement* [multiple vitamins; ferrous gluconate; folic acid]
iron *element (Fe)*
iron carbohydrate complex [see: polyferose]
iron dextran USP *hematinic*
iron heptonate [see: gleptoferron]
iron perchloride [see: ferric chloride]
iron polymalether [see: ferropolimaler]
iron sorbitex USAN, USP *hematinic*
Irospan timed-release capsules, timed-release tablets OTC *hematinic* [ferrous sulfate; ascorbic acid]
irsogladine INN
irtemazole USAN, INN, BAN *uricosuric*
IS 5-MN (isosorbide 5-mononitrate) [see: isorbide mononitrate]
isaglidole INN
isamfazone INN
isamoltan INN
isamoxole USAN, INN, BAN *antiasthmatic*
isaxonine INN
isbogrel INN
iscador *investigational antiviral for AIDS*
I-Scrub solution OTC *hygienic management agent of blepharitis; general eyelid cleaning*
isepamicin USAN, INN, BAN *antibacterial; aminoglycoside*
isethionate [see: amicarbalide]
ISG (immune serum globulin) [see: globulin, immune]
ISIS 2105 ℞ *investigational antiviral for genital warts*
Ismelin Sulfate tablets ℞ *antihypertensive; (orphan: reflex sympathetic*

dystrophy and causalgia) [guanethidine monosulfate]

ISMO film-coated tablets ℞ *angina preventative* [isosorbide mononitrate]

Ismotic solution ℞ *osmotic diuretic* [isosorbide]

iso-alcoholic elixir NF

isoaminile INN, BAN

isoamyl nitrate [see: amyl nitrite]

Iso-B capsules OTC *vitamin supplement* [multiple B vitamins; folic acid; biotin]

Iso-Bid sustained-release capsules ℞ *antianginal* [isosorbide dinitrate]

isobromindione INN

isobucaine HCl USP

isobutamben USAN, INN *topical anesthetic*

isobutane NF *aerosol propellant*

isobutyl *p*-aminobenzoate [see: isobutamben]

isobutyl 2-cyanoacrylate (IBC) [see: bucrylate]

isobutyl α-phenylcyclohexaneglycolate [see: ibuverine]

***p*-isobutylhydratropohydroxamic acid** [see: ibuproxam]

isobutylhydrochlorothiazide [see: buthiazide]

isobuzole BAN [also: glysobuzole]

Isocaine HCl injection ℞ *injectable local anesthetic* [mepivacaine HCl]

Isocal; Isocal HCN; Isocal HN liquid OTC *total enteral nutrition*

isocarboxazid USP, INN, BAN *antidepressant; MAO inhibitor*

Isocet tablets ℞ *analgesic; anti-inflammatory; sedative* [acetaminophen; caffeine; butalbital]

Isoclor Expectorant liquid ℞ *decongestant; antitussive; expectorant* [pseudoephedrine HCl; codeine phosphate; guaifenesin; alcohol]

Isoclor Timesules (sustained-release capsules), tablets, liquid OTC *decongestant; antihistamine* [pseudoephedrine HCl; chlorpheniramine maleate]

Isocom capsules ℞ *vasoconstrictor; sedative; analgesic (for migraine)* [isometheptene mucate; dichloralphenazone; acetaminophen]

isoconazole USAN, INN, BAN *antibacterial; antifungal*

isocromil INN

Isocult for Bacteriuria culture test for urine OTC *in vitro diagnostic aid for bacteriuria*

Isocult for *Candida* culture test OTC *in vitro diagnostic aid for vaginal candida*

Isocult for *N gonorrhoeae* and *Candida* culture test OTC *in vitro diagnostic aid for gonorrhea and candida*

Isocult for *Neisseria gonorrhoeae* culture test OTC *in vitro diagnostic aid for gonorrhea*

Isocult for *Pseudomonas aeruginosa* culture test for exudate or urine OTC *in vitro diagnostic aid for pseudomonas*

Isocult for *Staphylococcus aureus* culture test for exudate OTC *in vitro diagnostic aid for staphylococcus*

Isocult for *T vaginalis* and *Candida* culture test OTC *in vitro diagnostic aid for trichomonas and candida*

Isocult for *Trichomonas vaginalis* culture test OTC *in vitro diagnostic aid for trichomonas*

Isocult Throat Streptococci culture test ℞ *in vitro diagnostic test for streptococci*

isodapamide [see: zidapamide]

Isodine solution (discontinued 1991) OTC *broad-spectrum antimicrobial* [povidone-iodine]

***d*-isoephedrine HCl** [see: pseudoephedrine HCl]

isoetarine INN *bronchodilator* [also: isoetharine]

isoethadione [see: paramethadione]

isoetharine USAN, BAN *bronchodilator* [also: isoetarine]

isoetharine HCl USP, BAN *bronchodilator*

isoetharine mesylate USP, BAN *bronchodilator*

isofezolac INN

isoflupredone INN, BAN *anti-inflammatory* [also: isoflupredone acetate]

isoflupredone acetate USAN *anti-inflammatory* [also: isoflupredone]

isoflurane USAN, USP, INN, BAN *inhalation general anesthetic*

isoflurophate USP *antiglaucoma agent; irreversible cholinesterase inhibitor miotic* [also: dyflos]

Isoject (delivery system) *unit dose syringe*

I-Sol ophthalmic solution (discontinued 1992) OTC *extraocular irrigating solution* [balanced saline solution]

Isolan liquid OTC *oral nutritional supplement*

isoleucine (L-isoleucine) USAN, USP, INN *essential amino acid; symbols: Ile, I*

Isollyl Improved tablets, capsules ℞ *analgesic; antipyretic; sedative* [acetaminophen; caffeine; butalbital]

Isolyte E (G; H; M; P; R; S) with 5% Dextrose IV infusion ℞ *intravenous nutritional/electrolyte therapy* [combined electrolyte solution; dextrose]

Isolyte E; Isolyte S; Isolyte S pH 7.4 IV infusion ℞ *intravenous electrolyte therapy* [combined electrolyte solution]

Isolyte G with 10% Dextrose IV infusion (discontinued 1991) ℞ *intravenous nutritional/electrolyte therapy* [combined electrolyte solution; dextrose]

Isolyte S pH 7.4 IV infusion ℞ *intravenous electrolyte therapy* [combined electrolyte solution]

isomazole INN *cardiotonic* [also: isomazole HCl]

isomazole HCl USAN *cardiotonic* [also: isomazole]

isomeprobamate [see: carisoprodol]

isomerol USAN *antiseptic*

isometamidium BAN [also: isometamidium chloride]

isometamidium chloride INN [also: isometamidium]

isomethadone INN, BAN

isomethepdrine chloride [see: isometheptene]

isometheptene INN, BAN

isometheptene HCl [see: isometheptene]

isometheptene mucate *cerebral vasoconstrictor; "possibly effective" for migraine headaches*

Isomil; Isomil SF liquid OTC *hypoallergenic infant food* [soybean protein formula]

isomylamine HCl USAN *smooth muscle relaxant*

isoniazid USP, INN, BAN *bactericidal; primary tuberculostatic*

isonicophen [see: aconiazide]

isonicotinic acid hydrazide (INH) [see: isoniazid]

isonicotinic acid vanillylidenehydrazide [see: ftivazide]

1-isonicotinoyl-2-salicylidenehydrazine (INSH) [see: salinazid]

isonicotinylhydrazine [see: isoniazid]

isonixin INN

isooctadecanol [see: isostearyl alcohol]

isooctadecyl alcohol [see: isostearyl alcohol]

Isopap capsules ℞ *vasoconstrictor; sedative; analgesic (for migraine)* [isometheptene mucate; dichloralphenazone; acetaminophen]

isopentyl nitrite [see: amyl nitrite]

Iso-PH tablets OTC *dietary supplement* [plum pulp]

isophane insulin BAN *antidiabetic* [also: insulin, isophane]

isophenethanol [see: nifenalol]

isoprazone INN, BAN

isoprednidene INN, BAN

isopregnenone [see: dydrogesterone]

isoprenaline INN, BAN *bronchodilator; vasopressor for shock* [also: isoproterenol HCl]
L-**isoprenaline** [see: levisoprenaline]
isoprenaline HCl [see: isoproterenol HCl]
Isoprinosine *investigational immunomodulator; (orphan: subacute sclerosing panencephalitis)* [inosine pranobex]
isoprofen INN
isopropamide iodide USP, INN, BAN *peptic ulcer adjunct*
isopropanol [see: isopropyl alcohol]
isopropicillin INN
isoproponum iodide [see: isopropamide iodide]
7-**isopropoxyisoflavone** [see: ipriflavone]
isopropyl alcohol USP *topical anti-infective/antiseptic; solvent*
isopropyl alcohol, rubbing USP *rubefacient*
N-**isopropyl meprobamate** [see: carisoprodol]
isopropyl myristate NF *emollient*
isopropyl palmitate NF *oleaginous vehicle*
isopropyl sebacate
isopropylantipyrine [see: propyphenazone]
isopropylarterenol HCl [see: isoproterenol HCl]
isopropylarterenol sulfate [see: isoproterenol sulfate]
isoproterenol HCl USP *bronchodilator; vasopressor for shock* [also: isoprenaline]
isoproterenol sulfate USP *bronchodilator*
Isoptin film-coated tablets ℞ *antianginal; antiarrhythmic; antihypertensive* [verapamil HCl]
Isoptin IV injection ℞ *antitachyarrhythmic* [verapamil HCl]
Isoptin SR film-coated sustained-release tablets ℞ *antihypertensive* [verapamil HCl]

Isopto Alkaline; Isopto Plain; Isopto Tears Drop-Tainers (eye drops) OTC *ocular moisturizer/lubricant*
Isopto Atropine eye drops ℞ *cycloplegic; mydriatic* [atropine sulfate]
Isopto Carbachol Drop-Tainers (eye drops) ℞ *antiglaucoma agent; direct-acting miotic* [carbachol]
Isopto Carpine Drop-Tainers (eye drops) ℞ *antiglaucoma agent; direct-acting miotic* [pilocarpine HCl]
Isopto Cetamide eye drops ℞ *ophthalmic bacteriostatic* [sodium sulfacetamide]
Isopto Cetapred eye drop suspension ℞ *topical ophthalmic corticosteroidal anti-inflammatory; bacteriostatic* [prednisolone acetate; sodium sulfacetamide]
Isopto Eserine eye drops ℞ *antiglaucoma agent; reversible cholinesterase inhibitor miotic* [physostigmine salicylate]
Isopto Frin eye drops OTC *topical ocular decongestant* [phenylephrine HCl]
Isopto Homatropine eye drops ℞ *cycloplegic; mydriatic* [homatropine hydrobromide]
Isopto Hyoscine eye drops ℞ *cycloplegic; mydriatic* [scopolamine hydrobromide]
Isopto P-ES Drop-Tainers (eye drops) ℞ *antiglaucoma agent* [pilocarpine HCl; physostigmine salicylate]
Isordil Titradose (tablets), Tembid (capsules, tablets), sublingual ℞ *antianginal* [isosorbide dinitrate]
isosorbide USAN, USP, INN, BAN *osmotic diuretic*
isosorbide dinitrate USAN, USP, INN, BAN *coronary vasodilator; antianginal*
isosorbide mononitrate USAN, INN, BAN *coronary vasodilator*
Isosource; Isosource HN liquid OTC *oral nutritional supplement*

isospaglumic acid INN
isospirilene [see: spirilene]
isostearyl alcohol USAN *emollient; solvent*
isosulfamerazine [see: sulfaperin]
isosulfan blue USAN *lymphangiography aid* [also: sulphan blue]
isosulpride INN
Isotein HN powder OTC *oral nutritional supplement*
isothipendyl INN, BAN
isothipendyl HCl [see: isothipendyl]
isotiquimide USAN, INN, BAN *antiulcerative*
Isotrate Timecelles (sustained-release capsules) ℞ *antianginal* [isosorbide dinitrate]
isotretinoin USAN, USP, INN, BAN *keratolytic*
Isovex capsules ℞ *peripheral vasodilator* [ethaverine HCl]
Isovorin (*orphan: colorectal adenocarcinoma*) [L-leucovorin]
Isovue-128; Isovue-200; Isovue-300; Isovue-370 injection ℞ *parenteral radiopaque agent* [iopamidol]
Isovue-M 200; Isovue-M 300 intrathecal injection ℞ *parenteral myelographic radiopaque agent* [iopamidol]
isoxaprolol INN
isoxepac USAN, INN, BAN *anti-inflammatory*
isoxicam USAN, INN, BAN *nonsteroidal anti-inflammatory drug (NSAID); antiarthritic; analgesic; antipyretic*
isoxsuprine INN, BAN *peripheral vasodilator* [also: isoxsuprine HCl]
isoxsuprine HCl USP *peripheral vasodilator* [also: isoxsuprine]
I-Soyalac liquid OTC *hypoallergenic infant food* [soybean protein formula]
isradipine USAN, INN, BAN *calcium channel antagonist; calcium channel blocker*
isrodipine [see: isradipine]
Istin (European name for U.S. product Norvasc)

Isuprel intracardiac, IV, subcu or IM injection ℞ *vasopressors in acute heart block* [isoproterenol HCl]
Isuprel Mistometer (metered-dose inhalation aerosol), Glossets (sublingual tablets), solution for inhalation ℞ *bronchodilator for bronchial asthma and bronchospasm* [isoproterenol HCl]
itanoxone INN
itazigrel USAN, INN *platelet antiaggregatory agent*
itazogrel [see: itazigrel]
Itch-X gel OTC *topical local anesthetic* [pramoxine HCl]
itobarbital [see: butalbital]
itraconazole USAN, INN, BAN *antifungal*
itramin tosilate INN [also: itramin tosylate]
itramin tosylate BAN [also: itramin tosilate]
itrocainide INN
I-Tropine eye drops (discontinued 1991) ℞ *cycloplegic; mydriatic* [atropine sulfate]
Ivarest cream, lotion OTC *topical poison ivy treatment* [calamine; benzocaine]
ivarimod INN
Iveegam powder for IV infusion ℞ *passive immunizing agent* [immune globulin]
ivermectin USAN, INN, BAN *antiparasitic*
ivermectin component B$_{1a}$
ivermectin component B$_{1b}$
Ivomec-SR bolus ℞ *investigational antiparasitic* [ivermectin]
ivoqualine INN
Ivy Shield cream OTC *skin protectant*
Ivy-Chex spray OTC *topical poison ivy treatment* [polyvinylpyrrolidone-vinylacetate copolymers; methyl salicylate; benzalkonium chloride]

Ivy-Rid spray OTC *topical poison ivy treatment* [polyvinylpyrrolidone-vinylacetate copolymers; benzalkonium chloride]

J

Janimine Filmtabs (film-coated tablets) ℞ *tricyclic antidepressant; treatment for childhood enuresis* [imipramine HCl]
Japanese encephalitis vaccine *investigational vaccine*
Jenamicin IV or IM injection ℞ *aminoglycoside-type antibiotic* [gentamicin sulfate]
Jenest-28 tablets ℞ *oral contraceptive* [norethindrone; ethinyl estradiol]
Jeri-Bath Oil (discontinued 1992) OTC *bath emollient*
Jeri-Lotion (discontinued 1991) OTC *moisturizer; emollient*
Jets chewable tablets OTC *dietary supplement* [lysine; multiple vitamins]
JE-Vax powder for subcu injection ℞ *Japanese encephalitis vaccine* [inactivated Japanese encephalitis virus]
Jevity liquid OTC *total enteral nutrition*
Jiffy Toothache Drops OTC *topical oral anesthetic; analgesic; antipruritic/counterirritant* [benzocaine; eugenol; menthol]
jodphthalein sodium [see: iodophthalein sodium]
jofendylate [see: iophendylate]
jopanoic acid [see: iopanoic acid]
josamycin USAN, INN *antibacterial*
jotrizoic acid [see: iotrizoic acid]
juniper tar USP *antieczematic*
Just Tears eye drops OTC *ocular moisturizer/lubricant*

K

K + 10 film-coated extended-release tablets ℞ *potassium supplement* [potassium chloride]
K + Care ET effervescent tablets ℞ *potassium supplement* [potassium bicarbonate]
K + Care powder packets ℞ *potassium supplement* [potassium chloride]
⁴²K [see: potassium chloride K 42]
Kabikinase powder for IV or intracoronary infusion ℞ *thrombolytic enzyme for lysis of thrombi and catheter clearance* [streptokinase]
Kainair eye drops ℞ *topical ophthalmic anesthetic* [proparacaine HCl]
kainic acid INN
kalafungin USAN, INN *antifungal*
Kalcinate IV injection or infusion (discontinued 1992) ℞ *calcium replenishment for hypocalcemia or hyperkalemia* [calcium gluconate]
kallidinogenase INN, BAN
kalmopyrin [see: calcium acetylsalicylate]
kalsetal [see: calcium acetylsalicylate]
kanamycin INN, BAN *aminoglycoside bactericidal antibiotic; tuberculosis retreatment* [also: kanamycin sulfate]
kanamycin B [see: bekanamycin]
kanamycin sulfate USP *aminoglycoside bactericidal antibiotic; tuberculosis retreatment* [also: kanamycin]
Kank-a liquid OTC *topical anesthetic; oral antiseptic* [benzocaine; cetylpyridinium chloride]

Kantrex IV or IM injection, pediatric injection, capsules ℞ *aminoglycoside-type antibiotic* [kanamycin sulfate]

Kanulase tablets (discontinued 1991) OTC *digestive enzymes; gastric acidifier* [amylase; protease; lipase; pepsin; ox bile extract; cellulase; glutamic acid]

Kaochlor; Kaochlor S-F liquid ℞ *potassium supplement* [potassium chloride; alcohol]

Kaochlor-Eff tablets (discontinued 1991) ℞ *potassium supplement* [potassium chloride]

Kaodene Non-Narcotic liquid OTC *antidiarrheal; GI adsorbent; antacid* [kaolin; pectin; carboxymethylcellulose sodium; bismuth salicylate]

kaolin USP *GI adsorbent*

Kaon elixir ℞ *potassium supplement* [potassium gluconate]

Kaon tablets (discontinued 1991) ℞ *potassium supplement* [potassium gluconate]

Kaon-Cl 20% liquid ℞ *potassium supplement* [potassium chloride; alcohol]

Kaon-Cl; Kaon Cl-10 extended-release tablets ℞ *potassium supplement* [potassium chloride]

Kao-Nor tablets (discontinued 1991) ℞ *potassium supplement* [potassium gluconate]

Kaopectate, Children's chewable tablets, liquid OTC *antidiarrheal; GI adsorbent* [attapulgite]

Kaopectate II caplets OTC *antidiarrheal* [loperamide HCl]

Kaopectate Advanced Formula concentrated liquid OTC *antidiarrheal; GI adsorbent* [attapulgite]

Kaopectate concentrated liquid, caplets, chewable tablets OTC *antidiarrheal; GI adsorbent* [attapulgite]

Kaopectate Maximum Strength caplets OTC *antidiarrheal; GI adsorbent* [attapulgite; pectin]

Kao-Spen oral suspension OTC *GI adsorbent; antidiarrheal* [kaolin; pectin]

Kapectolin liquid OTC *GI adsorbent; antidiarrheal* [kaolin; pectin]

Kapectolin PG liquid ℞ *GI adsorbent; not generally regarded as safe and effective as an antidiarrheal* [opium; kaolin; pectin; hyoscyamine sulfate; atropine sulfate; scopolamine hydrobromide]

Kapectolin with Paregoric liquid (discontinued 1992) ℞ *GI adsorbent; (not generally regarded as safe and effective as an antidiarrheal)* [opium (paregoric); kaolin; pectin]

Kapseals (trademarked form) *capsules*

Karbozyme enteric-coated tablets OTC *dietary supplement* [pancreatin; sodium bicarbonate; potassium bicarbonate]

Karidium tablets, chewable tablets, drops ℞ *dental caries preventative* [sodium fluoride]

Karigel; Karigel-N gel ℞ *topical dental caries preventative* [sodium fluoride]

kasal USAN *food additive*

Kasdenol powder OTC *germicidal mouthwash* [monoxychlorosene]

Kasof capsules OTC *stool softener* [docusate potassium]

Kato powder packets ℞ *potassium supplement* [potassium chloride]

Kay Ciel liquid, powder packets ℞ *potassium supplement* [potassium chloride]

Kaybovite-1000 injection ℞ *antianemic; vitamin supplement* [cyanocobalamin]

Kayexalate powder ℞ *potassium-removing agent for hyperkalemia* [sodium polystyrene sulfonate]

Kaylixir liquid ℞ *potassium supplement* [potassium gluconate; alcohol]

Kaysine injection ℞ *treatment for varicose veins with stasis dermatitis* [adenosine phosphate]

K-C oral suspension OTC *antidiarrheal; GI adsorbent; antacid* [kaolin; pectin; bismuth subcarbonate]
KCl (potassium chloride) [q.v.]
K-DEC tablets OTC *vitamin/mineral/iron supplement* [multiple vitamins & minerals; ferrous fumarate; folic acid; biotin]
K-Dur 10; K-Dur 20 controlled-release tablets ℞ *potassium supplement* [potassium chloride]
kebuzone INN
Keflet tablets (discontinued 1993) ℞ *cephalosporin-type antibiotic* [cephalexin monohydrate]
Keflex Pulvules (capsules), oral suspension, pediatric drops ℞ *cephalosporin-type antibiotic* [cephalexin monohydrate]
Keflin, Neutral powder for IV or IM injection ℞ *cephalosporin-type antibiotic* [cephalothin sodium]
Keftab tablets ℞ *cephalosporin-type antibiotic* [cephalexin HCl monohydrate]
Kefurox powder for IV or IM injection, ADD-vantage vials, Faspaks ℞ *cephalosporin-type antibiotic* [cefuroxime sodium]
Kefzol powder for IV or IM injection ℞ *cephalosporin-type antibiotic* [cefazolin sodium]
K-Electrolyte effervescent tablets ℞ *potassium supplement* [potassium bicarbonate; potassium citrate]
K-Electrolyte/Cl effervescent tablets ℞ *potassium supplement* [potassium chloride]
kellofylline [see: visnafylline]
Kemadrin tablets ℞ *anticholinergic; antiparkinsonian agent* [procyclidine HCl]
Kenacort tablets, syrup ℞ *glucocorticoids* [triamcinolone]
Kenaject-40 IM, intra-articular, intrabursal, intradermal injection ℞ *glucocorticoids* [triamcinolone acetonide]

Kenalog in Orabase oral paste ℞ *topical oral corticosteroid* [triamcinolone acetonide]
Kenalog ointment, cream, lotion, aerosol spray ℞ *topical corticosteroid* [triamcinolone acetonide]
Kenalog-10; Kenalog-40 IM, intra-articular, intrabursal, intradermal injection ℞ *glucocorticoids* [triamcinolone acetonide]
Kenalog-H cream ℞ *topical corticosteroid* [triamcinolone acetonide]
Kendall's compound A [see: dehydrocorticosterone]
Kendall's compound B [see: corticosterone]
Kendall's compound E [see: cortisone acetate]
Kendall's compound F [see: hydrocortisone]
Kendall's desoxy compound B [see: desoxycorticosterone acetate]
Kenonel cream ℞ *topical corticosteroid* [triamcinolone acetonide]
Kenwood Therapeutic liquid OTC *vitamin/mineral supplement* [multiple vitamins & minerals]
keoxifene HCl [now: raloxifene HCl]
keracyanin INN
Keralyt gel ℞ *topical keratolytic* [salicylic acid]
Kerasol Therapeutic Bath Oil (discontinued 1991) OTC *bath emollient*
Keri Creme OTC *moisturizer; emollient*
Keri Facial Cleanser liquid OTC *soap-free cleanser*
Keri; Keri Light lotion OTC *moisturizer; emollient*
Kerid Ear Drops (discontinued 1991) OTC *agent to emulsify and disperse ear wax* [urea; glycerin]
Kerledex ℞ *investigational antihypertensive β-blocker and diuretic combination* [betaxolol HCl; chlorthalidone]
Kerlone tablets ℞ *antihypertensive; β-blocker* [betaxolol HCl]

Kerodex #51 cream OTC *skin protectant for dry or oily work*

Kerodex #71 cream OTC *water repellant skin protectant for wet work*

Kestrin Aqueous IM injection (discontinued 1991) ℞ *estrogen replacement therapy; antineoplastic for prostatic and breast cancer* [estrone]

Kestrone 5 IM injection ℞ *estrogen replacement therapy; antineoplastic for prostatic and breast cancer* [estrone]

Ketalar IV or IM injection ℞ *general anesthetic* [ketamine HCl]

ketamine INN, BAN *anesthetic* [also: ketamine HCl]

ketamine HCl USAN, USP *general anesthetic* [also: ketamine]

ketanserin USAN, INN, BAN *serotonin antagonist*

ketazocine USAN, INN *analgesic*

ketazolam USAN, INN, BAN *minor tranquilizer*

kethoxal USAN *antiviral* [also: ketoxal]

ketimipramine INN *antidepressant* [also: ketipramine fumarate]

ketimipramine fumarate [see: ketipramine fumarate]

ketipramine fumarate USAN *antidepressant* [also: ketimipramine]

ketobemidone INN, BAN

ketocaine INN

ketocainol INN

ketocholanic acid [see: dehydrocholic acid]

ketoconazole USAN, USP, INN, BAN *broad-spectrum antifungal; (orphan: cyclosporine-induced nephrotoxicity)*

Keto-Diastix reagent strips OTC *in vitro diagnostic aid for multiple urine products*

ketohexazine [see: cetohexazine]

ketoprofen USAN, INN, BAN *antiarthritic; nonsteroidal anti-inflammatory drug (NSAID); analgesic*

ketorfanol USAN, INN *analgesic*

ketorolac INN, BAN *analgesic; nonsteroidal anti-inflammatory drug (NSAID); antipyretic* [also: ketorolac tromethamine]

ketorolac tromethamine USAN *analgesic; nonsteroidal anti-inflammatory drug (NSAID); antipyretic* [also: ketorolac]

Ketostix reagent strips OTC *in vitro diagnostic aid for ketones in the urine*

ketotifen INN, BAN *antiasthmatic* [also: ketotifen fumarate]

ketotifen fumarate USAN *antiasthmatic* [also: ketotifen]

ketotrexate INN

ketoxal INN *antiviral* [also: kethoxal]

Key-E Kaps capsules OTC *vitamin supplement* [vitamin E]

Key-E tablets, caplets, cream, ointment, suppositories, powder, spray OTC *vitamin supplement; topical antioxidant* [vitamin E]

Key-Min cellulose-coated caplet OTC *mineral supplement* [multiple minerals; vitamin D$_3$]

Key-Plex injection ℞ *parenteral vitamin therapy* [multiple B vitamins; vitamin C]

Key-Pred 25; Key-Pred 50 IM injection ℞ *glucocorticoids* [prednisolone acetate]

Key-Pred-SP IV or IM injection ℞ *glucocorticoids* [prednisolone sodium phosphate]

Key-Ron cellulose-coated caplet OTC *iron supplement* [ferrous fumarate; vitamin B$_{12}$; vitamin C; bovine liver]

K-Feron IV, IM injection (discontinued 1992) ℞ *antianemic* [iron dextran]

K-Flex IV or IM injection ℞ *skeletal muscle relaxant* [orphenadrine citrate]

K-Forte Regular; K-Forte Maximum Strength chewable tablets (discontinued 1991) ℞ *potassium supplement* [potassium gluconate; po-

tassium chloride; potassium citrate; vitamin C]
K-G Elixir ℞ *potassium supplement* [potassium gluconate]
khellin INN
khelloside INN
Kiddy Chews chewable tablets OTC *vitamin supplement* [multiple vitamins; folic acid]
Kiddy Chews with Iron chewable tablets OTC *vitamin/iron supplement* [multiple vitamins; iron; folic acid]
KIE syrup ℞ *decongestant; expectorant* [ephedrine HCl; potassium iodide]
Kinesed tablets ℞ *anticholinergic; sedative* [atropine sulfate; scopolamine hydrobromide; hyoscyamine hydrobromide; phenobarbital]
Kinevac powder for IV injection ℞ *in vivo gallbladder function test* [sincalide]
kitasamycin USAN, INN, BAN *antibacterial*
KLB6 Complete tablets (discontinued 1992) OTC *dietary supplement* [multiple vitamins & food supplements]
KLB6; Ultra KLB6 softgels OTC *dietary supplement* [vitamin B$_6$; multiple food supplements]
K-Lease extended-release capsules ℞ *potassium supplement* [potassium chloride]
Klebcil IV or IM injection (discontinued 1991) ℞ *aminoglycoside-type antibiotic* [kanamycin sulfate]
Klerist-D sustained-release capsules, tablets ℞ *decongestant; antihistamine* [pseudoephedrine HCl; chlorpheniramine maleate]
Klonopin tablets, Rx Pak (prescription package), Tel-E-Dose (unit dose package) ℞ *anticonvulsant* [clonazepam]
K-Lor powder packets ℞ *potassium supplement* [potassium chloride]
Klor-10% liquid (discontinued 1991) ℞ *potassium* [potassium chloride]

Klor-Con 8; Klor-Con 10 film-coated extended-release tablets ℞ *potassium supplement* [potassium chloride]
Klor-Con; Klor-Con/25 powder packets ℞ *potassium supplement* [potassium chloride]
Klor-Con liquid (discontinued 1991) ℞ *potassium supplement* [potassium chloride]
Klor-Con/EF effervescent tablets ℞ *potassium supplement* [potassium bicarbonate; potassium citrate]
Kloromin tablets OTC *antihistamine* [chlorpheniramine maleate]
Klorvess liquid, effervescent granules, effervescent tablets ℞ *potassium supplement* [potassium chloride]
Klotrix film-coated controlled-release tablets ℞ *potassium supplement* [potassium chloride]
K-Lyte; K-Lyte DS effervescent tablets ℞ *potassium supplement* [potassium bicarbonate; potassium citrate]
K-Lyte/Cl; K-Lyte/Cl 50 effervescent tablets ℞ *potassium supplement* [potassium chloride]
K-Lyte/Cl powder ℞ *potassium supplement* [potassium chloride]
K-Norm controlled-release capsules ℞ *potassium supplement* [potassium chloride]
Koāte-HT IV (discontinued 1991) ℞ *antihemophilic; correct coagulation deficiency* [antihemophilic factor]
Koāte-HS; Koāte-HP powder for IV injection ℞ *antihemophilic; correct coagulation deficiency* [antihemophilic factor]
KoGENate powder for IV injection ℞ *antihemophilic for hemophilia A* [antihemophilic factor VIII, recombinant]
KOH (potassium hydroxide) [q.v.]
Kolantyl gel (discontinued 1991) OTC *antacid* [aluminum hydroxide; magnesium hydroxide]

Kolephrin caplets OTC *decongestant; antihistamine; analgesic* [pseudoephedrine HCl; chlorpheniramine maleate; acetaminophen]

Kolephrin GG/DM liquid OTC *antitussive; expectorant* [dextromethorphan hydrobromide; guaifenesin]

Kolephrin/DM caplets OTC *decongestant; antihistamine; antitussive; analgesic* [pseudoephedrine HCl; chlorpheniramine maleate; dextromethorphan hydrobromide; acetaminophen]

kolfocon A USAN *hydrophobic contact lens material*

kolfocon B USAN *hydrophobic contact lens material*

kolfocon C USAN *hydrophobic contact lens material*

kolfocon D USAN *hydrophobic contact lens material*

Kolyum liquid, powder ℞ *potassium supplement* [potassium gluconate; potassium chloride]

Komed lotion OTC *topical acne treatment* [salicylic acid; sodium thiosulfate; isopropyl alcohol]

Komex scrub (discontinued 1992) OTC *abrasive cleanser for acne* [sodium tetraborate decahydrate dissolving particles]

Konakion IM injection ℞ *coagulant; vitamin K deficiency* [phytonadione]

Kondon's Nasal jelly OTC *nasal decongestant* [ephedrine]

Kondremul emulsion, liquid OTC *emollient laxative* [mineral oil]

Kondremul with Phenolphthalein emulsion OTC *laxative* [mineral oil; phenolphthalein]

Konsyl powder OTC *bulk laxative* [psyllium]

Konsyl-D powder OTC *bulk laxative* [psyllium hydrophilic mucilloid]

Konȳne 80 IV infusion ℞ *factor IX deficiency; correct anticoagulant-induced hemorrhage* [factor IX complex, human]

Konȳne-HT (name changed to Konȳne 80 in 1992)

Kool Foot cream (discontinued 1991) ℞ *topical antifungal* [zinc undecylenate]

Kophane Cough & Cold Formula liquid OTC *decongestant; antihistamine; antitussive* [phenylpropanolamine HCl; chlorpheniramine maleate; dextromethorphan hydrobromide]

Korigesic tablets ℞ *decongestant; antihistamine; analgesic* [phenylephrine HCl; chlorpheniramine maleate; acetaminophen; caffeine]

Koromex condom, vaginal jelly OTC *spermicidal contraceptive* [nonoxynol 9]

Koromex Crystal Clear vaginal gel OTC *spermicidal contraceptive* [nonoxynol 9]

Koromex vaginal cream OTC *spermicidal contraceptive* [octoxynol 9]

Koromex vaginal foam (discontinued 1992) OTC *spermicidal contraceptive* [nonoxynol 9]

Kovitonic liquid OTC *hematinic* [ferric pyrophosphate; multiple B vitamins; lysine; folic acid]

K-P suspension (discontinued 1992) OTC *antidiarrheal; GI adsorbent* [kaolin; pectin]

K-Pek oral suspension OTC *antidiarrheal; GI adsorbent* [attapulgite]

K-Phen-50 injection ℞ *anthistamine; motion sickness; sleep aid; antiemetic; sedative* [promethazine HCl]

K-Phos Neutral film-coated tablets ℞ *phosphorus supplement* [dibasic potassium phosphate; monobasic sodium phosphate; monobasic potassium phosphate]

K-Phos No. 2; K-Phos M.F. tablets ℞ *urinary acidifier* [potassium acid phosphate; sodium acid phosphate]

K-Phos Original tablets ℞ *urinary acidifier* [potassium acid phosphate]

K.P.N. tablets OTC *vitamin/mineral/ calcium/iron supplement* [multiple vitamins & minerals; calcium; iron; folic acid]

⁸¹ᵐKr [see: krypton Kr 81m]

⁸⁵Kr [see: krypton clathrate Kr 85]

Kreo-Benz liquid (discontinued 1991) OTC *topical local anesthetic; counterirritant; antifungal* [benzocaine; amyl metacresol; myrrh; phenol]

Kronocaps (dosage form) *sustained-release capsules*

Kronofed-A Jr. Kronocaps (sustained-release capsules) ℞ *pediatric decongestant and antihistamine* [pseudoephedrine HCl; chlorpheniramine maleate]

Kronofed-A sustained-release capsules ℞ *decongestant; antihistamine* [pseudoephedrine HCl; chlorpheniramine maleate]

krypton *element (Kr)*

krypton clathrate Kr 85 USAN *radioactive agent*

krypton Kr 81m USAN, USP *radioactive agent*

K-Tab film-coated extended-release tablets ℞ *potassium supplement* [potassium chloride]

Kudrox liquid OTC *antacid* [aluminum hydroxide; magnesium hydroxide; simethicone]

Kutapressin subcu or IM injection ℞ *management of multiple dermatoses* [liver derivative complex]

Kutrase capsules ℞ *digestive enzymes; antispasmodic; sedative* [amylase; protease; lipase; cellulase; hyoscyamine sulfate; phenyltoloxamine citrate]

Ku-Zyme capsules ℞ *digestive enzymes* [amylase; protease; lipase; cellulase]

Ku-Zyme HP capsules ℞ *digestive enzymes* [pancrelipase]

Kwelcof liquid ℞ *antitussive; expectorant* [hydrocodone bitartrate; guaifenesin]

Kwell cream, lotion, shampoo ℞ *scabicide; pediculicide* [lindane]

Kwildane lotion, shampoo ℞ *scabicide; pediculicide* [lindane]

K-Y vaginal jelly OTC *lubricant*

kyamepromazin [see: cyamemazine]

Kybernin *(orphan: prevent and treat thromboembolism in AT-III deficiency)* [antithrombin III concentrate IV]

Kynacyte ℞ *investigational cancer chemotherapy enhancer*

Kytril ℞ *invetigational antiemetic*

L

L-5 hydroxytryptophan (L-5HTP) *(orphan: postanoxic intention myoclonus)*

L-696,229; L-697,661 *investigational antiviral for AIDS* [also: non-nucleoside reverse transcriptase inhibitor]

LA-12 IM injection ℞ *antianemic; vitamin supplement* [hydroxocobalamin]

LAAM (*l*-acetyl-α-methadol [or] *l*-alpha-acetyl-methadol) [see: levomethadyl acetate]

labetalol INN, BAN *antiadrenergic (α- and β-receptor)* [also: labetalol HCl]

labetalol HCl USAN, USP *antiadrenergic (α- and β-receptor)* [also: labetalol]

Labstix reagent strips OTC *in vitro diagnostic aid for multiple urine products*

Lac-Hydrin Five lotion OTC *moisturizer; emollient* [lactic acid]

Lac-Hydrin lotion ℞ *moisturizer; emollient* [lactic acid]

lacidipine USAN, INN, BAN *antihypertensive*

Lacril eye drops OTC *ocular moisturizer/lubricant*

Lacri-Lube NP; Lacri-Lube S.O.P. ophthalmic ointment OTC *ocular moisturizer/lubricant*
Lacri-Lube S.O.P. ointment OTC *ophthalmic lubricant*
Lacrisert ophthalmic insert OTC *ocular moisturizer/lubricant* [hydroxypropyl cellulose]
LactAid liquid, caplets OTC *digestive aid for lactose intolerance* [lactase enzyme]
lactalfate INN
lactase enzyme *digestive enzyme for lactose intolerance*
lactated potassic saline [see: potassic saline, lactated]
lactated Ringer's (LR) solution [see: Ringer's injection, lactated]
lactated Ringer's injection [see: Ringer's injection, lactated]
lactic acid USP *pH adjusting agent*
LactiCare lotion OTC *emollient; moisturizer* [lactic acid]
LactiCare-HC lotion ℞ *topical corticosteroid* [hydrocortisone]
Lactinex granules, chewable tablets OTC *dietary supplement; fever blister treatment; not generally regarded as safe and effective as an antidiarrheal* [Lactobacillus acidophilus; Lactobacillus bulgaricus]
Lactisol; Lactisol-Forte liquid ℞ *topical keratolytic* [salicylic acid; lactic acid]
lactitol INN, BAN
Lactobacillus acidophilus *dietary supplement; not generally regarded as safe and effective as an antidiarrheal*
Lactobacillus bulgaricus *dietary supplement; not generally regarded as safe and effective as an antidiarrheal*
lactobin *(orphan: AIDS-related diarrhea)*
lactobionic acid, calcium salt dihydrate [see: calcium lactobionate]
Lactocal-F film-coated tablets ℞ *vitamin/mineral/calcium/iron supplement* [multiple vitamins & minerals; calcium; iron; folic acid]
lactoflavin [see: riboflavin]
Lactogest soft gel capsules OTC *digestive aid for lactose intolerance* [lactase enzyme]
β-lactone [see: propiolactone]
γ-lactone D-glucofuranuronic acid [see: glucurolactone]
lactose NF *tablet and capsule diluent; dietary supplement*
Lactrase capsules OTC *digestive aid for lactose intolerance* [lactase enzyme]
lactulose USAN, USP, INN, BAN *laxative*
ladakamycin [now: azacitidine]
L.A.E. 20 IM injection (discontinued 1992) ℞ *estrogen replacement therapy; antineoplastic for prostatic cancer* [estradiol valerate in oil]
laidlomycin INN *veterinary growth stimulant* [also: laidlomycin propionate potassium]
laidlomycin propionate potassium USAN *veterinary growth stimulant* [also: laidlomycin]
Laki-Lorand factor [see: factor XIII]
Lamictal ℞ *investigational anticonvulsant*
Lamisil cream ℞ *topical antifungal* [terbinafine]
lamivudine USAN *antiviral*
lamotrigine USAN, INN, BAN *anticonvulsant*
Lampit (available only from the Centers for Disease Control) ℞ *investigational anti-infective for Chagas disease* [nifurtimox]
Lamprene capsules ℞ *(orphan: leprosy)* [clofazimine]
lamtidine INN, BAN
Lanabiotic ointment OTC *topical antibiotic; anesthetic* [polymyxin B sulfate; neomycin sulfate; bacitracin; lidocaine]
Lanacaine spray, cream OTC *topical anesthetic; antiseptic* [benzocaine; benzethonium chloride]

Lanacaps (dosage form) *timed-release capsules*
Lanacort 5; Lanacort 10 cream, ointment OTC *topical corticosteroid* [hydrocortisone acetate]
Lanaphilic OTC *ointment base*
Lanaphilic cream OTC *moisturizer; emollient; keratolytic* [urea]
Lanaphilic with Urea OTC *ointment base* [urea]
Lanatabs (dosage form) *sustained-release tablets*
lanatoside NF, INN, BAN
Lanatuss Expectorant liquid OTC *decongestant; antihistamine; expectorant* [phenylpropanolamine HCl; chlorpheniramine maleate; guaifenesin]
Lanazets Improved lozenges (discontinued 1993) OTC *topical anesthetic; oral antiseptic* [benzocaine; cetylpyridinium chloride]
Laniazid C.T. tablets ℞ *tuberculostatic* [isoniazid]
Laniazid tablets, syrup ℞ *tuberculostatic* [isoniazid]
lanolin USP *ointment base; water-in-oil emulsion; emollient/protectant*
lanolin, anhydrous USP *absorbent ointment base*
lanolin alcohols *ointment base ingredient*
Lanoline cream (discontinued 1992) OTC *moisturizer; emollient*
Lanolor cream OTC *moisturizer; emollient*
Lanophyllin elixir ℞ *bronchodilator* [theophylline]
Lanophyllin-GG capsules ℞ *antiasthmatic; expectorant* [theophylline; bronchodilator; guaifenesin]
Lanoplex elixir (discontinued 1993) OTC *vitamin supplement* [multiple B vitamins]
Lanorinal tablets, capsules ℞ *analgesic; antipyretic; sedative* [acetaminophen; caffeine; butalbital]

Lanoxicaps capsules ℞ *increase cardiac output; antiarrhythmic* [digoxin]
Lanoxin tablets, pediatric elixir, IV, IM injection ℞ *increase cardiac output; antiarrhythmic* [digoxin]
lansoprazole USAN, INN, BAN *antiulcerative*
lanthanum *element (La)*
Lanvisone cream (discontinued 1993) ℞ *topical corticosteroid; antifungal; antibacterial* [hydrocortisone; clioquinol]
lapirium chloride INN *surfactant* [also: lapyrium chloride]
LAPOCA (L-asparaginase, Oncovin, cytarabine, Adriamycin) *chemotherapy protocol*
laprafylline INN
lapyrium chloride USAN *surfactant* [also: lapirium chloride]
laramycin [see: zorbamycin]
Largon IV or IM injection ℞ *sedative; analgesic adjunct* [propiomazine HCl]
Lariam tablets ℞ *antimalarial (orphan: chloroquine-resistant malaria)* [mefloquine HCl]
Larobec tablets ℞ *vitamin supplement* [multiple B vitamins; vitamin C; folic acid]
Larodopa capsules (discontinued 1991) ℞ *antiparkinsonian* [levodopa]
Larodopa tablets ℞ *antiparkinsonian* [levodopa]
laroxyl [see: amitriptyline]
Larylgan throat spray (discontinued 1991) OTC *topical analgesic; antihistamine* [antipyrine; pyrilamine maleate; sodium caprylate]
lasalocid USAN, INN, BAN *coccidiostat for poultry*
Lasan; Lasan HP-1 cream (discontinued 1991) ℞ *topical antipsoriatic* [anthralin]
Lasan ointment ℞ *topical antipsoriatic* [anthralin]
Lasix tablets, oral solution, injection ℞ *loop diuretic* [furosemide]

Lassar's paste [see: betanaphthol; zinc oxide]
latamoxef INN, BAN *anti-infective* [also: moxalactam disodium]
latamoxef disodium [see: moxalactam disodium]
laudexium methylsulfate [see: laudexium metilsulfate; laudexium methylsulphate]
laudexium methylsulphate BAN [also: laudexium metilsulfate]
laudexium metilsulfate INN [also: laudexium methylsulphate]
lauralkonium chloride INN
laureth 10S USAN *spermaticide*
laureth 4 USAN *surfactant*
laureth 9 USAN *spermaticide; surfactant*
laurixamine INN
Lauro eye wash OTC *ocular irrigation*
laurocapram USAN, INN *excipient*
lauroguadine INN
laurolinium acetate INN, BAN
lauromacrogol 400 INN
lauryl isoquinolinium bromide USAN *anti-infective*
lavender oil NF
lavoltidine INN *antiulcerative; histamine H₂-receptor blocker* [also: lavoltidine succinate; loxtidine]
lavoltidine succinate USAN *antiulcerative; histamine H₂-receptor blocker* [also: lavoltidine; loxtidine]
Lavoptik Eye Wash ophthalmic solution OTC *extraocular irrigating solution* [balanced saline solution]
lawrencium *element (Lr)*
Lax Pills tablets OTC *laxative* [yellow phenolphthalein]
Laxative Pills tablets OTC *laxative* [yellow phenolphthalein]
Lazer Creme OTC *moisturizer; emollient* [vitamins A & E]
Lazer Formalyde solution ℞ *for hyperhidrosis and bromhidrosis* [formaldehyde]
LazerSporin-C ear drops ℞ *topical corticosteroidal anti-inflammatory; antibiotic* [hydrocortisone; neomycin sulfate; polymyxin B sulfate]
LC-65 Daily Cleaner solution OTC *contact lens cleaning solution*
LC-65 solution OTC *contact lens surfactant cleaning solution*
L-Caine injection ℞ *injectable local anesthetic* [lidocaine HCl]
L-Caine Viscous solution (discontinued 1991) ℞ *topical anesthetic for mouth and pharynx* [lidocaine HCl]
LCD (liquor carbonis detergens) [see: coal tar]
LCR (leurocristine) [see: vincristine]
lead *element (Pb)*
lecithin NF *emulsifying agent; dietary lipotropic supplement*
Ledercillin VK tablets, powder for oral solution ℞ *bactericidal antibiotic* [penicillin V potassium]
Lederplex capsules OTC *vitamin supplement* [multiple B vitamins]
Lederplex liquid (discontinued 1992) OTC *vitamin supplement* [multiple B vitamins]
lefetamine INN
leflunomide INN
Legalon (*orphan: Amanita phalloides [mushroom] liver poisoning*) [disodium silibinin dihemisuccinate]
Legatrin Rub gel OTC *counterirritant; topical anesthetic* [menthol; benzocaine; alcohol]
Legatrin tablets OTC *prevention and treatment of nocturnal leg cramps* [quinine sulfate]
leiopyrrole INN
lemidosul INN
lemon oil NF
lenampicillin INN
Lenate oral solution (discontinued 1993) OTC *expectorant; oral anti-infective; minor topical anesthetic* [menthol; guaifenesin; strong iodine tincture; phenol]
leniquinsin USAN, INN *antihypertensive*
lenitzol [see: amitriptyline]

lenograstim USAN, INN *immunomodulator*
lenperone USAN, INN *antipsychotic*
Lens Clear solution OTC *contact lens surfactant cleaning solution*
Lens Drops solution OTC *contact lens rewetting solution*
Lens Fresh drops OTC *contact lens rewetting solution*
Lens Lubricant solution OTC *contact lens rewetting solution*
Lens Plus Daily Cleaner solution OTC *contact lens surfactant cleaning solution*
Lens Plus Oxysept 1; Lens Plus Oxysept 2 solution OTC *contact lens disinfectant* [hydrogen peroxide]
Lens Plus Oxysept 2 Neutralizing tablets OTC *contact lens disinfectant neutralizer* [catalase]
Lens Plus Oxysept System solution OTC *two-step contact lens disinfectant*
Lens Plus Preservative Free aerosol solution OTC *contact lens rinsing and storage solution* [saline solution]
Lens Plus Rewetting Drops OTC *contact lens rewetting solution*
Lensept solution OTC *two-step contact lens disinfectant*
Lensine solution (discontinued 1992) OTC *contact lens cleaning solution*
Lens-Mate solution (discontinued 1991) OTC *contact lens wetting/soaking solution*
Lensrins solution (discontinued 1992) OTC *contact lens rinsing and storage solution* [preserved saline solution]
Lens-Wet solution OTC *contact lens rewetting solution*
Lente Iletin I subcu injection OTC *antidiabetic* [insulin zinc (beef-pork)]
Lente Iletin II (beef) subcu injection OTC *antidiabetic* [insulin zinc]
Lente Iletin II (pork) subcu injection OTC *antidiabetic* [insulin zinc]
Lente Insulin suspension for injection OTC *antidiabetic* [insulin zinc (beef)]
Lente Purified Pork Insulin suspension for injection OTC *antidiabetic* [insulin zinc (pork)]
lentin [see: carbachol]
lentinan *investigational immunomodulator for AIDS*
leptacline INN
lergotrile USAN, INN *prolactin enzyme inhibitor*
lergotrile mesylate USAN *prolactin enzyme inhibitor*
Lescol ℞ *investigational cholesterol-lowering agent*
letimide INN *analgesic* [also: letimide HCl]
letimide HCl USAN *analgesic* [also: letimide]
letosteine INN
letrazuril INN
leucarsone [see: carbarsone]
leucine (L-leucine) USAN, USP, INN *essential amino acid*; symbols: Leu, L
leucinocaine INN
leucocianidol INN
Leucomax ℞ *investigational cytokine for AIDS; (orphan: neutropenia; aplastic anemia; leukemia; severe burns)* [molgramostim]
leucomycin [see: kitasamycin; spiramycin]
L-leucovorin (*orphan: metastatic colorectal adenocarcinoma*)
leucovorin calcium USP *antianemic; folate replenisher; antidote to folic acid antagonist; (orphan: colorectal carcinoma)* [also: calcium folinate]
Leukeran tablets ℞ *antineoplastic* [chlorambucil]
Leukine powder for IV infusion ℞ *myeloid reconstitution after autologous bone marrow transplant (orphan)* [sargramostim]
leukocyte interferon [now: interferon alfa-n3]
leukocyte protease inhibitor, secretory (*orphan: bronchopulmonary dysplasia*)

leukocyte protease inhibitor, secretory, recombinant (orphan: congenital alpha₁ antitryptsin deficiency; cystic fibrosis)
leukocyte typing serum USP in vitro blood test
leukopoietin [see: sargramostim]
leupeptin (orphan: aid in microsurgical peripheral nerve repair)
leuprolide acetate USAN antineoplastic; (orphan: central precocious puberty) [also: leuprorelin]
leuprorelin INN, BAN antineoplastic [also: leuprolide acetate]
leurocristine (LCR) [see: vincristine]
leurocristine sulfate [see: vincristine sulfate]
Leustatin IV infusion ℞ hairy cell leukemia (orphan); (orphan: chronic lymphocytic leukemia) [cladribine]
levacetylmethadol INN narcotic analgesic [also: levomethadyl acetate]
levallorphan INN, BAN [also: levallorphan tartrate]
levallorphan tartrate USP [also: levallorphan]
levamfetamine INN anorexic [also: levamfetamine succinate; levamphetamine]
levamfetamine succinate USAN anorexic [also: levamfetamine; levamphetamine]
levamisole INN, BAN veterinary anthelmintic [also: levamisole HCl]
levamisole HCl USAN antineoplastic; veterinary anthelmintic [also: levamisole]
levamphetamine BAN anorexic [also: levamfetamine succinate; levamfetamine]
levarterenol [see: norepinephrine]
levarterenol bitartrate [now: norepinephrine bitartrate]
Levatol tablets ℞ antihypertensive; β-blocker [penbutolol sulfate]
levcycloserine USAN, INN enzyme inhibitor; (orphan: Gaucher's disease)

levdobutamine INN cardiotonic [also: levdobutamine lactobionate]
levdobutamine lactobionate USAN cardiotonic [also: levdobutamine]
levdropropizine INN
levisoprenaline INN
Levlen tablets ℞ oral contraceptive [ethinyl estradiol; levonorgestrel]
levlofexidine INN
levobetaxolol INN antiadrenergic (β-receptor) [also: levobetaxolol HCl]
levobetaxolol HCl USAN antiadrenergic (β-receptor) [also: levobetaxolol]
levobunolol INN, BAN antiadrenergic (β-receptor); topical antiglaucoma agent [also: levobunolol HCl]
levobunolol HCl USAN, USP antiadrenergic (β-receptor); topical antiglaucoma agent [also: levobunolol]
levocabastine INN, BAN antihistamine [also: levocabastine HCl]
levocabastine HCl USAN antihistamine; (orphan: vernal keratoconjunctivitis) [also: levocabastine]
levocarbinoxamine tartrate [see: rotoxamine tartrate]
levocarnitine USAN, USP, INN dietary amino acid; (orphan: primary carnitine deficiency)
levodopa USAN, USP, INN, BAN antiparkinsonian
Levo-Dromoran subcu injection, tablets ℞ narcotic analgesic; anxiolytic [levorphanol tartrate]
levofacetoperane INN
levofenfluramine INN
levofuraltadone USAN, INN antibacterial; antiprotozoal
levoglutamide INN nonessential amino acid
levoleucovorin calcium USAN antidote to folic acid antagonists
levomenol INN
levomepate [see: atromepine]
levomepromazine INN analgesic [also: methotrimeprazine]
levomethadone INN

levomethadyl acetate USAN *narcotic analgesic* [also: levacetylmethadol]
levomethorphan INN, BAN
levometiomeprazine INN
levomoprolol INN
levomoramide INN, BAN
levonantradol INN, BAN *analgesic* [also: levonantradol HCl]
levonantradol HCl USAN *analgesic* [also: levonantradol]
levonordefrin USP *adrenergic; vasoconstrictor* [also: corbadrine]
levonorgestrel USAN, USP, INN, BAN *progestin; contraceptive implant*
Levophed Bitartrate IV infusion ℞ *blood pressure control for acute or profound hypotension* [norepinephrine bitartrate]
Levophed IV infusion ℞ *vasopressor used in shock* [norepinephrine]
levophenacylmorphan INN, BAN
Levoprome IM injection ℞ *central analgesic; CNS depressant* [methotrimeprazine]
levopropicillin INN *antibacterial* [also: levopropylcillin potassium]
levopropicillin potassium [see: levopropylcillin potassium]
levopropoxyphene INN, BAN *antitussive* [also: levopropoxyphene napsylate]
levopropoxyphene napsylate USAN *antitussive* [also: levopropoxyphene]
levopropylcillin potassium USAN *antibacterial* [also: levopropicillin]
levopropylhexedrine INN
levoprotiline INN
levorin INN
levorphanol INN, BAN *narcotic analgesic* [also: levorphanol tartrate]
levorphanol tartrate USP *narcotic analgesic* [also: levorphanol]
Levo-T tablets ℞ *thyroid replacement therapy* [levothyroxine sodium]
Levothroid tablets, powder for injection ℞ *hypothyroidism; myxedema coma; TSH suppression in thyroid cancer* [levothyroxine sodium]
levothyroxine sodium (T_4) USP, INN *thyroid hormone* [also: thyroxine]
levoxadrol INN *local anesthetic; smooth muscle relaxant* [also: levoxadrol HCl]
levoxadrol HCl USAN *local anesthetic; smooth muscle relaxant* [also: levoxadrol]
Levoxine tablets, powder for IV injection ℞ *thyroid replacement therapy* [levothyroxine sodium]
Levsin tablets, drops, IV, subcu or IM injection, elixir ℞ *GI anticholinergic; antispasmodic* [hyoscyamine sulfate]
Levsin with Phenobarbital elixir (discontinued 1991) ℞ *anticholinergic; sedative* [hyoscyamine sulfate; phenobarbital]
Levsin with Phenobarbital tablets ℞ *anticholinergic; sedative* [hyoscyamine sulfate; phenobarbital]
Levsinex Timecaps (timed-release capsules) ℞ *GI anticholinergic; antispasmodic* [hyoscyamine sulfate]
Levsinex with Phenobarbital Timecaps (timed-release capsules) (discontinued 1992) ℞ *anticholinergic; sedative* [hyoscyamine sulfate; phenobarbital]
Levsin-PB drops ℞ *anticholinergic; sedative* [hyoscyamine sulfate; phenobarbital; alcohol]
Levsin/SL sublingual tablets (also may be chewed or swallowed) ℞ *GI anticholinergic; antispasmodic* [hyoscyamine sulfate]
levulose BAN *nutrient; caloric replacement* [also: fructose]
lexithromycin USAN, INN *antibacterial*
lexofenac INN
Lextron; Lextron Ferrous Pulvules (discontinued 1991) ℞ *antianemic* [ferrous sulfate; intrinsic factor; multiple B vitamins]

LHRF (luteinizing hormone-releasing factor) acetate hydrate [see: gonadorelin acetate]
LHRF diacetate tetrahydrate [now: gonadorelin acetate]
LHRF dihydrochloride [now: gonadorelin HCl]
LHRF HCl [see: gonadorelin HCl]
libecillide INN
libenzapril USAN, INN *angiotensin-converting enzyme (ACE) inhibitor*
Librax capsules ℞ *anticholinergic; anxiolytic* [clidinium bromide; chlordiazepoxide HCl]
Libritabs film-coated tablets ℞ *anxiolytic* [chlordiazepoxide]
Librium capsules, powder for injection ℞ *anxiolytic* [chlordiazepoxide HCl]
Lice-Enz foam shampoo OTC *pediculicide* [pyrethrins; piperonyl butoxide]
Lice-Enz shampoo kit OTC *pediculicide* [pyrethrins; piperonyl butoxide]
Licetrol 400 liquid OTC *pediculicide* [pyrethrins; piperonyl butoxide; petroleum distillate]
Licoplex DS IM injection ℞ *hematinic* [ferrous gluconate; multiple B vitamins; procaine HCl]
licryfilcon A USAN *hydrophilic contact lens material*
licryfilcon B USAN *hydrophilic contact lens material*
Lid Wipes-SPF OTC *eyelid cleansing wipes*
Lida-Mantle-HC cream ℞ *local anesthetic; topical corticosteroid* [lidocaine; hydrocortisone acetate]
lidamidine INN *antiperistaltic* [also: lidamidine HCl]
lidamidine HCl USAN *antiperistaltic* [also: lidamidine]
Lidex cream, gel, ointment, topical solution ℞ *topical corticosteroid* [fluocinonide]
Lidex-E cream ℞ *topical corticosteroid; emollient* [fluocinonide]
lidimycin INN *antifungal* [also: lydimycin]

lidocaine USP, INN *topical anesthetic* [also: lignocaine]
lidocaine benzyl benzoate [see: denatonium benzoate]
lidocaine HCl USP *local anesthetic; antiarrhythmic* [also: lignocaine HCl]
lidofenin USAN, INN *hepatic function test*
lidofilcon A USAN *hydrophilic contact lens material*
lidofilcon B USAN *hydrophilic contact lens material*
lidoflazine USAN, INN, BAN *coronary vasodilator*
Lidoject-1; Lidoject-2 injection ℞ *injectable local anesthetic* [lidocaine HCl]
LidoPen auto-injector (automatic IM injection device) ℞ *emergency injection for cardiac arrhythmias* [lidocaine HCl]
Lidox capsules ℞ *anticholinergic; anxiolytic* [clidinium bromide; chlordiazepoxide HCl]
Lids-N-Lashes ℞ *investigational eyelid hygiene product*
lifarizine USAN *platelet aggregation inhibitor*
LifeStage Stress Formula for Women tablets (discontinued 1991) OTC *antianemic* [ferrous fumarate; vitamins E & C; multiple B vitamins; folic acid]
LifeStage Women's Formula tablets (discontinued 1991) OTC *antianemic* [ferrous fumarate; multiple vitamins]
lifibrate USAN, INN *antihyperlipoproteinemic*
Lifoject IM injection ℞ *antianemic; vitamin supplement* [liver extracts; vitamin B_{12}; folic acid]
Lifolbex injection ℞ *hematinic; vitamin supplement* [liver extracts; folic acid; cyanocobalamin]
Lifomin-R IM injection ℞ *antianemic; vitamin supplement* [liver extracts; vitamin B_{12}; folic acid]

light mineral oil [see: mineral oil, light]
lignocaine BAN *topical anesthetic* [also: lidocaine]
lignocaine HCl BAN *local anesthetic; antiarrhythmic* [also: lidocaine HCl]
lignosulfonic acid, sodium salt [see: polignate sodium]
lilopristone INN
limaprost INN
limarsol [see: acetarsone]
Limbitrol; Limbitrol DS tablets ℞ *antidepressant; anxiolytic* [chlordiazepoxide; amitryptyline HCl]
lime USP *pharmaceutic necessity*
lime, sulfurated (calcium polysulfide, calcium thiosulfate) USP *wet dressing/soak for cystic acne and seborrhea*
linarotene USAN, INN *antikeratinizing agent*
Lincocin capsules, IV or IM injection ℞ *antibiotic* [lincomycin HCl]
lincomycin USAN, INN, BAN *bactericidal antibiotic*
lincomycin HCl USP *bactericidal antibiotic*
Lincorex IV or IM injection ℞ *antibiotic* [lincomycin HCl]
lindane USAN, USP, INN, BAN *pediculicide; scabicide*
Linguets (trademarked form) *buccal tablets*
linogliride USAN, INN *antidiabetic*
linogliride fumarate USAN *antidiabetic*
linolexamide [see: clinolamide]
Linomide ℞ *investigational immunomodulator for AIDS* [roquinimex]
linsidomine INN
Lioresal intrathecal injection ℞ *skeletal muscle relaxant (orphan: intractable spasticity)* [baclofen]
Lioresal tablets ℞ *skeletal muscle relaxant (orphan: spasticity)* [baclofen]
liothyronine INN, BAN *radioactive agent* [also: liothyronine I 125]

liothyronine I 125 USAN *radioactive agent* [also: liothyronine]
liothyronine I 131 USAN *radioactive agent*
liothyronine sodium (T_3) USP, BAN *thyroid hormone; (orphan: myxedema coma/precoma)*
liotrix USAN, USP *thyroid hormone*
Lip Medex ointment OTC *topical analgesic, anesthetic and antimicrobial* [camphor; phenol]
lipancreatin [see: pancrelipase]
lipase of pancreas [see: pancrelipase]
lipase triacylglycerol [see: pancrelipase]
Lipisorb powder OTC *enteral nutritional therapy* [protein; multiple vitamins & minerals; electrolytes]
Lipoflavonoid capsules OTC *dietary lipotropic with vitamin supplementation* [choline; inositol; multiple B vitamins; vitamin C; lemon bioflavonoids]
Lipogen capsules OTC *dietary lipotropic with vitamin supplementation* [choline; inositol; multiple B vitamins]
Lipomul liquid OTC *dietary fat supplement* [corn oil]
Lipo-Nicin/100; Lipo-Nicin/250 tablets ℞ *peripheral vasodilator* [niacin; niacinamide; multiple vitamins]
Lipo-Nicin/300 timed-release capsules ℞ *peripheral vasodilator* [niacin; niacinamide; multiple vitamins]
Liponol capsules OTC *dietary lipotropic with vitamin supplementation* [choline; inositol; methionine; multiple B vitamins; desiccated liver; liver concentrate]
Lipo-Plus soft capsules OTC *dietary supplement* [choline; inositol; L-methionine; porcine liver concentrate; lecithin]
liposomal gentamicin [see: gentamicin liposome]
liposome-encapsulated recombinant interleukin-2 [see: interleu-

kin-2, liposome-encapsulated recombinant]
liposome-encapsulated T4 endonuclease V [see: T4 endonuclease V, liposome encapsulated]
Liposyn II 10%; Liposyn II 20%; Liposyn III 10%; Liposyn III 20% IV infusion ℞ *nutritional therapy* [intravenous fat emulsion]
Lipo-Tears eye drops (discontinued 1993) OTC *ocular moisturizer/lubricant*
Lipotriad liquid, capsules OTC *dietary lipotropic with vitamin supplementation* [choline; inositol; multiple B vitamins]
Lipovite capsules OTC *vitamin supplement* [multiple B vitamins]
Liquaemin Sodium IV or deep subcu injection ℞ *anticoagulant* [heparin sodium]
liquefied phenol [see: phenol, liquefied]
Liquibid sustained-release tablet ℞ *expectorant* [guaifenesin]
Liqui-Cal softgels OTC *calcium supplement* [calcium carbonate]
Liqui-Char liquid OTC *adsorbent poisoning antidote* [activated charcoal]
Liquid Barosperse suspension ℞ *GI contrast radiopaque agent* [barium sulfate]
Liquid Cal-600 soft capsule OTC *calcium supplement* [calcium carbonate]
liquid glucose [see: glucose, liquid]
Liquid Lather body wash OTC *bath emollient*
liquid petrolatum [see: mineral oil]
Liquid Pred syrup ℞ *glucocorticoids* [prednisone]
Liqui-Doss emulsion OTC *emollient laxative* [mineral oil]
Liquifilm Tears; Liquifilm Forte eye drops OTC *ocular moisturizer/lubricant*
Liquifilm Wetting solution OTC *contact lens wetting solution*

Liquimat lotion OTC *antibacterial; exfoliant* [sulfur; alcohol]
Liquipake suspension ℞ *GI contrast radiopaque agent* [barium sulfate]
Liquiprin elixir, drops OTC *analgesic; antipyretic* [acetaminophen]
liquor carbonis detergens (LCD) [see: coal tar]
liroldine INN
lisadimate USAN, INN *sunscreen*
lisinopril USAN, INN, BAN *antihypertensive; angiotensin-converting enzyme inhibitor*
Listerex Scrub lotion OTC *topical acne cleanser* [salicylic acid]
Listerine; Cool-Mint Listerine mouthwash OTC *oral antiseptic* [thymol; eucalyptol; methyl salicylate; menthol; alcohol]
Listerine Throat Lozenges; Listerine Antiseptic Lozenges OTC *oral antiseptic* [hexylresorcinol]
Listermint with Fluoride oral rinse OTC *topical dental caries preventative* [sodium fluoride]
lisuride INN [also: lysuride]
Lithane tablets ℞ *psychotherapeutic* [lithium carbonate]
lithium element (Li)
lithium benzoate NF
lithium carbonate USAN, USP *antimanic; immunity booster in chemotherapy and AIDS*
lithium citrate USP *antimanic; immunity booster in chemotherapy and AIDS*
lithium hydroxide USP *antimanic*
lithium hydroxide monohydrate [see: lithium hydroxide]
lithium salicylate NF
Lithobid slow-release tablets ℞ *antipsychotic* [lithium carbonate]
Lithonate capsules ℞ *antipsychotic* [lithium carbonate]
Lithostat tablets ℞ *adjunctive therapy in urea-splitting urinary tract infections* [acetohydroxamic acid]

Lithotabs film-coated tablets ℞ *antipsychotic* [lithium carbonate]
litracen INN
Liver Combo No. 5 IM injection ℞ *antianemic; vitamin supplement* [liver extracts; vitamin B$_{12}$; folic acid]
liver derivative complex *claimed to be an anti-inflammatory*
liver extracts *source of vitamin B$_{12}$*
lividomycin INN
Livifol IM injection ℞ *antianemic; vitamin supplement* [liver extracts; vitamin B$_{12}$; folic acid]
Livitamin capsules OTC *hematinic* [ferrous fumarate; desiccated liver; multiple vitamins]
Livitamin chewable tablets OTC *hematinic* [ferrous fumarate; multiple B vitamins; vitamin C]
Livitamin liquid OTC *hematinic* [peptonized iron; liver fraction 1; multiple B vitamins]
Livitamin with Intrinsic Factor capsules ℞ *hematinic* [ferrous fumarate; multiple B vitamins; desiccated liver; vitamin C; intrinsic factor concentrate]
Livitrinsic-f capsules ℞ *hematinic* [ferrous fumarate; vitamins B$_{12}$ & C; intrinsic factor concentrate; folic acid]
Livostin ℞ *investigational drug for allergic conjunctivitis*
Livroben IM injection ℞ *antianemic; vitamin supplement* [liver extracts; vitamin B$_{12}$; folic acid]
lixazinone sulfate USAN *cardiotonic; phosphodiesterase inhibitor*
LKV-Drops powder + liquid OTC *vitamin supplement* [multiple vitamins; biotin]
LLD factor [see: cyanocobalamin]
LM 427 *investigational anti-infective for mycobacterial disease and AIDS* [rifabutin]
LMD (low molecular weight dextran) [see: dextran 40]

10% LMD IV injection ℞ *plasma volume expander; shock due to hemorrhage, burns, surgery* [dextran 40]
LMF (Leukeran, methotrexate, fluorouracil) *chemotherapy protocol*
LMWD (low molecular weight dextran) [see: dextran 40]
Lobac capsules ℞ *skeletal muscle relaxant; analgesic* [salicylamide; phenyltoloxamine; acetaminophen]
Lobana Body lotion OTC *moisturizer; emollient*
Lobana Body Shampoo liquid OTC *soap-free cleanser*
Lobana Derm-Ade cream OTC *moisturizer; emollient* [vitamins A, D & E]
Lobana Peri-Garde ointment OTC *moisturizer; emollient; antiseptic* [vitamins A, D & E; chloroxylenol]
lobeline INN *smoking deterrent*
lobendazole USAN, INN *veterinary anthelmintic*
lobenzarit INN *antirheumatic* [also: lobenzarit sodium]
lobenzarit sodium USAN *antirheumatic* [also: lobenzarit]
lobuprofen INN
locicortolone dicibate INN
locicortone [see: locicortolone dicibate]
Locoid ointment, cream (discontinued 1993) ℞ *topical corticosteroid* [hydrocortisone butyrate]
Locoid solution ℞ *topical corticosteroid; antiseptic* [hydrocortisone butyrate; alcohol]
lodaxaprine INN
lodazecar INN
lodelaben USAN, INN *antiarthritic; emphysema therapy adjunct*
Lodine capsules ℞ *nonsteroidal anti-inflammatory drug (NSAID); analgesic; antiarthritic* [etodolac]
lodinixil INN
lodiperone INN

Lodosyn tablets ℞ *antiparkinsonian agent (used with levodopa only)* [carbidopa]
lodoxamide INN, BAN *antiallergic; antiasthmatic* [also: lodoxamide ethyl]
lodoxamide ethyl USAN *antiallergic; antiasthmatic* [also: lodoxamide]
lodoxamide trometamol BAN *antiallergic; antiasthmatic* [also: lodoxamide tromethamine]
lodoxamide tromethamine USAN *antiallergic; antiasthmatic; (orphan: vernal keratoconjunctivitis)* [also: lodoxamide trometamol]
Loestrin 21 1/20; Loestrin 21 1.5/30 tablets ℞ *oral contraceptive* [norethindrone acetate; ethinyl estradiol]
Loestrin Fe 1/20; Loestrin Fe 1.5/30 tablets ℞ *oral contraceptive* [norethindrone acetate; ethinyl estradiol; ferrous fumarate]
lofemizole INN *anti-inflammatory; analgesic; antipyretic* [also: lofemizole HCl]
lofemizole HCl USAN *anti-inflammatory; analgesic; antipyretic* [also: lofemizole]
Lofenalac powder OTC *special diet for infants with phenylketonuria*
lofendazam INN, BAN
Lofene tablets ℞ *antidiarrheal* [diphenoxylate HCl; atropine sulfate]
lofentanil INN, BAN *narcotic analgesic* [also: lofentanil oxalate]
lofentanil oxalate USAN *narcotic analgesic* [also: lofentanil]
lofepramine INN, BAN *antidepressant* [also: lofepramine HCl]
lofepramine HCl USAN *antidepressant* [also: lofepramine]
lofexidine INN, BAN *antihypertensive* [also: lofexidine HCl]
lofexidine HCl USAN *antihypertensive* [also: lofexidine]
loflucarban INN
Logen tablets ℞ *antidiarrheal* [diphenoxylate HCl; atropine sulfate]

Lomanate liquid ℞ *antidiarrheal* [diphenoxylate HCl; atropine sulfate]
lombazole INN, BAN
lomefloxacin USAN, INN, BAN *antibacterial*
lomefloxacin HCl USAN *broad-spectrum bactericidal antibiotic*
lomefloxacin mesylate USAN *antibacterial*
lometraline INN *antipsychotic; antiparkinsonian* [also: lometraline HCl]
lometraline HCl USAN *antipsychotic; antiparkinsonian* [also: lometraline]
lometrexol INN *antineoplastic* [also: lometrexol sodium]
lometrexol sodium USAN *antineoplastic* [also: lometrexol]
lomevactone INN
lomifylline INN
Lomodix tablets ℞ *antidiarrheal* [diphenoxylate HCl; atropine sulfate]
lomofungin USAN *antifungal*
Lomotil liquid, tablets ℞ *antidiarrheal* [diphenoxylate HCl; atropine sulfate]
lomustine USAN, INN, BAN *antineoplastic*
Lonalac powder OTC *protein supplement*
lonapalene USAN *antipsoriatic*
lonaprofen INN
lonazolac INN
lonidamine INN
Loniten tablets ℞ *antihypertensive; vasodilator* [minoxidil]
Lonox tablets ℞ *antidiarrheal* [diphenoxylate HCl; atropine sulfate]
Lo/Ovral tablets ℞ *oral contraceptive* [ethinyl estradiol; norgestrel]
loperamide INN, BAN *antiperistaltic* [also: loperamide HCl]
loperamide HCl USAN, USP *antiperistaltic* [also: loperamide]
loperamide oxide INN, BAN
Lopid capsules (discontinued 1991) ℞ *antihyperlipidemic agent (cholesterol-lowering)* [gemfibrozil]

Lopid tablets ℞ *antihyperlipidemic agent (cholesterol-lowering)* [gemfibrozil]
Lopid-SR ℞ *investigational cholesterol-lowering agent*
lopirazepam INN
loprazolam INN, BAN
lopremone [now: protirelin]
Lopressor HCT 50/25; Lopressor HCT 100/25; Lopressor HCT 100/50 tablets ℞ *antihypertensive* [metoprolol tartrate; hydrochlorothiazide]
Lopressor tablets, IV injection ℞ *antianginal; antihypertensive; β-blocker* [metoprolol tartrate]
loprodiol INN
Loprox cream, lotion ℞ *topical antifungal* [ciclopirox olamine]
Lopurin tablets ℞ *uricosuric for gout* [allopurinol]
Lorabid Pulvules (capsules), powder for oral suspension ℞ *carbacephem-type antibiotic* [loracarbef]
loracarbef USAN, INN *antibacterial*
lorajmine INN *antiarrhythmic* [also: lorajmine HCl]
lorajmine HCl USAN *antiarrhythmic* [also: lorajmine]
lorapride INN
loratadine USAN, INN, BAN *antihistamine*
lorazepam USAN, USP, INN, BAN *anxiolytic; minor tranquilizer*
lorbamate USAN, INN *muscle relaxant*
lorcainide INN, BAN *antiarrhythmic* [also: lorcainide HCl]
lorcainide HCl USAN *antiarrhythmic* [also: lorcainide]
Lorcet; Lorcet Plus; Lorcet 10/650 tablets ℞ *narcotic analgesic* [hydrocodone bitartrate; acetaminophen]
Lorcet-HD capsules ℞ *narcotic analgesic* [hydrocodone bitartrate; acetaminophen]
lorcinadol USAN, INN, BAN *analgesic*

loreclezole USAN, INN, BAN *antiepileptic*
Lorelco tablets ℞ *serum cholesterol reduction* [probucol]
lorglumide INN
lormetazepam USAN, INN, BAN *sedative; hypnotic*
lornoxicam INN, BAN
Lorothidol (available only from the Centers for Disease Control) ℞ *investigational anti-infective for paragonimiasis and fascioliasis* [bithionol]
Loroxide lotion OTC *keratolytic for acne* [benzoyl peroxide]
lorpiprazole INN
Lortab 2.5/500; Lortab 5/500; Lortab 7.5/500 tablets ℞ *narcotic analgesic* [hydrocodone bitartrate; acetaminophen]
Lortab ASA tablets ℞ *narcotic analgesic* [hydrocodone bitartrate; aspirin]
Lortab liquid ℞ *narcotic analgesic* [hydrocodone bitartrate; acetaminophen; alcohol]
lortalamine USAN, INN *antidepressant*
lorzafone USAN, INN *minor tranquilizer*
losartan potassium USAN *antihypertensive*
Losec (name changed to Prilosec in 1991)
losigamone INN
losindole INN
losmiprofen INN
Losotron Plus liquid OTC *antacid; antiflatulent* [magaldrate; simethicone]
losulazine INN *antihypertensive* [also: losulazine HCl]
losulazine HCl USAN *antihypertensive* [also: losulazine]
Lotensin HCT 5/6.25; Lotensin HCT 10/12.5; Lotensin HCT 20/12.5; Lotensin HCT 20/25 tablets ℞ *antihypertensive; diuretic; angiotensin-converting enzyme inhibitor* [benazepril HCl; hydrochlorothiazide]

Lotensin tablets ℞ *antihypertensive; angiotensin-converting enzyme inhibitor* [benazepril HCl]
loteprednol INN *topical anti-inflammatory* [also: loteprednol etabonate]
loteprednol etabonate USAN *topical anti-inflammatory* [also: loteprednol]
lotifazole INN
lotrifen INN
Lotrimin AF cream, solution OTC *topical antifungal* [clotrimazole]
Lotrimin cream, solution, lotion ℞ *topical antifungal* [clotrimazole]
Lotrisone cream ℞ *topical corticosteroid; antifungal* [betamethasone dipropionate; clotrimazole]
lotucaine INN
Lotusate tablets (discontinued 1991) ℞ *hypnotic* [talbutal]
Lovan ℞ *investigational obesity and bulimia treatment* [fluoxetine]
lovastatin USAN, INN, BAN *antihypercholesterolemic; HMG-CoA reductase inhibitor*
low molecular weight dextran (LMD; LMWD) [see: dextran 40]
Lowila cake OTC *soap-free cleanser*
Low-Quel tablets ℞ *antidiarrheal* [diphenoxylate HCl; atropine sulfate]
Lowsium chewable tablets, oral suspension OTC *antacid; antiflatulent* [magaldrate; simethicone]
Lowsium Plus tablets, suspension OTC *antacid; antiflatulent* [magaldrate; simethicone]
loxanast INN
loxapine USAN, INN, BAN *minor tranquilizer; antipsychotic*
loxapine HCl *minor tranquilizer; antipsychotic*
loxapine succinate USAN *minor tranquilizer; antipsychotic*
loxiglumide INN
Loxitane C oral concentrate ℞ *antipsychotic* [loxapine HCl]
Loxitane capsules ℞ *antipsychotic* [loxapine succinate]
Loxitane IM injection ℞ *antipsychotic* [loxapine HCl]
loxoprofen INN
loxoribine USAN, INN *immunostimulant; vaccine adjuvant; (orphan: common variable immunodeficiency)*
loxotidine [now: lavoltidine succinate]
loxtidine BAN *antiulcerative; histamine H₂-receptor blocker* [also: lavoltidine succinate; lavoltidine]
lozilurea INN
Lozi-Tabs (trademarked form) *lozenges*
Lozol film-coated tablets ℞ *antihypertensive; diuretic* [indapamide]
L-PAM (L-phenylalanine mustard) [see: melphalan]
LR (lactated Ringer's) solution [see: Ringer's injection, lactated]
LSD (lysergic acid diethylamide) [see: lysergide]
Lubraseptic jelly OTC *topical antibacterial; topical anesthetic; lubricant*
LubraSol Bath Oil OTC *bath emollient*
Lubriderm Bath Oil OTC *bath emollient*
Lubriderm cream, lotion OTC *moisturizer; emollient*
Lubrin vaginal inserts OTC *vaginal lubricant*
lucanthone INN, BAN *antischistosomal* [also: lucanthone HCl]
lucanthone HCl USAN, USP *antischistosomal* [also: lucanthone]
lucartamide INN
lucensomycin [see: lucimycin]
lucimycin INN
Ludiomil coated tablets ℞ *tetracyclic antidepressant* [maprotiline HCl]
lufuradom INN
Lufyllin tablets, elixir, IM injection ℞ *bronchodilator* [dyphylline]
Lufyllin-400 tablets ℞ *bronchodilator* [dyphylline]
Lufyllin-EPG tablets, elixir ℞ *antiasthmatic; bronchodilator; decongestant; expectorant; sedative* [dyphyl-

line; ephedrine HCl; guaifenesin; phenobarbital]

Lufyllin-GG tablets, elixir ℞ *antiasthmatic; bronchodilator; expectorant* [dyphylline; guaifenesin]

Lugol solution ℞ *thyroid-blocking therapy; topical antimicrobial* [iodine; potassium iodide]

Luminal Sodium IV or IM injection ℞ *barbiturate sedative; hypnotic; anticonvulsant* [phenobarbital sodium]

Lung Check sputum test (discontinued 1993) OTC *in vitro diagnostic aid for precancerous lung cells*

lung surfactant, synthetic [see: colfosceril palmitate]

2,6-lupetidine [see: nanofin]

lupitidine INN *veterinary antagonist to histamine H_2 receptors* [also: lupitidine HCl]

lupitidine HCl USAN *veterinary antagonist to histamine H_2 receptors* [also: lupitidine]

Lupron; Lupron Depot subcu or IM injection ℞ *prostatic cancer; endometriosis; (orphan: central precocious puberty)* [leuprolide acetate]

luprostiol INN, BAN

Luramide tablets ℞ *loop diuretic* [furosemide]

Luride Lozi-Tabs (chewable tablets), drops ℞ *dental caries preventative* [sodium fluoride]

Luride SF Lozi-Tabs (lozenges) ℞ *dental caries preventative* [sodium fluoride]

Luride topical gel ℞ *dental caries preventative* [acidulated phosphate fluoride]

Lurline PMS tablets OTC *analgesic; antipyretic; diuretic* [acetaminophen; pamabrom; pyridoxine]

luteinizing hormone-releasing factor acetate hydrate [see: gonadorelin acetate]

luteinizing hormone-releasing factor diacetate tetrahydrate [now: gonadorelin acetate]

luteinizing hormone-releasing factor dihydrochloride [now: gonadorelin HCl]

luteinizing hormone-releasing factor HCl [see: gonadorelin HCl]

lutetium *element (Lu)*

lutrelin INN *luteinizing hormone-releasing hormone (LHRH) agonist* [also: lutrelin acetate]

lutrelin acetate USAN *luteinizing hormone-releasing hormone (LHRH) agonist* [also: lutrelin]

Lutrepulse powder for continuous ambulatory infusion ℞ *gonadotropin-releasing hormone for hypothalamic amenorrhea (orphan)* [gonadorelin acetate]

LuVax ℞ *investigational treatment for small cell lung cancer* [monoclonal antibodies]

Luvox ℞ *investigational anxiolytic*

luxabendazole INN, BAN

lyapolate sodium USAN *anticoagulant* [also: sodium apolate]

lycetamine USAN *topical antimicrobial*

lycine HCl [see: betaine HCl]

Lycolan elixir (discontinued 1993) OTC *oral amino acid supplement* [L-lysine]

lydimycin USAN *antifungal* [also: lidimycin]

lymecycline INN, BAN

Lymphazurin 1% injection ℞ *adjunct radiopaque agent for lymphography* [isosulfan blue]

lymphocyte immune globulin, antithymocyte *passive immunizing agent*

lymphogranuloma venereum antigen USP

lynestrenol USAN, INN *progestin* [also: lynoestrenol]

lynoestrenol BAN *progestin* [also: lynestrenol]

Lyphocin powder for IV or IM injection ℞ *glycopeptide-type antibiotic* [vancomycin HCl]

Lypholyte; Lypholyte II IV admixture ℞ *intravenous electrolyte therapy* [combined electrolyte solution]

lypressin USAN, USP, INN, BAN *posterior pituitary hormone; antidiuretic; vasoconstrictor*

lysergic acid diethylamide (LSD) [see: lysergide]

lysergide INN, BAN

lysine (L-lysine) USAN, INN *essential amino acid; symbols: Lys, K*

lysine acetate USP *amino acid*

lysine acetylsalicylate (*orphan status withdrawn 1993*)

lysine HCl USAN, USP *amino acid*

L-lysine monoacetate [see: lysine acetate]

L-lysine monohydrochloride [see: lysine HCl]

8-L-lysine vasopressin [see: lypressin]

Lysmins tablets (discontinued 1991) OTC *dietary supplement* [multiple minerals & amino acids]

Lysodren tablets ℞ *antineoplastic for inoperable adrenal cortical carcinoma* [mitotane]

lysostaphin USAN *antibacterial enzyme*

lysuride BAN [also: lisuride]

Lytren oral solution, Nursette (discontinued 1991) OTC *fluid and electrolyte replacement* [dextrose; potassium citrate; sodium chloride; sodium citrate; citric acid]

M

M2 3 + E tablets OTC *vitamin/mineral supplement* [calcium aspartate; magnesium aspartate; potassium aspartate; vitamin E]

M2 B125 timed-release tablets OTC *vitamin supplement* [multiple B vitamins]

M2 B60 timed-release capsules OTC *vitamin/mineral supplement* [multiple B vitamins; vitamin C; magnesium]

M2 C timed-release capsules OTC *vitamin supplement* [ascorbic acid; rutin]

M-2 protocol (vincristine, carmustine, cyclophosphamide, melphalan, prednisone) *chemotherapy protocol*

MAA (macroaggregated albumin) [see: albumin, aggregated]

Maalox HRF liquid OTC *antacid* [aluminum hydroxide; magnesium carbonate]

Maalox oral suspension, tablets, chewable tablets OTC *antacid* [magnesium hydroxide; aluminum hydroxide]

Maalox Plus chewable tablets, liquid OTC *antacid; antiflatulent* [aluminum hydroxide; magnesium hydroxide; simethicone]

Maalox TC chewable tablets, suspension OTC *antacid* [aluminum hydroxide; magnesium hydroxide]

Maalox Whip (discontinued 1991) OTC *antacid* [aluminum hydroxide; magnesium hydroxide]

MABOP (Mustargen, Adriamycin, bleomycin, Oncovin, prednisone) *chemotherapy protocol*

mabuterol INN

MAC (methotrexate, actinomycin D, cyclophosphamide) *chemotherapy protocol*

MAC (mitomycin, Adriamycin, cyclophosphamide) *chemotherapy protocol*

MACC (methotrexate, Adriamycin, cyclophosphamide, CCNU) *chemotherapy protocol*

MACHO (methotrexate, asparaginase, cyclophosphamide, hydroxydaunomycin, Oncovin) chemotherapy protocol

MACOP-B (methotrexate, Adriamycin, cyclophosphamide, Oncovin, prednisone, bleomycin) chemotherapy protocol

macroaggregated albumin (MAA) [see: albumin, aggregated]

macroaggregated iodinated (^{131}I) human albumin [see: macrosalb (^{131}I)]

Macrobid capsules ℞ *urinary antibacterial* [nitrofurantoin macrocrystals; nitrofurantoin monohydrate]

Macrodantin capsules, MACPAC (box of 7 cards of 4 capsules each) ℞ *urinary antibacterial* [nitrofurantoin macrocrystals]

Macrodex IV infusion ℞ *plasma-volume expander* [dextran 70]

macrogol 4000 INN, BAN [also: polyethylene glycol 4000]

macrogol ester 2000 INN *surfactant* [also: polyoxyl 40 stearate]

macrogol ester 400 INN *surfactant* [also: polyoxyl 8 stearate]

Macrolin ℞ *investigational agent for fungal disease and advanced cancer* [macrophage colony-stimulating factor]

macrophage colony-stimulating factor (M-CSF) *investigational antiviral for AIDS*

macrosalb (^{131}I) INN

macrosalb (^{99m}Tc) INN

Macroscint ℞ *investigational inflammation and infection imaging aid*

MAD (MeCCNU, Adriamycin) chemotherapy protocol

MADDOC (mechlorethamine, Adriamycin, dacarbazine, DDP, Oncovin, cyclophosphamide) chemotherapy protocol

maduramicin USAN, INN *anticoccidal*

mafenide USAN, INN, BAN *bacteriostatic; adjunct to burn therapy*

mafenide acetate USP *bacteriostatic;* (orphan: meshed autograft loss in burns)

mafenide HCl

mafilcon A USAN *hydrophilic contact lens material*

mafoprazine INN

mafosfamide INN

Mag-200 tablets OTC *magnesium supplement* [magnesium oxide]

magaldrate USAN, USP, INN *antacid*

Magan tablets ℞ *analgesic; antirheumatic* [magnesium salicylate]

Mag-Cal tablets OTC *dietary supplement* [calcium carbonate; vitamin D; multiple minerals]

Magnacal liquid OTC *oral nutritional supplement*

Magnagel chewable tablets OTC *antacid* [aluminum hydroxide; magnesium carbonate]

Magnalox liquid OTC *antacid* [aluminum hydroxide; magnesium hydroxide]

Magnalox Plus liquid OTC *antacid; antiflatulent* [aluminum hydroxide; magnesium hydroxide; simethicone]

Magnaprin; Magnaprin Arthritis Strength Captabs film-coated tablets OTC *analgesic; antipyretic; antiinflammatory; antirheumatic* [aspirin, buffered with aluminum hydroxide, magnesium hydroxide, and calcium carbonate]

Magnate tablets (discontinued 1991) OTC *magnesium supplement* [magnesium gluconate]

Magnatril chewable tablets OTC *antacid* [aluminum hydroxide; magnesium hydroxide; magnesium trisilicate]

Magnatril oral suspension OTC *antacid* [aluminum hydroxide; calcium carbonate; magnesium trisilicate]

magnesia, milk of USP *antacid; laxative* [also: magnesium hydroxide]

magnesia magma [now: magnesia, milk of]
magnesium *element (Mg)*
magnesium aluminosilicate hydrate [see: almasilate]
magnesium aluminum silicate NF *suspending agent*
magnesium amino acid chelate *dietary magnesium supplement*
magnesium aspartate [see: potassium aspartate & magnesium aspartate]
magnesium carbonate USP *antacid; dietary magnesium supplement*
magnesium carbonate hydrate [see: magnesium carbonate]
magnesium chloride USP *electrolyte replenisher*
magnesium chloride hexahydrate [see: magnesium chloride]
magnesium citrate USP *saline laxative*
magnesium clofibrate INN
magnesium gluconate USP *magnesium replenisher*
magnesium D-gluconate dihydrate [see: magnesium gluconate]
magnesium D-gluconate hydrate [see: magnesium gluconate]
magnesium glycinate USAN
magnesium hydroxide USP *antacid; saline laxative* [also: magnesia, milk of]
magnesium oxide USP *antacid; sorbent*
magnesium phosphate USP *antacid*
magnesium phosphate pentahydrate [see: magnesium phosphate]
magnesium salicylate USP *analgesic; antipyretic; anti-inflammatory; antirheumatic*
magnesium salicylate tetrahydrate [see: magnesium salicylate]
magnesium silicate NF *tablet excipient*
magnesium silicate hydrate [see: magnesium trisilicate]
magnesium stearate NF *tablet and capsule lubricant*

magnesium sulfate USP *anticonvulsant; saline laxative; electrolyte replenisher*
magnesium sulfate heptahydrate [see: magnesium sulfate]
magnesium trisilicate USP *antacid*
Magnevist injection ℞ *parenteral radiopaque agent* [gadopentetate dimeglumine]
Magonate tablets, liquid OTC *magnesium supplement* [magnesium gluconate]
Mag-Ox 400 tablets OTC *antacid; magnesium supplement* [magnesium oxide]
Magsal tablets ℞ *analgesic; antipyretic; anti-inflammatory; antihistamine* [magnesium salicylate; phenyltoloxamine citrate]
Mag-Tab SR sustained-release caplets OTC *magnesium supplement* [magnesium lactate]
Magtrate tablets OTC *magnesium supplement* [magnesium gluconate]
Maigret-50 tablets (discontinued 1991) ℞ *nasal decongestant* [phenylpropanolamine HCl]
MainStream ℞ *investigational IV system*
maitansine INN *antineoplastic* [also: maytansine]
Major-Con chewable tablets OTC *antiflatulent* [simethicone]
Major-gesic tablets OTC *antihistamine; analgesic* [phenyltoloxamine citrate; acetaminophen]
Malatal tablets ℞ *anticholinergic; sedative* [atropine sulfate; scopolamine hydrobromide; hyoscyamine hydrobromide; phenobarbital]
malathion USP, BAN *pediculicide*
maletamer INN *antiperistaltic* [also: malethamer]
malethamer USAN *antiperistaltic* [also: maletamer]
maleylsulfathiazole INN
malic acid NF *acidifying agent*
malidone [see: aloxidone]

Mallamint chewable tablets OTC *antacid* [calcium carbonate]

Mallazine eye drops OTC *topical ocular decongestant* [tetrahydrozoline HCl]

Mallergan VC Cough syrup ℞ *decongestant; antihistamine; antitussive* [phenylephrine HCl; promethazine HCl; codeine phosphate; alcohol]

Mallisol ointment OTC *broad-spectrum antimicrobial* [povidone-iodine]

Mallisol surgical scrub (discontinued 1992) OTC *broad-spectrum antimicrobial* [povidone-iodine]

Mallopress tablets (discontinued 1991) ℞ *antihypertensive* [hydrochlorothiazide; reserpine]

malonal [see: barbital]

malotilate USAN, INN *liver disorder treatment*

Malotuss syrup (discontinued 1992) OTC *expectorant* [guaifenesin; alcohol]

Maltsupex tablets, powder, liquid OTC *bulk laxative* [nondiastatic barley malt extract]

Mammol ointment OTC *emollient for nipples of nursing mothers* [bismuth subnitrate]

m-AMSA (acridinylamine methanesulphon anisidide) [see: amsacrine]

Mandameth enteric-coated tablets ℞ *urinary antibacterial* [methenamine mandelate]

Mandelamine film-coated tablets, oral suspension, suspension forte, granules ℞ *urinary antibacterial* [methenamine mandelate]

mandelic acid NF

Mandex enteric-coated tablets (discontinued 1991) ℞ *urinary anti-infective; analgesic; antispasmodic* [methenamine mandelate; salicylamide; belladonna extract]

Mandol powder for IV or IM injection, ADD-vantage vials, Faspaks ℞ *cephalosporin-type antibiotic* [cefamandole nafate]

manganese *element* (Mn)

manganese chloride USP *dietary manganese supplement*

manganese chloride tetrahydrate [see: manganese chloride]

manganese gluconate (manganese D-gluconate) USP *dietary manganese supplement*

manganese glycerophosphate NF

manganese hypophosphite NF

manganese phosphinate [see: manganese hypophosphite]

manganese sulfate USP *dietary manganese supplement*

manganese sulfate monohydrate [see: manganese sulfate]

Manganese Trace Metal Additive IV injection (discontinued 1991) ℞ *intravenous nutritional therapy* [manganese sulfate]

Manga-Pak IV injection (discontinued 1992) ℞ *intravenous nutritional therapy* [manganese sulfate]

manidipine 6300 INN

manna sugar [see: mannitol]

Mannest tablets (discontinued 1992) ℞ *estrogen hormone replacement* [conjugated estrogens]

mannite [see: mannitol]

mannitol (D-mannitol) USP *renal function test aid; osmotic diuretic; urologic irrigant*

mannitol hexanitrate INN

mannityl nitrate [see: mannitol hexanitrate]

mannomustine INN, BAN

mannosulfan INN

Manoplax film-coated tablets ℞ *vasodilator for congestive heart failure* [flosequinan]

manozodil INN

Mantadil cream ℞ *topical corticosteroid; antihistamine* [hydrocortisone acetate; chlorcyclizine HCl]

Mantoux test [see: tuberculin]

Maolate tablets ℞ *skeletal muscle relaxant* [chlorphenesin carbamate]

Maox tablets OTC *antacid* [magnesium oxide]

maprotiline USAN, INN *antidepressant*

maprotiline HCl USP *tetracyclic antidepressant*

Marax tablets ℞ *antiasthmatic; bronchodilator; decongestant; anxiolytic* [theophylline; ephedrine sulfate; hydroxyzine HCl]

Marax-DF pediatric syrup ℞ *antiasthmatic; bronchodilator; decongestant; expectorant; anxiolytic* [theophylline; ephedrine sulfate; hydroxyzine HCl]

Marazide tablets (discontinued 1991) ℞ *diuretic; antihypertensive* [benzthiazide]

Marbaxin 750 tablets ℞ *skeletal muscle relaxant* [methocarbamol]

Marbec tablets OTC *dietary supplement* [multiple B vitamins; vitamin C; brewer's yeast]

Marblen tablets, oral suspension OTC *antacid* [calcium carbonate; magnesium carbonate]

Marcaine HCl; Marcaine Spinal injection ℞ *injectable local anesthetic* [bupivacaine HCl]

Marcaine HCl with Epinephrine injection ℞ *injectable local anesthetic* [bupivacaine HCl; epinephrine bitartrate]

Marcillin capsules, powder for oral suspension ℞ *penicillin-type antibiotic* [ampicillin trihydrate]

Marcof Expectorant liquid ℞ *antitussive; expectorant* [hydrocodone bitartrate; potassium guaiacolsulfonate]

Marezine IM injection (discontinued 1993) ℞ *antiemetic; anticholinergic; antihistamine; motion sickness preventative* [cyclizine lactate]

Marezine tablets OTC *antiemetic; anticholinergic; antihistamine; motion sickness preventative* [cyclizine HCl]

Marflex tablets ℞ *skeletal muscle relaxant* [orphenadrine citrate]

Margesic capsules ℞ *analgesic; anti-inflammatory; sedative* [acetaminophen; caffeine; butalbital]

Margesic H capsules ℞ *narcotic analgesic* [hydrocodone bitartrate; acetaminophen]

Margesic No. 3 tablets ℞ *analgesic* [acetaminophen; codeine phosphate]

maridomycin INN

Marine Lipid Concentrate softgels OTC *dietary supplement* [omega-3 fatty acids; vitamin E]

Marinol capsules ℞ *antiemetic for cancer chemotherapy; appetite stimulant for AIDS patients (orphan)* [dronabinol]

mariptiline INN

Marlin Salt System; Marlin Salt System II tablets OTC *contact lens rinsing and storage solution* [sodium chloride for normal saline solution]

Marlipids III capsules (discontinued 1993) OTC *dietary supplement* [omega-3 fatty acids; vitamin E]

Marmine IV or IM injection ℞ *antinauseant; antiemetic; antivertigo; motion sickness preventative* [dimenhydrinate]

Marmine tablets OTC *antinauseant; antiemetic; antivertigo; motion sickness preventative* [dimenhydrinate]

Marnal tablets, capsules ℞ *analgesic; antipyretic; anti-inflammatory; sedative* [acetaminophen; caffeine; butalbital]

Marnatal-F film-coated tablets ℞ *vitamin/mineral/calcium/iron supplement* [multiple vitamins & minerals; calcium; iron; folic acid]

Marogen *(orphan: anemia of end-stage renal disease)* [epoetin beta]

maroxepin INN

Marplan tablets ℞ *monoamine oxidase (MAO) inhibitor antidepressant* [isocarboxazid]

Marpres tablets ℞ *antihypertensive* [hydrochlorothiazide; reserpine; hydralazine HCl]

Marthritic tablets ℞ *analgesic; antipyretic; anti-inflammatory; antirheumatic* [salsalate]

masoprocol USAN, INN *antineoplastic*

Massé Breast cream OTC *moisturizer and emollient for nipples of nursing women*

Massengill Baking Soda Freshness solution OTC *vaginal cleanser and deodorizer* [sodium bicarbonate]

Massengill Disposable Douche; Massengill Unscented solution OTC *antiseptic/germicidal; vaginal cleanser and deodorizer; acidity modifier* [cetylpyridinium chloride; lactic acid; sodium lactate]

Massengill Disposable Douche; Massengill Vinegar & Water Extra Mild solution OTC *vaginal cleanser and deodorizer; acidity modifier* [vinegar (acetic acid)]

Massengill Douche powder OTC *astringent; antipruritic/counterirritant; vaginal cleanser and deodorizer* [ammonium alum; phenol; methyl salicylate; menthol; thymol]

Massengill Douche solution concentrate OTC *vaginal cleanser and deodorizer; acidity modifier* [lactic acid; sodium lactate; sodium bicarbonate]

Massengill Medicated Douche with Cepticin; Massengill Medicated Disposable Douche with Cepticin solution OTC *antiseptic/germicidal; vaginal cleanser and deodorizer* [povidone-iodine]

Massengill Medicated towelettes OTC *topical corticosteriodal anti-inflammatory* [hydrocortisone]

Massengill Vinegar & Water Extra Cleansing with Puraclean solution OTC *vaginal cleanser and deodorizer; antiseptic; acidity modifier* [vinegar (acetic acid); cetylpyridinium chloride]

Materna tablets ℞ *vitamin/mineral/calcium/iron supplement* [multiple vitamins & minerals; calcium; iron; folic acid; biotin]

matrix metalloproteinase inhibitor *(orphan: corneal ulcers)*

Matulane capsules ℞ *antineoplastic adjunct for stages III and IV Hodgkin's disease* [procarbazine HCl]

Maxair Autohaler (breath-activated metered-dose inhaler) ℞ *bronchodilator for bronchospasm* [pirbuterol acetate]

Maxaquin film-coated tablets ℞ *broad-spectrum fluoroquinolone-type antibiotic* [lomefloxacin HCl]

Max-Caro capsules OTC *to reduce photosensitivity reaction* [beta-carotene]

MaxEPA soft capsules OTC *dietary supplement* [omega-3 fatty acids; multiple vitamins & minerals]

Maxicam ℞ *investigational nonsteroidal anti-inflammatory drug (NSAID); antiarthritic; analgesic; antipyretic* [isoxicam]

Maxidex Drop-Tainers (eye drop suspension) ℞ *ophthalmic topical corticosteroidal anti-inflammatory* [dexamethasone]

Maxidex ophthalmic ointment ℞ *ophthalmic topical corticosteroidal anti-inflammatory* [dexamethasone sodium phosphate]

Maxiflor cream, ointment ℞ *topical corticosteroidal anti-inflammatory* [diflorasone diacetate]

Maxilube Personal Lubricant jelly OTC *vaginal lubricant*

Maximum Blue Label; Maximum Green Label; Maximum Red Label tablets OTC *dietary supplement* [multiple vitamins & minerals; biotin; choline; bioflavonoids; inositol; SOD; lysine]

Maxitrol eye drop suspension, ophthalmic ointment ℞ *topical ophthalmic corticosteroidal anti-inflammatory; antibiotic* [dexamethasone; neomycin sulfate; polymyxin B sulfate]

Maxivate ointment, cream, lotion ℞ *topical corticosteroid* [betamethasone diproprionate]

Maxolon tablets ℞ *antidopaminergic; antiemetic for chemotherapy; peristaltic* [metoclopramide monohydrochloride monohydrate]

Maxovite sustained-release tablets OTC *vitamin/mineral supplement* [multiple vitamins & minerals; folic acid; biotin]

Maxzide tablets ℞ *diuretic* [triamterene; hydrochlorothiazide]

Mayotic ear drop suspension (discontinued 1992) ℞ *topical corticosteroidal anti-inflammatory; antibiotic* [hydrocortisone; neomycin sulfate; polymyxin B sulfate]

maytansine USAN *antineoplastic* [also: maitansine]

May-Vita elixir ℞ *vitamin supplement* [multiple B vitamins; folic acid]

Mazanor tablets ℞ *anorexiant* [mazindol]

mazaticol INN

MAZE (*m*-AMSA, azacitidine, etoposide) *chemotherapy protocol*

Mazicon IV injection ℞ *benzodiazepine antagonist to reverse anesthesia or treat overdose* [flumazenil]

mazindol USAN, USP, INN, BAN *anorexiant; (orphan: Duchenne's muscular dystrophy)*

mazipredone INN

Mazon cream (discontinued 1991) OTC *topical antipsoriatic; antiseborrheic; keratolytic; antifungal* [coal tar; salicylic acid; resorcinol; benzoic acid]

MB (methylene blue) [q.v.]

M-BACOD (methotrexate, bleomycin, Adriamycin, cyclophosphamide, Oncovin, dexamethasone) *chemotherapy protocol*

M-BACOS (methotrexate, bleomycin, Adriamycin, cyclophosphamide, Oncovin, Solu-Medrol) *chemotherapy protocol*

MBD (methotrexate, bleomycin, DDP) *chemotherapy protocol*

MBR (methylene blue, reduced) [see: methylene blue]

M-Caps capsules ℞ *urinary acidifier to control ammonia production* [racemethionine]

MCBP (melphalan, cyclophosphamide, BCNU, prednisone) *chemotherapy protocol*

MCH (microfibrillar collagen hemostat) [q.v.]

MCP (melphalan, cyclophosphamide, prednisone) *chemotherapy protocol*

M-CSF (macrophage colony-stimulating factor) [q.v.]

MCT (medium chain triglycerides) [q.v.]

MCT oil OTC *dietary fat supplement* [medium chain triglycerides from coconut oil]

MCV (methotrexate, cisplatin, vinblastine) *chemotherapy protocol*

MD-60; MD-76 injection ℞ *parenteral radiopaque agent* [diatrizoate meglumine; diatrizoate sodium]

MD-Gastroview solution ℞ *GI contrast radiopaque agent* [diatrizoate meglumine; diatrizoate sodium]

MDP (methylene diphosphonate) [now: medronate disodium]

MEA (mercaptoethylamine) [see: mercaptamine]

measles, mumps & rubella virus vaccine, live USP *active immunizing agent for measles (rubeola), mumps and rubella*

measles immune globulin USP

measles & rubella virus vaccine, live USP *active immunizing agent for measles (rubeola) and rubella*

measles virus vaccine live USP *active immunizing agent for measles (rubeola)*
Measurin timed-release tablets (discontinued 1992) OTC *analgesic; antipyretic; anti-inflammatory* [aspirin]
Mebadin (available only from the Centers for Disease Control) ℞ *investigational anti-infective for amebiasis and amebic dysentery* [dehydroemetine]
meballymal [see: secobarbital]
mebamoxine [see: benmoxin]
mebanazine INN, BAN
Mebaral tablets ℞ *sedative; anticonvulsant* [mephobarbital]
mebendazole USAN, USP, INN *anthelmintic*
mebenoside INN
mebeverine INN *smooth muscle relaxant* [also: mebeverine HCl]
mebeverine HCl USAN *smooth muscle relaxant* [also: mebeverine]
mebezonium iodide INN, BAN
mebhydrolin INN, BAN
mebiquine INN
mebolazine INN
mebrofenin USAN, INN *hepatobiliary function test*
mebrophenhydramine HCl [see: embramine HCl]
mebubarbital [see: pentobarbital]
mebumal [see: pentobarbital]
mebutamate USAN, INN *antihypertensive*
mebutizide INN
mecamylamine INN *antihypertensive* [also: mecamylamine HCl]
mecamylamine HCl USP *antihypertensive* [also: mecamylamine]
mecarbinate INN
mecarbine [see: mecarbinate]
MeCCNU (methyl chloroethyl-cyclohexyl-nitrosourea) [see: semustine]
mecetronium ethylsulfate USAN *antiseptic* [also: mecetronium etilsulfate]

mecetronium etilsulfate INN *antiseptic* [also: mecetronium ethylsulfate]
mechlorethamine HCl USP *antineoplastic* [also: chlormethine; mustine]
Mechol tablets OTC *dietary supplement* [multiple B vitamins; vitamin C; soy protein; brewer's yeast]
meciadanol INN
mecillinam INN, BAN *antibacterial* [also: amdinocillin]
mecinarone INN
Meclan cream ℞ *topical antibiotic for acne vulgaris* [meclocycline sulfosalicylate]
meclizine *antiemetic; antihistamine; anticholinergic; motion sickness relief*
meclizine HCl USP *antiemetic; antihistamine; anticholinergic; motion sickness relief* [also: meclozine]
meclocycline USAN, INN, BAN *antibacterial*
meclocycline sulfosalicylate USAN, USP *antibacterial antibiotic*
meclofenamate sodium USAN, USP *analgesic; antiarthritic; nonsteroidal anti-inflammatory drug (NSAID)*
meclofenamic acid USAN, INN *nonsteroidal anti-inflammatory drug (NSAID)*
meclofenoxate INN, BAN
Meclomen capsules ℞ *nonsteroidal anti-inflammatory drug (NSAID); antiarthritic; analgesic* [meclofenamate sodium]
meclonazepam INN
mecloqualone USAN, INN *sedative; hypnotic*
mecloralurea INN
meclorisone INN, BAN *topical anti-inflammatory* [also: meclorisone dibutyrate]
meclorisone dibutyrate USAN *topical anti-inflammatory* [also: meclorisone]
mecloxamine INN

meclozine INN, BAN *antiemetic; antihistamine; anticholinergic; motion sickness relief* [also: meclizine HCl]

mecobalamin USAN, INN *vitamin; hematopoietic*

mecrilate INN *tissue adhesive* [also: mecrylate]

mecrylate USAN *tissue adhesive* [also: mecrilate]

Mectizan ℞ *investigational antiparasitic*

MECY (methotrexate, cyclophosphamide) *chemotherapy protocol*

mecysteine INN

Meda Cap capsules OTC *analgesic; antipyretic* [acetaminophen]

Meda Syrup Forte (discontinued 1992) OTC *decongestant; antihistamine; antitussive; expectorant* [phenylephrine HCl; chlorpheniramine maleate; dextromethorphan hydrobromide; guaifenesin]

Meda Tab tablets OTC *analgesic; antipyretic* [acetaminophen]

Medacote lotion OTC *topical antihistamine; astringent; antipruritic* [pyrilamine maleate; zinc oxide; menthol; camphor]

Medadyne liquid OTC *topical anesthetic; oral antiseptic; astringent* [benzocaine; methylbenzethonium chloride; tannic acid; camphor; menthol]

Medadyne throat spray OTC *topical anesthetic; oral antiseptic* [lidocaine; cetalkonium chloride]

Medalone 40; Medalone 80 [see: depMedalone 40; depMedalone 80]

Medamint throat lozenges OTC *oral anesthetic* [benzocaine]

Medatussin Plus syrup ℞ *decongestant; antihistamine; antitussive; expectorant* [phenylpropanolamine HCl; chlorpheniramine maleate; phenyltoloxamine citrate; dextromethorphan hydrobromide; guaifenesin]

Medatussin syrup, pediatric syrup OTC *antitussive; expectorant; demulcent* [dextromethorphan hydrobromide; guaifenesin; potassium citrate; citric acid]

medazepam INN *minor tranquilizer* [also: medazepam HCl]

medazepam HCl USAN *minor tranquilizer* [also: medazepam]

medazomide INN

medazonamide [see: medazomide]

Medazyme chewable tablets (discontinued 1992) OTC *digestive enzymes; antiflatulent* [amylase; protease; lipase; cellulase; simethicone]

medetomidine INN, BAN *veterinary analgesic; veterinary sedative* [also: medetomidine HCl]

medetomidine HCl USAN *veterinary analgesic; veterinary sedative* [also: medetomidine]

MEDI 488 ℞ *investigational HIV vaccine*

Mediatric capsules (discontinued 1993) ℞ *geriatric dietary supplement with hormones* [multiple B vitamins; iron; methyltestosterone; conjugated estrogens; methamphetamine HCl]

medibazine INN

medical air [see: air, medical]

medicinal zinc peroxide [see: zinc peroxide, medicinal]

Medicone Derma ointment OTC *topical local anesthetic; antibacterial; counterirritant* [benzocaine; zinc oxide; hydroxyquinoline sulfate; ichthammol]

Medicone Derma-HC ointment (discontinued 1992) ℞ *topical corticosteroid; anesthetic; antifungal; vasoconstrictor* [hydrocortisone acetate; benzocaine; oxyquinoline sulfate; ephedrine; menthol; ichthammol; zinc oxide]

Medicone Dressing cream OTC *topical local anesthetic; antibacterial; astringent* [benzocaine; hydroxyquinoline sulfate; cod liver oil; zinc oxide; menthol]

Medicone Rectal ointment OTC *topical local anesthetic; antibacterial; as-*

tringent [benzocaine; hydroxyquinoline sulfate; castor oil; zinc oxide; menthol; balsam Peru]

Medicone suppositories OTC *emollient; protectant* [live yeast cell derivative; shark liver oil]

Mediconet anorectal wipes (discontinued 1992) OTC *astringent; antiseptic; antifungal* [witch hazel; glycerin; benzalkonium chloride; ethoxylated lanolin; methylparaben]

Medi-Flu caplets, liquid OTC *decongestant; antihistamine; antitussive; analgesic* [pseudoephedrine HCl; chlorpheniramine maleate; dextromethorphan hydrobromide; acetaminophen]

medifoxamine INN

Medigesic capsules, tablets ℞ *analgesic; antipyretic; anti-inflammatory; sedative* [acetaminophen; caffeine; butalbital]

Medihaler Ergotamine inhaler (discontinued 1992) ℞ *migraine-specific vasoconstrictor* [ergotamine tartrate]

Medihaler-Epi inhalation aerosol OTC *bronchodilator for bronchial asthma* [epinephrine bitartrate]

Medihaler-Iso inhalation aerosol ℞ *bronchodilator* [isoproterenol sulfate]

Medikets troches (discontinued 1991) OTC *topical anesthetic; oral antiseptic* [benzocaine; cetylpyridinium chloride]

Medilax tablets, chewable tablets OTC *laxative* [phenolphthalein]

medinal [see: barbital sodium]

Mediplast plaster OTC *topical keratolytic* [salicylic acid]

Mediplex Tabules (tablets) OTC *vitamin/mineral supplement* [multiple vitamins & minerals]

Medipren tablets, caplets OTC *nonsteroidal anti-inflammatory drug (NSAID); antiarthritic; analgesic* [ibuprofen]

Mediquell chewy squares (discontinued 1991) OTC *antitussive* [dextromethorphan hydrobromide]

Medi-Quick aerosol OTC *topical local anesthetic; antiseptic* [lidocaine HCl; benzalkonium chloride]

Medi-Quick ointment OTC *topical antibiotic* [polymyxin B sulfate; neomycin; bacitracin]

Medi-Quick spray OTC *topical local anesthetic; antiseptic* [lidocaine; benzalkonium chloride]

medium chain triglycerides (MCT) *dietary lipid supplement*

medorinone USAN, INN *cardiotonic*

medorubicin INN

Medotar ointment OTC *topical antipsoriatic; antiseborrheic; astringent; antiseptic* [coal tar; zinc oxide]

Medralone 40; Medralone 80 intralesional, soft tissue, and IM injection ℞ *glucocorticoids* [methylprednisolone acetate]

medrogestone USAN, INN, BAN *progestin*

Medrol Acetate Topical ointment (discontinued 1993) ℞ *topical corticosteroid* [methylprednisolone acetate]

Medrol tablets, Dosepak (unit of use package) ℞ *glucocorticoids* [methylprednisolone]

medronate disodium USAN *pharmaceutic aid*

medronic acid USAN, INN, BAN *pharmaceutic aid*

medroxalol USAN, INN, BAN *antihypertensive*

medroxalol HCl USAN *antihypertensive*

medroxiprogesterone acetate [see: medroxyprogesterone acetate]

medroxyprogesterone INN, BAN *progestin; antineoplastic* [also: medroxyprogesterone acetate]

medroxyprogesterone acetate USP *progestin; antineoplastic* [also: medroxyprogesterone]

medrylamine INN
medrysone USAN, USP, INN *glucocorticoid; ophthalmic anti-inflammatory*
mefeclorazine INN
mefenamic acid USAN, USP, INN, BAN *analgesic; nonsteroidal anti-inflammatory drug (NSAID)*
mefenidil USAN, INN *cerebral vasodilator*
mefenidil fumarate USAN *cerebral vasodilator*
mefenidramium metilsulfate INN
mefenorex INN *anorexic* [also: mefenorex HCl]
mefenorex HCl USAN *anorexic* [also: mefenorex]
mefeserpine INN
mefexamide USAN, INN *CNS stimulant*
mefloquine USAN, INN, BAN *antimalarial*
mefloquine HCl USAN *antimalarial schizonticide (orphan)*
Mefoxin powder for IV or IM injection, ADD-Vantage vials ℞ *cephalosporin-type antibiotic* [cefoxitin sodium]
mefruside USAN, INN *diuretic*
Mega B with C tablets OTC *vitamin supplement* [multiple B vitamins; vitamin C; folic acid; biotin]
Mega VM-80 tablets OTC *geriatric vitamin/mineral supplement* [multiple vitamins & minerals; folic acid; biotin]
Mega-B tablets OTC *vitamin supplement* [multiple B vitamins; folic acid; biotin]
Megace OS oral suspension ℞ *investigational agent for cachexia (orphan)* [megestrol acetate]
Megace tablets ℞ *antineoplastic; (orphan: AIDS-related anorexia and cachexia)* [megestrol acetate]
Megadose tablets OTC *geriatric vitamin/mineral supplement* [multiple vitamins & minerals; folic acid; biotin]

megalomicin INN *antibacterial* [also: megalomicin potassium phosphate]
megalomicin potassium phosphate USAN *antibacterial* [also: megalomicin]
Megaton elixir ℞ *vitamin/mineral supplement* [multiple B vitamins & minerals; folic acid]
megestrol INN, BAN *antineoplastic* [also: megestrol acetate]
megestrol acetate USAN, USP *antineoplastic; (orphan: AIDS-related anorexia and cachexia)* [also: megestrol]
meglitinide INN
meglucycline INN
meglumine USP, INN *radiopaque medium*
meglumine diatrizoate BAN *radiopaque medium* [also: diatrizoate meglumine]
meglumine iocarmate BAN *radiopaque medium* [also: iocarmate meglumine]
meglumine iothalamate BAN *radiopaque medium* [also: iothalamate meglumine]
meglumine ioxaglate BAN *radiopaque medium* [also: ioxaglate meglumine]
meglutol USAN, INN *antihyperlipoproteinemic*
mel B [see: melarsoprol]
mel W [see: melarsonyl potassium]
Melacine ℞ *(orphan: stages III–IV melanoma)* [melanoma vaccine]
meladrazine INN, BAN
melafocon A USAN *hydrophobic contact lens material*
Melanex solution ℞ *hyperpigmentation bleaching agent* [hydroquinone]
melanoma vaccine *(orphan: stages III-IV melanoma)*
melarsonyl potassium INN, BAN
melarsoprol INN, BAN *investigational anti-infective for trypanosomiasis*
melengestrol INN *antineoplastic; progestin* [also: melengestrol acetate]

melengestrol acetate USAN *antineoplastic; progestin* [also: melengestrol]
meletimide INN
melfalan [see: melphalan]
Melfiat tablets (discontinued 1991) ℞ *anorexiant* [phendimetrazine tartrate]
Melfiat-105 Unicelles sustained-release capsules ℞ *anorexiant* [phendimetrazine tartrate]
Melimmune-1; Melimmune-2 ℞ *investigational treatment for malignant melanoma* [monoclonal antibodies]
melinamide INN
melitracen INN *antidepressant* [also: melitracen HCl]
melitracen HCl USAN *antidepressant* [also: melitracen]
melizame USAN, INN *sweetener*
Mellaril tablets, oral concentrate ℞ *antipsychotic* [thioridazine HCl]
Mellaril-S oral suspension ℞ *antipsychotic* [thioridazine HCl]
meloxicam INN
melperone INN, BAN
melphalan (MPL) USAN, USP, INN, BAN *antineoplastic; (orphan: multiple myeloma; metastatic melanoma)*
MelVax ℞ *investigational treatment for malignant melanoma* [monoclonal antibodies]
memantine INN
memotine INN *antiviral* [also: memotine HCl]
memotine HCl USAN *antiviral* [also: memotine]
menabitan INN *analgesic* [also: menabitan HCl]
menabitan HCl USAN *analgesic* [also: menabitan]
menadiol BAN *vitamin K_4; prothrombogenic* [also: menadiol sodium diphosphate]
menadiol sodium diphosphate USP *vitamin K_4; prothrombogenic* [also: menadiol]
menadiol sodium sulfate INN

menadione USP *vitamin K_3; prothrombogenic*
menadione sodium bisulfite USP, INN
Menadol tablets OTC *nonsteroidal anti-inflammatory drug (NSAID); antiarthritic; analgesic* [ibuprofen]
menaphthene [see: menadione]
menaphthone [see: menadione]
menaphthone sodium bisulfite [see: menadione sodium bisulfite]
menaquinone *vitamin K_2; prothrombogenic*
menatetrenone INN
menbutone INN, BAN
mendelevium *element (Md)*
Menest tablets ℞ *estrogen replacement therapy* [esterified estrogens]
menfegol INN
menglytate INN
menichlopholan [see: niclofolan]
Meni-D capsules ℞ *anticholinergic; antivertigo agent; motion sickness preventative* [meclizine]
meningococcal polysaccharide vaccine, group A USP *active bacterin for meningitis (Neisseria meningitidis)*
meningococcal polysaccharide vaccine, group C USP *active bacterin for meningitis (Neisseria meningitidis)*
meningococcal polysaccharide vaccine, group W-135 *active bacterin for meningitis (Neisseria meningitidis)*
meningococcal polysaccharide vaccine, group Y *active bacterin for meningitis (Neisseria meningitidis)*
menitrazepam INN
menoctone USAN, INN *antimalarial*
menogaril USAN, INN *antineoplastic*
Menomune-A/C/Y/W-135 powder for subcu injection ℞ *meningitis vaccine* [meningococcal polysaccharide vaccine, groups A, C, Y & W-135]
Menoplex tablets OTC *analgesic; antipyretic; antihistamine* [acetaminophen; phenyltoloxamine citrate]
menotropins USAN, USP *gonad-stimulating principle; gonadotropin*

Menrium 5-2; Menrium 5-4; Menrium 10-4 tablets ℞ *estrogen deficiency; menopausal symptoms* [esterified estrogens; chlordiazepoxide]

Mentane ℞ *investigational agent for Alzheimer's disease* [velnacrine]

menthol USP *topical antipruritic/antiseptic; mild local anesthetic*

MenthoRub vaporizing ointment OTC *counterirritant* [menthol; camphor; eucalyptus oil; oil of turpentine]

meobentine INN *antiarrhythmic* [also: meobentine sulfate]

meobentine sulfate USAN *antiarrhythmic* [also: meobentine]

mepacrine INN *anthelmintic; antimalarial* [also: quinacrine HCl]

mepacrine HCl [see: quinacrine HCl]

meparfynol [see: methylpentynol]

mepartricin USAN, INN *antifungal; antiprotozoal*

mepazine acetate [see: pecazine]

mepenzolate bromide USP, INN *peptic ulcer adjunct*

mepenzolate methylbromide [see: mepenzolate bromide]

mepenzolone bromide [see: mepenzolate bromide]

Mepergan Fortis capsules ℞ *narcotic analgesic; sedative* [meperidine HCl; promethazine HCl]

Mepergan injection ℞ *narcotic analgesic; sedative* [meperidine HCl; promethazine HCl]

meperidine HCl USP *narcotic analgesic* [also: pethidine]

Mephaquin (*orphan: chloroquine-resistant malaria*) [mefloquine HCl]

mephenesin NF, INN

mephenhydramine [see: moxastine]

mephenoxalone INN

mephentermine INN *adrenergic; vasoconstrictor* [also: mephentermine sulfate]

mephentermine sulfate USP *adrenergic; vasoconstrictor; vasopressor for shock* [also: mephentermine]

mephenytoin USAN, USP, INN *anticonvulsant* [also: methoin]

mephobarbital USP *anticonvulsant; sedative* [also: methylphenobarbital; methylphenobarbitone]

Mephyton tablets ℞ *coagulant; vitamin K deficiency* [phytonadione]

mepicycline [see: pipacycline]

Mepig (*orphan: pulmonary infections of cystic fibrosis*) [mucoid exopolysaccharide Pseudomonas hyperimmune globulin]

mepindolol INN, BAN

mepiperphenidol bromide

mepiprazole INN, BAN

mepirizole [see: epirizole]

mepiroxol INN

mepitiostane INN

mepivacaine INN *local anesthetic* [also: mepivacaine HCl]

mepivacaine HCl USP *local anesthetic* [also: mepivacaine]

mepixanox INN

mepramidil INN

meprednisone USAN, USP, INN

meprobamate USP, INN *anxiolytic; minor tranquilizer*

Meprogesic Q tablets ℞ *analgesic; antipyretic; anti-inflammatory; anxiolytic* [aspirin; meprobamate]

Mepron film-coated tablets ℞ *antiprotozoal for AIDS-related Pneumocystis carinii pneumonia (PCP)* [atovaquone]

meproscillarin INN, BAN

Meprospan sustained-release capsules ℞ *anxiolytic* [meprobamate]

meprothixol BAN [also: meprotixol]

meprotixol INN [also: meprothixol]

meprylcaine INN *local anesthetic* [also: meprylcaine HCl]

meprylcaine HCl USP *local anesthetic* [also: meprylcaine]

meptazinol INN, BAN *analgesic* [also: meptazinol HCl]

meptazinol HCl USAN *analgesic* [also: meptazinol]

mepyramine INN, BAN *antihistamine* [also: pyrilamine maleate]
mepyramine maleate [see: pyrilamine maleate]
mepyrium [see: amprolium]
mepyrrotazine [see: dimelazine]
mequidox USAN, INN *antibacterial*
mequinol INN
mequitamium iodide INN
mequitazine INN, BAN
mequitazium iodide [see: mequitamium iodide]
meragidone sodium
meralein sodium USAN, INN *topical anti-infective*
meralluride NF, INN
merbaphen USP
merbromin NF, INN *general antiseptic*
mercaptamine INN *antiurolithic* [also: cysteamine]
mercaptoarsenical [see: arsthinol]
mercaptoarsenol [see: arsthinol]
mercaptoethylamine (MEA) [see: mercaptamine]
mercaptomerin (MT6) INN [also: mercaptomerin sodium]
mercaptomerin sodium USP [also: mercaptomerin]
mercaptopurine USP, INN *antineoplastic*
mercuderamide INN
mercufenol chloride USAN *topical anti-infective*
mercumatilin sodium INN
mercuric oxide, yellow NF *ophthalmic antiseptic*
mercuric salicylate NF
mercuric succinimide NF
mercurobutol INN
Mercurochrome II liquid, spray (discontinued 1991) OTC *topical local anesthetic; antiseptic; counterirritant* [lidocaine HCl; benzalkonium chloride; menthol; isopropyl alcohol]
Mercurochrome solution OTC *antiseptic* [merbromin]
mercurophylline NF, INN
mercurous chloride [see: calomel]

mercury *element (Hg)*
mercury, ammoniated USP *topical anti-infective; antipsoriatic*
mercury amide chloride [see: mercury, ammoniated]
mercury oleate NF
merethoxylline procaine
mergocriptine INN
merisoprol acetate Hg 197 USAN *radioactive agent*
merisoprol acetate Hg 203 USAN *radioactive agent*
merisoprol Hg 197 USAN *renal function test; radioactive agent*
Meritene liquid, powder OTC *total enteral nutrition; nutritional supplement*
Merlenate ointment ℞ *topical antifungal* [zinc undecylenate; caprylic acid; sodium propionate]
meropenem INN, BAN *broad-spectrum antibiotic*
Merrem ℞ *investigational broad-spectrum antibiotic* [meropenem]
mersalyl INN
mersalyl sodium [see: mersalyl]
Mersol solution, tincture OTC *antiseptic; antibacterial; antifungal* [thimerosal]
Merthiolate Aeropump (discontinued 1991) OTC *antiseptic; antibacterial; antifungal* [thimerosal]
Merthiolate solution, tincture (discontinued 1992) OTC *antiseptic; antibacterial; antifungal* [thimerosal]
mertiatide INN
Meruvax II subcu injection ℞ *rubella vaccine* [rubella virus vaccine, live]
mesabolone INN
mesalamine USAN *anti-inflammatory; treatment of ulcerative colitis and proctitis* [also: mesalazine]
mesalazine INN, BAN *anti-inflammatory; treatment of ulcerative colitis and proctitis* [also: mesalamine]
Mesantoin tablets ℞ *anticonvulsant* [mephenytoin]

meseclazone USAN, INN *anti-inflammatory*
mesifilcon A USAN *hydrophilic contact lens material*
mesna USAN, INN, BAN *detoxifying agent;* (*orphan: hemorrhagic cystitis; cyclophosphamide-induced urotoxicity*)
Mesnex IV injection ℞ (*orphan: hemorrhagic cystitis prophylaxis; cyclophosphamide-induced urotoxicity*) [mesna]
mesocarb INN
meso-inositol [see: inositol]
meso-NDGA (nordihydroguaiaretic acid) [see: masoprocol]
meso-nordihydroguaiaretic acid (NDGA) [see: masoprocol]
mesoridazine USAN, INN *antipsychotic*
mesoridazine besylate USP *antipsychotic*
mespirenone INN
mestanolone INN, BAN
mestenediol [see: methandriol]
mesterolone USAN, INN *androgen*
Mestinon tablets, syrup, Timespan (sustained-release tablets), IM or IV injection ℞ *anticholinesterase muscle stimulant; muscle relaxant reversal* [pyridostigmine bromide]
mestranol USAN, USP, INN *estrogen*
mesudipine INN
mesulergine INN
mesulfamide INN
mesulfen INN [also: mesulphen]
mesulphen BAN [also: mesulfen]
mesuprine INN *vasodilator; smooth muscle relaxant* [also: mesuprine HCl]
mesuprine HCl USAN *vasodilator; smooth muscle relaxant* [also: mesuprine]
mesuximide INN *anticonvulsant* [also: methsuximide]
metabromsalan USAN, INN *disinfectant*
metabutethamine HCl NF
metabutoxycaine HCl NF

metacetamol INN, BAN
metaclazepam INN
metacycline INN *antibacterial* [also: methacycline]
metaglycodol INN
metahexamide INN
metahexanamide [see: metahexamide]
Metahydrin tablets ℞ *diuretic* [trichlormethiazide]
metalkonium chloride INN
metallibure INN *anterior pituitary activator for swine* [also: methallibure]
metalol HCl USAN *antiadrenergic (β-receptor)*
metamelfalan INN
metamfazone INN [also: methamphazone]
metamfepramone INN [also: dimepropion]
metamfetamine INN CNS *stimulant* [also: methamphetamine HCl]
metamizole sodium INN *analgesic; antipyretic* [also: dipyrone]
metampicillin INN
Metamucil effervescent powder OTC *bulk laxative; antacid* [psyllium hydrophilic mucilloid; sodium bicarbonate; potassium bicarbonate]
Metamucil powder, wafers OTC *bulk laxative* [psyllium hydrophilic mucilloid]
metandienone INN [also: methandrostenolone; methandienone]
Metandren Linguets (discontinued 1991) ℞ *androgen for male hypogonadism, impotence and breast cancer* [methyltestosterone]
Metandren tablets (discontinued 1992) ℞ *androgen for male hypogonadism, impotence and breast cancer* [methyltestosterone]
metanixin INN
metaoxedrine chloride [see: phenylephrine HCl]
metaphosphoric acid, potassium salt [see: potassium metaphosphate]

metaphosphoric acid, trisodium salt [see: sodium trimetaphosphate]
metaphyllin [see: aminophylline]
metapramine INN
Metaprel inhalation aerosol powder, solution for inhalation, tablets, syrup ℞ *bronchodilator* [metaproterenol sulfate]
metaproterenol polistirex USAN *bronchodilator* [also: orciprenaline]
metaproterenol sulfate USAN, USP *bronchodilator*
metaradrine bitartrate [see: metaraminol bitartrate]
metaraminol INN *adrenergic; vasopressor for shock* [also: metaraminol bitartrate]
metaraminol bitartrate USP *adrenergic; vasopressor for shock* [also: metaraminol]
Metasep shampoo OTC *antibacterial; antiseborrheic* [parachlorometaxylenol]
Metastron ℞ *investigational imaging agent*
Metatensin #2; Metatensin #4 tablets ℞ *diuretic; antihypertensive* [trichlormethiazide; reserpine]
metaterol INN
metaxalone USAN, INN *skeletal muscle relaxant*
metazamide INN
metazepium iodide [see: buzepide metiodide]
metazide INN
metazocine INN, BAN
metbufen INN
metcaraphen HCl
Meted; Meted-2 shampoo (discontinued 1991) OTC *antiseborrheic; keratolytic* [sulfur; salicylic acid]
meteneprost USAN, INN *oxytocic; prostaglandin*
metenolone INN *anabolic* [also: methenolone acetate]
metenolone acetate [see: methenolone acetate]
metergoline INN, BAN

metergotamine INN
metescufylline INN
metesculetol INN
metethoheptazine INN
metetoin INN *anticonvulsant* [also: methetoin]
metformin USAN, INN *antidiabetic*
methacholine bromide NF
methacholine chloride USP, INN *cholinergic*
methacrylic acid copolymer NF *tablet-coating agent*
methacycline USAN *antibacterial* [also: metacycline]
methacycline HCl USP *gram-negative and gram-positive bacteriostatic; antirickettsial*
methadol [see: dimepheptanol]
methadone INN *narcotic analgesic* [also: methadone HCl]
methadone HCl USP *narcotic analgesic* [also: methadone]
methadonium chloride [see: methadone HCl]
methadyl acetate USAN *narcotic analgesic* [also: acetylmethadol]
methafilcon B USAN *hydrophilic contact lens material*
Methagual OTC *counterirritant* [methyl salicylate; guaiacol]
Methalgen cream OTC *counterirritant* [methyl salicylate; menthol; camphor; mustard oil]
methallenestril INN
methallenestrol [see: methallenestril]
methallibure USAN *anterior pituitary activator for swine* [also: metallibure]
methalthiazide USAN *diuretic; antihypertensive*
methamoctol
methamphazone BAN [also: metamfazone]
methamphetamine HCl USP *CNS stimulant* [also: metamfetamine]
methampyrone [now: dipyrone]
methanabol [see: methandriol]
methandienone BAN [also: methandrostenolone; metandienone]

methandriol
methandrostenolone USP [also: metandienone; methandienone]
methaniazide INN
methanol [see: methyl alcohol]
methantheline bromide USP *peptic ulcer adjunct* [also: methanthelinium bromide]
methanthelinium bromide INN, BAN *anticholinergic* [also: methantheline bromide]
methaphenilene INN, BAN [also: methaphenilene HCl]
methaphenilene HCl NF [also: methaphenilene]
methapyrilene INN [also: methapyrilene fumarate]
methapyrilene fumarate USP [also: methapyrilene]
methapyrilene HCl USP
methaqualone USAN, USP, INN *hypnotic; sedative*
methaqualone HCl USP
metharbital USP, INN *anticonvulsant* [also: metharbitone]
metharbitone BAN *anticonvulsant* [also: metharbital]
methastyridone INN
Methatropic capsules OTC *dietary lipotropic with vitamin supplementation* [choline; inositol; methionine; multiple B vitamins; desiccated liver; liver concentrate]
methazolamide USP, INN *carbonic anhydrase inhibitor*
Meth-Choline caplets (discontinued 1992) OTC *dietary lipotropic with vitamin supplementation* [choline; inositol; methionine; multiple B vitamins; desiccated liver; liver concentrate]
methdilazine USP, INN *antipruritic*
methdilazine HCl USP *antipruritic; antihistamine*
methenamine USP, INN *urinary antibacterial*

methenamine hippurate USAN, USP *urinary antibacterial* [also: hexamine hippurate]
methenamine mandelate USP *urinary antibacterial*
methenolone acetate USAN *anabolic* [also: metenolone]
methenolone enanthate USAN *anabolic*
metheptazine INN
Methergine tablets, IV, IM injection ℞ *control postpartum uterine atony; postpartum hemorrhage* [methylergonovine maleate]
methestrol INN
methetharimide [see: bemegride]
methetoin USAN *anticonvulsant* [also: metetoin]
methicillin sodium USAN, USP *bactericidal antibiotic* [also: meticillin]
methimazole USP *thyroid inhibitor* [also: thiamazole]
methindizate BAN [also: metindizate]
methiodal sodium USP, INN
methiomeprazine INN
methiomeprazine HCl [see: methiomeprazine]
methionine (L-methionine) USAN, USP, INN *essential amino acid; symbols:* Met, M
methionine (DL-methionine) USP, INN *urinary acidifier* [also: racemethionine]
methionine-enkephalin *investigational immunomodulator for AIDS*
methionyl granulocyte CSF, recombinant (orphan: *myelodysplastic syndrome*)
methionyl human granulocyte CSF, recombinant (orphan: *neutropenia in bone marrow transplants*)
methiothepin [see: metitepine]
methisazone USAN *antiviral* [also: metisazone]
methitural INN
methixene HCl USAN *smooth muscle relaxant* [also: metixene]

methocamphone methylsulfate [see: trimethidinium methosulfate]
methocarbamol USP, INN *skeletal muscle relaxant*
methocidin INN
methohexital USP, INN
methohexital sodium USP *general anesthetic*
methoin BAN *anticonvulsant* [also: mephenytoin]
methonaphthone [see: menbutone]
methophedrine [see: methoxyphedrine]
methophenazine [see: metofenazate]
methopholine USAN *analgesic* [also: metofoline]
methoprene INN
methopromazine INN
methopromazine maleate [see: methopromazine]
methopyrimazole [see: epirizole]
***d*-methorphan** [see: dextromethorphan]
***d*-methorphan hydrobromide** [see: dextromethorphan hydrobromide]
methoserpidine INN, BAN
methotrexate (MTX) USAN, USP, INN, BAN *antineoplastic; antirheumatic; systemic antipsoriatic*
methotrexate & laurocapram (*orphan: topical mycosis fungoides*)
Methotrexate LPF Sodium preservative-free injection ℞ *antineoplastic for leukemia, psoriasis and rheumatoid arthritis* [methotrexate sodium]
methotrexate sodium USP *antineoplastic; antirheumatic; (orphan: osteogenic sarcoma)*
Methotrexate/Azone ℞ (*orphan: topical mycosis fungoides*) [methotrexate; laurocapram]
methotrimeprazine USAN, USP *central analgesic; CNS depressant* [also: levomepromazine]
methoxamine INN *adrenergic; vasoconstrictor* [also: methoxamine HCl]

methoxamine HCl USP *adrenergic; vasoconstrictor; vasopressor for shock* [also: methoxamine]
methoxiflurane [see: methoxyflurane]
methoxsalen USP *pigmentation agent for vitiligo; antipsoriatic*
methoxy polyethylene glycol [see: polyethylene glycol monomethyl ether]
methoxyfenoserpin [see: mefeserpine]
methoxyflurane USAN, USP, INN, BAN *inhalation general anesthetic*
methoxyphedrine INN
methoxyphenamine INN [also: methoxyphenamine HCl]
methoxyphenamine HCl USP [also: methoxyphenamine]
4-methoxyphenol [see: mequinol]
***o*-methoxyphenyl salicylate acetate** [see: guacetisal]
methoxypromazine maleate [see: methopromazine]
8-methoxypsoralen (8-MOP) [see: methoxsalen]
5-methoxyresorcinol [see: flamenol]
methphenoxydiol [see: guaifenesin]
methscopolamine bromide USP *peptic ulcer adjunct* [also: hyoscine methobromide]
methsuximide USP, BAN *anticonvulsant* [also: mesuximide]
methyclothiazide USAN, USP, INN *diuretic; antihypertensive*
methydromorphine [see: methyldihydromorphine]
methyl alcohol NF *solvent*
methyl benzoquate BAN *coccidiostat for poultry* [also: nequinate]
methyl cresol [see: cresol]
methyl cysteine [see: mecysteine]
methyl *p*-hydroxybenzoate [see: methylparaben]
methyl isobutyl ketone NF *alcohol denaturant*
methyl nicotinate USAN
methyl palmoxirate USAN *antidiabetic*

methyl phthalate [see: dimethyl phthalate]
methyl salicylate NF *flavoring agent; counterirritant; topical anesthetic*
methyl sulfoxide [see: dimethyl sulfoxide]
methyl violet [see: gentian violet]
***l*-methylaminoethanolcatechol** [see: epinephrine]
methylaminopterin [see: methotrexate]
methylandrostenediol [see: methandriol]
methylatropine nitrate USAN *anticholinergic* [also: atropine methonitrate]
methylbenactyzium bromide INN
methylbenzethonium chloride USP, INN *topical anti-infective/antiseptic*
α-methylbenzylhydrazine [see: mebanazine]
methylcarbamate of salicylanilide [see: anilamate]
methyl-CCNU (chloroethyl-cyclohexyl-nitrosourea) [see: semustine]
methylcellulose USP, INN *suspending and viscosity-increasing agent*
methylcellulose, propylene glycol ether of [see: hydroxypropyl methylcellulose]
methylchromone INN, BAN
methyldesorphine INN, BAN
methyldigoxin [see: metildigoxin]
methyldihydromorphine INN
methyldihydromorphinone HCl [see: metopon]
methyldinitrobenzamide [see: dinitolmide]
methyldioxatrine [see: meletimide]
***N*-methyldiphenethylamine** [see: demelverine]
methyldopa USAN, USP, INN *antihypertensive*
α-methyldopa [now: methyldopa]
methyldopate HCl USAN, USP *antihypertensive*

6-methylenandrosta-1,4-diene-3,17-dione (*orphan: hormonal therapy for metastatic carcinoma of the breast*)
methylene blue (MB) USP *antimethemoglobinemic; GU antiseptic; cyanide poisoning antidote* [also: methylthioninium chloride]
methylene chloride NF *solvent*
methylene diphosphonate (MDP) [now: medronate disodium]
6-methyleneoxytetracycline (MOTC) [see: methacycline]
methylene prednisolone [see: prednylidene]
methylergometrine INN *oxytocic* [also: methylergonovine maleate]
methylergometrine maleate [see: methylergonovine maleate]
methylergonovine maleate USP *oxytocic* [also: methylergometrine]
methylergonovinium bimaleate [see: methylergonovine maleate]
methylergotamine [see: metergotamine]
methylestrenolone [see: normethandrone]
methyl-GAG [see: methylglyoxal-bis-guanylhydrazone]
Methylgesic liquid (discontinued 1992) OTC *counterirritant* [methyl salicylate; menthol; camphor; methyl nicotinate; dipropylene glycol salicylate]
methylglyoxal-*bis*-guanylhydrazone (methyl-GAG; MGBG)
1-methylhexylamine [see: tuaminoheptane]
1-methylhexylamine sulfate [see: tuaminoheptane sulfate]
***N*-methylhydrazine** [see: procarbazine]
methylmorphine [see: codeine]
methyl-nitro-imidazole [see: carnidazole]
methylnortestosterone [see: normethandrone]

methylparaben USAN, NF *antifungal agent; preservative*
methylparaben sodium USAN, NF *antimicrobial preservative*
methylparafynol [see: meparfynol]
methylpentynol INN, BAN
methylperidol [see: moperone]
(+)-methylphenethylamine [see: dextroamphetamine]
(–)-methylphenethylamine [see: levamphetamine]
methylphenethylamine HCl [see: amphetamine HCl]
methylphenethylamine phosphate [see: amphetamine phosphate]
(–)-methylphenethylamine succinate [see: levamfetamine succinate]
methylphenethylamine sulfate [see: amphetamine sulfate]
(+)-methylphenethylamine sulfate [see: dextroamphetamine sulfate]
methylphenidate INN CNS *stimulant* [also: methylphenidate HCl]
methylphenidate HCl USP CNS *stimulant for attention deficit disorders and narcolepsy* [also: methylphenidate]
methylphenobarbital INN *anticonvulsant; sedative* [also: mephobarbital; methylphenobarbitone]
methylphenobarbitone BAN *anticonvulsant; sedative* [also: mephobarbital; methylphenobarbital]
d-**methylphenylamine sulfate** [see: dextroamphetamine sulfate]
methylphytyl napthoquinone [see: phytonadione]
methylprednisolone USP, INN, BAN *glucocorticoid*
methylprednisolone aceponate INN
methylprednisolone acetate USP *topical corticosteroid*
methylprednisolone hemisuccinate USP *adrenocortical steroid*
methylprednisolone sodium phosphate USAN *glucocorticoid*
methylprednisolone sodium succinate USP *glucocorticoid*

methylprednisolone suleptanate USAN, INN *anti-inflammatory*
methylpromazine
4-methylpyrazole (4-MP) [see: fomepizole]
methylrosaniline chloride [now: gentian violet]
methylrosanilinium chloride INN *topical anti-infective* [also: gentian violet]
methylscopolamine bromide [see: methscopolamine bromide]
methyltestosterone USP, INN, BAN *oral androgen*
methyltheobromine [see: caffeine]
methylthionine chloride [see: methylene blue]
methylthionine HCl [see: methylene blue]
methylthioninium chloride INN *antimethemoglobinemic; antidote to cyanide poisoning* [also: methylene blue]
methylthiouracil USP, INN
α-**methyl-DL-thyroxine ethyl ester** [see: etiroxate]
methyltrienolone [see: metribolone]
methynodiol diacetate USAN *progestin* [also: metynodiol]
methyprylon USP, INN *sedative; hypnotic* [also: methprylone]
methyprylone BAN *sedative* [also: methyprylon]
methyridene BAN [also: metyridine]
methysergide USAN, INN, BAN *migraine-specific vasoconstrictor*
methysergide maleate USP *migraine-specific vasoconstrictor*
metiamide USAN, INN *antagonist to histamine H_2 receptors*
metiapine USAN, INN *antipsychotic*
metiazinic acid INN
metibride INN
meticillin INN *antibacterial* [also: methicillin sodium]
meticillin sodium [see: methicillin sodium]
Meticorten tablets ℞ *glucocorticoids* [prednisone]

meticrane INN
metildigoxin INN
Metimyd eye drop suspension, ophthalmic ointment ℞ *topical ophthalmic corticosteroidal anti-inflammatory; bacteriostatic* [prednisolone acetate; sodium sulfacetamide]
metindizate INN [also: methindizate]
metioprim USAN, INN, BAN *antibacterial*
metioxate INN
metipirox INN
metipranolol USAN, INN, BAN *ophthalmic antihypertensive (β-blocker)*
metipranolol HCl *topical antiglaucoma agent (β-blocker)*
metiprenaline INN
metirosine INN *antihypertensive* [also: metyrosine]
metisazone INN *antiviral* [also: methisazone]
metitepine INN
metixene INN *smooth muscle relaxant* [also: methixene HCl]
metixene HCl [see: methixene HCl]
Metizol tablets (discontinued 1991) ℞ *bactericidal antibiotic; amebicide* [metronidazole]
metizoline INN *adrenergic; vasoconstrictor* [also: metizoline HCl]
metizoline HCl USAN *adrenergic; vasoconstrictor* [also: metizoline]
metkefamide INN *analgesic* [also: metkephamid acetate]
metkefamide acetate [see: metkephamid acetate]
metkephamid acetate USAN *analgesic* [also: metkefamide]
metochalcone INN
metocinium iodide INN
metoclopramide INN *antiemetic for chemotherapy; GI stimulant; antidopaminergic* [also: metoclopramide HCl]
metoclopramide HCl USAN, USP *antiemetic for chemotherapy; GI stimulant; antidopaminergic* [also: metoclopramide]

metoclopramide monohydrochloride monohydrate *antiemetic for chemotherapy; GI stimulant; antidopaminergic*
metocurine iodide USAN, USP *neuromuscular blocker; muscle relaxant*
metofenazate INN
metofoline INN *analgesic* [also: methopholine]
metogest USAN, INN *hormone*
metolazone USAN, INN *diuretic; antihypertensive*
metomidate INN, BAN
metopimazine USAN, INN *antiemetic*
Metopirone tablets ℞ *pituitary function test* [metyrapone]
metopon INN
metopon HCl [see: metopon]
metoprine USAN *antineoplastic*
metoprolol USAN, INN, BAN *antiadrenergic (β-receptor)*
metoprolol fumarate USAN *antihypertensive*
metoprolol succinate USAN *antianginal; antihypertensive*
metoprolol tartrate USAN, USP *antiadrenergic (β-receptor)*
metoquizine USAN, INN *anticholinergic*
metoserpate INN *veterinary sedative* [also: metoserpate HCl]
metoserpate HCl USAN *veterinary sedative* [also: metoserpate]
metostilenol INN
metoxepin INN
metoxiestrol [see: moxestrol]
Metra tablets ℞ *anorexiant* [phendimetrazine tartrate]
metrafazoline INN
metralindole INN
metrazifone INN
metrenperone USAN, INN, BAN *veterinary myopathic*
Metreton Ophthalmic eye drops ℞ *ophthalmic topical corticosteroidal anti-inflammatory* [prednisolone sodium phosphate]

metribolone INN
Metric 21 tablets ℞ *antiprotozoal* [metronidazole]
metrifonate INN [also: metriphonate]
metrifudil INN
metriphonate BAN [also: metrifonate]
metrizamide USAN, INN *radiopaque medium*
metrizoate sodium USAN *radiopaque medium* [also: sodium metrizoate]
Metro I.V. ready-to-use injection ℞ *antibiotic; antiprotozoal; amebicide* [metronidazole]
Metrodin HP ℞ *investigational infertility treatment* [urofollitropin]
Metrodin powder for IM injection ℞ *(orphan: induction of ovulation in polycystic ovarian disease)* [urofollitropin]
MetroGel topical gel ℞ *antibacterial; antiprotozoal; (orphan: decubitus ulcers; acne rosacea; perioral dermatitis)* [metronidazole]
MetroGel Vaginal gel ℞ *antibacterial; antiprotozoal* [metronidazole]
metronidazole USAN, USP, INN, BAN *antibiotic; antiprotozoal; amebicide; (orphan: decubitus ulcers; acne rosacea; perioral dermatitis)*
metronidazole benzoate *antiprotozoal (Trichomonas)*
metronidazole HCl USAN *antibiotic; antiprotozoal; amebicide*
metronidazole phosphate USAN *antibacterial; antiprotozoal*
Metryl tablets (discontinued 1992) ℞ *antibiotic; antiprotozoal; amebicide* [metronidazole]
Metubine Iodide IV injection ℞ *anesthesia adjunct* [metocurine iodide]
metuclazepam [see: metaclazepam]
meturedepa USAN, INN *antineoplastic*
metynodiol INN *progestin* [also: methynodiol diacetate]
metynodiol diacetate [see: methynodiol diacetate]

metyrapone USAN, USP, INN *pituitary function test*
metyrapone tartrate USAN *pituitary function test*
metyridine INN [also: methyridene]
metyrosine USAN, USP *antihypertensive; pheochromocytomic agent*
Mevacor tablets ℞ *cholesterol-lowering antihyperlipidemic* [lovastatin]
Mevanin-C capsules (discontinued 1992) OTC *vitamin/mineral/iron supplement* [multiple vitamins & minerals; iron; folic acid; hesperidin complex]
mevastatin INN
mevinolin [now: lovastatin]
mexafylline INN
Mexate powder for IV or IM injection (discontinued 1991) ℞ *systemic antipsoriatic; antineoplastic* [methotrexate sodium]
mexazolam INN
mexenone INN, BAN
mexiletine INN, BAN *antiarrhythmic* [also: mexiletine HCl]
mexiletine HCl USAN, USP *antiarrhythmic* [also: mexiletine]
mexiprostil INN
Mexitil capsules ℞ *antiarrhythmic* [mexiletine HCl]
mexoprofen INN
mexrenoate potassium USAN, INN *aldosterone antagonist*
Mexsana Medicated powder OTC *topical diaper rash treatment* [kaolin; zinc oxide; eucalyptus oil; camphor; corn starch]
mezacopride INN
mezepine INN
mezilamine INN
Mezlin powder for IV or IM injection, ADD-vantage vials ℞ *extended-spectrum penicillin-type antibiotic* [mezlocillin sodium]
mezlocillin USAN, INN *antibacterial*
mezlocillin sodium USP *bactericidal antibiotic*

MF (mitomycin, fluorouracil) *chemotherapy protocol*

MFP (melphalan, fluorouracil, medroxyprogesterone acetate) *chemotherapy protocol*

MG Cold Sore Formula solution (discontinued 1991) OTC *topical oral anesthetic; antipruritic/counterirritant* [menthol; lidocaine]

MG217 Dual Treatment lotion OTC *topical antipsoriatic; antiseborrheic* [coal tar solution]

MG217 Medicated conditioner OTC *topical antipsoriatic; antiseborrheic* [coal tar solution]

MG217 Medicated ointment, shampoo OTC *topical antipsoriatic; antiseborrheic; antifungal; keratolytic* [coal tar solution; colloidal sulfur; salicylic acid]

MG400 shampoo OTC *antiseborrheic; keratolytic* [salicylic acid; sulfur]

MGA (melengestrol acetate) [q.v.]

MGBG (methylglyoxal-*bis*-guanylhydrazone)

MGW (magnesium sulfate + glycerin + water) enema [q.v.]

Miacalcic ℞ *investigational osteoporosis treatment*

Miacalcin nasal spray, subcu or IM injection ℞ *calcium regulator; (orphan: Paget's disease; osteitis deformans)* [calcitonin (salmon)]

Mi-Acid liquid OTC *antacid; antiflatulent* [aluminum hydroxide; magnesium hydroxide; simethicone]

mianserin INN *serotonin inhibitor; antihistamine* [also: mianserin HCl]

mianserin HCl USAN *serotonin inhibitor; antihistamine* [also: mianserin]

mibolerone USAN, INN *anabolic; androgen*

Micatin cream, powder, aerosol powder, liquid spray OTC *topical antifungal* [miconazole nitrate]

Mi-Cebrin; Mi-Cebrin T tablets (discontinued 1993) OTC *vitamin/mineral/iron supplement* [multiple vitamins & minerals; iron]

micinicate INN

miconazole USP, INN, BAN *fungicidal*

miconazole nitrate USAN, USP *antifungal*

Micrainin tablets ℞ *analgesic; antipyretic; anti-inflammatory; anxiolytic* [aspirin; meprobamate]

MICRhoGAM IM injection ℞ *obstetric Rh factor immunity suppressant* [Rh$_o$(D) immune globulin]

microbubble contrast agent *(orphan: diagnostic aid for intracranial tumors)*

microcrystalline cellulose [see: cellulose, microcrystalline]

microcrystalline wax [see: wax, microcrystalline]

microfibrillar collagen hemostat (MCH) *topical hemostatic*

Micro-K LS extended-release powder packets ℞ *potassium supplement* [potassium chloride]

Micro-K; Micro-K 10 Extencaps (controlled-release capsules) ℞ *potassium supplement* [potassium chloride]

Microlipid emulsion OTC *dietary fat supplement* [safflower oil]

Micronase tablets ℞ *antidiabetic* [glyburide]

microNefrin solution for inhalation OTC *bronchodilator for bronchial asthma and COPD* [racepinephrine]

micronized aluminum *astringent*

micronomicin INN

Micronor tablets ℞ *oral contraceptive (progestin only)* [norethindrone]

Microstix-3 reagent strips OTC *in vitro diagnostic aid for nitrate in urine and bacterial growth*

MicroTrak Chlamydia trachomatis Direct Specimen Test slide test OTC *in vitro diagnostic aid for Chlamydia trachomatis*

MicroTrak HSV 1/HSV 2 Culture Identification/Typing Test kit

OTC *in vitro diagnostic aid for herpes simplex virus in tissue cultures*
MicroTrak HSV 1/HSV 2 Direct Specimen Identification/Typing Test kit OTC *in vitro diagnostic aid for herpes simplex virus in external lesions*
MicroTrak Neisseria gonorrhoeae Culture Test slide test OTC *in vitro diagnostic aid for gonorrhea*
Microx (name changed to Mykrox in 1990)
mictine [see: aminometradine]
Mictrin (name changed to Ezide in 1991)
Micturin ℞ *investigational agent for urinary incontinence* [terodiline HCl]
midaflur USAN, INN *sedative*
midaglizole INN
midalcipran [see: milnacipran]
midamaline INN
Midamine ℞ *(orphan: idiopathic orthostatic hypotension)* [midodrine HCl]
Midamor tablets ℞ *potassium-sparing diuretic* [amiloride HCl]
midazogrel INN
midazolam INN *general anesthetic* [also: midazolam HCl]
midazolam HCl USAN *general anesthetic* [also: midazolam]
midazolam maleate USAN *intravenous anesthetic*
Midchlor capsules ℞ *vasoconstrictor; sedative; analgesic (for migraine)* [isometheptene mucate; dichloralphenazone; acetaminophen]
midecamycin INN
midodrine INN, BAN *antihypertensive; vasoconstrictor* [also: midodrine HCl]
midodrine HCl USAN *antihypertensive; vasoconstrictor; (orphan: idiopathic orthostatic hypotension)* [also: midodrine]
Midol, Teen caplets OTC *analgesic; anti-inflammatory; diuretic* [acetaminophen; pamabrom]

Midol 200 tablets OTC *nonsteroidal anti-inflammatory drug (NSAID); antiarthritic; analgesic* [ibuprofen]
Midol IB tablets OTC *nonsteroidal anti-inflammatory drug (NSAID); antiarthritic; analgesic* [ibuprofen]
Midol; Midol for Cramps caplets OTC *analgesic; antipyretic; anti-inflammatory; muscle relaxant* [aspirin; caffeine; cinnamedrine HCl]
Midol Multi-Symptom Formula caplets OTC *analgesic; anti-inflammatory; antihistaminic sleep aid* [acetaminophen; pyrilamine maleate]
Midol Multi-Symptom Menstrual caplets OTC *analgesic; anti-inflammatory; antihistaminic sleep aid* [acetaminophen; caffeine; pyrilamine maleate]
Midol PM caplets OTC *analgesic; antipyretic; antihistaminic sleep aid* [acetaminophen; diphenhydramine]
Midol PMS capsules OTC *analgesic; anti-inflammatory; diuretic; antihistaminic sleep aid* [acetaminophen; pamabrom; pyrilamine maleate]
Midrin capsules ℞ *vasoconstrictor; sedative; analgesic (for migraine)* [isometheptene mucate; dichloralphenazone; acetaminophen]
MIFA (mitomycin, fluorouracil, Adriamycin) *chemotherapy protocol*
mifentidine INN
mifepristone INN, BAN *progesterone antagonist; abortifacient*
Miflex capsules (discontinued 1991) ℞ *skeletal muscle relaxant; analgesic* [chlorzoxazone; acetaminophen]
mifobate USAN, INN *antiatherosclerotic*
Migergot P-B suppositories (discontinued 1991) ℞ *migraine treatment; vasoconstrictor; anticholinergic; sedative* [ergotamine tartrate; caffeine; pentobarbital; belladonna extract]
Mighty Vite T tablets OTC *vitamin/mineral supplement* [multiple vitamins & minerals]

miglitol USAN, INN, BAN α-glucosidase inhibitor

Migranol nasal spray ℞ investigational antimigraine agent

Migratine capsules ℞ vasoconstrictor; sedative; analgesic (for migraine) [isometheptene mucate; dichloralphenazone; acetaminophen]

mikamycin INN, BAN

Mil Adrene; Mil Adrene Forte tablets OTC dietary supplement [raw adrenal concentrate]

milacemide INN anticonvulsant; antidepressant [also: milacemide HCl]

milacemide HCl USAN anticonvulsant; antidepressant [also: milacemide]

Mil-Adregen tablets OTC dietary supplement [multiple glandular concentrates; multiple vitamins; zinc]

Mil-A-Mulsion drops OTC vitamin supplement [vitamin A palmitate; vitamin E]

Milco B tablets OTC vitamin supplement [multiple B vitamins]

Milco-B-Forte tablets OTC vitamin/mineral supplement [multiple B vitamins; vitamin C; zinc]

Milco-Zyme timed-release tablets OTC dietary supplement [multiple enzymes]

mild silver protein [see: silver protein, mild]

Mild-C chewable tablets, capsules, timed-release caplets OTC vitamin supplement [calcium ascorbate]

milenperone USAN, INN, BAN antipsychotic

milipertine USAN, INN antipsychotic

milk of bismuth [see: bismuth, milk of]

milk of magnesia [see: magnesia, milk of]

Milkinol emulsion OTC emollient laxative [mineral oil]

milnacipran INN

Milontin Kapseals (capsules) ℞ anticonvulsant [phensuximide]

Milophene tablets ℞ ovulation stimulant [clomiphene citrate]

miloxacin INN

Milprem-400 tablets (discontinued 1991) ℞ estrogen deficiency; menopausal symptoms [conjugated estrogens; meprobamate]

milrinone USAN, INN, BAN cardiotonic

milrinone lactate vasodilator for congestive heart failure

Miltab #1 tablets OTC dietary supplement [multiple vitamins; levoglutamide; magnesium aspartate]

miltefosine INN

Miltown-200; Miltown-400; Miltown-600 tablets ℞ anxiolytic [meprobamate]

milverine INN

Mil-V-Zyme capsules OTC dietary supplement [multiple enzymes]

mimbane INN analgesic [also: mimbane HCl]

mimbane HCl USAN analgesic [also: mimbane]

minaprine USAN, INN, BAN psychotropic

minaprine HCl USAN antidepressant

minaxolone USAN, INN anesthetic

mindodilol INN

mindolic acid [see: clometacin]

mindoperone INN

MINE (mesna, ifosfamide, Novantrone, etoposide) chemotherapy protocol

minepentate INN, BAN

Mineral Compleet caplets OTC mineral supplement [multiple minerals; kelp]

Mineral Ice [see: Therapeutic Mineral Ice]

mineral oil USP emollient/protectant; laxative; solvent

mineral oil, light NF tablet and capsule lubricant; vehicle

mini-COAP (cyclophosphamide, Oncovin, ara-C, prednisone) chemotherapy protocol

Minidyne solution OTC *broad-spectrum antimicrobial* [povidone-iodine]

Mini-Gamulin Rh IM injection ℞ *obstetric Rh factor immunity suppressant* [Rh₀(D) immune globulin]

Min-I-Mix (delivery system) *dual-chambered prefilled syringe*

Minipress capsules ℞ *antihypertensive; antiadrenergic* [prazosin HCl]

Minipress XL extended-release tablets ℞ *antihypertensive* [prazosin HCl]

Minitran transdermal patch ℞ *antiarrhythmic* [nitroglycerin]

Minit-Rub OTC *counterirritant* [methyl salicylate; menthol; camphor]

Minizide 1; Minizide 2; Minizide 5 capsules ℞ *antihypertensive* [prazosin HCl; polythiazide]

Minocin pellet-filled capsules, oral suspension, powder for IV injection ℞ *tetracycline-type antibiotic; (orphan: chronic malignant pleural effusion)* [minocycline HCl]

Minocin tablets (discontinued 1991) ℞ *tetracycline-type antibiotic* [minocycline HCl]

minocromil USAN, INN, BAN *prophylactic antiallergic*

minocycline USAN, INN, BAN *gram-negative and gram-positive bacteriostatic; antirickettsial*

minocycline HCl USP *antibacterial; (orphan: chronic malignant pleural effusion)*

Minodyl tablets ℞ *antihypertensive; vasodilator* [minoxidil]

minoxidil USAN, USP, INN, BAN *antihypertensive; peripheral vasodilator; hair growth stimulant*

Mintezol chewable tablets, oral suspension ℞ *anthelmintic* [thiabendazole]

Mintox oral suspension OTC *antacid* [aluminum hydroxide; magnesium hydroxide]

Mintox Plus liquid OTC *antacid; antiflatulent* [aluminum hydroxide; magnesium hydroxide; simethicone]

Minulet ℞ *investigational oral contraceptive*

Minute-Gel ℞ *topical dental caries preventative* [acidulated phosphate fluoride]

Miochol solution ℞ *direct-acting miotic for ophthalmic surgery* [acetylcholine chloride]

mioflazine INN, BAN *coronary vasodilator* [also: mioflazine HCl]

mioflazine HCl USAN *coronary vasodilator* [also: mioflazine]

Mio-Rel injection ℞ *muscle relaxant* [orphenadrine citrate]

Miostat solution ℞ *direct-acting miotic for ophthalmic surgery* [carbachol]

mipimazole INN

Miradon tablets ℞ *anticoagulant* [anisindione]

MiraFlow solution OTC *contact lens cleaning solution*

MiraSept System solution OTC *two-step contact lens disinfectant*

mirfentanil INN *analgesic* [also: mirfentanil HCl]

mirfentanil HCl USAN *analgesic* [also: mirfentanil]

mirincamycin INN *antibacterial; antimalarial* [also: mirincamycin HCl]

mirincamycin HCl USAN *antibacterial; antimalarial* [also: mirincamycin]

miristalkonium chloride INN

miroprofen INN

mirosamicin INN

mirtazapine USAN, INN *antidepressant*

misonidazole USAN, INN *antiprotozoal (Trichomonas)*

misoprostol USAN, INN, BAN *prevention of NSAID-induced gastric ulcers*

Mission Prenatal; Mission Prenatal F.A.; Mission Prenatal H.P. tablets OTC *vitamin/iron supplement*

[multiple vitamins; ferrous gluconate; folic acid]

Mission Prenatal Rx film-coated tablets ℞ *vitamin/calcium/iron supplement* [multiple vitamins; calcium; iron; folic acid]

Mission Pre-Surgical tablets OTC *antianemic* [ferrous gluconate; multiple vitamins]

Mission Surgical Supplement tablets OTC *vitamin/iron supplement* [multiple vitamins; ferrous gluconate]

Mistometer (trademarked form) *metered-dose inhalation aerosol*

Mithracin powder for IV infusion ℞ *antineoplastic for testicular cancer* [plicamycin]

mithramycin [now: plicamycin]

mitindomide USAN, INN *antineoplastic*

mitobronitol INN, BAN

mitocarcin USAN, INN *antineoplastic*

mitoclomine INN, BAN

mitocromin USAN *antineoplastic*

mitoflaxone INN

mitogillin USAN, INN *antineoplastic*

mitoguazone INN *investigational antineoplastic for non-Hodgkin's lymphoma*

mitolactol INN *(orphan: cervical squamous carcinoma)*

mitomalcin USAN, INN *antineoplastic*

mitomycin USAN, USP, INN, BAN *antineoplastic*

mitomycin C (MTC) [see: mitomycin]

mitonafide INN

mitopodozide INN, BAN

mitoquidone INN, BAN

mitosper USAN, INN *antineoplastic*

mitotane USAN, USP, INN *antineoplastic*

mitotenamine INN, BAN

mitoxantrone INN *antineoplastic* [also: metoxantrone HCl; mitozantrone]

mitoxantrone HCl USAN *antineoplastic; (orphan: acute myelogenous leukemia; acute nonlymphocytic leukemia)* [also: mitoxantrone; mitozantrone]

mitozantrone BAN *antineoplastic* [also: mitoxantrone HCl; mitoxantrone]

mitozolomide INN, BAN

Mitran capsules ℞ *anxiolytic* [chlordiazepoxide HCl]

Mitrolan chewable tablets OTC *bulk laxative; antidiarrheal* [calcium polycarbophil]

mitronal [see: cinnarizine]

Mity-Mycin ointment (discontinued 1991) OTC *topical antibiotic; antihistamine* [polymyxin B sulfate; neomycin sulfate; bacitracin; diperodon HCl]

Mivacron IV infusion ℞ *muscle relaxant; adjunct to anesthesia* [mivacurium chloride]

mivacurium chloride USAN, INN, BAN *neuromuscular blocking agent*

mixed respiratory vaccine (MRV) *active bacterin for respiratory tract infections*

mixed tocopherols [see: vitamin E]

mixidine USAN, INN *coronary vasodilator*

Mixtard 70/30 suspension for injection OTC *antidiabetic* [isophane insulin (pork); insulin (pork)]

Mixtard Human 70/30 suspension for injection OTC *antidiabetic* [isophane insulin (human); insulin (human)]

mizoribine INN

M-KYA capsules OTC *prevention and treatment of nocturnal leg cramps* [quinine sulfate]

MMOPP (methotrexate, mechlorethamine, Oncovin, procarbazine, prednisone) *chemotherapy protocol*

MMP injection ℞ *diagnosis and treatment of allergies* [mold allergenic extracts]

MMR (measles, mumps & rubella vaccines) [q.v.]
M-M-R II subcu injection ℞ *measles, mumps and rubella vaccine* [measles, mumps & rubella virus vaccine]
MM-Zyme tablets OTC *dietary supplement* [multiple enzymes]
MOB (mechlorethamine, Oncovin, bleomycin) *chemotherapy protocol*
MOB-III (mitomycin, Oncovin, bleomycin, cisplatin) *chemotherapy protocol*
Moban tablets, oral concentrate ℞ *antipsychotic* [molindone HCl]
mobecarb INN
mobenzoxamine INN
Mobidin tablets ℞ *analgesic; antipyretic; anti-inflammatory; antirheumatic* [magnesium salicylate]
Mobigesic tablets OTC *analgesic; antipyretic; anti-inflammatory; antihistamine* [magnesium salicylate; phenyltoloxamine citrate]
Mobisyl Creme OTC *topical analgesic* [trolamine salicylate]
moccasin snake antivenin [see: antivenin (Crotalidae) polyvalent]
mocimycin INN
mociprazine INN
moclobemide USAN, INN, BAN *antidepressant*
moctamide INN
Moctanin biliary infusion ℞ *anticholelithogenic; (orphan: dissolution of cholesterol gallstones)* [monoctanoin]
modafinil INN *antinarcoleptic*
modaline INN *antidepressant* [also: modaline sulfate]
modaline sulfate USAN *antidepressant* [also: modaline]
Modane Bulk liquid OTC *bulk laxative* [psyllium hydrophilic mucilloid]
Modane Plus tablets OTC *laxative; stool softener* [white phenolphthalein; docusate sodium]
Modane Soft capsules OTC *stool softener* [docusate sodium]

Modane tablets OTC *laxative* [white phenolphthalein]
modecainide USAN, INN *antiarrhythmic*
Moderil tablets ℞ *antihypertensive* [rescinnamine]
Modicon tablets ℞ *oral contraceptive* [ethinyl estradiol; norethindrone]
modified bovine lung surfactant extract [see: beractant]
modified Burow solution [see: aluminum acetate solution]
modified cellulose gum [now: croscarmellose sodium]
modified Shohl solution (sodium citrate & citric acid) *urinary alkalinizer; compounding agent*
Modrastane capsules ℞ *adrenal steroid inhibitor* [trilostane]
Modual powder OTC *carbohydrate caloric supplement* [glucose polymers]
Moduretic tablets ℞ *diuretic* [amiloride HCl; hydrochlorothiazide]
moexipril INN
MOF (MeCCNU, Oncovin, fluorouracil) *chemotherapy protocol*
mofebutazone INN
mofedione [see: oxazidione]
mofloverine INN
mofoxime INN
MOF-STREP; MOF-Strep (MeCCNU, Oncovin, fluorouracil, streptozocin) *chemotherapy protocol*
Mogadon ℞ *investigational benzodiazepine-type tranquilizer; anxiolytic; anticonvulsant; hypnotic* [nitrazepam]
moguisteine INN
Moi-Stir; Moi-Stir 10 oral spray, Swabsticks OTC *saliva substitute*
Moisture Derm lotion OTC *emollient* [mineral oil; stearic acid; petrolatum; lanolin; lanolin alcohol; trolamine; cetyl alcohol]
Moisture Drops eye drops OTC *ocular moisturizer/lubricant*
Moisturel lotion OTC *moisturizer; emollient* [dimethicone]

molecusol & carbamazepine (orphan: emergency rescue of grand mal status epilepticus)
molfarnate INN
molgramostim USAN, INN, BAN antineutropenic; investigational cytokine for AIDS; (orphan: neutropenia; anemia; leukemia; burns)
molinazone USAN, INN analgesic
molindone INN antipsychotic [also: molindone HCl]
molindone HCl USAN antipsychotic [also: molindone]
Mol-Iron tablets OTC hematinic [ferrous sulfate]
Mol-Iron with Vitamin C tablets OTC hematinic [ferrous sulfate; ascorbic acid]
Mollifene Ear Drops OTC agent to emulsify and disperse ear wax [carbamide peroxide]
molracetam INN
molsidomine USAN, INN antianginal; coronary vasodilator
Moly-B capsule OTC dietary supplement [molybdenum]
molybdenum element (Mo)
Moly-Pak IV injection (discontinued 1992) ℞ intravenous nutritional therapy [ammonium molybdate tetrahydrate]
Molypen IV injection ℞ intravenous nutritional therapy [ammonium molybdate tetrahydrate]
Momentum caplets OTC analgesic; antipyretic; anti-inflammatory; antihistamine [aspirin; phenyltoloxamine citrate]
mometasone INN, BAN topical corticosteroid [also: mometasone furoate]
mometasone furoate USAN topical corticosteroid [also: mometasone]
MOMP (mechlorethamine, Oncovin, methotrexate, prednisone) chemotherapy protocol
monalazone disodium INN
monalium hydrate [see: magaldrate]

monensin USAN, INN antiprotozoal; antibacterial; antifungal
Monistat 3 vaginal suppositories ℞ antifungal [miconazole nitrate]
Monistat 7 vaginal suppositories, vaginal cream OTC antifungal [miconazole nitrate]
Monistat Dual-Pak vaginal suppositories + cream ℞ antifungal [miconazole nitrate]
Monistat i.v. intrathecal or IV injection ℞ systemic antifungal [miconazole]
Monistat-Derm cream ℞ topical antifungal [miconazole nitrate]
Monistat-Derm lotion (discontinued 1991) ℞ topical antifungal [miconazole nitrate]
mono- & di-acetylated monoglycerides NF plasticizer
mono- & di-glycerides NF emulsifying agent
monobasic potassium phosphate [see: potassium phosphate, monobasic]
monobasic sodium phosphate [see: sodium phosphate, monobasic]
monobenzone USP, INN depigmenting agent for vitiligo
monobenzyl ether of hydroquinone [see: monobenzone]
monobromated camphor [see: camphor, monobromated]
monocalcium phosphate [see: calcium phosphate, dibasic]
Monocaps tablets OTC vitamin/mineral/iron supplement [multiple vitamins & minerals; ferrous fumarate; folic acid; biotin]
Monocete liquid ℞ cauterant; keratolytic [monochloroacetic acid]
Mono-Chlor liquid ℞ cauterant; keratolytic [monochloroacetic acid]
monochloroacetic acid strong keratolytic/cauterant
monochlorothymol [see: chlorothymol]

monochlorphenamide [see: clofenamide]
Monocid powder for IV or IM injection ℞ *cephalosporin-type antibiotic* [cefonicid sodium]
Monoclate; Monoclate P powder for IV injection ℞ *antihemophilic* [antihemophilic factor VIII:C]
monoclonal antibodies (murine or human) recognizing B-cell lymphoma idiotypes *(orphan: B-cell lymphoma)*
monoclonal antibody (human) against hepatitis B virus *(orphan: hepatitis B prophylaxis)*
monoclonal antibody 17-1A *(orphan: pancreatic cancer)*
monoclonal antibody MSL-109 *investigational antiviral for AIDS*
monoclonal antibody PM-81 *(orphan: acute myelogenous leukemia)*
monoclonal antibody PM-81 & AML-2-23 *(orphan: bone marrow transplant for acute myelogenous leukemia)*
monoclonal antiendotoxin antibody XMMEN-OE5 *(orphan: gram-negative sepsis)*
monoclonal factor IX *(orphan: hemophilia B complications)*
Monocor (name changed to Probeta in 1992)
monoctanoin USAN, BAN *anticholelithogenic; (orphan: cholesterol gallstones)*
monoctanoin component A
monoctanoin component B
monoctanoin component C
monoctanoin component D
Mono-Diff test kit ℞ *in vitro diagnostic aid for mononucleosis*
Monodox capsules ℞ *antibiotic* [doxycycline monohydrate]
monoethanolamine NF *surfactant*
monoethanolamine oleate INN *sclerosing agent* [also: ethanolamine oleate]

Monogen ℞ *investigational treatment for T-cell leukemia* [monoclonal antibodies]
Mono-Gesic film-coated tablets ℞ *analgesic; antipyretic; anti-inflammatory; antirheumatic* [salsalate]
Monoket ℞ *investigational antianginal*
Mono-Latex test kit ℞ *in vitro diagnostic aid for mononucleosis*
Mono-Lisa test kit (discontinued 1992) ℞ *in vitro diagnostic aid for mononucleosis*
monomercaptoundecahydro-closo-DQ decaborate sodium *(orphan: boron neutron capture therapy for glioblastoma multiforme)*
monometacrine INN
Mononine ℞ *(orphan: hemophilia B complications)* [monoclonal factor IX]
Mononine powder for IV infusion ℞ *factor IX deficiency; control bleeding in factor VII deficiency* [factor IX complex]
monooctanoin [see: monoctanoin]
monophenylbutazone [see: mofebutazone]
monophosphothiamine INN
Mono-Plus test kit ℞ *in vitro diagnostic aid for mononucleosis*
monopotassium 4-aminosalicylate [see: aminosalicylate potassium]
monopotassium carbonate [see: potassium bicarbonate]
monopotassium D-gluconate [see: potassium gluconate]
monopotassium monosodium tartrate tetrahydrate [see: potassium sodium tartrate]
monopotassium phosphate [see: potassium phosphate, monobasic]
Monopril tablets ℞ *antihypertensive; angiotensin-converting enzyme inhibitor* [fosinopril sodium]
monosodium *p*-aminohippurate [see: aminohippurate sodium]
monosodium 4-aminosalicylate dihydrate [see: aminosalicylate sodium]

monosodium L-ascorbate [see: sodium ascorbate]
monosodium carbonate [see: sodium bicarbonate]
monosodium D-gluconate [see: sodium gluconate]
monosodium glutamate NF *flavoring agent; perfume*
monosodium phosphate dihydrate [see: sodium phosphate, monobasic]
monosodium phosphate monohydrate [see: sodium phosphate, monobasic]
monosodium salicylate [see: sodium salicylate]
monosodium sulfite [see: sodium bisulfite]
monosodium D-thyroxine hydrate [see: dextrothyroxine sodium]
monosodium L-thyroxine hydrate [see: levothyroxine sodium]
Monospot test kit ℞ *in vitro diagnostic aid for mononucleosis*
monostearin [see: glyceryl monostearate]
Monosticon Dri-Dot test kit ℞ *in vitro diagnostic aid for mononucleosis*
Monosticon test kit (discontinued 1991) ℞ *in vitro diagnostic aid for mononucleosis*
monosulfiram BAN [also: sulfiram]
Mono-Sure test kit ℞ *in vitro diagnostic aid for mononucleosis*
Mono-Test; Mono-Test (FTB) test kit ℞ *in vitro diagnostic aid for mononucleosis*
monothioglycerol NF *preservative*
Mono-Vacc Test (O.T.) single-use intradermal puncture test device ℞ *tuberculosis skin test* [old tuberculin]
monoxerutin INN
montirelin INN
8-MOP (8-methoxypsoralen) [see: methoxsalen]
MOP (Mustargen, Oncovin, prednisone) *chemotherapy protocol*

8-MOP capsules ℞ *to increase tolerance to sunlight and enhance pigmentation* [methoxsalen]
MOP-BAP (mechlorethamine, Oncovin, procarbazine, bleomycin, Adriamycin, prednisone) *chemotherapy protocol*
moperone INN
mopidamol INN
mopidralazine INN
MOPP (mechlorethamine, Oncovin, procarbazine, prednisone) *chemotherapy protocol*
MOPP (mustine HCl, Oncovin, procarbazine, prednisone) *chemotherapy protocol*
MOPP/ABV (mechlorethamine, Oncovin, procarbazine, prednisone, Adriamycin, bleomycin, vinblastine) *chemotherapy protocol*
MOPP-BLEO; MOPP-Bleo (mechlorethamine, Oncovin, procarbazine, prednisone, bleomycin) *chemotherapy protocol*
MOPPHDB (mechlorethamine, Oncovin, procarbazine, prednisone, high-dose bleomycin) *chemotherapy protocol*
MOPPLDB (mechlorethamine, Oncovin, procarbazine, prednisone, low-dose bleomycin) *chemotherapy protocol*
MOPr (mechlorethamine, Oncovin, procarbazine) *chemotherapy protocol*
moprolol INN
moquizone INN
moracizine INN, BAN *antiarrhythmic* [also: moricizine]
morantel INN *anthelmintic* [also: morantel tartrate]
morantel tartrate USAN *anthelmintic* [also: morantel]
Moranyl (available only from the Centers for Disease Control) ℞ *investigational anti-infective for trypanosomiasis and onchocerciasis* [suramin sodium]

morazone INN, BAN
morclofone INN
More-Dophilus powder OTC *dietary supplement; fever blister treatment; not generally regarded as safe and effective as an antidiarrheal* [Lactobacillus]
morforex INN
moricizine USAN *antiarrhythmic* [also: moracizine]
moricizine HCl *antiarrhythmic*
morinamide INN
morniflumate USAN, INN *anti-inflammatory*
morocromen INN
moroxydine INN, BAN
morphazinamide [see: morinamide]
morpheridine INN, BAN
morphine BAN *narcotic analgesic* [also: morphine sulfate]
morphine dinicotinate ester [see: nicomorphine]
morphine HCl USP
morphine sulfate (MS) USP *narcotic analgesic; (orphan: intraspinal microinfusion)* [also: morphine]
4-morpholinecarboximidoylguanidine [see: moroxydine]
2-morpholinoethylrutin [see: ethoxazorutoside]
3-morpholinosydnoneimine [see: linsidomine]
morpholinyl succinimide [see: morsuximide]
morpholinylethyl morphine [see: pholcodine]
morrhuate sodium USP *sclerosing agent* [also: sodium morrhuate]
morsuximide INN
morsydomine [see: molsidomine]
Morton Salt Substitute; Morton Seasoned Salt Substitute OTC *salt substitute* [potassium chloride]
Mosco liquid OTC *topical keratolytic* [salicylic acid]
Mosco Nail-A-Cain liquid (discontinued 1991) OTC *analgesic for ingrown toenails*
motapizone INN

MOTC (methyleneoxytetracycline) [see: methacycline]
Motilium ℞ *investigational antiemetic* [domperidone]
Motofen tablets ℞ *antidiarrheal* [difenoxin HCl; atropine sulfate]
motrazepam INN
motretinide USAN, INN *keratolytic*
Motrin IB caplets, tablets OTC *nonsteroidal anti-inflammatory drug (NSAID); antiarthritic; analgesic* [ibuprofen]
Motrin tablets ℞ *nonsteroidal anti-inflammatory drug (NSAID); antiarthritic; analgesic* [ibuprofen]
MouthKote spray OTC *saliva substitute*
moveltipril INN
moxadolen INN
moxalactam disodium USAN, USP *bactericidal antibiotic* [also: latamoxef]
Moxam powder for IV or IM injection (discontinued 1992) ℞ *cephalosporin-type antibiotic* [moxalactam disodium]
moxaprindine INN
moxastine INN
moxaverine INN, BAN
moxazocine USAN, INN *analgesic; antitussive*
moxestrol INN
moxicoumone INN
moxidectin USAN, INN *veterinary antiparasitic*
moxipraquine INN, BAN
moxiraprine INN
moxisylyte INN [also: thymoxamine]
moxnidazole USAN, INN *antiprotozoal (Trichomonas)*
moxonidine INN
Moxy Compound tablets ℞ *antiasthmatic; bronchodilator; dencongestant; anxiolytic* [theophylline; ephedrine sulfate; hydroxyzine HCl]
4 MP *(orphan: methanol or ethylene glycol poisoning)* [4-methylpyrazole]
MP (melphalan, prednisone) *chemotherapy protocol*

4-MP (4-methylpyrazole) [see: fomepizole]
6-MP (6-mercaptopurine) [see: mercaptopurine]
MPF [see: Mucoprotective Factor]
MPL (melphalan) [q.v.]
MPL + PRED (melphalan, prednisone) *chemotherapy protocol*
M-Prednisol-40; M-Prednisol-80 intralesional, soft tissue, and IM injection ℞ *glucocorticoids* [methylprednisolone acetate]
MRV (mixed respiratory vaccine) [q.v.]
MRV subcu injection ℞ *active respiratory bacteria immunizing agent* [mixed respiratory vaccine]
M-R-Vax II subcu injection ℞ *measles and rubella vaccine* [measles & rubella virus vaccine, live]
MS (morphine sulfate) [q.v.]
MS Contin controlled-release tablets ℞ *narcotic analgesic; preoperative sedative and anxiolytic* [morphine sulfate]
MSIR immediate-release tablets, oral solution, oral concentrate ℞ *narcotic analgesic; preoperative sedative and anxiolytic* [morphine sulfate]
MSL-109 ℞ *investigational antiviral for AIDS*
MSTA (Mumps Skin Test Antigen) suspension for intradermal injection ℞ *mumps skin test* [killed mumps virus]
MT6 (mercaptomerin) [q.v.]
MTC (mitomycin C) [see: mitomycin]
M.T.E.-4; M.T.E.-5; M.T.E.-6; M.T.E.-7; M.T.E.-4 Concentrated; M.T.E.-5 Concentrated; M.T.E.-6 Concentrated IV injection ℞ *intravenous nutritional therapy* [multiple trace elements (metals)]
MTX (methotrexate) [q.v.]
MTX + MP (methotrexate, mercaptopurine) *chemotherapy protocol*
MTX + MP + CTX (methotrexate, mercaptopurine, cyclophosphamide) *chemotherapy protocol*
mucoid exopolysaccharide pseudomonas hyperimmune globulin *(orphan: pulmonary infections of cystic fibrosis)*
Mucomyst solution for nebulization or intratracheal instillation ℞ *mycolytic; (orphan: severe acetaminophen overdose)* [acetylcysteine sodium]
Mucoplex tablets OTC *dietary supplement* [vitamins B_2 & B_{12}; liver fraction]
Mucoprotective Factor (MPF) (trademarked ingredient) *aromatic flavored syrup* [eriodictyon]
Mucosil-10; Mucosil-20 solution for nebulization or intratracheal instillation ℞ *mycolytic* [acetylcysteine sodium]
Mucosol solution ℞ *mycolytic; (orphan: severe acetaminophen overdose)* [acetylcysteine]
Mudrane GG tablets, elixir ℞ *antiasthmatic; decongestant; expectorant; sedative* [theophylline; ephedrine HCl; guaifenesin; phenobarbital]
Mudrane GG-2 tablets ℞ *antiasthmatic; bronchodilator; expectorant* [theophylline; guaifenesin]
Mudrane tablets ℞ *antiasthmatic; bronchodilator; decongestant; expectorant; sedative* [aminophylline; ephedrine HCl; potassium iodide; phenobarbital]
Mudrane-2 tablets ℞ *antiasthmatic; expectorant* [theophylline; potassium iodide]
Multa-Gen 12 + E capsules (discontinued 1992) OTC *vitamin supplement* [multiple vitamins; folic acid]
MulTE-Pak-4; MulTE-Pak-5 IV injection ℞ *intravenous nutritional therapy* [multiple trace elements (metals)]
Multi 75 timed-release tablets OTC *vitamin/mineral supplement* [multiple

vitamins & minerals; folic acid; biotin]

Multi Vit drops (discontinued 1993) OTC *vitamin supplement* [multiple vitamins]

Multi Vit with Fluoride drops *vitamin supplement; dental caries prophylaxis* [multiple vitamins; fluoride]

Multi Vit with Iron drops OTC *vitamin/iron supplement* [multiple vitamins; iron]

Multi Vitamin Concentrate injection ℞ *parenteral vitamin supplement* [multiple vitamins]

Multibret-500 Hematinic timed-release tablets ℞ *hematinic* [ferrous sulfate; multiple B vitamins; sodium ascorbate]

Multibret-Folic-500 timed-release tablets ℞ *hematinic* [ferrous sulfate; multiple B vitamins; sodium ascorbate; folic acid]

Multicebrin tablets (discontinued 1991) OTC *vitamin supplement* [multiple vitamins]

Multi-Day Plus Iron tablets OTC *vitamin/iron supplement* [multiple vitamins; iron; folic acid]

Multi-Day Plus Minerals tablets OTC *vitamin/mineral/iron supplement* [multiple vitamins & minerals; iron; folic acid; biotin]

Multi-Day tablets OTC *vitamin supplement* [multiple vitamins; folic acid]

Multi-Day with Calcium and Extra Iron tablets OTC *vitamin/calcium/iron supplement* [multiple vitamins; calcium; iron; folic acid]

Multi-Gel soft capsules OTC *vitamin/mineral supplement* [multiple vitamins & minerals; papaya concentrate; bioflavonoids; lecithin]

Multi-Glan tablets OTC *dietary supplement* [multiple glandular concentrates]

Multilex; Multilex-T & M tablets OTC *vitamin/mineral/iron supplement* [multiple vitamins & minerals; iron]

Multilyte effervescent tablets (discontinued 1993) OTC *vitamin/mineral supplement* [multiple vitamins & minerals; folic acid; biotin; phenylalanine]

Multilyte-20; Multilyte-40 IV admixture ℞ *intravenous electrolyte therapy* [combined electrolyte solution]

Multi-Mineral tablets OTC *mineral supplement* [multiple minerals]

Multiple Electrolyte 2 with 5% Invert Sugar; Multiple Electrolyte 2 with 10% Invert Sugar IV infusion (discontinued 1991) ℞ *intravenous nutritional/electrolyte therapy* [combined electrolyte solution; invert sugar (50% dextrose + 50% fructose)]

Multiple Trace Element; Multiple Trace Element Concentrated; Multiple Trace Element Neonatal; Multiple Trace Element Pediatric IV injection ℞ *intravenous nutritional therapy* [multiple trace elements (metals)]

Multiple Trace Element with Selenium; Multiple Trace Element with Selenium Concentrated IV injection ℞ *intravenous nutritional therapy* [multiple trace elements (metals)]

Multistix; Multistix SG; Multistix 2; Multistix 7; Multistix 8 SG; Multistix 9; Multistix 9 SG; Multistix 10 SG reagent strips OTC *in vitro diagnostic aid for multiple urine products*

Multitest CMI single-use intradermal skin test device ℞ *skin test for multiple allergen sensitivity* [skin test antigens (seven different); glycerin (one for test control)]

Multi-Vita-Drops OTC *vitamin supplement* [multiple vitamins]

Multi-Vita-Drops with Fluoride (discontinued 1993) ℞ *pediatric vitamin supplement and dental caries preventative* [multiple vitamins; fluoride]

Multi-Vita-Drops with Iron OTC *vitamin/iron supplement* [multiple vitamins; iron]

multivitamin infusion *(orphan: total parenteral nutrition for very low birth-weight infants)*

Multivitamin with Fluoride drops ℞ *pediatric vitamin supplement and dental caries preventative* [multiple vitamins; fluoride]

Multivitamins Rowell capsules OTC *vitamin supplement* [multiple vitamins]

Mulvidren-F Softabs (chewable tablets) ℞ *pediatric vitamin supplement and dental caries preventative* [multiple vitamins; fluoride]

mumps skin test antigen USP *dermal mumps immune test*

Mumps Skin Test Antigen [see: MSTA]

mumps vaccine [see: mumps virus vaccine, inactivated]

mumps virus vaccine, inactivated NF

mumps virus vaccine, live USP *active immunizing agent for mumps*

Mumpsvax subcu injection ℞ *mumps vaccine* [mumps virus vaccine, live]

mupirocin USAN, INN, BAN *topical antibacterial antibiotic*

murabutide INN

muramyl-tripeptide *investigational immunomodulator for AIDS*

Murine Contact Lens Cleaner solution (discontinued 1992) OTC *contact lens surfactant cleaning solution*

Murine Ear Drops OTC *agent to emulsify and disperse ear wax* [carbamide peroxide; alcohol]

Murine eye drops OTC *ocular moisturizer/lubricant*

murine monoclonal antibody [see: muromonab-CD3]

Murine Plus eye drops OTC *topical ocular decongestant* [tetrahydrozoline HCl]

Murine Preserved All-Purpose Saline solution (discontinued 1992) OTC *contact lens rinsing and storage solution* [preserved saline solution]

Murine Regular Formula ophthalmic solution OTC *extraocular irrigating solution* [balanced saline solution]

Murine Sterile Lubricating and Rewetting Drops (discontinued 1992) OTC *contact lens rewetting solution*

Muro Tears eye drops OTC *ocular moisturizer/lubricant*

Muro-128 Ophthalmic eye drops, ophthalmic ointment OTC *corneal edema reducing adjunct; diagnostic aid* [hypertonic saline solution]

murocainide INN

Murocel eye drops OTC *ocular moisturizer/lubricant*

Murocoll-2 Ophthalmic eye drops ℞ *mydriatic; cycloplegic* [scopolamine hydrobromide; phenylephrine HCl]

murodermin INN

muromonab-CD3 USAN, INN *monoclonal antibody immunosuppressive for renal transplants*

MuscleRub ointment OTC *counterirritant* [methyl salicylate; menthol]

Mus-Lax capsules ℞ *skeletal muscle relaxant; analgesic* [chlorzoxazone; acetaminophen]

mustaral oil [see: allyl isothiocyanate]

mustard oil [see: allyl isothiocyanate]

Mustargen powder for IV or intracavitary injection ℞ *antineoplastic* [mechlorethamine HCl]

Musterole Deep Strength Rub OTC *counterirritant* [methyl salicylate; methyl nicotinate; menthol]

Musterole Extra Strength OTC *counterirritant* [camphor; menthol]

mustine BAN *antineoplastic* [also: mechlorethamine HCl; chlormethine]

mustine HCl [see: mechlorethamine HCl]

Mutamycin powder for IV injection ℞ *antineoplastic antibiotic for acute stomach and pancreas cancer* [mitomycin]

muzolimine USAN, INN *diuretic; antihypertensive*

M-VAC (methotrexate, vinblastine, Adriamycin, cisplatin) *chemotherapy protocol*

M.V.C. 9 + 3 injection ℞ *parenteral vitamin supplement* [multiple vitamins; folic acid; biotin]

M.V.C. 9+4 Pediatric powder for injection ℞ *vitamin therapy* [multiple vitamins; folic acid; biotin]

MVF (mitoxantrone, vincristine, fluorouracil) *chemotherapy protocol*

M.V.I. Neonatal IV infusion ℞ *(orphan: total parenteral nutrition for very low birthweight infants)* [multiple vitamins]

M.V.I. Pediatric powder for injection ℞ *parenteral vitamin supplement* [multiple vitamins; folic acid; biotin]

M.V.I.-12 injection ℞ *parenteral vitamin supplement* [multiple vitamins; folic acid; biotin]

M.V.M. capsules OTC *vitamin/mineral/iron supplement* [multiple vitamins & minerals; iron; folic acid; biotin]

MVPP (mechlorethamine, vinblastine, procarbazine, prednisone) *chemotherapy protocol*

MVT (mitoxantrone, VePesid, thiotepa) *chemotherapy protocol*

MVVPP (mechlorethamine, vincristine, vinblastine, procarbazine, prednisone) *chemotherapy protocol*

My Cort Otic #1-20 ear drops (discontinued 1991) ℞ *topical corticosteroidal anti-inflammatory; antibiotic* [hydrocortisone; neomycin sulfate; polymyxin B sulfate]

Myadec tablets OTC *vitamin/mineral/iron supplement* [multiple vitamins & minerals; iron; folic acid; biotin]

Myambutol film-coated tablets ℞ *tuberculostatic* [ethambutol HCl]

Myapap drops ℞ *analgesic; antipyretic* [acetaminophen]

Mycelex cream, solution ℞ *topical antifungal* [clotrimazole]

Mycelex OTC cream, solution OTC *topical antifungal* [clotrimazole]

Mycelex Twin Pack cream + tablets ℞ *topical antifungal* [clotrimazole]

Mycelex-7 vaginal cream, vaginal tablets OTC *antifungal* [clotrimazole]

Mycelex-G vaginal cream, vaginal tablets, troches ℞ *antifungal* [clotrimazole]

Mycifradin Sulfate oral solution ℞ *aminoglycoside-type antibiotic* [neomycin sulfate]

Mycifradin Sulfate tablets, powder for IM injection (discontinued 1991) ℞ *aminoglycoside-type antibiotic* [neomycin sulfate]

Myciguent ointment, cream OTC *topical antibiotic* [neomycin sulfate]

Mycinette spray OTC *topical anesthetic; oral antiseptic; astringent* [phenol; alum]

Mycinettes lozenges OTC *topical anesthetic; oral antiseptic; expectorant* [benzocaine; cetylpyridinium chloride; terpin hydrate]

Myci-Spray nasal spray OTC *nasal decongestant; antihistamine* [phenylephrine HCl; pyrilamine maleate]

Mycitracin Plus ointment OTC *topical antibiotic; local anesthetic* [polymyxin B sulfate; neomycin sulfate; bacitracin; lidocaine]

Mycitracin Triple Antibiotic ointment OTC *topical antibiotic* [polymyxin B sulfate; neomycin sulfate; bacitracin]

Myco-Biotic II cream ℞ *topical corticosteroid; antifungal* [triamcinolone acetonide; nystatin]

Mycobutin capsules ℞ *prevention of Mycobacterium avium complex (MAC) in advanced HIV patients (orphan)* [rifabutin]

Mycogen II cream, ointment ℞ *topical corticosteroid; antifungal* [triamcinolone acetonide; nystatin]

Mycolog-II cream, ointment ℞ *topical corticosteroid; antifungal* [triamcinolone acetonide; nystatin]

Myconel cream ℞ *topical corticosteroid; antifungal* [triamcinolone acetonide; nystatin]

mycophenolate mofetil USAN *immunomodulator*

mycophenolic acid USAN, INN *antineoplastic*

Mycostatin cream, ointment, powder, vaginal tablets ℞ *topical antifungal* [nystatin]

Mycostatin film-coated tablets ℞ *systemic antifungal* [nystatin]

Mycostatin oral suspension, Pastilles (troches) ℞ *antifungal; oral candidiasis treatment* [nystatin]

Myco-Triacet II cream, ointment ℞ *topical corticosteroid; antifungal* [triamcinolone acetonide; nystatin]

mydeton [see: tolperisone]

Mydfrin Ophthalmic 2.5% eye drops ℞ *ophthalmic decongestant/vasoconstrictor; mydriatic* [phenylephrine HCl]

Mydrapred Drop-Tainers (eye drop suspension) ℞ *ophthalmic topical corticosteroidal anti-inflammatory; cycloplegic; mydriatic* [prednisolone acetate; atropine sulfate]

Mydriacyl Ophthalmic eye drops ℞ *cycloplegic; mydriatic* [tropicamide]

myelin *(orphan: multiple sclerosis)*

myelosan [see: busulfan]

myfadol INN

Myfedrine liquid (discontinued 1993) OTC *nasal decongestant* [pseudoephedrine HCl]

Myfedrine Plus liquid OTC *decongestant; antihistamine* [pseudoephedrine HCl; chlorpheniramine maleate]

Mygel oral suspension OTC *antacid; antiflatulent* [aluminum hydroxide; magnesium hydroxide; simethicone]

Mygel II oral suspension (discontinued 1991) OTC *antacid; antiflatulent* [aluminum hydroxide; magnesium hydroxide; simethicone]

Myidone tablets ℞ *anticonvulsant* [primidone]

Myidyl syrup ℞ *anthistamine* [triprolidine HCl]

My-K Elixir (discontinued 1992) ℞ *potassium supplement* [potassium gluconate]

Mykinac cream ℞ *topical antifungal* [nystatin]

Mykrox tablets ℞ *antihypertensive* [metolazone]

Mylanta Gas chewable tablets OTC *antiflatulent* [simethicone]

Mylanta gelcaps OTC *antacid* [calcium carbonate; magnesium carbonate]

Mylanta; Mylanta-II chewable tablets, liquid OTC *antacid; antiflatulent* [aluminum hydroxide; magnesium hydroxide; simethicone]

Mylaxen IV (discontinued 1991) ℞ *succinylcholine neuromuscular blockade adjunct* [hexafluorenium bromide]

Myleran tablets ℞ *antineoplastic for palliation in chronic myelogenous leukemia* [busulfan]

Mylicon drops OTC *antiflatulent* [simethicone]

Mylicon; Mylicon-80; Mylicon-125 chewable tablets (name changed to Mylanta Gas in 1992)

Myminic Expectorant liquid OTC *decongestant; expectorant* [phenylpropanolamine HCl; guaifenesin; alcohol]

Myminic syrup OTC *antihistamine; decongestant* [phenylpropanolamine HCl; chlorpheniramine maleate]

Myminicol liquid OTC *decongestant; antihistamine; antitussive* [phenylpropanolamine HCl; chlorpheniramine maleate; dextromethorphan hydrobromide]

Mynatal capsules ℞ *vitamin/mineral/calcium/iron supplement* [multiple vitamins & minerals; calcium; iron; folic acid; biotin]

Mynatal FC; Mynatal P.N. Forte; Mynatal Rx caplets ℞ *vitamin/mineral/iron supplement* [multiple vitamins & minerals; iron; folic acid]

Mynate 90 Plus caplets ℞ *vitamin/mineral supplement* [multiple vitamins & minerals; folic acid; docusate sodium]

Myochrysine IM injection ℞ *antirheumatic* [gold sodium thiomalate]

Myoflex Creme OTC *topical analgesic* [trolamine salicylate]

Myolin IV or IM injection ℞ *skeletal muscle relaxant* [orphenadrine citrate]

Myoscint ℞ *(orphan: diagnostic aid for cardiac necrosis and myocarditis)* [indium In 111 murine monoclonal antibody Fab to myosin; imicromab pentetate]

Myotonachol tablets ℞ *postsurgical cholinergic bladder muscle stimulant* [bethanechol chloride]

Myotrophin ℞ *(orphan: amyotrophic lateral sclerosis)* [insulin-like growth factor-1]

Myoview ℞ *investigational cardiovascular imaging aid*

Myphetane DC Cough syrup ℞ *decongestant; antihistamine; antitussive* [phenylpropanolamine HCl; brompheniramine maleate; codeine phosphate; alcohol]

Myphetane DX syrup ℞ *decongestant; antihistamine; antitussive* [pseudoephedrine HCl; brompheniramine maleate; dextromethorphan hydrobromide]

Myphetapp elixir OTC *decongestant; antihistamine* [phenylpropanolamine HCl; brompheniramine maleate]

myralact INN, BAN

myricodine [see: myrophine]

myristica oil [see: nutmeg oil]

myristyl alcohol NF *stiffening agent*

myristyltrimethylammonium bromide *antiseborrheic*

myrophine INN, BAN

myrtecaine INN

Mysoline tablets, oral suspension ℞ *anticonvulsant* [primidone]

myspamol [see: proquamezine]

Mytelase caplets ℞ *anticholinesterase muscle stimulant; myasthenia gravis treatment* [ambenonium chloride]

Mytrex cream, ointment ℞ *topical corticosteroid; antifungal* [triamcinolone acetonide; nystatin]

Mytussin AC Cough syrup ℞ *antitussive; expectorant* [codeine phosphate; guaifenesin; alcohol]

Mytussin DAC syrup ℞ *decongestant; antitussive; expectorant* [pseudoephedrine HCl; codeine phosphate; guaifenesin; alcohol]

Mytussin DM syrup OTC *antitussive; expectorant* [dextromethorphan hydrobromide; guaifenesin; alcohol]

Mytussin syrup OTC *expectorant* [guaifenesin; alcohol]

myuizone [see: thioacetazone; thiacetazone]

N

N₂ (nitrogen) [q.v.]
N-3 polyunsaturated fatty acids [see: doconexent; icosapent; omega-3 marine triglycerides]
²²Na [see: sodium chloride Na 22]
nabazenil USAN, INN *anticonvulsant*
nabilone USAN, INN, BAN *minor tranquilizer*
nabitan INN *analgesic* [also: nabitan HCl]
nabitan HCl USAN *analgesic* [also: nabitan]
naboctate INN *antiglaucoma agent; antinauseant* [also: naboctate HCl]
naboctate HCl USAN *antiglaucoma agent; antinauseant* [also: naboctate]
nabumetone USAN, INN, BAN *nonsteroidal anti-inflammatory drug (NSAID); antiarthritic*
nabutan HCl [now: nabitan HCl]
NAC (nitrogen mustard, Adriamycin, CCNU) *chemotherapy protocol*
nacartocin INN
NaCl (sodium chloride) [q.v.]
NAD (nicotinamide-adenine dinucleotide) [see: nadide]
nadide USAN, INN *antagonist to alcohol and narcotics*
nadisan [see: carbutamide]
nadolol USAN, USP, INN, BAN *antianginal; antihypertensive; antiadrenergic (β-receptor)*
nadoxolol INN
naepaine HCl NF
nafamostat INN
nafarelin INN, BAN *luteinizing hormone-releasing hormone (LHRH) agonist* [also: nafarelin acetate]
nafarelin acetate USAN *luteinizing hormone-releasing hormone (LHRH) agonist; (orphan: central precocious puberty)* [also: nafarelin]
Nafazair eye drops ℞ *topical ocular vasoconstrictor* [naphazoline HCl]
nafazatrom INN, BAN
nafcaproic acid INN

Nafcil powder for IV or IM injection ℞ *bactericidal antibiotic (penicillinase-resistant penicillin)* [nafcillin sodium]
nafcillin INN *antibacterial* [also: nafcillin sodium]
nafcillin sodium USAN, USP *bactericidal antibiotic* [also: nafcillin]
nafenodone INN
nafenopin USAN, INN *antihyperlipoproteinemic*
nafetolol INN
nafimidone INN *anticonvulsant* [also: nafimidone HCl]
nafimidone HCl USAN *anticonvulsant* [also: nafimidone]
nafiverine INN
naflocort USAN, INN *topical adrenocortical steroid*
nafomine INN *muscle relaxant* [also: nafomine malate]
nafomine malate USAN *muscle relaxant* [also: nafomine]
nafoxadol INN
nafoxidine HCl USAN, INN *antiestrogen*
nafronyl oxalate USAN *vasodilator* [also: naftidrofuryl]
naftalofos USAN, INN *veterinary anthelmintic*
naftazone INN, BAN
naftidrofuryl INN *vasodilator* [also: nafronyl oxalate]
naftifine INN, BAN *antifungal* [also: naftifine HCl]
naftifine HCl USAN *antifungal* [also: naftifine]
Naftin cream, gel ℞ *topical antifungal* [naftifine HCl]
naftopidil INN
naftoxate INN
naftypramide INN
Naganol (available only from the Centers for Disease Control) ℞ *investigational anti-infective for trypanosomiasis and onchocerciasis* [suramin sodium]

nalazosulfamide [see: salazosulfamide]
nalbuphine INN, BAN *narcotic agonist-antagonist analgesic; narcotic antagonist* [also: nalbuphine HCl]
nalbuphine HCl USAN *narcotic agonist-antagonist analgesic; narcotic antagonist* [also: nalbuphine]
Naldec Pediatric syrup ℞ *decongestant; antihistamine* [phenylpropanolamine HCl; phenylephrine HCl; phenyltoloxamine citrate; chlorpheniramine maleate]
Naldecon CX Adult liquid ℞ *decongestant; antitussive; expectorant* [phenylpropanolamine HCl; codeine phosphate; guaifenesin]
Naldecon DX Adult liquid OTC *decongestant; antitussive; expectorant* [phenylpropanolamine HCl; dextromethorphan hydrobromide; guaifenesin]
Naldecon DX children's syrup, pediatric drops OTC *pediatric decongestant, antitussive and expectorant* [phenylpropanolamine HCl; dextromethorphan hydrobromide; guaifenesin]
Naldecon EX children's syrup, pediatric drops OTC *decongestant; expectorant* [phenylpropanolamine HCl; guaifenesin]
Naldecon Senior DX liquid OTC *antitussive; expectorant* [dextromethorphan hydrobromide; guaifenesin]
Naldecon Senior EX liquid OTC *expectorant* [guaifenesin]
Naldecon sustained-release tablets, syrup, pediatric syrup, pediatric drops ℞ *decongestant; antihistamine* [phenylpropanolamine HCl; phenylephrine HCl; chlorpheniramine maleate; phenyltoloxamine citrate]
Naldegesic tablets OTC *decongestant; analgesic* [pseudoephedrine HCl; acetaminophen]
Naldelate syrup, pediatric syrup ℞ *decongestant; antihistamine* [phenylpropanolamine HCl; phenylephrine HCl; phenyltoloxamine citrate; chlorpheniramine maleate]
Nalfon Pulvules (capsules), tablets ℞ *nonsteroidal anti-inflammatory drug (NSAID); antiarthritic; analgesic* [fenoprofen calcium]
Nalgest sustained-release tablets, syrup, pediatric syrup, pediatric drops ℞ *decongestant; antihistamine* [phenylpropanolamine HCl; phenylephrine HCl; chlorpheniramine maleate; phenyltoloxamine citrate]
nalidixane [see: nalidixic acid]
nalidixate sodium USAN *antibacterial*
nalidixic acid USAN, USP, INN *urinary bactericidal*
Nallpen IV or IM injection ℞ *bactericidal antibiotic (penicillinase-resistant penicillin)* [nafcillin sodium]
nalmefene USAN, INN, BAN *narcotic antagonist*
nalmetrene [now: nalmefene]
nalmexone INN *analgesic; narcotic antagonist* [also: nalmexone HCl]
nalmexone HCl USAN *analgesic; narcotic antagonist* [also: nalmexone]
nalorphine INN [also: nalorphine HCl]
nalorphine HCl USP [also: nalorphine]
naloxiphane tartrate [see: levallorphan tartrate]
naloxone INN *narcotic antagonist* [also: naloxone HCl]
naloxone HCl USAN, USP *narcotic antagonist* [also: naloxone]
Nalspan syrup ℞ *decongestant; antihistamine* [phenylpropanolamine HCL; phenylephrine HCl; chlorpheniramine maleate; phenyltoloxamine citrate]
naltrexone USAN, INN, BAN *narcotic antagonist*
naltrexone HCl *(orphan: opiate blockage and maintenance in formerly opiate-dependent individuals)*

naminterol INN
[¹³N]ammonia [see: ammonia N 13]
namoxyrate USAN, INN *analgesic*
namuron [see: cyclobarbitone]
nanafrocin INN
Nandrobolic IM injection ℞ *anabolic steroid for metastatic breast cancer in women* [nandrolone phenpropionate]
nandrolone BAN *anabolic* [also: nandrolone cyclotate]
nandrolone cyclotate USAN *anabolic* [also: nandrolone]
nandrolone decanoate USAN, USP *androgen; anabolic steroid*
nandrolone phenpropionate USP *androgen; anabolic steroid*
naniopine [see: nanofin]
nanofin INN
nanterinone INN, BAN
nantradol INN *analgesic* [also: nantradol HCl]
nantradol HCl USAN *analgesic* [also: nantradol]
Napa ℞ *investigational antiarrhythmic* [acecainide HCl]
NAPA (*N*-acetyl-*p*-aminophenol) [see: acetaminophen]
NAPA (*N*-acetylprocainamide) [q.v.]
napactadine INN *antidepressant* [also: napactadine HCl]
napactadine HCl USAN *antidepressant* [also: napactadine]
napamezole INN *antidepressant* [also: napamezole HCl]
napamezole HCl USAN *antidepressant* [also: napamezole]
Napamide capsules ℞ *antiarrhythmic* [disopyramide phosphate]
naphazoline INN, BAN *topical ocular vasoconstrictor; nasal decongestant* [also: naphazoline HCl]
naphazoline HCl USP *topical ocular vasoconstrictor; nasal decongestant* [also: naphazoline]
Naphazoline-A ophthalmic solution ℞ *topical ocular vasoconstrictor* [naphazoline HCl; pheniramine maleate]

Naphcon Drop-Tainers (eye drops) OTC *topical ocular vasoconstrictor* [naphazoline HCl]
Naphcon Forte Drop-Tainers (eye drops) ℞ *topical ocular vasoconstrictor* [naphazoline HCl]
Naphcon-A eye drops ℞ *topical ocular decongestant/antihistamine* [naphazoline HCl; pheniramine maleate]
2-naphthol [see: betanaphthol]
naphthonone INN
naphthypramide [see: naftypramide]
Naphuride (available only from the Centers for Disease Control) ℞ *investigational anti-infective for trypanosomiasis and onchocerciasis* [suramin sodium]
napirimus INN
Napril tablets OTC *decongestant; antihistamine* [pseudoephedrine HCl; chlorpheniramine maleate]
naprodoxime INN
Naprosyn SR ℞ *investigational nonsteroidal anti-inflammatory drug (NSAID); antiarthritic; analgesic* [naproxen]
Naprosyn tablets, oral suspension ℞ *nonsteroidal anti-inflammatory drug (NSAID); antiarthritic; analgesic* [naproxen]
naproxen USAN, USP, INN, BAN *analgesic; antiarthritic; nonsteroidal anti-inflammatory drug (NSAID); antipyretic*
naproxen sodium USAN, USP *analgesic; antiarthritic; nonsteroidal anti-inflammatory drug (NSAID); antipyretic*
naproxol USAN, INN *anti-inflammatory; analgesic; antipyretic*
Naqua tablets ℞ *diuretic; antihypertensive* [trichlormethiazide]
Naquival tablets (discontinued 1991) ℞ *antihypertensive* [trichlormethiazide; reserpine]
naranol INN *antipsychotic* [also: naranol HCl]
naranol HCl USAN *antipsychotic* [also: naranol]

narasin USAN, INN, BAN *coccidiostat; veterinary growth stimulant*

Narcan IV, subcu or IM injection, neonatal injection ℞ *narcotic antagonist; hypotension treatment* [naloxone HCl]

narcotine [see: noscapine]

narcotine HCl [see: noscapine HCl]

Nardil tablets ℞ *monoamine oxidase (MAO) inhibitor antidepressant* [phenelzine sulfate]

Nasacort nasal spray ℞ *intranasal corticosteroidal anti-inflammatory* [triamcinolone acetonide]

Nasahist B subcu or IM injection ℞ *anthistamine; anaphylaxis* [brompheniramine maleate]

Nasahist sustained-release capsules ℞ *decongestant; antihistamine* [phenylpropanolamine HCl; phenylephrine HCl; chlorpheniramine maleate]

Nasal Moist nasal spray OTC *nasal moisturizer* [sodium chloride (saline)]

NāSal nasal spray, nose drops OTC *nasal moisturizer* [sodium chloride (saline)]

Nasal Relief nasal spray OTC *nasal decongestant* [oxymetazoline HCl]

Nasalcrom nasal spray ℞ *bronchodilator for bronchial asthma and bronchospasm* [cromolyn sodium]

Nasalide nasal spray ℞ *intranasal steroidal anti-inflammatory* [flunisolide]

Nasostat disposable nasal balloon (discontinued 1991) OTC *control of nosebleeds*

Natabec FA Kapseals (capsules) (discontinued 1992) OTC *vitamin/mineral/iron supplement* [multiple vitamins & minerals; iron; folic acid]

Natabec Kapseals (capsules) (discontinued 1992) OTC *vitamin/mineral/iron supplement* [multiple vitamins & minerals; iron]

Natabec Rx Kapseals (capsules) ℞ *vitamin/calcium/iron supplement* [multiple vitamins; calcium; iron; folic acid]

Natabec with Fluoride capsules (discontinued 1992) ℞ *pediatric vitamin deficiency and dental caries prevention* [multiple vitamins; fluoride; iron]

Natacomp-FA film-coated tablets ℞ *vitamin/mineral/iron supplement* [multiple vitamins & minerals; iron; folic acid]

Natacyn eye drop suspension ℞ *ophthalmic antifungal agent* [natamycin]

Natafort Filmseal (film-coated tablets) ℞ *vitamin/calcium/iron supplement* [multiple vitamins; calcium; iron; folic acid]

Nata-Key coated caplets OTC *vitamin/mineral supplement* [multiple vitamins & minerals; bioflavonoids]

Natalins Rx tablets ℞ *vitamin/calcium/iron supplement* [multiple vitamins; calcium; iron; folic acid; biotin]

Natalins tablets OTC *vitamin/mineral/calcium/iron supplement* [multiple vitamins & minerals; calcium; iron; folic acid]

natamycin USAN, USP, INN *ophthalmic antibacterial/antifungal antibiotic*

Natarex Prenatal tablets ℞ *vitamin/calcium/iron supplement* [multiple vitamins; calcium; iron; folic acid]

Natural Vegetable powder OTC *bulk laxative* [psyllium hydrophilic mucilloid]

Nature's Bounty 1 timed-release tablets OTC *vitamin/mineral/calcium/iron supplement* [multiple vitamins & minerals; calcium; iron; folic acid; biotin]

Nature's Remedy tablets OTC *laxative* [cascara sagrada]

Naturetin tablets ℞ *diuretic; antihypertensive* [bendroflumethiazide]

Naus-A-Way solution OTC *antinauseant; antiemetic* [phosphorated carbohydrate solution]

Nausetrol solution OTC *antinauseant; antiemetic* [phosphorated carbohydrate solution]

Navane capsules ℞ *antipsychotic* [thiothixene]

Navane oral concentrate, IM solution, powder for IM injection ℞ *antipsychotic* [thiothixene HCl]

naxagolide INN *antiparkinsonian; dopamine agonist* [also: naxagolide HCl]

naxagolide HCl USAN *antiparkinsonian; dopamine agonist* [also: naxagolide]

naxaprostene INN

N-B-P ointment OTC *topical antibiotic* [polymyxin B sulfate; neomycin sulfate; bacitracin]

ND Clear sustained-release capsules ℞ *decongestant; antihistamine* [pseudoephedrine HCl; chlorpheniramine maleate]

ND Stat subcu or IM injection ℞ *antihistamine; anaphylaxis* [brompheniramine maleate]

ND-Gesic tablets OTC *decongestant; antihistamine; analgesic* [phenylephrine HCl; chlorpheniramine maleate; pyrilamine maleate; acetaminophen]

nealbarbital INN [also: nealbarbitone]

nealbarbitone BAN [also: nealbarbital]

nebacumab (*orphan: gram-negative bacteremia in endotoxin shock*)

Nebcin IV or IM injection, pediatric injection, powder for injection ℞ *aminoglycoside-type antibiotic* [tobramycin sulfate]

nebidrazine INN

nebivolol USAN, INN *antihypertensive* (β-blocker)

nebracetam INN

nebramycin USAN, INN *antibacterial*

nebramycin factor 6 [see: tobramycin]

NebuPent inhalation aerosol ℞ *antiprotozoal; (orphan: Pneumocystis carinii pneumonia)* [pentamidine isethionate]

nedocromil USAN, INN, BAN *prophylactic antiallergic*

nedocromil calcium USAN *prophylactic antiallergic*

nedocromil sodium USAN *prophylactic antiallergic; antiasthmatic*

N.E.E. 1/35 tablets ℞ *oral contraceptive* [ethinyl estradiol; norethindrone]

nefazodone INN *antidepressant* [also: nefazodone HCl]

nefazodone HCl USAN *antidepressant* [also: nefazodone]

neflumozide INN *antipsychotic* [also: neflumozide HCl]

neflumozide HCl USAN *antipsychotic* [also: neflumozide]

nefocon A USAN *hydrophobic contact lens material*

nefopam INN *analgesic* [also: nefopam HCl]

nefopam HCl USAN *analgesic* [also: nefopam]

nefrolan [see: clorexolone]

NegGram caplets, oral suspension ℞ *urinary anti-infective* [nalidixic acid]

neldazosin INN

nelezaprine INN *muscle relaxant* [also: nelezaprine maleate]

nelezaprine maleate USAN *muscle relaxant* [also: nelezaprine]

Nelova 1/35E; Nelova 0.5/35E; Nelova 10/11 tablets ℞ *oral contraceptive* [ethinyl estradiol; norethindrone]

Nelova 1/50M tablets ℞ *oral contraceptive* [mestranol; norethindrone]

Nelulen 1/35E; Nelulen 1/50E tablets ℞ *oral contraceptive* [ethynodiol diacetate; ethinyl estradiol]

nemadectin USAN, INN *veterinary antiparasitic*

Nembutal elixir ℞ *sedative; hypnotic* [pentobarbital]

Nembutal Sodium capsules, IV or IM injection, suppositories ℞ *sedative; hypnotic* [pentobarbital sodium]
neoarsphenamine NF, INN
Neobiotic tablets (discontinued 1991) ℞ *aminoglycoside-type antibiotic* [neomycin sulfate]
Neocaf *(orphan: apnea of prematurity)* [caffeine]
Neo-Calglucon syrup OTC *calcium supplement* [calcium glubionate]
neocarzinostatin [now: zinostatin]
Neo-Castaderm liquid OTC *topical antifungal; astringent; antiseptic* [resorcinol; boric acid; acetone; sodium bisulfite; phenol; alcohol]
Neocera (trademarked ingredient) *suppository base* [PEG 400, 1450, 8000; polysorbate 60]
neocid [see: chlorophenothane]
Neocidin eye drops ℞ *ophthalmic antibiotic* [polymyxin B sulfate; neomycin sulfate; gramicidin]
neocinchophen NF, INN
Neo-Cort-Dome (discontinued 1991) [see: Otic Neo-Cort-Dome]
Neo-Cortef cream (discontinued 1993) ℞ *topical corticosteroid; antibiotic* [hydrocortisone; neomycin sulfate]
Neo-Cortef eye drop suspension (discontinued 1991) ℞ *topical ophthalmic corticosteroidal anti-inflammatory; antibiotic* [hydrocortisone acetate; neomycin sulfate]
Neo-Cortef ointment ℞ *topical corticosteroid; antibiotic* [hydrocortisone; neomycin sulfate]
Neo-Cultol jelly OTC *emollient laxative* [mineral oil]
Neocyten IV or IM injection ℞ *skeletal muscle relaxant* [orphenadrine citrate]
NeoDecadron cream ℞ *topical corticosteroid; antibiotic* [dexamethasone phosphate; neomycin sulfate]
NeoDecadron eye drops, ophthalmic ointment ℞ *topical ophthalmic corticosteroidal anti-inflammatory; antibiotic* [dexamethasone sodium phosphate; neomycin sulfate]
Neo-Durabolic IM injection ℞ *anabolic steroid for anemia of renal insufficiency* [nandrolone decanoate]
neodymium *element (Nd)*
Neofed tablets (discontinued 1991) OTC *nasal decongestant* [pseudoephedrine HCl]
Neo-fradin oral solution ℞ *aminoglycoside-type antibiotic* [neomycin sulfate]
Neoloid emulsion OTC *laxative* [castor oil]
Neomac ointment OTC *topical antibiotic* [polymyxin B sulfate; neomycin sulfate; bacitracin]
Neo-Medrol Acetate liquid ℞ *topical corticosteroid; antibiotic* [methylprednisolone acetate; neomycin sulfate]
neo-mercazole [see: carbimazole]
Neomixin ointment OTC *topical antibiotic* [polymyxin B sulfate; neomycin sulfate; bacitracin zinc]
neomycin INN, BAN *antibacterial* [also: neomycin palmitate]
neomycin B [see: framycetin]
neomycin palmitate USAN *antibacterial* [also: neomycin]
neomycin sulfate USP *aminoglycoside antibacterial antibiotic*
neomycin undecenoate [see: neomycin undecylenate]
neomycin undecylenate USAN *antibacterial; antifungal*
Neomycin-Dex ophthalmic solution ℞ *topical corticosteroid; antibiotic* [neomycin sulfate; dexamethasone sodium phosphate]
neon *element (Ne)*
Neopap suppositories OTC *analgesic; antipyretic* [acetaminophen]
neopenyl [see: clemizole penicillin]
Neo-Polycin ointment (discontinued 1991) OTC *topical antibiotic* [polymyxin B sulfate; neomycin sulfate; bacitracin zinc]

neoquate [see: nequinate]
Neoquess IM injection ℞ *gastrointestinal antispasmodic* [dicyclomine HCl]
Neoquess tablets ℞ *gastrointestinal antispasmodic* [hyoscyamine sulfate]
NeoRespin timed-release capsules OTC *bronchodilator for bronchial asthma and bronchospasm* [ephedrine HCl]
Neosar powder for IV injection ℞ *antineoplastic* [cyclophosphamide]
Neosporin cream OTC *topical antibiotic* [polymyxin B sulfate; neomycin sulfate]
Neosporin G.U. Irrigant solution ℞ *bactericidal* [neomycin sulfate; polymyxin B sulfate]
Neosporin ointment OTC *topical antibiotic* [polymyxin B sulfate; neomycin sulfate; bacitracin]
Neosporin Ophthalmic eye drops ℞ *ophthalmic antibiotic* [polymyxin B sulfate; neomycin sulfate; gramicidin]
Neosporin Ophthalmic ointment ℞ *ophthalmic antibiotic* [polymyxin B sulfate; neomycin sulfate; bacitracin]
Neosporin Plus cream OTC *topical antibiotic; anesthetic* [polymyxin B sulfate; neomycin; lidocaine]
Neosporin Plus ointment OTC *topical antibiotic; anesthetic* [polymyxin B sulfate; neomycin; bacitracin zinc; lidocaine]
neostigmine BAN *cholinergic muscle stimulant* [also: neostigmine bromide]
neostigmine bromide USP, INN, BAN *cholinergic muscle stimulant* [also: neostigmine]
neostigmine methylsulfate USP *cholinergic muscle stimulant*
Neo-Synalar cream ℞ *topical corticosteroid; antibacterial* [fluocinolone acetonide; neomycin sulfate]
Neo-Synephrine 12 Hour nasal spray OTC *nasal decongestant* [oxymetazoline HCl]

Neo-Synephrine 12 Hour nose drops (discontinued 1992) OTC *nasal decongestant* [oxymetazoline HCl]
Neo-Synephrine 2.5% Ophthalmic; Neo-Synephrine 10% Plain Ophthalmic eye drops ℞ *ophthalmic decongestant/vasoconstrictor; mydriatic* [phenylephrine HCl]
Neo-Synephrine HCl IV, subcu or IM injection ℞ *vasopressor used in shock* [phenylephrine HCl]
Neo-Synephrine HCl ophthalmic solution ℞ *vasoconstrictor; mydriatic* [phenylephrine HCl]
Neo-Synephrine jelly (discontinued 1992) OTC *nasal decongestant* [phenylephrine HCl]
Neo-Synephrine nasal spray, nose drops OTC *nasal decongestant* [phenylephrine HCl]
Neo-Synephrine Viscous Ophthalmic eye drops ℞ *ophthalmic decongestant/vasoconstrictor; mydriatic* [phenylephrine HCl]
Neo-Tabs tablets ℞ *aminoglycoside-type antibiotic* [neomycin sulfate]
Neotal Ophthalmic ointment ℞ *ophthalmic antibiotic* [polymyxin B sulfate; neomycin sulfate; bacitracin]
Neo-Tears eye drops (discontinued 1991) OTC *ocular moisturizer/lubricant*
Neo-Thrycex ointment (discontinued 1991) OTC *topical antibiotic* [polymyxin B sulfate; neomycin sulfate; bacitracin]
Neothylline tablets ℞ *bronchodilator* [dyphylline]
Neothylline-GG tablets ℞ *bronchodilator; expectorant* [dyphylline; guaifenesin]
Neotrace-4 IV injection ℞ *intravenous nutritional therapy* [multiple trace elements (metals)]
Neotricin ointment, eye drops (name changed to Ocutricin in 1992)
NeoVadrin Advanced Formula Centurion A to Zinc capsules (dis-

continued 1991) OTC *vitamin/mineral/iron supplement* [multiple vitamins & minerals; iron; biotin; folic acid]

NeoVadrin B Complex "50"; NeoVadrin B Complex "100" tablets (discontinued 1992) OTC *vitamin B supplement* [multiple B vitamins; folic acid; biotin; inositol; choline bitartrate]

NeoVadrin Centurion tablets (discontinued 1991) OTC *antianemic* [ferrous fumarate; multiple vitamins]

NeoVadrin Children's Chewable Tablets (discontinued 1992) OTC *vitamin supplement* [multiple vitamins; folic acid]

NeoVadrin Children's Chewable Tablets with Iron (discontinued 1991) OTC *vitamin/iron supplement* [multiple vitamins; iron; folic acid]

NeoVadrin Oystershell Calcium with Vitamin D tablets (discontinued 1992) OTC *dietary supplement* [calcium carbonate; vitamin D]

NeoVadrin Prenatal tablets (discontinued 1991) OTC *vitamin/mineral/iron supplement* [multiple vitamins & minerals; iron; folic acid]

NeoVadrin Therapeutic M tablets (discontinued 1992) OTC *vitamin/mineral/iron supplement* [multiple vitamins & minerals; iron; biotin; folic acid]

NeoVicaps timed-release capsules (discontinued 1991) OTC *vitamin/zinc supplement* [multiple B vitamins; vitamin C; zinc]

NephrAmine 5.4% IV infusion ℞ *nutritional therapy for renal failure* [multiple essential amino acids; cysteine; electrolytes]

Nephro-Calci tablets OTC *calcium supplement* [calcium carbonate]

Nephrocaps capsules ℞ *vitamin supplement* [multiple B vitamins; vitamin C; folic acid; biotin]

Nephro-Derm cream OTC *moisturizer; emollient; antipruritic; counterirritant* [camphor; menthol]

Nephro-Fer tablets OTC *hematinic* [ferrous fumarate]

Nephro-Mag tablets (discontinued 1991) OTC *magnesium supplement* [magnesium carbonate]

Nephron solution for inhalation OTC *bronchodilator for bronchial asthma* [racepinephrine]

Nephro-Vite Rx + Fe film-coated tablets ℞ *hematinic* [multiple B vitamins; vitamin C; iron; folic acid; biotin]

Nephro-Vite Rx film-coated tablets ℞ *vitamin supplement* [multiple B vitamins; vitamin C; folic acid; biotin]

Nephro-Vite tablets OTC *vitamin supplement* [multiple B vitamins; vitamin C]

Nephro-Vite Vitamin B Complex and C Supplement tablets OTC *vitamin supplement* [multiple B vitamins; vitamin C; folic acid; biotin]

Nephrox oral suspension OTC *antacid; laxative* [aluminum hydroxide; mineral oil]

neptamustine INN *antineoplastic* [also: pentamustine]

Neptazane tablets ℞ *carbonic anhydrase inhibitor; diuretic* [methazolamide]

neptunium *element (Np)*

nequinate USAN, INN *coccidiostat for poultry* [also: methyl benzoquate]

neraminol INN

nerbacadol INN

neridronic acid INN

nerve growth factor *investigational agent for chemotherapy-induced peripheral neuropathy*

Nervine Nighttime Sleep-Aid tablets OTC *antihistaminic sleep aid* [diphenhydramine HCl]

Nervocaine 1%; Nervocaine 2% injection ℞ *injectable local anesthetic* [lidocaine HCl]

Nesacaine; Nesacaine MPF injection ℞ *injectable local anesthetic* [chloroprocaine HCl]
nesapidil INN
nesosteine INN
Nestabs FA tablets ℞ *vitamin/calcium/iron supplement* [multiple vitamins; calcium; ferrous fumarate; folic acid]
Nestabs tablets OTC *vitamin/calcium/iron supplement* [multiple vitamins; calcium; ferrous fumarate; folic acid]
Nestrex tablets OTC *vitamin supplement* [pyridoxine HCl]
nethalide [see: pronetalol]
netilmicin INN, BAN *aminoglycoside bactericidal antibiotic* [also: netilmicin sulfate]
netilmicin sulfate USAN, USP *aminoglycoside bactericidal antibiotic* [also: netilmicin]
netobimin USAN, INN, BAN *veterinary anthelmintic*
netrafilcon A USAN *hydrophilic contact lens material*
Netromicina (Mexican name for U.S. product Netromycin)
Netromycin IV or IM injection ℞ *aminoglycoside-type antibiotic* [netilmicin sulfate]
Neupogen injection ℞ *(orphan: severe chronic neutropenia; myelodysplastic syndrome)* [filgrastim]
Neuramate tablets ℞ *anxiolytic* [meprobamate]
NeuRecover-DA; NeuRecover-LT; NeuRecover-SA capsules OTC *dietary supplement* [multiple vitamins, minerals & amino acids; folic acid; biotin]
Neurodep injection OTC *parenteral vitamin therapy* [multiple B vitamins, vitamin C]
Neurodep-Caps capsules OTC *vitamin supplement* [vitamins B_1, B_6 and B_{12}]
Neuroforte-R injection ℞ *vitamin B_{12} therapy* [cyanocobalamin]

Neuroforte-Six injection ℞ *vitamin therapy* [multiple B vitamins; vitamin C]
Neurolite ℞ *investigational brain imaging aid*
Neurontin ℞ *investigational anticonvulsant* [gabapentin]
neurosin [see: calcium glycerophosphate]
NeuroSlim capsules OTC *dietary supplement* [multiple vitamins, minerals & amino acids; folic acid; biotin]
neurotrophic growth factor *investigational treatment for neurological conditions*
neustab [see: thioacetazone; thiacetazone]
Neut IV or subcu injection ℞ *pH buffer for metabolic acidosis; urinary alkalinizer* [sodium bicarbonate]
neutral acriflavine [see: acriflavine]
neutral insulin INN, BAN *antidiabetic* [also: insulin, neutral]
neutramycin USAN, INN *antibacterial*
Neutra-Phos capsules, powder OTC *phosphorus supplement* [monobasic sodium phosphate; monobasic potassium phosphate; dibasic sodium phosphate; dibasic potassium phosphate]
Neutra-Phos-K capsules, powder OTC *phosphorus supplement* [monobasic potassium phosphate; dibasic potassium phosphate]
NeuTrexin ℞ *investigational antineoplastic for AIDS-related Pneumocystis carinii pneumonia* [trimetrexate]
neutroflavine [see: acriflavine]
Neutrogena Acne Mask OTC *topical keratolytic cleaning mask for acne* [benzoyl peroxide]
Neutrogena Body lotion, oil OTC *moisturizer; emollient*
Neutrogena Drying gel OTC *astringent; antiseptic* [hamamelis water; isopropyl alcohol]

Neutrogena Moisture lotion OTC *moisturizer; emollient*

Neutrogena Norwegian Formula Hand cream OTC *moisturizer; emollient*

Neutrogena Soap; Neutrogena Acne Cleansing; Neutrogena Baby Cleansing Formula; Neutrogena Dry Skin bar OTC *therapeutic skin cleanser*

Neutrogena T/Derm oil OTC *topical antipsoriatic; antiseborrheic* [coal tar]

Neutrogena T/Gel Scalp Solution gel (discontinued 1992) OTC *antiseborrheic; antipsoriatic* [coal tar]

Neutrogena T/Gel shampoo, conditioner OTC *antiseborrheic; antipsoriatic; antipruritic; antibacterial* [coal tar]

Neutrogena T/Sal shampoo OTC *antiseborrheic; antipsoriatic; antipruritic; antibacterial* [salicylic acid; coal tar]

nevirapine USAN *antiviral*

Nevrotose No. 3 tablets (discontinued 1991) ℞ *anticholinergic; sedative* [hyoscyamus; phenobarbital]

New Decongest syrup, pediatric syrup, pediatric drops ℞ *decongestant; antihistamine* [phenylpropanolamine HCl; phenylephrine HCl; chlorpheniramine maleate; phenyltoloxamine citrate]

New Decongestant sustained-release tablets ℞ *decongestant; antihistamine* [phenylpropanolamine HCl; phenylephrine HCl; chlorpheniramine maleate; phenyltoloxamine citrate]

New Freshness Douche solution (discontinued 1991) OTC *vaginal cleanser and deodorizer; acidity modifier* [vinegar (acetic acid)]

new-estranol 1 [see: diethylstilbestrol]

new-oestranol 1 [see: diethylstilbestrol]

new-oestranol 11 [see: diethylstilbestrol dipropionate]

New-Skin liquid, spray OTC *skin protectant; antiseptic* [hydroxyquinoline]

nexeridine INN *analgesic* [also: nexeridine HCl]

nexeridine HCl USAN *analgesic* [also: nexeridine]

NG-29 (*orphan: diagnostic aid for pituitary release of growth hormone*)

N.G.T. cream ℞ *topical corticosteroid; antifungal* [triamcinolone acetonide; nystatin]

Nia-Bid sustained-action capsules OTC *vitamin supplement* [niacin]

Niac timed-release capsules OTC *vitamin supplement* [niacin]

Niacels timed-release capsules OTC *vitamin supplement* [niacin]

niacin USP *vitamin B_3; vasodilator; antihyperlipidemic* [also: nicotinic acid]

niacinamide USP *vitamin B_3; enzyme cofactor* [also: nicotinamide]

niacinamide hydroiodide *expectorant*

Niacin-Time time-release wax-matrix tablet OTC *vitamin supplement* [niacin]

Niacor immediate-release tablets ℞ *antihyperlipidemic* [niacin]

nialamide NF, INN

niaprazine INN

Niazide tablets ℞ *diuretic; antihypertensive* [trichlormethiazide]

nibroxane USAN, INN *topical antimicrobial*

Nicabate (European name for U.S. product Nicoderm)

nicafenine INN

nicainoprol INN

nicametate INN, BAN

nicaraven INN

nicarbazin BAN

nicardipine INN, BAN *vasodilator; calcium channel blocker* [also: nicardipine HCl]

nicardipine HCl USAN *vasodilator; calcium channel blocker* [also: nicardipine]

N'Ice lozenges OTC *topical antipruritic/counterirritant; mild local anesthetic* [menthol]

N'Ice Vitamin C Drops (lozenges) OTC *vitamin supplement* [ascorbic acid; menthol; sorbitol]
nicergoline USAN, INN *vasodilator*
niceritrol INN, BAN
nicethamide BAN [also: nikethamide]
niceverine INN
nickel *element (Ni)*
Niclocide chewable tablets ℞ *anthelmintic (tapeworm)* [niclosamide]
niclofolan INN, BAN
niclosamide USAN, INN *anthelmintic*
Nico-400 timed-release capsules OTC *vitamin supplement* [niacin]
Nicobid Tempules (timed-release capsules) OTC *niacin therapy* [niacin]
nicoboxil INN
nicoclonate INN
nicocodine INN, BAN
nicocortonide INN
Nicoderm transdermal patch ℞ *smoking deterrent; nicotine withdrawal aid* [nicotine]
nicodicodine INN, BAN
nicoduozide (isoniazid + nicothiazone)
nicofibrate INN
nicofuranose INN
nicofurate INN
nicogrelate INN
Nicolar tablets ℞ *niacin therapy; antihyperlipidemic* [niacin]
nicomol INN
nicomorphine INN, BAN
nicopholine INN
nicorandil USAN, INN *coronary vasodilator*
Nicorette; Nicorette DS chewing pieces ℞ *smoking deterrent; nicotine withdrawal aid* [nicotine polacrilex]
nicothiazone INN
nicotinaldehyde thiosemicarbazone [see: nicothiazone]
nicotinamide INN, BAN *vitamin B₃; enzyme cofactor* [also: niacinamide]
nicotinamide-adenine dinucleotide (NAD) [now: nadide]

nicotine polacrilex USAN *smoking deterrent; nicotine withdrawal aid*
nicotine resin complex [see: nicotine polacrilex]
Nicotinex elixir OTC *vitamin supplement* [niacin]
nicotinic acid INN, BAN *vitamin B₃; vasodilator; antihyperlipidemic* [also: niacin]
nicotinic acid amide [see: niacinamide]
nicotinic acid 1-oxide [see: oxiniacic acid]
nicotinohydroxamic acid [see: nicoxamat]
6-nicotinoyl dihydrocodeine [see: nicodicodine]
6-nicotinoylcodeine [see: nicocodine]
4-nicotinoylmorpholine [see: nicopholine]
nicotinyl alcohol USAN, BAN *peripheral vasodilator*
nicotinyl tartrate
Nicotrol transdermal patch ℞ *smoking deterrent; nicotine withdrawal aid* [nicotine]
nicotylamide [see: niacinamide]
nicoumalone BAN [also: acenocoumarol]
Nico-Vert capsules ℞ *anticholinergic; antiemetic; antivertigo agent; motion sickness preventative* [dimenhydrinate]
nicoxamat INN
nictiazem INN
nictindole INN
nidroxyzone INN
Nidryl elixir OTC *antihistamine; antitussive* [diphenhydramine HCl]
nifedipine USAN, USP, INN, BAN *coronary vasodilator; calcium channel blocker; (orphan: interstitial cystitis)*
nifenalol INN
nifenazone INN, BAN
Niferex Daily tablets OTC *vitamin/mineral supplement* [multiple vitamins & minerals]

Niferex elixir, film-coated tablets OTC *hematinic* [polysaccharide-iron complex]

Niferex Forte elixir ℞ *hematinic* [polysaccharide-iron complex; folic acid; cyanocobalamin]

Niferex with Vitamin C chewable tablets OTC *hematinic* [polysaccharide-iron complex; ascorbic acid; sodium ascorbate]

Niferex-150 capsules OTC *hematinic* [polysaccharide-iron complex]

Niferex-150 Forte capsules ℞ *hematinic* [polysaccharide-iron complex; folic acid; cyanocobalamin]

Niferex-PN film-coated tablets ℞ *prenatal vitamin/iron supplement* [multiple vitamins; polysaccharide-iron complex; folic acid]

Niferex-PN Forte film-coated tablets ℞ *prenatal vitamin/mineral/calcium/iron supplement* [multiple vitamins & minerals; calcium; polysaccharide-iron complex; folic acid]

niflumic acid INN

nifluridide USAN *ectoparasiticide*

nifungin USAN, INN

nifuradene USAN, INN *antibacterial*

nifuralazine [see: furalazine]

nifuraldezone USAN, INN *antibacterial*

nifuralide INN

nifuramizone [see: nifurethazone]

nifuratel USAN, INN *antibacterial; antifungal; antiprotozoal (Trichomonas)*

nifuratrone USAN, INN *antibacterial*

nifurazolidone [see: furazolidone]

nifurdazil USAN, INN *antibacterial*

nifurethazone INN

nifurfoline INN

nifurhydrazone [see: nihydrazone]

nifurimide USAN, INN *antibacterial*

nifurizone INN

nifurmazole INN

nifurmerone USAN, INN *antifungal*

nifuroquine INN

nifuroxazide INN

nifuroxime NF, INN

nifurpipone (NP) INN

nifurpirinol USAN, INN *antibacterial*

nifurprazine INN

nifurquinazol USAN, INN *antibacterial*

nifursemizone USAN, INN *antiprotozoal for poultry (Histomonas)*

nifursol USAN, INN *antiprotozoal for poultry (Histomonas)*

nifurthiazole USAN, INN *antibacterial*

nifurthiline [see: thiofuradene]

nifurtimox INN, BAN *investigational anti-infective for Chagas disease*

nifurtoinol INN

nifurvidine INN

nifurzide INN

niguldipine INN

nihydrazone INN

nikethamide NF, INN [also: nicethamide]

Nil vaginal cream (discontinued 1992) ℞ *bacteriostatic; antiseptic; vulnerary* [sulfanilamide; aminacrine HCl; allantoin]

nileprost INN

nilestriol INN *estrogen* [also: nylestriol]

Niloric sublingual tablets (discontinued 1991) ℞ *for age-related mental capacity decline* [ergoloid mesylates]

nilprazole INN

Nilstat cream, ointment, vaginal tablets ℞ *topical antifungal* [nystatin]

Nilstat film-coated tablets ℞ *systemic antifungal* [nystatin]

Nilstat oral suspension, powder for oral suspension ℞ *antifungal; oral candidiasis treatment* [nystatin]

niludipine INN

nilutamide INN

nilvadipine USAN, INN *calcium channel antagonist*

nimazone USAN, INN *anti-inflammatory*

Nimbus test kit ℞ *in vitro diagnostic aid for urine pregnancy test*

Nimbus II test kit (discontinued 1992) ℞ *in vitro diagnostic aid for urine pregnancy test*
nimesulide INN, BAN
nimetazepam INN
nimidane USAN, INN *veterinary acaricide*
nimodipine USAN, INN, BAN *vasodilator; calcium channel blocker*
nimorazole INN, BAN
Nimotop soft liquid-filled capsules ℞ *calcium channel blocker for subarachnoid hemorrhage* [nimodipine]
nimustine INN
niobium *element (Nb)*
niometacin INN
Nion B Plus C caplets OTC *vitamin supplement* [multiple B vitamins; vitamin C]
Nipent IV injection ℞ *antineoplastic antibiotic; (orphan: hairy cell and chronic lymphocytic leukemias)* [pentostatin]
niperotidine INN
nipradilol INN
Nipride powder for IV infusion (discontinued 1992) ℞ *antihypertensive for hypertensive crisis* [sodium nitroprusside]
niprofazone INN
niridazole USAN, INN *antischistosomal*
Nisaval tablets (discontinued 1992) ℞ *antihistamine* [pyrilamine maleate]
nisbuterol INN *bronchodilator* [also: nisbuterol mesylate]
nisbuterol mesylate USAN *bronchodilator* [also: nisbuterol]
nisobamate USAN, INN *minor tranquilizer*
nisoldipine USAN, INN *coronary vasodilator*
nisoxetine USAN, INN *antidepressant*
nisterime INN *androgen* [also: nisterime acetate]
nisterime acetate USAN *androgen* [also: nisterime]

nitarsone USAN, INN *antiprotozoal (Histomonas)*
nitazoxanide INN
Nite Time Cold Formula liquid OTC *analgesic; decongestant; antihistamine; antitussive* [acetaminophen; doxylamine succinate; pseudoephedrine HCl; dextromethorphan hydrobromide; alcohol]
NiteLite OTC *investigational cough/cold medication*
nithiamide USAN *veterinary antibacterial* [also: aminitrozole; acinitrazole]
nitracrine INN
nitrafudam INN *antidepressant* [also: nitrafudam HCl]
nitrafudam HCl USAN *antidepressant* [also: nitrafudam]
nitralamine HCl USAN *antifungal*
nitramisole INN *anthelmintic* [also: nitramisole HCl]
nitramisole HCl USAN *anthelmintic* [also: nitramisole]
nitraquazone INN
nitratophenylmercury [see: phenylmercuric nitrate]
nitrazepam USAN, INN, BAN *anticonvulsant; hypnotic*
Nitrazine Paper rolls OTC *in vitro diagnostic aid for urine pH determination*
nitre, sweet spirit of [see: ethyl nitrite]
nitrefazole INN, BAN
nitrendipine USAN, INN, BAN *antihypertensive; calcium channel blocker*
nitric acid NF *acidifying agent*
nitricholine perchlorate INN
p-**nitrobenzenearsonic acid** [see: nitarsone]
Nitro-Bid IV infusion ℞ *antianginal; perioperative antihypertensive; for congestive heart failure with myocardial infarction* [nitroglycerin]
Nitro-Bid ointment, Plateau Caps (controlled-release capsules) ℞ *angina pectoris* [nitroglycerin]

Nitrocine Timecaps (timed-release capsules), transdermal patch ℞ antianginal [nitroglycerin]
nitroclofene INN
nitrocycline USAN, INN *antibacterial*
nitrodan USAN, INN *anthelmintic*
Nitrodisc transdermal patch ℞ antianginal [nitroglycerin]
Nitro-Dur transdermal patch ℞ antianginal [nitroglycerin]
nitroethanolamine [see: aminoethyl nitrate]
Nitrofan capsules ℞ *urinary antibacterial* [nitrofurantoin]
nitrofuradoxadone [see: furmethoxadone]
nitrofural INN *topical anti-infective* [also: nitrofurazone]
nitrofurantoin USP, INN *urinary bacteriostatic*
nitrofurantoin sodium
nitrofurazone USP *broad-spectrum bactericidal; adjunct to burn treatments* [also: nitrofural]
nitrofurmethone [see: furaltadone]
nitrofuroxizone [see: nidroxyzone]
Nitrogard transmucosal extended-release tablets *antianginal* [nitroglycerin]
nitrogen (N$_2$) NF *air displacement agent; element (N)*
nitrogen monoxide [see: nitrous oxide]
nitrogen mustard [see: mechlorethamine HCl]
nitrogen oxide (N$_2$O) [see: nitrous oxide]
nitroglycerin USP *coronary vasodilator; antianginal* [also: glyceryl trinitrate]
Nitroglyn extended-release capsules ℞ *antianginal* [nitroglycerin]
nitrohydroxyquinoline [see: nitroxoline]
Nitrol ointment, Appli-Kit (ointment & adhesive dosage covers) ℞ *antianginal* [nitroglycerin]

Nitrolan liquid OTC *oral nutritional supplement*
Nitrolingual Spray lingual aerosol ℞ *antianginal* [nitroglycerin]
nitromannitol [see: mannitol hexanitrate]
nitromersol USP *topical anti-infective*
nitromide USAN *coccidiostat for poultry; antibacterial*
nitromifene INN
nitromifene citrate USAN *antiestrogen*
Nitrong ointment, tablets ℞ *antianginal* [nitroglycerin]
Nitropress powder for IV injection, ADD-Vantage vials, Univials ℞ *antihypertensive for hypertensive crisis* [sodium nitroprusside]
nitroprusside sodium [see: sodium nitroprusside]
nitroscanate USAN, INN *veterinary anthelmintic*
Nitrostat IV infusion (discontinued 1992) ℞ *antianginal* [nitroglycerin]
Nitrostat sublingual tablets ℞ *antianginal* [nitroglycerin]
nitrosulfathiazole INN [also: para-nitrosulfathiazole]
nitrous acid, sodium salt [see: sodium nitrite]
nitrous oxide (N$_2$O) USP *inhalation general anesthetic*
nitroxinil INN
nitroxoline INN, BAN
nivacortol INN *glucocorticoid* [also: nivazol]
nivadipine [see: nilvadipine]
nivaquine [see: chloroquine phosphate]
nivazol USAN *glucocorticoid* [also: nivacortol]
Nivea After Tan; Nivea Moisturizing; Nivea Moisturizing Extra Enriched lotion OTC *moisturizer; emollient*
Nivea Creme Soap bar OTC *therapeutic skin cleanser*

Nivea Moisturizing; Nivea Skin oil OTC *moisturizer; emollient*
Nivea Ultra Moisturizing Creme OTC *moisturizer; emollient*
nivimedone sodium USAN *antiallergic*
Nix creme rinse OTC *pediculicide; scabicide* [permethrin; alcohol]
nixylic acid INN
nizatidine USAN, USP, INN, BAN *treatment of duodenal ulcers; histamine H₂ antagonist*
nizofenone INN
Nizoral cream, shampoo ℞ *topical antifungal* [ketoconazole]
Nizoral tablets ℞ *systemic antifungal* [ketoconazole]
N-Multistix; N-Multistix SG reagent strips OTC *in vitro diagnostic aid for multiple urine products*
nobelium *element (No)*
noberastine USAN, INN, BAN *antihistaminic*
nocloprost INN
nocodazole USAN, INN *antineoplastic*
Noctec capsules, syrup (discontinued 1992) ℞ *sedative; hypnotic* [chloral hydrate]
N'Odor softgels OTC *urinary and fecal odor control* [chlorophyllin copper complex]
NōDōz tablets (discontinued 1993) OTC *CNS stimulant; analeptic* [caffeine]
nofecainide INN
nogalamycin USAN, INN *antineoplastic*
No-Hist capsules ℞ *nasal decongestant* [phenylephrine HCl; phenylpropanolamine HCl; pseudoephedrine HCl]
Nolahist tablets OTC *antihistamine* [phenindamine tartrate]
Nolamine timed-release tablets ℞ *decongestant; antihistamine* [phenylpropanolamine HCl; chlorpheniramine maleate; phenindamine tartrate]

Nolex LA long-acting tablets ℞ *decongestant; expectorant* [phenylpropanolamine HCl; guaifenesin]
nolinium bromide USAN, INN *antisecretory; antiulcerative*
Noludar 200 tablets (discontinued 1991) ℞ *sedative; hypnotic* [methyprylon]
Noludar 300 capsules ℞ *sedative; hypnotic* [methyprylon]
Nolvadex tablets ℞ *hormonal therapy for breast cancer* [tamoxifen citrate]
nomegestrol INN
nomelidine INN
nomifensine INN *antidepressant* [also: nomifensine maleate]
nomifensine maleate USAN *antidepressant* [also: nomifensine]
nonabine INN, BAN
nonabsorbable surgical suture [see: suture, nonabsorbable surgical]
nonachlazine [now: azaclorzine HCl]
nonaperone INN
nonapyrimine INN
nonathymulin INN
nondestearinated cod liver oil [see: cod liver oil, nondestearinated]
nonivamide INN
non-nucleoside reverse transcriptase inhibitor *investigational antiviral for AIDS* [also: L-696,229; L-697-661]
nonoxinol 15 INN *surfactant* [also: nonoxynol 15]
nonoxinol 30 INN *surfactant* [also: nonoxynol 30]
nonoxinol 4 INN *surfactant* [also: nonoxynol 4]
nonoxinol 9 INN *wetting and solubilizing agent; spermaticide* [also: nonoxynol 9]
nonoxynol 10 NF *surfactant*
nonoxynol 15 USAN *surfactant* [also: nonoxinol 15]
nonoxynol 30 USAN *surfactant* [also: nonoxinol 30]
nonoxynol 4 USAN *surfactant* [also: nonoxinol 4]

nonoxynol 9 USAN, USP *wetting and solubilizing agent; spermicide* [also: nonoxinol 9]
nonylphenoxypolyethoxyethanol [see: nonoxynol 4, 9, 15, & 30]
Nootropil *(orphan: myoclonus)* [piracetam]
noracymethadol INN *analgesic* [also: noracymethadol HCl]
noracymethadol HCl USAN *analgesic* [also: noracymethadol]
Noradex tablets ℞ *skeletal muscle relaxant* [orphenadrine citrate]
noradrenaline bitartrate [see: norepinephrine bitartrate]
Noralac chewable tablets OTC *antacid* [calcium carbonate; magnesium carbonate; bismuth subnitrate]
noramidopyrine methanesulfonate sodium [see: dipyrone]
norandrostenolone phenylpropionate [see: nandrolone phenpropionate]
norbolethone USAN *anabolic* [also: norboletone]
norboletone INN *anabolic* [also: norbolethone]
norbudrine INN [also: norbutrine]
norbutrine BAN [also: norbudrine]
Norcept-E 1/35 tablets ℞ *oral contraceptive* [ethinyl estradiol; norethindrone]
Norcet 7 capsules, tablets (discontinued 1991) ℞ *narcotic analgesic* [hydrocodone bitartrate; acetaminophen]
Norcet capsules ℞ *narcotic analgesic* [hydrocodone bitartrate; acetaminophen]
norclostebol INN
norcodeine INN, BAN
Norcuron powder for IV injection ℞ *neuromuscular blocker* [vecuronium bromide]
norcycline [see: sancycline]
nordazepam INN
nordefrin HCl NF

Nordette-21; Nordette-28 tablets ℞ *oral contraceptive* [ethinyl estradiol; levonorgestrel]
nordinone INN
Norditropin ℞ *(orphan: growth failure; Turner syndrome; anovulation; severe burns)* [somatropin]
Nordryl capsules, elixir, cough syrup, injection ℞/OTC *antihistamine; motion sickness preventative; sleep aid; antiparkinsonian* [diphenhydramine HCl]
Nordryl Cough Syrup OTC *antitussive* [diphenhydramine HCl]
Norel Plus capsules ℞ *decongestant; antihistamine; analgesic* [phenylpropanolamine HCl; chlorpheniramine maleate; phenyltoloxamine citrate; acetaminophen]
norephedrine HCl [see: phenylpropanolamine HCl]
norepinephrine INN *adrenergic; vasoconstrictor; vasopressor for shock* [also: norepinephrine bitartrate]
norepinephrine bitartrate USAN, USP *adrenergic; vasoconstrictor; vasopressor for shock* [also: norepinephrine]
norethandrolone NF, INN
Norethin 1/35 E tablets ℞ *oral contraceptive* [ethinyl estradiol; norethindrone]
Norethin 1/50 M tablets ℞ *oral contraceptive* [mestranol; norethindrone]
norethindrone USP *progestin* [also: norethisterone]
norethindrone acetate USP *progestin*
norethisterone INN, BAN *progestin* [also: norethindrone]
norethynodrel USAN, USP *progestin* [also: noretynodrel]
noretynodrel INN *progestin* [also: norethynodrel]
noreximide INN
norfenefrine INN
Nor-Feran IM, IV ℞ *antianemic* [iron dextran]

Norflex sustained-release tablets, IV or IM injection ℞ *muscle relaxant* [orphenadrine citrate]
norfloxacin USAN, USP, INN, BAN *broad-spectrum bactericidal antibiotic*
norfloxacin succinil INN
norflurane USAN, INN *inhalation anesthetic*
Norgesic; Norgesic Forte tablets ℞ *skeletal muscle relaxant; analgesic; CNS stimulant* [orphenadrine citrate; aspirin; caffeine]
norgesterone INN
norgestimate USAN, INN, BAN *progestin*
norgestomet USAN, INN *progestin*
***d*-norgestrel** *(incorrect enantiomer designation)* [now: levonorgestrel]
norgestrel USAN, USP, INN *progestin*
D-norgestrel [see: levonorgestrel]
norgestrienone INN
Norinyl 1 + 35 tablets ℞ *oral contraceptive* [norethindrone; ethinyl estradiol]
Norinyl 1 + 50 tablets ℞ *oral contraceptive* [norethindrone; mestranol]
Norisodrine Aerotrol (inhalation aerosol) ℞ *bronchodilator* [isoproterenol HCl]
Norisodrine with Calcium Iodide syrup ℞ *bronchodilator; expectorant* [isoproterenol sulfate; calcium iodide; alcohol]
Norlac Rx tablets ℞ *vitamin/mineral/calcium/iron supplement* [multiple vitamins & minerals; calcium; iron; folic acid]
Norlestrin 1/50; Norlestrin 21 2.5/50 tablets ℞ *oral contraceptive* [ethinyl estradiol; norethindrone acetate]
Norlestrin Fe 1/50; Norlestrin Fe 2.5/50 tablets ℞ *oral contraceptive* [ethinyl estradiol; norethindrone acetate; ferrous fumarate]
norletimol INN
norleusactide INN [also: pentacosactride]

norlevorphanol INN, BAN
Norlutate tablets ℞ *progestin; amenorrhea; functional uterine bleeding; endometriosis* [norethindrone acetate]
Norlutin tablets ℞ *progestin; amenorrhea; functional uterine bleeding* [norethindrone]
½ normal saline (½ NS; 0.45% sodium chloride) *electrolyte replacement*
line solution]
normal serum albumin [see: albumin, human]
normethadone INN, BAN
normethandrolone [see: normethandrone]
normethandrone
normethisterone [see: normethandrone]
Normiflo ℞ *investigational anticoagulant for hip and knee surgery*
Normodyne tablets, IV ℞ *antihypertensive; alpha- and beta-andrenergic blocking agent* [labetalol HCl]
normorphine INN, BAN
Normosang *(orphan: acute symptomatic porphyria)* [heme arginate]
Normosol-M 900 Cal IV infusion (discontinued 1991) ℞ *intravenous nutritional/electrolyte therapy* [combined electrolyte solution; fructose]
Normosol-M and 5% Dextrose; Normosol-R and 5% Dextrose IV infusion ℞ *intravenous nutritional/electrolyte therapy* [combined electrolyte solution; dextrose]
Normosol-R; Normosol-R pH 7.4 IV infusion ℞ *intravenous electrolyte therapy* [combined electrolyte solution]
Normozide film-coated tablets ℞ *antihypertensive* [labetalol; hydrochlorothiazide]
Nor-O.D. tablets ℞ *oral contraceptive (progestin only)* [norethindrone]
Noroxin film-coated tablets ℞ *broad-spectrum fluoroquinolone-type antibiotic* [norfloxacin]

Norpace capsules ℞ *antiarrhythmic* [disopyramide phosphate]
Norpace CR controlled-release capsules ℞ *antiarrhythmic* [disopyramide phosphate]
norpipanone INN, BAN
Norplant implant Silastic capsules ℞ *implant contraceptive system* [levonorgestrel]
Norpramin film-coated tablets ℞ *tricyclic antidepressant* [desipramine HCl]
norpseudoephedrine [see: cathine]
Nor-QD tablets ℞ *oral contraceptive* [norethindrone]
nortestosterone phenylpropionate [see: nandrolone phenpropionate]
Nor-Tet capsules ℞ *broad-spectrum antibiotic* [tetracycline HCl]
nortetrazepam INN
nortriptyline HCl USAN, USP, INN *tricyclic antidepressant*
Norvasc tablets ℞ *antianginal; antihypertensive; calcium channel blocker* [amlodipine]
norvinisterone INN
norvinodrel [see: norgesterone]
Norwich Aspirin tablets (discontinued 1992) OTC *analgesic; antipyretic; anti-inflammatory; antirheumatic* [aspirin]
Norwich Extra Strength tablets OTC *analgesic; antipyretic; anti-inflammatory; antirheumatic* [aspirin]
Norzine IM injection, suppositories, tablets ℞ *antiemetic* [thiethylperazine maleate]
NoSalt; NoSalt Seasoned OTC *salt substitute* [potassium chloride]
nosantine INN, BAN
noscapine USP, INN *antitussive*
noscapine HCl NF
nosiheptide USAN, INN *veterinary growth stimulant*
Nōstril; Children's Nōstril nasal spray OTC *nasal decongestant* [phenylephrine HCl]

Nōstrilla nasal spray OTC *nasal decongestant* [oxymetazoline HCl]
notensil maleate [see: acepromazine]
Nova-Dec tablets OTC *vitamin/mineral/iron supplement* [multiple vitamins & minerals; iron; folic acid; biotin]
Novafed A sustained-release capsules ℞ *decongestant; antihistamine* [pseudoephedrine HCl; chlorpheniramine maleate]
Novafed timed-release capsules ℞ *nasal decongestant* [pseudoephedrine HCl]
Novagest Expectorant with Codeine liquid ℞ *decongestant; antitussive; expectorant* [pseudoephedrine HCl; codeine phosphate; guaifenesin; alcohol]
Novahistine DH liquid ℞ *antitussive; decongestant; antihistamine* [pseudoephedrine HCl; codeine phosphate; chlorpheniramine maleate; alcohol]
Novahistine DMX liquid OTC *antitussive; decongestant; antihistamine* [pseudoephedrine HCl; guaifenesin; dextromethorphan hydrobromide; alcohol]
Novahistine elixir OTC *decongestant; antihistamine* [chlorpheniramine maleate; phenylephrine HCl]
Novahistine Expectorant liquid ℞ *expectorant; antitussive; decongestant* [pseudoephedrine HCl; guaifenesin; codeine phosphate; alcohol]
novamidon [see: aminopyrine]
Novamine; Novamine 15% IV infusion ℞ *total parenteral nutrition; peripheral parenteral nutrition* [multiple essential & nonessential amino acids]
Novantrone IV injection ℞ *antineoplastic antibiotic; (orphan: acute myelogenous leukemia; acute nonlymphocytic leukemia)* [mitoxantrone HCl]
Novapren ℞ *investigational antiviral for AIDS*

novobiocin INN, BAN *bacteriostatic antibiotic* [also: novobiocin calcium]

novobiocin calcium USP *bacteriostatic antibiotic* [also: novobiocin]

novobiocin sodium USP *bacteriostatic antibiotic*

Novocain injection ℞ *injectable local anesthetic* [procaine HCl]

Novolin 70/30 suspension for injection, PenFill (cartridge) OTC *antidiabetic* [isophane insulin (human); insulin (human)]

Novolin L suspension for injection, PenFill (cartridge) OTC *antidiabetic* [insulin zinc (human)]

Novolin N suspension for injection, PenFill (cartridge) OTC *antidiabetic* [isophane insulin (human)]

Novolin R injection, PenFill (cartridge) OTC *antidiabetic* [insulin (human)]

noxiptiline INN [also: noxiptyline]

noxiptyline BAN [also: noxiptiline]

noxythiolin BAN [also: noxytiolin]

noxytiolin INN [also: noxythiolin]

NP (nifurpipone) [q.v.]

NP-27 solution, powder, spray powder, cream OTC *topical antifungal* [tolnaftate]

NPA (novel plasminogen activator) ℞ *investigational treatment for heart attack and blood clot disorders*

NPH (neutral protamine Hagedorn) insulin [see: insulin, isophane]

NPH Iletin I (beef) subcu injection OTC *antidiabetic* [isophane insulin]

NPH Iletin I (pork) subcu injection OTC *antidiabetic* [isophane insulin]

NPH Iletin I subcu injection OTC *antidiabetic* [isophane insulin (beef-pork)]

NPH Iletin II (beef) subcu injection OTC *antidiabetic* [isophane insulin]

NPH Iletin II (pork) subcu injection OTC *antidiabetic* [isophane insulin]

NPH Insulin suspension for injection OTC *antidiabetic* [isophane insulin (beef)]

NPH Purified Pork Isophane Insulin suspension for injection OTC *antidiabetic* [isophane insulin (pork)]

NS (normal saline) [q.v.]

NTS transdermal patches ℞ *antianginal* [nitroglycerin]

NTZ Long Acting nasal spray, nose drops OTC *nasal decongestant* [oxymetazoline HCl]

Nu Soap *hypoallergenic soap substitute*

Nubain IV, subcu or IM injection ℞ *narcotic agonist-antagonist analgesic* [nalbuphine HCl]

nuclomedone INN

nuclotixene INN

Nucofed Expectorant; Nucofed Pediatric Expectorant syrup ℞ *antitussive; decongestant; expectorant* [codeine phosphate; pseudoephedrine HCl; guaifenesin; alcohol]

Nucofed syrup, capsules ℞ *antitussive; decongestant* [codeine phosphate; pseudoephedrine HCl]

Nucotuss Expectorant; Nucotuss Pediatric Expectorant liquid *antitussive; decongestant; expectorant* [codeine phosphate; pseudoephedrine HCl; guaifenesin; alcohol]

Nudit cream OTC *depilatory*

nufenoxole USAN, INN *antiperistaltic*

Nu-Iron 150 capsules OTC *hematinic* [polysaccharide-iron complex]

Nu-Iron elixir OTC *hematinic* [polysaccharide-iron complex]

Nu-Iron Plus elixir ℞ *hematinic* [polysaccharide iron complex; vitamin B_{12}; folic acid]

Nu-Iron V film-coated tablets ℞ *vitamin/iron supplement* [multiple vitamins; polysaccharide iron complex; folic acid]

Nu'Leven enteric-coated tablets (discontinued 1991) OTC *digestive enzymes* [pancreatic enzyme concentrate; ox bile extract; cellulase; pepsin]

Nulicaine injection ℞ *injectable local anesthetic* [lidocaine HCl]

Nullo tablets OTC *vulnerary; fecal and urinary odor control* [chlorophyllin copper complex]

NuLytely powder for oral solution ℞ *pre-procedure bowel cleansing* [sodium bicarbonate; sodium chloride; potassium chloride]

Numorphan IV, subcu or IM injection ℞ *narcotic analgesic; preoperative support of anesthesia; (orphan: narcotic-tolerant pain)* [oxymorphone HCl]

Numzident gel OTC *topical oral anesthetic* [benzocaine]

Num-zit lotion, gel OTC *topical oral anesthetic; antipruritic/counterirritant* [benzocaine; menthol]

Nupercainal ointment, cream OTC *topical local anesthetic* [dibucaine]

Nupercainal suppositories OTC *astringent; adsorbent* [zinc oxide; bismuth subgallate]

Nuprin tablets, caplets OTC *nonsteroidal anti-inflammatory drug (NSAID); antiarthritic; analgesic* [ibuprofen]

Nuromax IV ℞ *neuromuscular blocker* [doxacurium chloride]

Nursette (trademarked form) *prefilled disposable bottle*

Nursoy liquid OTC *hypoallergenic infant food* [soybean protein formula]

Nu-Salt OTC *salt substitute* [potassium chloride]

nutmeg oil NF

Nutracort cream, lotion ℞ *topical corticosteroid* [hydrocortisone]

Nutraderm OTC *lotion base*

Nutraderm Bath Oil OTC *bath emollient*

Nutraderm cream, lotion OTC *moisturizer; emollient*

Nutraloric powder OTC *oral nutritional supplement*

Nutramigen liquid, Nursette (prefilled disposable bottle) OTC *hypoallergenic infant food* [protein hydrolysate formula]

Nutraplus cream, lotion OTC *moisturizer; emollient; keratolytic* [urea]

Nutra-Soothe bath oil OTC *bath emollient* [colloidal oatmeal; light mineral oil]

Nutra-Support capsules OTC *dietary supplement* [multiple vitamins & minerals]

NutraTear eye drops OTC *ocular moisturizer/lubricant*

Nutren 1.0; Nutren 1.5; Nutren 2.0 liquid OTC *oral nutritional supplement*

Nutrex tablets (discontinued 1992) OTC *vitamin/mineral/iron supplement* [multiple vitamins & minerals; iron; biotin]

Nutricon tablets OTC *vitamin/mineral/calcium/iron supplement* [multiple vitamins & minerals; calcium; iron; folic acid; biotin]

Nutrilan liquid OTC *oral nutritional supplement*

NutriLipid 10%; NutriLipid 20% IV infusion (discontinued 1992) ℞ *nutritional therapy* [intravenous fat emulsion]

Nutrilyte; Nutrilyte II IV admixture ℞ *intravenous electrolyte therapy* [combined elecrolyte solution]

Nutrineal PD-2 Peritoneal Dialysis Solution with 1.1% Amino Acid ℞ *(orphan: malnourishment of continuous ambulatory peritoneal dialysis)*

Nutropin ℞ *(orphan: growth failure; Turner syndrome; anovulation; severe burns)* [somatropin]

Nutrox capsules OTC *dietary supplement* [multiple vitamins, minerals & amino acids]

nuvenzepine INN

nyctal [see: carbromal]

nydrane [see: benzchlorpropamide]

Nydrazid IM injection ℞ *tuberculostatic* [isoniazid]
nylestriol USAN *estrogen* [also: nilestriol]
nylidrin HCl USP *peripheral vasodilator* [also: buphenine]
NyQuil Cough/Cold, Children's liquid OTC *pediatric decongestant, antihistamine and antitussive* [pseudoephedrine HCl; chlorpheniramine maleate; dextromethorphan hydrobromide]
NyQuil LiquiCaps (liquid-filled capsules) OTC *decongestant; antihistamine; antitussive; analgesic* [pseudoephedrine HCl; diphenhydramine HCl; dextromethorphan hydrobromide; acetaminophen]
NyQuil Nighttime Cold/Flu Medicine liquid OTC *decongestant; antihistamine; antitussive; analgesic* [pseudoephedrine HCl; doxylamine succinate; dextromethorphan hydrobromide; acetaminophen; alcohol]
NyQuil Nighttime Head Cold, Allergy Formula, Children's liquid OTC *pediatric decongestant and antihistamine* [pseudoephedrine HCl; chlorpheniramine maleate]
Nystaform ointment (discontinued 1991) ℞ *topical antifungal* [nystatin; iodochlorhydroxyquin]
nystatin USP, INN, BAN *antifungal*
Nystatin-LF I.V. ℞ *investigational antiviral for AIDS* [AR-121 (drug code—generic name not yet approved)]
Nystex cream, ointment, oral suspension ℞ *topical antifungal* [nystatin]
Nytcold Medicine liquid OTC *decongestant; antihistamine; antitussive; analgesic* [pseudoephedrine HCl; doxylamine succinate; dextromethorphan hydrobromide; acetaminophen; alcohol]
NyteTime liquid OTC *analgesic; antipyretic; antitussive; antihistamine; decongestant* [acetaminophen; dextromethorphan hydrobromide; doxylamine succinate; pseudoephedrine HCl]
Nytol tablets OTC *antihistaminic sleep aid* [diphenhydramine HCl]
Nytyme liquid OTC *analgesic; decongestant; antihistamine; antitussive* [acetaminophen; doxylamine succinate; pseudoephedrine HCl; dextromethorphan hydrobromide; alcohol]

O

O₂ (oxygen) [q.v.]
OAP (Oncovin, ara-C, prednisone) *chemotherapy protocol*
oatmeal, colloidal *demulcent*
Obalan tablets ℞ *anorexiant* [phendimetrazine tartrate]
obecalp *placebo (spelled backward)*
Obe-nix capsules ℞ *appetite suppressant* [phentermine HCl]
Obephen capsules ℞ *anorexiant* [phentermine HCl]
Obermine capsules (discontinued 1992) ℞ *anorexiant* [phentermine HCl]
Obestin-30 capsules (discontinued 1992) ℞ *anorexiant* [phentermine HCl]
Obetrol-10; Obetrol-20 tablets ℞ *CNS stimulant* [dextroamphetamine sulfate; dextroamphetamine saccharate; amphetamine aspartate; amphetamine sulfate]

Obeval tablets (discontinued 1991) ℞ *anorexiant* [phendimetrazine tartrate]
obidoxime chloride USAN, INN *cholinesterase reactivator*
Ob-tinic tablets (discontinued 1991) ℞ *antianemic* [ferrous fumarate; multiple vitamins]
Obtundia Calamine cream OTC *astringent; antiseptic; topical anesthetic* [camphor; metacresol; zinc oxide; calamine]
Obtundia topical spray, swab pads, liquid, cream OTC *germicide; fungicide; topical anesthetic* [camphor; metacresol]
O-Cal f.a. tablets ℞ *vitamin/mineral/calcium/iron supplement and dental caries preventative* [multiple vitamins & minerals; calcium; iron; folic acid; sodium fluoride]
Occlusal; Occlusal-HP liquid OTC *topical keratolytic* [salicylic acid]
Occucoat ophthalmic solution ℞ *ophthalmic surgical aid; gonioscopic examination aid* [hydroxypropyl methylcellulose]
Occusoft V.M.S. film-coated tablets OTC *vitamin/mineral supplement* [vitamins A, C & E; multiple minerals]
Ocean Mist nasal spray OTC *nasal moisturizer* [sodium chloride (saline)]
ocfentanil INN *narcotic analgesic* [also: ocfentanil HCl]
ocfentanil HCl USAN *narcotic analgesic* [also: ocfentanil]
ociltide INN
OCL oral solution ℞ *pre-procedure bowel evacuant* [polyethylene glycol-electrolyte solution]
ocrase INN
ocrilate INN *tissue adhesive* [also: ocrylate]
ocrylate USAN *tissue adhesive* [also: ocrilate]
octabenzone USAN, INN *ultraviolet screen*
octacaine INN
octacosactrin BAN [also: tosactide]

octadecafluorodecehydronaphthalene [see: perflunafene]
octadecanoic acid, calcium salt [see: calcium stearate]
octadecanoic acid, sodium salt [see: sodium stearate]
octadecanoic acid, zinc salt [see: zinc stearate]
1-octadecanol [see: stearyl alcohol]
9-octadecenylamine hydrofluoride [see: dectaflur]
octafonium chloride INN
Octamide PFS IV or IM injection ℞ *antiemetic for chemotherapy; GI stimulant; peristaltic* [metoclopramide monohydrochloride monohydrate]
Octamide tablets (discontinued 1992) ℞ *antidopaminergic; antiemetic; peristaltic* [metoclopramide HCl]
octamoxin INN
octamylamine INN
octanoic acid USAN, INN *antifungal*
octapinol INN
octastine INN
octatropine methylbromide INN, BAN *anticholinergic* [also: anisotropine methylbromide]
octatropone bromide [see: anisotropine methylbromide]
octaverine INN, BAN
octazamide USAN, INN *analgesic*
octenidine INN, BAN *topical anti-infective* [also: octenidine HCl]
octenidine HCl USAN *topical anti-infective* [also: octenidine]
octenidine saccharin USAN *dental plaque inhibitor*
Octicare ear drops, ear drop suspension ℞ *topical corticosteroidal anti-inflammatory; antibiotic* [hydrocortisone; neomycin sulfate; polymyxin B sulfate]
octicizer USAN *plasticizer*
octimibate INN
octisamyl [see: octamylamine]
Octocaine HCl injection ℞ *injectable local anesthetic* [lidocaine HCl]
octoclothepine [see: clorotepine]

octocrilene INN *ultraviolet screen* [also: octocrylene]
octocrylene USAN *ultraviolet screen* [also: octocrilene]
octodecactide [see: codactide]
octodrine USAN, INN *adrenergic; vasoconstrictor; local anesthetic*
octopamine INN
octotiamine INN
octoxinol INN *surfactant/wetting agent* [also: octoxynol 9]
octoxynol 9 USAN, NF *surfactant/wetting agent; spermicide* [also: octoxinol]
octreotide USAN, INN, BAN *gastric antisecretory*
octreotide acetate USAN *gastric antisecretory*
octriptyline INN *antidepressant* [also: octriptyline phosphate]
octriptyline phosphate USAN *antidepressant* [also: octriptyline]
octrizole USAN, INN *ultraviolet screen*
S-octyl thiobenzoate [see: tioctilate]
octyl-2-cyanoacrylate [see: ocrylate]
octyldodecanol NF *oleaginous vehicle*
Ocu-Bath Eye Lotion ophthalmic solution (discontinued 1992) OTC *extraocular irrigating solution* [balanced saline solution]
OcuCaps caplets OTC *vitamin/mineral supplement* [vitamins A, C & E; multiple minerals]
Ocu-Carpine eye drops ℞ *antiglaucoma agent; direct-acting miotic* [pilocarpine HCl]
Ocuclear eye drops OTC *topical ocular vasoconstrictor* [oxymetazoline HCl]
OcuClenz solution OTC *eyelid cleanser*
Ocudose (trademarked delivery device) *single-use eye drop dispenser*
Ocu-Drop ophthalmic solution (discontinued 1992) OTC *extraocular irrigating solution* [balanced saline solution]

Ocufen eye drops ℞ *ocular nonsteroidal anti-inflammatory; intraoperative miosis inhibitor* [flurbiprofen sodium]
ocufilcon A USAN *hydrophilic contact lens material*
ocufilcon B USAN *hydrophilic contact lens material*
ocufilcon C USAN *hydrophilic contact lens material*
ocufilcon D USAN *hydrophilic contact lens material*
ocufilcon E USAN *hydrophilic contact lens material*
Ocuflox ℞ *investigational ophthalmic antibiotic*
Oculinum powder for extraocular muscle injection ℞ *(orphan: blepharospasm and strabismus of dystonia; cervical dystonia; pediatric cerebral palsy)* [botulinum toxin type A]
Ocumeter (trademarked delivery device) *eye drop dispenser*
Ocupress eye drops ℞ *antiglaucoma agent (β-blocker)* [carteolol HCl]
Ocusert Pilo-20; Ocusert Pilo-40 continuous-release ocular wafer ℞ *antiglaucoma agent; direct-acting miotic* [pilocarpine]
Ocutricin Ophthalmic eye drops ℞ *ophthalmic antibiotic* [polymyxin B sulfate; neomycin sulfate; gramicidin]
Ocutricin ophthalmic ointment ℞ *ophthalmic antibiotic* [polymyxin B sulfate; neomycin sulfate; bacitracin]
Ocuvite film-coated tablets OTC *vitamin/mineral supplement* [vitamins A, C & E; multiple minerals]
OCuZIN tablets OTC *vitamin/mineral supplement* [vitamins A, C & E; zinc; copper; selenium]
Odor Free ArthriCare [see: ArthriCare, Odor Free]
Odor-Scrip capsules (discontinued 1991) ℞ *urinary acidifier to control ammonia production* [racemethionine]
oestradiol BAN *estrogen* [also: estradiol]

oestradiol benzoate BAN [also: estradiol benzoate]
oestradiol valerate BAN *estrogen* [also: estradiol valerate]
oestriol succinate BAN *estrogen* [also: estriol; estriol succinate]
oestrogenine [see: diethylstilbestrol]
oestromenin [see: diethylstilbestrol]
oestrone BAN *estrogen* [also: estrone]
Off-Ezy Wart Remover liquid OTC *topical keratolytic* [salicylic acid]
O-Flex IV or IM injection ℞ *skeletal muscle relaxant* [orphenadrine citrate]
ofloxacin USAN, INN, BAN *broad-spectrum bactericidal antibiotic; (orphan: bacterial corneal ulcers)*
ofornine USAN, INN *antihypertensive*
oftasceine INN
Ogen Divide-Tabs (scored tablets) ℞ *hormone for estrogen replacement therapy and osteoporosis prevention* [estropipate sulfate]
Ogen vaginal cream ℞ *hormone; estrogen replacement* [estropipate]
oil of mustard [see: allyl isothiocyanate]
oil ricini [see: castor oil]
Oilatum Soap bar OTC *therapeutic skin cleanser* [polyunsaturated vegetable oil]
ointment, hydrophilic USP *ointment base; oil-in-water emulsion*
ointment, white USP *oleaginous ointment base*
ointment, yellow USP *ointment base*
olaflur USAN, INN, BAN *dental caries prophylactic*
olanzapine USAN *antipsychotic*
olaquindox INN, BAN
old tuberculin (OT) [see: tuberculin]
oleandomycin INN [also: oleandomycin phosphate]
oleandomycin, triacetate ester [see: troleandomycin]
oleandomycin phosphate NF [also: oleandomycin]
oleic acid NF *emulsion adjunct*

oleic acid I 125 USAN *radioactive agent*
oleic acid I 131 USAN *radioactive agent*
oleovitamin A [now: vitamin A]
oleovitamin A & D USP *source of vitamins A and D*
oleovitamin D, synthetic [now: ergocalciferol]
olethytan 20 [see: polysorbate 80]
oletimol INN
oleum caryophylii [see: clove oil]
oleum gossypii seminis [see: cottonseed oil]
oleum maydis [see: corn oil]
oleum ricini [see: castor oil]
oleyl alcohol NF *emulsifying agent; emollient*
oligomycin D [see: rutamycin]
olive oil NF *pharmaceutic aid*
olivomycin INN
olmidine INN
olpimedone INN
olsalazine INN, BAN *GI anti-inflammatory* [also: olsalazine sodium]
olsalazine sodium USAN *GI anti-inflammatory; treatment of ulcerative colitis* [also: olsalazine]
oltipraz INN
olvanil USAN, INN *analgesic*
OM 401 *(orphan: sickle cell disease)*
OMAD (Oncovin, methotrexate/citrovorum factor, Adriamycin, dactinomycin) *chemotherapy protocol*
Omega Oil (discontinued 1992) OTC *counterirritant; topical antiseptic* [methyl salicylate; methyl nicotinate; capsicum oleoresin; histamine dihydrochloride; alcohol]
omega-3 fatty acids [see: doconexent; icosapent; omega-3 marine triglycerides]
omega-3 marine triglycerides BAN [also: doconexent; icosapent]
omeprazole USAN, INN, BAN *gastric acid secretion depressant*
omidoline INN

Omniflox film-sealed tablets (discontinued 1992) ℞ *broad-spectrum fluoroquinolone-type antibiotic* [temafloxacin HCl]

OmniHist L.A. long-acting tablets ℞ *decongestant; antihistamine; anticholinergic* [phenylephrine HCl; chlorpheniramine maleate; methscopolamine nitrate]

Omnipaque injection ℞ *parenteral radiopaque agent* [iohexol]

Omnipen capsules ℞ *penicillin-type antibiotic* [ampicillin, anhydrous]

Omnipen powder for oral suspension ℞ *penicillin-type antibiotic* [ampicillin trihydrate]

Omnipen-N powder for IV or IM injection, ADD-vantage vials ℞ *penicillin-type antibiotic* [ampicillin sodium]

Omniscan ℞ *investigational magnetic resonance imaging agent for the central nervous system* [gadodiamide]

omoconazole INN

omonasteine INN

OMS Concentrate oral solution ℞ *analgesic* [morphine sulfate]

onapristone INN

Oncoject ℞ *investigational antineoplastic*

Oncolysin B ℞ *investigational antineoplastic for B-cell lymphoma, leukemia, AIDS lymphoma and myeloma* [monoclonal antibodies]

OncoRad OV103 ℞ *(orphan: ovarian cancer)*

OncoScint CR/OV ℞ *investigational imaging aid for ovarian and colorectal cancers* [monoclonal antibodies]

OncoScint OV103 *(orphan: diagnostic aid in ovarian carcinoma)* [indium In 111 murine monoclonal antibody B72.3]

OncoScint PR ℞ *investigational imaging aid for prostate cancer* [monoclonal antibodies]

OncoTrac ℞ *investigational diagnostic aid for melanoma and small cell lung cancer* [monoclonal antibodies]

Oncovin IV injection, Hyporets (prefilled syringes) ℞ *antineoplastic* [vincristine sulfate]

ondansetron INN *antiemetic for chemotherapy; antischizophrenic; anxiolytic* [also: ondansetron HCl]

ondansetron HCl USAN *antiemetic for chemotherapy; antischizophrenic; anxiolytic* [also: ondansetron]

1 + 1-F Creme ℞ *topical corticosteroid; antifungal; antibacterial; local anesthetic* [hydrocortisone; iodochlorhydroxyquin; pramoxine]

1% HC ointment ℞ *topical corticosteroid* [hydrocortisone]

One Tablet Daily OTC *vitamin supplement* [multiple vitamins; folic acid]

One Tablet Daily with Iron film-coated tablets OTC *vitamin/iron supplement* [multiple vitamins; iron; folic acid]

One-A-Day Essential; One-A-Day Plus Extra C tablets OTC *vitamin supplement* [multiple vitamins; folic acid]

One-A-Day Maximum Formula tablets OTC *vitamin/mineral/iron supplement* [multiple vitamins & minerals; iron; folic acid; biotin]

One-A-Day Stressgard tablets OTC *vitamin/mineral/iron supplement* [multiple vitamins & minerals; iron; folic acid]

One-A-Day Within (name changed to One-A-Day Women's Formula in 1993)

One-A-Day Women's Formula tablets OTC *vitamin/calcium/iron supplement* [multiple vitamins; calcium; iron; folic acid]

ontianil INN

Ony-Clear Nail aerosol spray ℞ *topical antifungal; antibacterial* [triacetin;

cetylpyridinium chloride; chloroxylenol; benzalkonium chloride]
Onysin liquid OTC *vitamin supplement* [multiple vitamins]
OPAL (Oncovin, prednisone, L-asparaginase) *chemotherapy protocol*
Opcon eye drops ℞ *topical ocular vasoconstrictor* [naphazoline HCl]
Opcon-A eye drops ℞ *topical ocular decongestant/antihistamine* [naphazoline HCl; pheniramine maleate]
Operand solution, prep pads, swab sticks, surgical scrub, perineal wash concentrate, aerosol, Iofoam skin cleanser, ointment, douche OTC *broad-spectrum antimicrobial* [povidone-iodine]
Ophtha P/S Ophthalmic eye drop suspension (discontinued 1992) ℞ *topical ophthalmic corticosteroidal anti-inflammatory; bacteriostatic* [prednisolone acetate; sodium sulfacetamide]
Ophthacet eye drops ℞ *ophthalmic bacteriostatic* [sodium sulfacetamide]
Ophthaine eye drops ℞ *topical ophthalmic anesthetic* [proparacaine HCl]
Ophthalgan Ophthalmic eye drops ℞ *agent to clear edematous cornea for ophthalmoscopic examination* [glycerin]
Ophthetic eye drops ℞ *topical ophthalmic anesthetic* [proparacaine HCl]
Ophthochlor eye drops (discontinued 1992) ℞ *ophthalmic antibiotic* [chloramphenicol]
Ophthocort ophthalmic ointment ℞ *topical ophthalmic corticosteroidal anti-inflammatory; antibiotic* [hydrocortisone acetate; chloramphenicol; polymyxin B sulfate]
opiniazide INN
opipramol INN *antidepressant; antipsychotic* [also: opipramol HCl]
opipramol HCl USAN *antidepressant; antipsychotic* [also: opipramol]
opium USP *narcotic analgesic*
opium, powdered USP

OPP (Oncovin, procarbazine, prednisone) *chemotherapy protocol*
Opticare PMS tablets OTC *vitamin/mineral supplement; digestive enzymes* [multiple vitamins & minerals; iron; folic acid; biotin; pancrelipase]
Opti-Clean; Opti-Clean II solution OTC *contact lens cleaning solution*
Opticrom 4% eye drops ℞ *ocular antiallergin;* (*orphan: vernal keratoconjunctivitis*) [cromolyn sodium]
Opti-Free solution OTC *contact lens disinfectant*
Optigene 3 eye drops OTC *topical ocular decongestant* [tetrahydrozoline HCl]
Optilets-500 Filmtabs (film-coated tablets) OTC *vitamin supplement* [multiple vitamins]
Optilets-M-500 Filmtabs (film-coated tablets) OTC *vitamin/mineral/iron supplement* [multiple vitamins & minerals; iron]
Optimine tablets ℞ *antihistamine* [azatadine maleate]
Optimmune (*orphan: keratoconjunctivitis sicca in Sjögren syndrome*) [cyclosporine]
Optimox Prenatal tablets OTC *vitamin/mineral/calcium/iron supplement* [multiple vitamins & minerals; calcium; iron; folic acid]
Optimyd eye drops ℞ *topical ophthalmic corticosteroidal anti-inflammatory; bacteriostatic* [prednisolone sodium phosphate; sodium sulfacetamide]
Optinaps individually wrapped OTC *disposable hand towelettes*
OptiPranolol eye drops ℞ *antiglaucoma agent (β-blocker)* [metipranolol HCl]
Opti-Pure aerosol solution OTC *contact lens rinsing and storage solution* [saline solution]
Optiray 160; Optiray 240; Optiray 320; Optiray 350 injection ℞ *parenteral radiopaque agent* [ioversol]

Optised eye drops OTC *topical ocular decongestant; astringent; antiseptic* [phenylephrine HCl; zinc sulfate]

Opti-Soft solution OTC *contact lens rinsing and storage solution* [preserved saline solution]

Opti-Tears solution OTC *contact lens rewetting solution*

Optivite P.M.T. tablets OTC *geriatric vitamin/mineral supplement* [multiple vitamins & minerals; folic acid; biotin]

Opti-zyme Enzymatic Cleaner tablets OTC *contact lens enzymatic cleaner*

ORA5 oral liquid OTC *oral anti-infective* [copper sulfate; iodine; potassium iodide]

Orabase Baby teething gel OTC *oral topical anesthetic and analgesic* [benzocaine]

Orabase HCA oral paste ℞ *topical corticosteroid* [hydrocortisone acetate]

Orabase Lip Healer cream OTC *topical anesthetic and analgesic* [benzocaine; allantoin; menthol]

Orabase-B oral paste OTC *oral topical anesthetic* [benzocaine]

Orabase-O orthodontic gel OTC *oral topical anesthetic* [benzocaine]

Orabase-Plain oral paste OTC *relief from minor oral irritations*

Oracin lozenges OTC *topical anesthetic; antipruritic/counterirritant* [benzocaine; menthol]

Oracit solution ℞ *urinary alkalinizing agent* [sodium citrate; citric acid]

Oradex-C troches OTC *topical anesthetic; oral antiseptic* [benzocaine; cetylpyridinium chloride]

Ora-Fresh mouthwash OTC *oral antiseptic/antifungal* [methylparaben; zinc chloride]

Oragest SR sustained-release capsules ℞ *decongestant; antihistamine* [phenylpropanolamine HCl; chlorpheniramine maleate]

Oragrafin Calcium granules for oral suspension ℞ *oral cholecystographic radiopaque agent* [ipodate calcium]

Oragrafin Sodium capsules ℞ *oral cholecystographic radiopaque agent* [ipodate sodium]

Orajel Brace-aid gel OTC *topical oral anesthetic; vulnerary* [benzocaine; allantoin]

Orajel Brace-aid Rinse (discontinued 1993) OTC *topical oral anti-inflammatory/anti-infective for braces* [carbamide peroxide]

Orajel; Maximum Strength Orajel; Baby Orajel gel OTC *topical oral anesthetic* [benzocaine]

Orajel Mouth-Aid liquid OTC *topical oral anesthetic; antiseptic* [benzocaine; cetylpyridinium chloride; alcohol]

Orajel Teeth & Gum Cleanser, Baby gel OTC *removes plaque-like film*

Orajel/d gel OTC *topical anesthetic; analgesic* [benzocaine; eugenol]

Oralet lollypop ℞ *investigational pre-anesthesia narcotic*

Oralone Dental paste ℞ *topical oral corticosteroid* [triamcinolone acetonide]

Oramide tablets ℞ *antidiabetic* [tolbutamide]

Oraminic II subcu or IM injection ℞ *anthistamine; anaphylaxis* [brompheniramine maleate]

Oramorph SR sustained-release tablets ℞ *narcotic analgesic* [morphine sulfate]

orange flower oil NF *flavoring agent; perfume*

orange flower water NF

orange oil NF

orange peel tincture, sweet NF

orange spirit, compound NF

orange syrup NF

Oranyl Plus tablets OTC *decongestant; analgesic; antipyretic* [pseudoephedrine HCl; acetaminophen]

Oranyl tablets OTC *decongestant* [pseudoephedrine HCl]
Orap tablets ℞ *antipsychotic* [pimozide]
Oraphen-PD elixir OTC *analgesic; antipyretic* [acetaminophen]
orarsan [see: acetarsone]
Orasept liquid OTC *oral topical anesthetic; oral antiseptic* [tannic acid; methylbenzethonium chloride; benzocaine; alcohol]
Orasept throat spray OTC *oral anesthetic; oral antiseptic* [benzocaine; methylbenzethonium chloride; alcohol]
Orasone tablets ℞ *glucocorticoids* [prednisone]
Ora-stetic liquid OTC *topical anesthetic; antiseptic; antipruritic* [phenol; phenolate sodium]
Oratect gel OTC *oral topical anesthetic and analgesic* [benzocaine]
Oratrast powder for oral suspension ℞ *GI contrast medium* [barium sulfate]
orazamide INN
Orazinc capsules, tablets OTC *zinc supplement* [zinc sulfate]
orbutopril INN
orciprenaline INN, BAN *bronchodilator* [also: metaproterenol polistirex]
orciprenaline polistirex [see: metaproterenol polistirex]
orconazole INN *antifungal* [also: orconazole nitrate]
orconazole nitrate USAN *antifungal* [also: orconazole]
Ordrine AT extended-release capsules ℞ *antitussive; decongestant* [caramiphen edisylate; phenylpropanolamine HCl]
Ordrine S.R. sustained-release capsules ℞ *decongestant; antihistamine* [phenylpropanolamine HCl; chlorpheniramine maleate]
orestrate INN
orestrol [see: diethylstilbestrol dipropionate]
Oretic tablets ℞ *antihypertensive* [hydrochlorothiazide]

Oreticyl 25; Oreticyl 50; Oreticyl Forte tablets ℞ *antihypertensive* [hydrochlorothiazide; deserpidine]
Oreton Methyl tablets ℞ *androgen for male hypogonadism, impotence and breast cancer* [methyltestosterone]
Orex oral solution OTC *saliva substitute*
Orexin Softab (chewable tablets) (discontinued 1993) OTC *vitamin supplement* [vitamins B_1, B_6 & B_{12}]
Orflagen sustained-release tablets (discontinued 1991) ℞ *skeletal muscle relaxant* [orphenadrine citrate]
ORG 10172 ℞ *investigational antithrombotic for stroke and deep venous thrombosis*
Organidin tablets, elixir, solution ℞ *expectorant* [iodinated glycerol]
Orgaran ℞ *investigational therapy for stroke and deep venous thrombosis* [danaproid]
orgotein USAN, INN, BAN *anti-inflammatory; antirheumatic; (orphan: protection of organ donor tissue from free radicals)*
Orimune oral liquid ℞ *poliomyelitis vaccine* [poliovirus vaccine, live oral trivalent]
Orinase Diagnostic powder for IV injection ℞ *in vivo pancreas function test* [tolbutamide sodium]
Orinase tablets ℞ *antidiabetic* [tolbutamide]
orlipastat [see: orlistat]
orlistat USAN, INN *pancreatic lipase inhibitor*
ormaplatin USAN *antineoplastic*
Ormazine IV or IM injection ℞ *antipsychotic* [chlorpromazine HCl]
ormetroprim USAN, INN *antibacterial*
Ornade Spansules (sustained-release capsules) ℞ *decongestant; antihistamine* [phenylpropanolamine HCl; chlorpheniramine maleate]

Ornex caplets OTC *decongestant; analgesic* [pseudoephedrine HCl; acetaminophen]
ornidazole USAN, INN *anti-infective*
Ornidyl IV injection concentrate ℞ *antiprotozoal; (orphan: sleeping sickness; Pneumocystis carinii pneumonia)* [eflornithine HCl]
ornipressin INN
ornithine (L-ornithine) INN
ornithine vasopressin [see: ornipressin]
ornoprostil INN
orotic acid INN
orotirelin INN
orpanoxin USAN, INN *anti-inflammatory*
orphenadrine citrate [see: orphenadrine citrate]
orphenadrine INN *skeletal muscle relaxant; antihistamine* [also: orphenadrine citrate]
orphenadrine citrate USP *skeletal muscle relaxant; antihistamine* [also: orphenadrine]
Orphenate IV or IM injection ℞ *skeletal muscle relaxant* [orphenadrine citrate]
Orphengesic; Orphengesic Forte tablets ℞ *skeletal muscle relaxant; analgesic; CNS stimulant* [orphenadrine citrate; aspirin; caffeine]
orpressin [see: ornipressin]
Ortega Otic M ear drops ℞ *topical corticosteroidal anti-inflammatory; antibiotic* [hydrocortisone; neomycin sulfate; polymyxin B sulfate]
ortetamine INN
orthesin [see: benzocaine]
Ortho Dienestrol vaginal cream ℞ *estrogen deficiency in menopause* [dienestrol]
Ortho Drops eye drop suspension ℞ *topical ophthalmic corticosteroidal anti-inflammatory; antibiotic* [hydrocortisone acetate; neomycin sulfate]
Ortho-Cept tablets ℞ *oral contraceptive* [ethinyl estradiol; desogestrel]

Orthoclone OKT3 IV injection ℞ *immunosuppressant for organ transplantation* [muromonab-CD3]
Ortho-Creme vaginal cream OTC *spermicidal contraceptive* [nonoxynol 9]
orthocresol NF
Ortho-Cyclen; Ortho Tri-Cyclen tablets ℞ *oral contraceptive* [ethinyl estradiol; norgestimate]
Ortho-Est tablets ℞ *hormone for estrogen replacement therapy and osteoporosis prevention* [estropipate sulfate]
Ortho-Gynol vaginal jelly OTC *spermicidal contraceptive* [octoxynol 9]
Ortholinum *(orphan: spasmodic torticollis)* [botulinum toxin]
Ortho-Novum 1/35; Ortho-Novum 10/11 tablets ℞ *oral contraceptive* [norethindrone; ethinyl estradiol]
Ortho-Novum 1/50 tablets ℞ *oral contraceptive* [mestranol; norethindrone]
Ortho-Novum 7/7/7 tablets ℞ *oral contraceptive* [norethindrone; ethinyl estradiol]
orthotolidine
Ortho-Tricept ℞ *investigational oral contraceptive*
Orthoxicol Cough syrup OTC *decongestant; antihistamine; antitussive* [phenylpropanolamine HCl; chlorpheniramine maleate; dextromethorphan hydrobromide; alcohol]
Orthozyme-CD5+ ℞ *investigational graft-versus-host preventative* [immunoconjugate]
Or-Toptic M eye drop suspension ℞ *topical ophthalmic corticosteroidal anti-inflammatory; bacteriostatic* [prednisolone acetate; sodium sulfacetamide]
Or-Tyl IM injection ℞ *gastrointestinal antispasmodic* [dicyclomine HCl]
Orudis capsules ℞ *nonsteroidal anti-inflammatory drug (NSAID); antiarthritic; analgesic* [ketoprofen]
osalmid INN
osarsal [see: acetarsone]

Os-Cal 250 + D; Os-Cal 500 + D film-coated tablets OTC *dietary supplement* [calcium carbonate; vitamin D]

Os-Cal 500 tablets, chewable tablets OTC *calcium supplement* [calcium carbonate]

Os-Cal Fortified; Os-Cal Plus tablets OTC *vitamin/calcium/iron supplement* [multiple vitamins; calcium carbonate; iron]

osmadizone INN

Osmitrol IV infusion ℞ *osmotic diuretic* [mannitol]

osmium *element (Os)*

Osmoglyn solution ℞ *osmotic diuretic* [glycerin]

Osmolite; Osmolite HN liquid OTC *total enteral nutrition*

Osmovist injection ℞ *parenteral radiopaque agent* [iotrolan]

Osteon-D tablets (discontinued 1992) OTC *calcium supplement* [calcium; vitamin D; phosphorus; magnesium]

Ostiderm lotion OTC *for hyperhidrosis and bromhidrosis* [aluminum sulfate; phenol; zinc oxide]

Osto-K chewable tablets (discontinued 1992) OTC *potassium supplement* [potassium gluconate; potassium chloride; potassium citrate; vitamin C]

ostreogrycin INN, BAN

osvarsan [see: acetarsone]

OT (old tuberculin) [see: tuberculin]

Otic Domeboro ear drops ℞ *antibacterial/antifungal* [acetic acid; aluminum acetate]

Otic Neo-Cort-Dome (discontinued 1991) *antibiotic; topical corticosteroid; antimicrobial* [neomycin sulfate; hydrocortisone; acetic acid]

Otic Tridesilon ear drops ℞ *topical corticosteroidal anti-inflammatory; antibacterial/antifungal* [desonide; acetic acid]

Otic-Care ear drops, otic suspension ℞ *topical corticosteroidal anti-inflammatory; antibiotic* [hydrocortisone; neomycin sulfate; polymyxin B sulfate]

Otic-HC ear drops (discontinued 1992) ℞ *topical corticosteroid; antibacterial/antifungal; anesthetic* [hydrocortisone; pramoxine; chloroxylenol; acetic acid]

Otic-Plain ear drops (discontinued 1992) ℞ *anesthetic; antibacterial/antifungal; anesthetic* [pramoxine HCl; acetic acid; parachlorometaxylenol]

otilonium bromide INN, BAN

otimerate sodium INN

OtiTricin otic suspension ℞ *topical corticosteroidal anti-inflammatory; antibiotic* [hydrocortisone; neomycin sulfate; polymyxin B sulfate]

Oto Ear Drops ℞ *local anesthetic; analgesic* [benzocaine; antipyrine; glycerin]

Otobiotic Otic ear drops ℞ *topical corticosteroidal anti-inflammatory; antibiotic* [hydrocortisone; polymyxin B sulfate]

Otocain ear drops ℞ *topical local anesthetic; anitbacterial/antifungal* [benzocaine; benzethonium chloride]

Otocalm ear drops ℞ *topical local anesthetic; analgesic* [benzocaine; antipyrine]

Otocort ear drops, otic suspension ℞ *topical corticosteroidal anti-inflammatory; antibiotic* [neomycin sulfate; polymyxin B sulfate; hydrocortisone]

Otomycin-HPN Otic ear drops ℞ *topical corticosteroidal anti-inflammatory; antibiotic* [hydrocortisone; neomycin sulfate; polymyxin B sulfate]

Otoreid-HC ear drops (discontinued 1991) ℞ *topical corticosteroidal anti-inflammatory; antibiotic* [hydrocortisone; neomycin sulfate; polymyxin B sulfate]

Otosporin ear drops ℞ *topical corticosteroidal anti-inflammatory; antibiotic* [hydrocortisone; neomycin sulfate; polymyxin B sulfate]

Otrivin nasal spray, nose drops, pediatric drops OTC *nasal decongestant* [xylometazoline HCl]
ouabain USP
Outgro solution OTC *pain relief for ingrown toenails* [tannic acid; chlorobutanol; isopropyl alcohol]
O-V Statin package with both oral tablets & vaginal tablets (discontinued 1992) ℞ *antifungal* [nystatin]
ovandrotone albumin INN, BAN
Ovcon 50; Ovcon 35 tablets ℞ *oral contraceptive* [ethinyl estradiol; norethindrone]
Ovide lotion ℞ *pediculicide* [malathion; isopropyl alcohol]
ovine corticotropin-releasing hormone (*orphan: adrenocorticotropic hormone-dependent Cushing syndrome*)
Ovral tablets ℞ *oral contraceptive* [ethinyl estradiol; norgestrel]
Ovrette tablets ℞ *oral contraceptive (progestin only)* [norgestrel]
OvuGen kit OTC *in vitro diagnostic aid to predict ovulation time*
OvuKIT Self-Test kit OTC *in vitro diagnostic aid to predict ovulation time*
OvuQUICK Self-Test kit OTC *in vitro diagnostic aid to predict ovulation time*
ox bile extract [see: bile salts]
oxabolone cipionate INN
oxabrexine INN
oxaceprol INN
oxacillin INN *antibacterial* [also: oxacillin sodium]
oxacillin sodium USAN, USP *bactericidal antibiotic* [also: oxacillin]
oxadimedine INN
oxadimedine HCl [see: oxadimedine]
oxaflozane INN
oxaflumazine INN
oxafuradene [see: nifuradene]
oxagrelate USAN, INN *platelet antiaggregatory agent*
oxalinast INN
oxaliplatin INN

oxamarin INN *hemostatic* [also: oxamarin HCl]
oxamarin HCl USAN *hemostatic* [also: oxamarin]
oxametacin INN
oxamisole INN *immunoregulator* [also: oxamisole HCl]
oxamisole HCl USAN *immunoregulator* [also: oxamisole]
oxamniquine USAN, USP, INN *antischistosomal; anthelmintic*
oxamphetamine hydrobromide [see: hydroxyamphetamine hydrobromide]
oxamycin [see: cycloserine]
oxanamide INN
Oxandrin tablets ℞ *anabolic steroid for weight gain; (orphan: Turner syndrome; growth and puberty delay; AIDS)* [oxandrolone]
oxandrolone USAN, USP, INN, BAN *androgen; anabolic steroid; (orphan: Turner syndrome; growth and puberty delay; AIDS)*
oxantel INN *anthelmintic* [also: oxantel pamoate]
oxantel pamoate USAN *anthelmintic* [also: oxantel]
oxapadol INN
oxapium iodide INN
oxaprazine
oxapropanium iodide INN
oxaprotiline INN *antidepressant* [also: oxaprotiline HCl]
oxaprotiline HCl USAN *antidepressant* [also: oxaprotiline]
oxaprozin USAN, INN, BAN *nonsteroidal anti-inflammatory drug (NSAID)*
oxarbazole USAN, INN *antiasthmatic*
oxarutine [see: ethoxazorutoside]
oxatomide USAN, INN *antiallergic; antiasthmatic*
oxazafone INN
oxazepam USAN, USP, INN *anxiolytic; minor tranquilizer; alcohol withdrawal therapy*
oxazidione INN

oxazolam INN
oxazolidin [see: oxyphenbutazone]
oxazorone INN
oxcarbazepine INN
oxdralazine INN
oxeladin INN, BAN
oxendolone USAN, INN *antiandrogen for benign prostatic hypertrophy*
oxepinac INN
oxerutins BAN
oxetacaine INN *topical anesthetic* [also: oxethazaine]
oxetacillin INN
2-oxetanone [see: propiolactone]
oxethazaine USAN, BAN *topical anesthetic* [also: oxetacaine]
oxetorone INN *migraine-specific analgesic* [also: oxetorone fumarate]
oxetorone fumarate USAN *migraine-specific analgesic* [also: oxetorone]
oxfenamide [see: oxiramide]
oxfendazole USAN, INN *anthelmintic*
oxfenicine USAN, INN, BAN *vasodilator*
oxibendazole USAN, INN *anthelmintic*
oxibetaine INN
oxibuprocaine chloride [see: benoxinate HCl]
oxichlorochine sulfate [see: hydroxychloroquine sulfate]
oxicinchophen [see: oxycinchophen]
oxiconazole INN, BAN *antifungal* [also: oxiconazole nitrate]
oxiconazole nitrate USAN *antifungal* [also: oxiconazole]
oxicone [see: oxycodone]
oxidized cellulose [see: cellulose, oxidized]
oxidized cholic acid [see: dehydrocholic acid]
oxidized regenerated cellulose [see: cellulose, oxidized regenerated]
oxidopamine USAN, INN *ophthalmic adrenergic*
oxidronic acid USAN, INN, BAN *calcium regulator*
oxifenamate [see: hydroxyphenamate]

oxifentorex INN
Oxi-Freeda tablets OTC *dietary supplement* [multiple vitamins, minerals & amino acids]
oxifungin INN *antifungal* [also: oxifungin HCl]
oxifungin HCl USAN *antifungal* [also: oxifungin]
oxilorphan USAN, INN *narcotic antagonist*
oximetazoline HCl [see: oxymetazoline HCl]
oximetholone [see: oxymetholone]
oximonam USAN, INN *antibacterial*
oximonam sodium USAN *antibacterial*
oxindanac INN
oxiniacic acid INN
oxiperomide USAN, INN *antipsychotic*
oxipertine [see: oxypertine]
oxipethidine [see: hydroxypethidine]
oxiphenbutazone [see: oxyphenbutazone]
oxiphencyclimine chloride [see: oxyphencyclimine HCl]
Oxipor VHC lotion OTC *topical antipsoriatic; antiseborrheic; keratolytic; anesthetic* [coal tar solution; salicylic acid; benzocaine; alcohol]
oxiprocaine [see: hydroxyprocaine]
oxiprogesterone caproate [see: hydroxyprogesterone caproate]
oxipurinol INN *xanthine oxidase inhibitor* [also: oxypurinol]
oxiracetam INN, BAN
oxiramide USAN, INN *antiarrhythmic*
oxisopred INN
Oxistat cream, lotion ℞ *topical antifungal* [oxiconazole nitrate]
oxistilbamidine isethionate [see: hydroxystilbamidine isethionate]
oxisuran USAN, INN *antineoplastic*
oxitefonium bromide INN
oxitetracaine [see: hydroxytetracaine]
oxitetracycline [see: oxytetracycline]
oxitriptan INN
oxitriptyline INN

oxitropium bromide INN, BAN
oxmetidine INN, BAN *antagonist to histamine H₂ receptors* [also: oxmetidine HCl]
oxmetidine HCl USAN *antagonist to histamine H₂ receptors* [also: oxmetidine]
oxmetidine mesylate USAN *antagonist to histamine H₂ receptors*
oxodipine INN
oxogestone INN *progestin* [also: oxogestone phenpropionate]
oxogestone phenpropionate USAN *progestin* [also: oxogestone]
oxolamine INN
oxolinic acid USAN, INN *antibacterial*
oxomemazine INN
oxonazine INN
oxophenarsine INN [also: oxophenarsine HCl]
oxophenarsine HCl USP [also: oxophenarsine]
5-oxoproline [see: pidolic acid]
oxoprostol INN, BAN
oxothiazolidine carboxylate *investigational immunomodulator for AIDS*
oxozepam [see: oxazepam]
oxpentifylline BAN *vasodilator; hemorheologic agent* [also: pentoxifylline]
oxpheneridine INN
oxprenoate potassium INN
oxprenolol INN *coronary vasodilator* [also: oxprenolol HCl]
oxprenolol HCl USAN, USP *coronary vasodilator* [also: oxprenolol]
Oxsoralen lotion ℞ *repigmenting adjunct with ultraviolet A for vitiligo* [methoxsalen]
Oxsoralen; Oxsoralen-Ultra capsules ℞ *antipsoriatic* [methoxsalen]
oxtriphylline USP *bronchodilator* [also: choline theophyllinate]
Oxy 5; Oxy 5 Tinted lotion OTC *topical keratolytic for acne* [benzoyl peroxide]
Oxy 10 wash (liquid), lotion, cover cream OTC *topical keratolytic for acne* [benzoyl peroxide]
Oxy Clean Lathering Facial scrub OTC *abrasive cleanser for acne* [sodium tetraborate decahydrate dissolving particles]
Oxy Clean Medicated Cleanser & Pads OTC *topical acne cleanser* [salicylic acid; menthol]
Oxy Clean Medicated Pads for Sensitive Skin OTC *topical acne cleanser* [salicylic acid; alcohol]
Oxy Clean Soap bar OTC *medicated cleanser for acne* [salicylic acid; sodium borate]
Oxy Medicated Soap bar OTC *medicated cleanser for acne* [triclosan]
Oxy Night Watch lotion OTC *topical acne treatment* [salicylic acid; alcohol; silica]
oxybenzone USAN, USP, INN *ultraviolet screen*
oxybuprocaine INN, BAN *topical anesthetic* [also: benoxinate HCl]
oxybuprocaine HCl [see: benoxinate HCl]
oxybutynin INN, BAN *anticholinergic; urinary antispasmodic* [also: oxybutynin chloride]
oxybutynin chloride USAN, USP *anticholinergic; urinary antispasmodic* [also: oxybutynin]
Oxycel pads, pledgets, strips ℞ *topical hemostatic aid in surgical hemostasis* [oxidized cellulose]
oxychlorosene USAN *topical anti-infective*
oxychlorosene sodium USAN *topical anti-infective*
oxycinchophen INN, BAN
oxyclipine INN *anticholinergic* [also: propenzolate HCl]
oxyclipine HCl [see: propenzolate HCl]
oxyclozanide INN, BAN
oxycodone USAN, INN, BAN *narcotic analgesic*

oxycodone HCl USAN, USP *narcotic analgesic*
oxycodone terephthalate USP *narcotic analgesic*
Oxydess II tablets ℞ *CNS stimulant; amphetamine* [dextroamphetamine sulfate]
oxydimethylquinazine [see: antipyrine]
oxydipentonium chloride INN
oxyethyltheophylline [see: etofylline]
oxyfedrine INN, BAN
oxyfenamate INN *minor tranquilizer* [also: hydroxyphenamate]
oxyfilcon A USAN *hydrophilic contact lens material*
oxygen (O$_2$) USP *medicinal gas; element (O)*
oxygen, polymeric *(orphan: sickle cell anemia)*
oxygen 93 percent USP *medicinal gas*
oxymesterone INN, BAN
Oxymeta 12 nasal spray OTC *decongestant* [oxymetazoline HCl]
oxymetazoline INN, BAN *topical ocular vasoconstrictor; nasal decongestant* [also: oxymetazoline HCl]
oxymetazoline HCl USAN, USP *topical ocular vasoconstrictor; nasal decongestant* [also: oxymetazoline]
oxymetholone USAN, USP, INN, BAN *androgen; anabolic steroid*
oxymethylene urea [see: polynoxylin]
oxymorphone INN, BAN *narcotic analgesic* [also: oxymorphone HCl]
oxymorphone HCl USP *narcotic analgesic; (orphan: narcotic-tolerant pain)* [also: oxymorphone]
oxypendyl INN
oxypertine USAN, INN *antidepressant*
oxyphenbutazone USP, INN *anti-inflammatory; antirheumatic; antipyretic; analgesic*
oxyphencyclimine INN *anticholinergic* [also: oxyphencyclimine HCl]

oxyphencyclimine HCl USP *peptic ulcer adjunct* [also: oxyphencyclimine]
oxyphenhydrazine [see: carsalam]
oxyphenisatin acetate USAN *laxative* [also: oxyphenisatine]
oxyphenisatine INN *laxative* [also: oxyphenisatin acetate]
oxyphenonium bromide
oxyphylline [see: etofylline]
oxypurinol USAN *xanthine oxidase inhibitor* [also: oxipurinol]
oxypyrronium bromide INN
oxyquinoline USAN *disinfectant/antiseptic*
oxyquinoline benzoate [see: benzoxiquine]
oxyquinoline sulfate USAN, NF *complexing agent*
oxyridazine INN
oxysonium iodide INN
oxytetracycline USP, INN *bacteriostatic antibiotic; antirickettsial*
oxytetracycline calcium USP *antibacterial*
oxytetracycline HCl USP *bacteriostatic antibiotic; antirickettsial*
oxytocin USP, INN *oxytocic; posterior pituitary hormone*
Oxyzal Wet Dressing liquid OTC *antiseptic dressing for minor infections* [oxyquinoline sulfate; benzalkonium chloride]
Oysco 500 chewable tablets OTC *calcium supplement* [calcium carbonate]
Oysco D tablets (discontinued 1993) OTC *dietary supplement* [calcium carbonate; vitamin D]
Oyst-Cal 500 film-coated tablets OTC *calcium supplement* [calcium carbonate]
Oyst-Cal-D film-coated tablets OTC *dietary supplement* [calcium carbonate; vitamin D]
Oyster Calcium 500 + D tablets OTC *dietary supplement* [calcium carbonate; vitamin D]

Oyster Calcium tablets OTC *dietary supplement* [calcium carbonate]
Oyster Calcium with Vitamin D tablets OTC *dietary supplement* [calcium carbonate; vitamin D]
Oyster Shell Calcium with Vitamin D tablets OTC *calcium supplement* [calcium carbonate; vitamin D]
Oyster Shell Calcium-500 tablets OTC *calcium supplement* [calcium carbonate]
Oystercal 500 tablets OTC *calcium supplement* [calcium carbonate]
Oystercal-D 250 tablets OTC *dietary supplement* [calcium carbonate; vitamin D]
ozagrel INN
ozolinone USAN, INN *diuretic*

P

P & S liquid OTC *antimicrobial hair dressing* [phenol]
P & S Plus gel OTC *topical antipsoriatic; antiseborrheic; keratolytic* [coal tar solution; salicylic acid]
P & S shampoo OTC *antiseborrheic; keratolytic* [salicylic acid]
P₁E₁; P₂E₁; P₃E₁; P₄E₁; P₆E₁ Drop-Tainers (eye drops) ℞ *antiglaucoma agent* [pilocarpine HCl; epinephrine bitartrate]
³²**P** [see: chromic phosphate P 32]
³²**P** [see: polymetaphosphate P 32]
³²**P** [see: sodium phosphate P 32]
PAB (para-aminobenzoate) [see: aminobenzoic acid]
PABA (para-aminobenzoic acid) [now: aminobenzoic acid]
PABA sodium [see: aminobenzoate sodium]
Pabalate enteric-coated tablets OTC *analgesic; antipyretic; anti-inflammatory* [sodium salicylate; sodium aminobenzoate]
Pabalate-SF enteric-coated tablets ℞ *analgesic; antipyretic; anti-inflammatory* [potassium salicylate; potassium aminobenzoate]
PAB-Esc-C (Platinol, Adriamycin, bleomycin, escalating doses of cyclophosphamide) *chemotherapy protocol*

pabestrol D [see: diethylstilbestrol dipropionate]
PAC (Platinol, Adriamycin, cyclophosphamide) *chemotherapy protocol*
P-A-C tablets OTC *analgesic; antipyretic; anti-inflammatory; sedative* [aspirin; caffeine; tartrazine]
PACE (Platinol, Adriamycin, cyclophosphamide, etoposide) *chemotherapy protocol*
Packer's Pine Tar shampoo, soap OTC *antiseborrheic; antipsoriatic; antipruritic; antibacterial* [pine tar]
paclitaxel *antineoplastic for ovarian cancer*
pacrinolol INN
padimate INN *ultraviolet screen* [also: padimate A]
padimate A USAN *ultraviolet screen* [also: padimate]
padimate O USAN *ultraviolet screen*
pafenolol INN
PAH (para-aminohippurate) [see: aminohippuric acid]
PAHA (para-aminohippuric acid) [see: aminohippuric acid]
Pain Bust-R II cream OTC *counterirritant* [methyl salicylate; menthol]
Pain Reliever tablets OTC *analgesic; antipyretic; anti-inflammatory* [acetaminophen; aspirin; caffeine]

Pain-Alay spray, gargle OTC *oral analgesic*
palatrigine INN, BAN
paldimycin USAN, INN *antibacterial*
paldimycin A [see: paldimycin]
paldimycin B [see: paldimycin]
palestrol [see: diethylstilbestrol]
palinum [see: cyclobarbitone]
palladium *element (Pd)*
palmidrol INN
Palmiron tablets (discontinued 1991) OTC *antianemic* [ferrous fumarate]
Palmiron-C chewable tablets (discontinued 1991) OTC *antianemic* [ferrous fumarate; ascorbic acid]
palmoxirate sodium USAN *antidiabetic* [also: palmoxiric acid]
palmoxiric acid INN *antidiabetic* [also: palmoxirate sodium]
PALS coated tablets OTC *vulnerary; fecal and urinary odor control* [chlorophyllin copper complex]
PAM; L-PAM (phenylalanine mustard) [see: melphalan]
2-PAM (2-pyridine aldoxime methylchloride) [see: pralidoxime chloride]
pamabrom USAN *nonprescription diuretic*
pamaquine naphthoate NF
pamatolol INN *antiadrenergic (β-receptor)* [also: pamatolol sulfate]
pamatolol sulfate USAN *antiadrenergic (β-receptor)* [also: pamatolol]
Pamelor capsules, oral solution ℞ *tricyclic antidepressant* [nortriptyline HCl]
pamidronate disodium USAN *bone resorption suppressant*
pamidronic acid INN, BAN
Pamine tablets ℞ *anticholinergic; peptic ulcer treatment* [methscopolamine bromide]
Pamisyl *(orphan: ulcerative colitis)* [aminosalicylic acid]
Pamprin Maximum Cramp Relief caplets OTC *analgesic; antipyretic; diuretic; antihistaminic sleep aid* [acetaminophen; pamabrom; pyrilamine maleate]
Pamprin Maximum Cramp Relief capsules (discontinued 1992) OTC *analgesic; antipyretic; diuretic; antihistaminic sleep aid* [acetaminophen; pamabrom; pyrilamine maleate]
Pamprin; Multi-Symptom Relief Formula Pamprin tablets OTC *analgesic; antipyretic; diuretic; antihistaminic sleep aid* [acetaminophen; pamabrom; pyrilamine maleate]
Pamprin-IB coated tablets (discontinued 1993) OTC *nonsteroidal anti-inflammatory drug (NSAID); antiarthritic; analgesic* [ibuprofen]
Pan C-500 tablets OTC *dietary supplement* [vitamin C; hesperidin; citrus bioflavonoids]
panadiplon USAN, INN *anxiolytic*
Panadol, Children's chewable tablets, liquid OTC *analgesic; antipyretic* [acetaminophen]
Panadol, Infants' drops OTC *analgesic; antipyretic* [acetaminophen]
Panadol tablets OTC *analgesic; antipyretic* [acetaminophen]
Panadyl Forte sustained-release tablets (discontinued 1993) ℞ *decongestant; antihistamine* [phenylpropanolamine HCl; phenylephrine HCl; chlorpheniramine maleate]
Panadyl sustained-release tablets (discontinued 1992) ℞ *decongestant; antihistamine* [phenylpropanolamine HCl; pyrilamine maleate; pheniramine maleate]
Panafil ointment ℞ *topical enzyme for wound debridement; vulnerary; wound deodorant* [papain; urea; chlorophyllin copper complex]
Panafil White ointment ℞ *topical enzyme for wound debridement; vulnerary* [papain; urea]
Panalgesic cream OTC *counterirritant* [methyl salicylate; menthol]

Panalgesic liniment OTC *counterirritant; topical antiseptic* [methyl salicylate; camphor; menthol; alcohol]

Panasol-S tablets ℞ *glucocorticoids* [prednisone]

pancopride USAN, INN *antiemetic; anxiolytic; peristaltic stimulant*

Pancrease; Pancrease MT 4; Pancrease MT 10; Pancrease MT 16; Pancrease MT 25 capsules containing enteric-coated microtablets ℞ *digestive enzymes* [pancrelipase]

pancreatin USP *digestive enzyme*

Pancreatin, 4X; Pancreatin, 8X tablets OTC *digestive enzymes* [pancreatin]

pancrelipase USAN, USP *digestive enzyme*

Pancrezyme 4X tablets OTC *digestive enzymes* [pancreatin]

pancuronium bromide USAN, INN *neuromuscular blocker; muscle relaxant*

Panex; Panex 500 tablets OTC *analgesic; antipyretic* [acetaminophen]

Panhematin powder for IV injection ℞ *enzyme inhibitor; (orphan: acute intermittent porphyria; hereditary coproporphyria)* [hemin]

panidazole INN, BAN

Panmycin capsules ℞ *broad-spectrum antibiotic* [tetracycline HCl]

panomifene INN

Panorex ℞ *investigational antineoplastic for colorectal cancer; (orphan: pancreatic cancer)* [monoclonal antibody 17-1A]

Panoxyl 5; Panoxyl 10 gel, cleansing bar ℞ *keratolytic for acne* [benzoyl peroxide]

Panoxyl AQ 2.5; Panoxyl AQ 5; Panoxyl AQ 10 gel ℞ *keratolytic for acne* [benzoyl peroxide]

Panscol lotion, ointment OTC *topical keratolytic* [salicylic acid]

pantenicate INN

panthenol USAN, USP, INN *B complex vitamin*

D-panthenol [see: dexpanthenol]

Panthoderm cream OTC *antipruritic; vulnerary; emollient* [dexpanthenol]

Pantopon injection (discontinued 1993) ℞ *narcotic analgesic; sedative; hypnotic* [opium alkaloids HCl]

pantoprazole USAN, INN, BAN *antiulcerative*

DL-pantothenic acid [see: calcium pantothenate, racemic]

pantothenic acid BAN *vitamin B_5; enzyme cofactor* [also: calcium pantothenate]

pantothenol [see: dexpanthenol]

D-pantothenyl alcohol [see: dexpanthenol]

pantothenyl alcohol [see: panthenol]

panuramine INN, BAN

Panwarfin tablets ℞ *anticoagulant* [warfarin sodium]

Panzyme tablets (discontinued 1991) ℞ *digestive enzymes; antispasmodic; sedative* [pancreatin; pepsin; homatropine methylbromide; hyoscyamine sulfate; scopolamine hydrobromide; phenobarbital]

Papadeine #3 tablets ℞ *narcotic analgesic* [codeine phosphate; acetaminophen]

papain USP *topical proteolytic enzyme for necrotic tissue debridement*

papaverine BAN *smooth muscle relaxant; peripheral vasodilator; (orphan: sexual dysfunction in spinal cord injuries)* [also: papaverine HCl]

papaverine HCl USP *smooth muscle relaxant; peripheral vasodilator* [also: papaverine]

papaveroline INN, BAN

Papaya Enzyme chewable tablets OTC *digestive enzymes* [papain; amylase]

Paplex solution ℞ *topical keratolytic* [salicylic acid; lactic acid]

Paplex Ultra solution ℞ *topical keratolytic* [salicylic acid]

Par Decon sustained-action tablets (discontinued 1993) ℞ *decongestant;*

antihistamine [phenylpropanolamine HCl; phenylephrine HCl; phenyltoloxamine citrate; chlorpheniramine maleate]

Par Glycerol C liquid ℞ *expectorant; antitussive* [iodinated glycerol; codeine phosphate]

Par Glycerol DM liquid ℞ *expectorant; antitussive* [iodinated glycerol; dextromethorphan hydrobromide]

Par Glycerol elixir ℞ *expectorant* [iodinated glycerol]

Par vaginal cream (discontinued 1991) ℞ *bacteriostatic; antiseptic; vulnerary* [sulfanilamide; aminacrine HCl; allantoin]

para-aminobenzoate (PAB) [see: aminobenzoic acid]

para-aminobenzoic acid (PABA) [now: aminobenzoic acid]

para-aminohippurate (PAH) [see: aminohippuric acid]

para-aminohippurate sodium [see: aminohippurate sodium]

para-aminohippuric acid (PAHA) [see: aminohippuric acid]

para-aminosalicylate (PAS) [see: aminosalicylic acid]

para-aminosalicylic acid (PASA) [see: aminosalicylic acid]

parabromdylamine maleate [see: brompheniramine maleate]

paracetaldehyde [see: paraldehyde]

paracetamol INN, BAN *analgesic; antipyretic* [also: acetaminophen]

parachlorometaxylenol (PCMX) *topical antiseptic; broad-spectrum antibacterial*

parachlorophenol (PCP) USP *topical antibacterial*

parachlorophenol, camphorated USP *topical dental anti-infective*

paracodin [see: dihydrocodeine]

Paradione capsules, oral solution ℞ *anticonvulsant* [paramethadione]

paraffin NF *stiffening agent*

paraffin, liquid [see: mineral oil]

paraffin, synthetic NF *stiffening agent*

Paraflex tablets ℞ *muscle relaxant* [chlorzoxazone]

paraflutizide INN

Parafon Forte DSC caplets ℞ *muscle relaxant* [chlorzoxazone]

paraformaldehyde USP

ParaGard IUD ℞ *contraceptive* [copper]

Para-Hist HD liquid ℞ *decongestant; antihistamine; antitussive* [phenylephrine HCl; chlorpheniramine maleate; hydrocodone bitartrate]

Para-Hist syrup ℞ *decongestant; antihistamine; antitussive* [codeine phosphate; promethazine HCl; phenylephrine HCl; alcohol]

parahydrecin [now: isomerol]

Paral oral liquid, rectal liquid ℞ *sedative; hypnotic* [paraldehyde]

paraldehyde USP *hypnotic; sedative; anticonvulsant*

paramethadione USP, INN, BAN *anticonvulsant*

paramethasone INN *glucocorticoid* [also: paramethasone acetate]

paramethasone acetate USAN, USP *glucocorticoid* [also: paramethasone]

para-nitrosulfathiazole NF [also: nitrosulfathiazole]

paranyline HCl USAN *anti-inflammatory* [also: renytoline]

parapenzolate bromide USAN, INN *anticholinergic*

Paraplatin powder for IV injection ℞ *antineoplastic for ovarian cancer* [carboplatin]

parapropamol INN

pararosaniline embonate INN *antischistosomal* [also: pararosaniline pamoate]

pararosaniline pamoate USAN *antischistosomal* [also: pararosaniline embonate]

Parathar powder for IV injection ℞ *in vivo diagnostic aid for parathyroid-induced hypocalcemia (orphan)* [teriparatide acetate]

parathesin [see: benzocaine]

parathiazine INN
parathyroid USP *hormone*
paraxazone INN
parbendazole USAN, INN *anthelmintic*
parconazole INN *antifungal* [also: parconazole HCl]
parconazole HCl USAN *antifungal* [also: parconazole]
Par-Drix sustained-release tablets ℞ *decongestant; antihistamine* [pseudoephedrine sulfate; dexbrompheniramine maleate]
Paredrine eye drops ℞ *mydriatic* [hydroxyamphetamine hydrobromide]
paregoric (PG) (a preparation of opium, anise oil, benzoic acid, camphor, alcohol, and glycerin) USP *antiperistaltic; narcotic analgesic*
Paremyd eye drops ℞ *mydriatic* [hydroxyamphetamine hydrobromide; tropicamide]
parenabol [see: boldenone undecylenate]
Parepectolin concentrated liquid OTC *GI adsorbent; antidiarrheal* [attapulgite]
pareptide INN *antiparkinsonian* [also: pareptide sulfate]
pareptide sulfate USAN *antiparkinsonian* [also: pareptide]
parethoxycaine INN
parethoxycaine HCl [see: parethoxycaine]
Par-F tablets ℞ *vitamin/mineral/calcium/iron supplement* [multiple vitamins & minerals; calcium; iron; folic acid]
Pargen Fortified tablets (discontinued 1991) ℞ *skeletal muscle relaxant; analgesic* [chlorzoxazone; acetaminophen]
pargeverine INN
pargolol INN
pargyline INN *antihypertensive* [also: pargyline HCl]
pargyline HCl USAN, USP *antihypertensive* [also: pargyline]

Parhist SR sustained-release capsules ℞ *decongestant; antihistamine* [phenylpropanolamine HCl; chlorpheniramine maleate]
paridocaine INN
Parlodel SnapTabs (scored tablets), capsules ℞ *antiparkinsonian agent; lactation prevention; acromegaly therapy* [bromocriptine mesylate]
Parmine capsules (discontinued 1991) ℞ *anorexiant* [phentermine HCl]
Par-Natal Plus 1 Improved tablets ℞ *vitamin/calcium/iron supplement* [multiple vitamins; calcium; iron; folic acid]
Parnate tablets ℞ *monoamine oxidase (MAO) inhibitor antidepressant* [tranylcypromine sulfate]
parodilol INN
parodyne [see: antipyrine]
paroleine [see: mineral oil]
paromomycin INN, BAN *aminoglycoside bactericidal antibiotic; amebicide* [also: paromomycin sulfate]
paromomycin sulfate USP *aminoglycoside bactericidal antibiotic; amebicide* [also: paromomycin]
paroxetine USAN, INN, BAN *antidepressant*
paroxetine HCl *antidepressant*
paroxyl [see: acetarsone]
paroxypropione INN
parpanit HCl [see: caramiphen HCl]
parsalmide INN
Parsidol tablets ℞ *anticholinergic; antiparkinsonian* [ethopropazine HCl]
Partapp elixir OTC *decongestant; antihistamine* [phenylpropanolamine HCl; brompheniramine maleate]
Partapp TD timed-release tablets ℞ *decongestant; antihistamine* [phenylpropanolamine HCl; phenylephrine HCl; brompheniramine maleate]
particrin USAN, INN *antifungal; antiprotozoal*
Partuss LA long-acting tablets ℞ *decongestant; expectorant* [phenylpropanolamine HCl; guaifenesin]

Par-Vag vaginal suppositories (discontinued 1991) ℞ *bacteriostatic; antiseptic; vulnerary* [sulfanilamide; aminacrine HCl; allantoin]
parvaquone INN, BAN
Parvlex tablets OTC *hematinic* [ferrous fumarate; multiple B vitamins; vitamin C; folic acid]
PAS (para-aminosalicylate) [see: aminosalicylic acid]
PASA (para-aminosalicylic acid) [see: aminosalicylic acid]
pasiniazid INN
Pastilles (dosage form) *troches*
PATCO (prednisone, ara-C, thioguanine, cyclophosphamide, Oncovin) *chemotherapy protocol*
Pathilon film-coated tablets ℞ *peptic ulcer treatment adjunct* [tridihexethyl chloride]
Pathocil capsules, powder for oral suspension ℞ *bactericidal antibiotic (penicillinase-resistant penicillin)* [dicloxacillin sodium monohydrate]
paulomycin USAN, INN *antibacterial*
Pavabid HP capsulets (tablets) ℞ *cerebral and peripheral vasodilator* [papaverine HCl]
Pavabid Plateau Caps (controlled-release capsules) ℞ *cerebral and peripheral vasodilator* [papaverine HCl]
Pavased timed-release capsules ℞ *peripheral vasodilators* [papaverine HCl]
Pavasule timed-release tablets (discontinued 1991) ℞ *peripheral vasodilators* [papaverine HCl]
Pavatine timed-release capsules ℞ *peripheral vasodilators* [papaverine HCl]
Pavatym timed-release capsules (discontinued 1992) ℞ *muscle relaxant* [papaverine HCl]
PAVe (procarbazine, Alkeran, Velban) *chemotherapy protocol*
Paverolan Lanacaps (timed-release capsules) ℞ *peripheral vasodilators* [papaverine HCl]
Pavulon IM injection ℞ *neuromuscular blocker* [pancuronium bromide]

paxamate INN
Paxarel tablets ℞ *anxiolytic; sedative* [acetylcarbromal]
Paxil film-coated tablets ℞ *antidepressant* [paroxetine HCl]
Paxipam tablets ℞ *anxiolytic* [halazepam]
pazelliptine INN
Pazo Hemorrhoid ointment, suppositories OTC *topical anesthetic; vasoconstrictor; astringent* [benzocaine; ephedrine sulfate; camphor; zinc oxide]
pazoxide USAN, INN *antihypertensive*
PBV (Platinol, bleomycin, vinblastine) *chemotherapy protocol*
PBZ (pyribenzamine) [see: tripelennamine]
PBZ tablets, elixir ℞ *antihistamine* [tripelennamine HCl]
PBZ-SR sustained-release tablets ℞ *antihistamine* [tripelennamine HCl]
PC (phosphatidylcholine) [see: lecithin]
PCE (Platinol, cyclophosphamide, etoposide) *chemotherapy protocol*
PCE (polymer-coated erythromycin) [see: erythromycin]
PCE Dispertabs (delayed-release tablets) ℞ *macrolide antibiotic* [erythromycin]
PCMX (parachlorometaxylenol) [q.v.]
PCP (parachlorophenol) [q.v.]
PCP (phenylcyclohexyl piperidine) [see: phencyclidine HCl]
PCV (procarbazine, CCNU, vincristine) *chemotherapy protocol*
PDGA (pteroyldiglutamic acid)
PDLA (phosphinicodilactic acid) [see: foscolic acid]
PDP Liquid Protein OTC *dietary supplement* [hydrolyzed protein; L-tryptophan]
PE (phenylephrine) [q.v.]
PE (polyethylene) [q.v.]
peanut oil NF *solvent*

PEB (Platinol, etoposide, bleomycin) *chemotherapy protocol*
pecazine INN, BAN
pecazine acetate [see: pecazine]
pecilocin INN, BAN
pecocycline INN
pectin USP *suspending agent; protectant; GI adsorbent*
Pedameth capsules, liquid ℞ *urinary acidifier to control ammonia production* [racemethionine]
PediaCare 1 syrup (discontinued 1991) OTC *antitussive* [dextromethorphan hydrobromide]
PediaCare Allergy Formula liquid OTC *antihistamine* [chlorpheniramine maleate]
PediaCare Cold-Allergy chewable tablets OTC *pediatric decongestant and antihistamine* [pseudoephedrine HCl; chlorpheniramine maleate]
PediaCare Cough-Cold Formula; PediaCare Children's Cough-Cold Formula liquid, chewable tablets OTC *pediatric decongestant, antihistamine and antitussive* [pseudoephedrine HCl; chlorpheniramine maleate; dextromethorphan hydrobromide]
PediaCare Infant's Decongestant drops OTC *nasal decongestant* [pseudoephedrine HCl]
PediaCare NightRest liquid OTC *pediatric decongestant, antihistamine and antitussive* [pseudoephedrine HCl; chlorpheniramine maleate; dextromethorphan hydrobromide]
Pediacof syrup ℞ *decongestant; antihistamine; antitussive; expectorant* [phenylephrine HCl; chlorpheniramine maleate; codeine phosphate; potassium iodide; alcohol]
Pediaflor drops ℞ *dental caries preventative* [sodium fluoride]
Pedialyte oral solution OTC *electrolyte replacement* [sodium, potassium, and chloride electrolytes]

PediaPatch transdermal patch ℞ *topical keratolytic* [salicylic acid]
Pediapred oral liquid ℞ *glucocorticoids* [prednisolone sodium phosphate]
PediaProfen oral suspension ℞ *nonsteroidal anti-inflammatory drug (NSAID); antiarthritic; analgesic* [ibuprofen]
PediaSure liquid OTC *oral nutritional supplement*
Pediatric Maintenance Solution (discontinued 1992) ℞ *electrolyte replacement* [sodium chloride; dextrose; sodium lactate]
Pediazole oral suspension ℞ *antibiotic* [erythromycin ethylsuccinate; sulfisoxazole acetyl]
Pedi-Bath Salts OTC *bath emollient*
Pedi-Boro Soak Paks powder packets OTC *astringent wet dressing (modified Burow solution)* [aluminum sulfate; calcium acetate]
Pedi-Cort V Creme ℞ *topical corticosteroid; antifungal; antibacterial* [hydrocortisone; clioquinol]
Pedicran with Iron elixir (discontinued 1991) OTC *antianemic* [ferric pyrophosphate; multiple B vitamins]
Pedi-Dri powder ℞ *topical antifungal; anhidrotic* [zinc undecylenate; aluminum chlorhydroxide; menthol; formaldehyde]
Pediotic ear drop suspension ℞ *topical corticosteroidal anti-inflammatory; antibiotic* [hydrocortisone; neomycin sulfate; polymyxin B sulfate]
Pedi-Pro foot powder OTC *topical antifungal; anhidrotic* [zinc undecylenate; aluminum chlorhydroxide; menthol; chloroxylenol]
Pedituss Cough syrup ℞ *decongestant; antihistamine; antitussive; expectorant* [phenylephrine HCl; chlorpheniramine maleate; codeine phosphate; potassium iodide; alcohol]
Pedi-Vit-A Creme OTC *moisturizer; emollient* [vitamin A]

Pedotic otic suspension ℞ *topical corticosteroidal anti-inflammatory; antibiotic* [hydrocortisone; neomycin sulfate; polymyxin B sulfate]

PedTE-Pak-4 IV injection ℞ *intravenous nutritional therapy* [multiple trace elements (metals)]

Pedtrace-4 IV injection ℞ *intravenous nutritional therapy* [multiple trace elements (metals)]

PedvaxHIB powder for IM injection ℞ *Haemophilus influenzae type b (HIB) vaccine* [Hemophilus b conjugate vaccine]

PeeWee's Children's Vitamins chewable tablets OTC *vitamin/iron supplement* [multiple vitamins; iron; folic acid]

pefloxacin USAN, INN, BAN *antibacterial*

pefloxacin mesylate USAN *antibacterial*

PEG (polyethylene glycol) [q.v.]

P.E.G. Ointment OTC *ointment base* [polyethylene glycol 400; polyethylene glycol 3350]

PEG SOD ℞ *investigational agent to prevent irreversible brain damage following head trauma* [polyethylene glycol succinate conjugated superoxide dismutase]

PEG-ADA (polyethylene glycol-adenosine deaminase) [see: pegademase bovine]

pegademase INN *adenosine deaminase replacement* [also: pegademase bovine]

pegademase bovine USAN *adenosine deaminase replacement; (orphan: severe combined immunodeficiency disease)* [also: pegademase]

PEG-adenosine deaminase (PEG-ADA) [see: pegademase bovine]

Peganone tablets ℞ *anticonvulsant* [ethotoin]

PEG-L-asparaginase *(orphan: acute lymphocytic leukemia)*

pegaspargase USAN, INN *antineoplastic*

PEG-ES (polyethylene glycol-electrolyte solution) [q.v.]

PEG-hemoglobin (polyethylene glycol-hemoglobin) [in development 1992]

PEG-interleukin-2 (polyethylene glycol-interleukin-2) *investigational cytokine for AIDS; (orphan: primary immunodeficiencies)*

PEG-intron A (polyethylene glycol-intron A) [in development 1992]

peglicol 5 oleate USAN *emulsifying agent*

pegoterate USAN, INN *suspending agent*

pegoxol 7 stearate USAN *emulsifying agent*

PEG-SOD (polyethylene glycol-superoxide dismutase) *free-radical scavenger* [in clinical trials 1992]

Pelamine tablets ℞ *antihistamine* [tripelennamine HCl]

pelanserin INN *antihypertensive; vasodilator; serotonin adrenergic blocker* [also: pelanserin HCl]

pelanserin HCl USAN *antihypertensive; vasodilator; serotonin adrenergic blocker* [also: pelanserin]

peliomycin USAN, INN *antineoplastic*

pelretin USAN, INN *antikeratinizing agent*

pelrinone INN *cardiotonic* [also: pelrinone HCl]

pelrinone HCl USAN *cardiotonic* [also: pelrinone]

pemedolac USAN, INN *analgesic*

pemerid INN *antitussive* [also: pemerid nitrate]

pemerid nitrate USAN *antitussive* [also: pemerid]

pemirolast INN *antiallergic; mediator release inhibitor* [also: pemirolast potassium]

pemirolast potassium USAN *antiallergic; mediator release inhibitor* [also: pemirolast]
pemoline USAN, INN *stimulant for attention deficit disorders and narcolepsy*
pempidine INN, BAN
penamecillin USAN, INN, BAN *antibacterial*
penbutolol INN, BAN *antiadrenergic (β-receptor)* [also: penbutolol sulfate]
penbutolol sulfate USAN *antiadrenergic (β-receptor)* [also: penbutolol]
penciclovir INN, BAN
pendecamaine INN, BAN
pendiomide [see: azamethonium bromide]
Penecort cream, solution ℞ *topical corticosteroid* [hydrocortisone]
Penecort solution (discontinued 1991) ℞ *topical corticosteroid* [hydrocortisone]
Penetrex film-coated tablets ℞ *broad-spectrum fluoroquinolone-type antibiotic for GU infections* [enoxacin]
PenFill (trademarked form) *insulin injector refill cartridge*
penfluridol USAN, INN *antipsychotic*
penflutizide INN
pengitoxin INN
penicillamine USAN, USP, INN *metal chelating agent; antirheumatic*
penicillin aluminum
penicillin benzathine phenoxymethyl [now: penicillin V benzathine]
penicillin calcium USP
penicillin G benzathine USP *bactericidal antibiotic* [also: benzathine benzylpenicillin; benzathine penicillin]
penicillin G hydrabamine
penicillin G potassium USP *bactericidal antibiotic* [also: benzylpenicillin potassium]
penicillin G procaine USP *bactericidal antibiotic* [also: procaine penicillin]
penicillin G redox [see: redox-penicillin G]
penicillin G sodium USP *bactericidal antibiotic* [also: benzylpenicillin sodium]
penicillin hydrabamine phenoxymethyl [now: penicillin V hydrabamine]
penicillin N [see: adicillin]
penicillin O [see: almecillin]
penicillin O chloroprocaine
penicillin O potassium
penicillin O sodium
penicillin phenoxymethyl [now: penicillin V]
penicillin potassium G [see: penicillin G potassium]
penicillin potassium phenoxymethyl [now: penicillin V potassium]
penicillin V USAN, USP *bactericidal antibiotic* [also: phenoxymethylpenicillin]
penicillin V benzathine USAN, USP *antibacterial*
penicillin V hydrabamine USAN, USP *antibacterial*
penicillin V potassium USAN, USP *bactericidal antibiotic*
penicillin-152 potassium [see: phenethicillin potassium]
penicillinase INN, BAN
penicillinphenyrazine [see: phenyracillin]
Penicillin-VK oral solution, tablets ℞ *antibiotic* [penicillin V potassium]
penidural [see: benzathine penicillin]
penimepicycline INN
penimocycline INN
penirolol INN
Pen-Kera cream OTC *moisturizer; emollient*
penmesterol INN
penoctonium bromide INN
penprostene INN
pentabamate USAN, INN *minor tranquilizer*
Pentacef powder for IV or IM injection ℞ *cephalosporin-type antibiotic* [ceftazidime]

pentacosactride BAN [also: norleusactide]
pentacynium chloride INN
pentacyone chloride [see: pentacynium chloride]
pentaerithritol tetranicotinate [see: niceritrol]
pentaerithrityl tetranitrate INN *vasodilator* [also: pentaerythritol tetranitrate]
pentaerythritol tetranitrate (PETN) USP *vasodilator; "possibly effective" antianginal* [also: pentaerithrityl tetranitrate]
pentaerythritol trinitrate [see: pentrinitrol]
pentafilcon A USAN *hydrophilic contact lens material*
pentafluranol INN
pentagastrin USAN, INN *gastric secretion indicator*
pentagestrone INN
pentalamide INN, BAN
pentalyte USAN, USP, NF *electrolyte combination*
Pentam 300 IV or IM injection ℞ *antiprotozoal; (orphan: Pneumocystis carinii pneumonia)* [pentamidine isethionate]
pentamethazene [see: azamethonium bromide]
pentamethonium bromide INN, BAN
pentamethylenetetrazol [see: pentylenetetrazol]
pentamidine INN, BAN
pentamidine isethionate *antiprotozoal; (orphan: Pneumocystis carinii pneumonia)*
pentamin [see: azamethonium bromide]
pentamorphone USAN, INN *narcotic analgesic*
pentamoxane INN
pentamoxane HCl [see: pentamoxane]
pentamustine USAN *antineoplastic* [also: neptamustine]

pentanedial [see: glutaral]
pentanitrol [see: pentaerythritol tetranitrate]
pentaphonate
pentapiperide INN
pentapiperium methylsulfate USAN *anticholinergic* [also: pentapiperium metilsulfate]
pentapiperium metilsulfate INN *anticholinergic* [also: pentapiperium methylsulfate]
pentaquine INN [also: pentaquine phosphate]
pentaquine phosphate USP [also: pentaquine]
Pentasa ℞ *investigational anti-inflammatory for ulcerative colitis* [mesalamine]
pentasodium colistinmethanesulfonate [see: colistimethate sodium]
Pentaspan ℞ *(orphan: leukapheresis adjunct to improve leukocyte yield)* [pentastarch]
pentastarch USAN, BAN *leukapheresis adjunct; red cell sedimenting agent; (orphan: centrifugal harvesting of leukocytes)*
pentavalent gas gangrene antitoxin
Pentazine injection ℞ *antihistamine; motion sickness; sleep aid; antiemetic; sedative* [promethazine HCl]
pentazocine USAN, USP, INN, BAN *narcotic agonist-antagonist analgesic*
pentazocine HCl USAN, USP *analgesic*
pentazocine lactate USAN, USP *analgesic*
pentetate calcium trisodium USAN *plutonium-chelating agent* [also: calcium trisodium pentetate]
pentetate calcium trisodium Yb 169 USAN *radioactive agent*
pentetate disodium [see: pentetic acid, sodium salts]
pentetate indium disodium In 111 USAN *diagnostic aid; radioactive agent*

pentetate monosodium [see: pentetic acid, sodium salts]
pentetate pentasodium [see: pentetic acid, sodium salts]
pentetate tetrasodium [see: pentetic acid, sodium salts]
pentetate trisodium [see: pentetic acid, sodium salts]
pentetate trisodium calcium [see: pentetate calcium trisodium; calcium trisodium pentetate]
pentethylcyclanone [see: cyclexanone]
pentetic acid USAN, BAN *diagnostic aid*
pentetic acid, sodium salts *diagnostic aid*
pentetrazol INN [also: pentylenetetrazol]
penthanil diethylenetriamine pentaacetic acid (DTPA) [see: pentetic acid]
penthienate bromide NF
Penthrane liquid for vaporization ℞ *inhalation general anesthetic* [methoxyflurane]
penthrichloral INN, BAN
pentiapine INN *antipsychotic* [also: pentiapine maleate]
pentiapine maleate USAN *antipsychotic* [also: pentiapine]
penticide [see: chlorophenothane]
Pentids for Syrup; Pentids '400' for Syrup powder for oral solution ℞ *bactericidal antibiotic* [penicillin G potassium]
Pentids; Pentids '400'; Pentids '800' tablets ℞ *bactericidal antibiotic* [penicillin G potassium]
pentifylline INN, BAN
pentigetide USAN, INN *antiallergic*
pentisomicin USAN, INN *anti-infective*
pentisomide INN
pentizidone INN *antibacterial* [also: pentizidone sodium]
pentizidone sodium USAN *antibacterial* [also: pentizidone]

pentobarbital USP, INN *sedative; hypnotic*
pentobarbital sodium USP *hypnotic; sedative* [also: pentobarbitone sodium]
pentobarbitone sodium BAN *hypnotic; sedative* [also: pentobarbital sodium]
pentolinium tartrate NF [also: pentolonium tartrate]
pentolonium tartrate INN [also: pentolinium tartrate]
pentolonum bitartrate [see: pentolinium tartrate]
pentomone USAN, INN *prostate growth inhibitor*
pentopril USAN, INN *angiotensin-converting enzyme (ACE) inhibitor*
pentorex INN
pentosalen BAN
pentosan polysulfate sodium USAN, INN *anti-inflammatory for interstitial cystitis*
Pentostam (available only from the Centers for Disease Control) ℞ *investigational anti-infective for leishmaniasis* [sodium stibogluconate]
pentostatin USAN, INN *potentiator; antineoplastic antibiotic; (orphan: hairy cell and chronic lymphocytic leukemias)*
Pentothal IV, rectal suspension ℞ *general anesthetic* [thiopental sodium]
pentoxifylline USAN, INN *vasodilator; hemorheologic agent* [also: oxpentifylline]
pentoxiverine citrate [see: carbetapentane citrate]
pentoxyverine INN [also: carbetapentane citrate]
pentoxyverine citrate [see: carbetapentane citrate]
Pentrax shampoo OTC *antiseborrheic; antipsoriatic; antipruritic; antibacterial* [coal tar]
pentrinitrol USAN, INN *coronary vasodilator*
Pentylan tablets ℞ *antianginal* [pentaerythritol tetranitrate]

6-pentyl-*m*-cresol [see: amylmetacresol]
pentylenetetrazol NF [also: pentetrazol]
pentymal [see: amobarbital]
Pen-V tablets ℞ *bactericidal antibiotic* [penicillin V potassium]
Pen-Vee K tablets, powder for oral solution ℞ *bactericidal antibiotic* [penicillin V potassium]
Pepcid film-coated tablets, powder for oral suspension, IV injection (status change from ℞ to OTC pending) *gastric and duodenal ulcer treatment; histamine H_2 antagonist* [famotidine]
pepleomycin [see: peplomycin sulfate]
peplomycin INN *antineoplastic* [also: peplomycin sulfate]
peplomycin sulfate USAN *antineoplastic* [also: peplomycin]
peppermint NF *flavoring agent; perfume*
peppermint oil NF *flavoring agent*
peppermint spirit USP *flavoring agent; perfume*
peppermint water NF *flavored vehicle*
pepsin *digestive aid*
pepstatin USAN, INN *pepsin enzyme inhibitor*
Peptamen liquid OTC *oral nutritional supplement*
Peptavlon subcu injection ℞ *in vivo gastrointestinal function test* [pentagastrin]
peptide T *investigational antiviral for AIDS*
Pepto Diarrhea Control oral solution OTC *antidiarrheal* [loperamide HCl; alcohol]
Pepto-Bismol chewable tablets, liquid OTC *antidiarrheal; antinauseant* [bismuth subsalicylate]
peraclopone INN
peradoxime INN
perafensine INN
peralopride INN
peraquinsin INN
perastine INN

peratizole INN, BAN
perbufylline INN
Perchloracap capsules ℞ *pertechnetate Tc 99m accumulation blocker; for hyperthyroidism* [potassium perchlorate]
Percocet tablets ℞ *narcotic analgesic* [oxycodone HCl; acetaminophen]
Percodan; Percodan-Demi tablets ℞ *narcotic analgesic* [oxycodone HCl; oxycodone terephthalate; aspirin]
Percogesic tablets OTC *analgesic; antipyretic* [phenyltoloxamine citrate; acetaminophen]
Perdiem Fiber granules OTC *laxative* [psyllium; senna]
Perdiem granules OTC *laxative* [psyllium husk; senna]
perfilcon A USAN *hydrophilic contact lens material*
perfluamine INN, BAN
perflubron USAN *blood substitute*
perflunafene INN, BAN
perfluorochemical emulsion *synthetic blood oxygen carrier for PTCA*
perfomedil INN
perfosfamide USAN *antineoplastic; (orphan: ex vivo treatment of autologous bone marrow for leukemia)*
Pergamid ℞ *(orphan: ex vivo treatment of autologous bone marrow in leukemia)* [perfosfamide]
pergolide INN, BAN *dopamine agonist* [also: pergolide mesylate]
pergolide mesylate USAN *dopamine agonist; antiparkinsonian* [also: pergolide]
Pergonal powder for IM injection ℞ *induction of ovulation; stimulation of spermatogenesis* [menotropins]
perhexiline INN *coronary vasodilator* [also: perhexiline maleate]
perhexiline maleate USAN *coronary vasodilator* [also: perhexiline]
Periactin tablets, syrup ℞ *antihistamine; cold urticaria; anticholinergic* [cyproheptadine HCl]
periciazine INN [also: pericyazine]

Peri-Colace capsules, syrup OTC *laxative; stool softener* [docusate sodium; casanthranol]
pericyazine BAN [also: periciazine]
Peridex mouth rinse ℞ *antimicrobial; gingivitis treatment; (orphan: oral mucositis)* [chlorhexidine gluconate]
Peridin-C tablets OTC *vitamin supplement* [ascorbic acid; hesperidin complex; hesperidin methyl chalcone bioflavonoids]
Peri-Dos softgels OTC *laxative; stool softener* [docusate sodium; casanthranol]
Perifoam anorectal aerosol foam (discontinued 1991) OTC *topical anesthetic; antiseptic; sloughing agent* [pramoxine HCl; benzalkonium chloride; allantoin; lanolin; witch hazel]
Perihemin capsules (discontinued 1991) ℞ *antianemic* [ferrous fumarate; vitamins B$_{12}$ & C; intrinsic factor; folic acid]
Perimed oral rinse OTC *oral antibacterial* [hydrogen peroxide; povidone-iodine]
perimetazine INN
perindopril USAN, INN, BAN *angiotensin-converting enzyme (ACE) inhibitor*
perindopril erbumine USAN *antihypertensive*
perindoprilat INN, BAN
perisoxal INN
Peritinic tablets (discontinued 1991) OTC *antianemic* [ferrous fumarate; multiple B vitamins; vitamin C; folic acid]
Peritrate SA sustained-action tablets ℞ *antianginal* [pentaerythritol tetranitrate]
Peritrate tablets ℞ *antianginal* [pentaerythritol tetranitrate]
perlapine USAN, INN *hypnotic*
Perles (dosage form) *capsules*
permanganic acid, potassium salt [see: potassium permanganate]
Permapen Isoject (unit dose syringe) ℞ *bactericidal antibiotic* [penicillin G benzathine]
Permax tablets ℞ *antiparkinsonian agent* [pergolide mesylate]
permethrin USAN, INN, BAN *ectoparasiticide*
Permitil tablets, oral concentrate ℞ *antipsychotic* [fluphenazine HCl]
Pernivit-R injection ℞ *vitamin therapy* [liver concentrate; folic acid; cyanocobalamin]
Pernox Scrub; Pernox Lathering Lotion OTC *abrasive cleanser for acne* [sulfur; salicylic acid; aluminum oxide]
peroxide, dibenzoyl [see: benzoyl peroxide]
Peroxyl mouth rinse, oral gel OTC *cleansing of oral wounds* [hydrogen peroxide]
perphenazine USP, INN *antipsychotic; antiemetic; antidopaminergic; intractable hiccough relief*
Persa-Gel 5%; Persa-Gel 10%; Persa-Gel W 5%; Persa-Gel W 10% gel ℞ *topical keratolytic for acne* [benzoyl peroxide]
Persantine IV injection ℞ *in vivo coronary artery function test* [dipyridamole]
Persantine tablets ℞ *antiplatelet agent* [dipyridamole]
persic oil NF *vehicle*
persilic acid INN
Personal Lubricant vaginal gel (discontinued 1992) OTC *lubricant*
Pertofrane capsules ℞ *tricyclic antidepressant* [desipramine HCl]
Pertropin capsules OTC *dietary lipotropic agent* [linolenic acid; multiple essential fatty acids]
Pertussin (name changed to Pertussin ES in 1990)
Pertussin AM liquid OTC *decongestant; antitussive; expectorant* [pseudoephedrine HCl; dextromethorphan hydrobromide; guaifenesin; alcohol]

Pertussin CS; Pertussin ES syrup OTC *antitussive* [dextromethorphan hydrobromide]

Pertussin PM liquid OTC *decongestant; antihistamine; antitussive; analgesic* [pseudoephedrine HCl; doxylamine succinate; dextromethorphan hydrobromide; acetaminophen; alcohol]

pertussis immune globulin USP *passive immunizing agent*

pertussis immune human globulin [now: pertussis immune globulin]

pertussis vaccine USP *active immunizing agent*

pertussis vaccine adsorbed USP *active immunizing agent*

peruvian balsam NF *topical local protectant; rubefacient*

pethidine INN, BAN *narcotic analgesic* [also: meperidine HCl]

pethidine HCl [see: meperidine HCl]

PETN (pentaerythritol tetranitrate) [q.v.]

petrichloral INN

petrolatum USP *ointment base; emollient/protectant*

petrolatum, hydrophilic USP *absorbent ointment base; topical protectant*

petrolatum, liquid [see: mineral oil]

petrolatum, liquid emulsion [see: mineral oil emulsion]

petrolatum, white USP *oleaginous ointment base; topical protectant*

petrolatum gauze [see: gauze, petrolatum]

petroleum jelly [see: petrolatum]

pexantel INN

Pfeiffer's Allergy tablets OTC *antihistamine* [chlorpheniramine maleate]

Pfeiffer's Cold Sore lotion OTC *topical oral anesthetic; antipruritic/counterirritant* [gum benzoin; camphor; menthol; thymol; eucalyptol]

Pfizerpen powder for injection ℞ *bactericidal antibiotic* [penicillin G potassium]

Pfizerpen-AS IM injection ℞ *bactericidal antibiotic* [penicillin G procaine]

PFT (L-phenylalanine mustard, fluorouracil, tamoxifen) *chemotherapy protocol*

PG (paregoric) [q.v.]

PG (prostaglandin) [q.v.]

PGA (pteroylglutamic acid) [see: folic acid]

PGE₁ (prostaglandin E₁) [now: alprostadil]

PGE₂ (prostaglandin E₂) [now: dinoprostone]

PGF₂β (prostaglandin F₂β) [see: dinoprost]

PGF₂β (prostaglandin F₂β) THAM [see: dinoprost tromethamine]

PGI₂ (prostaglandin I₂) [now: epoprostenol]

PGX (prostaglandin X) [now: epoprostenol]

Phacotron Gold ℞ *investigational phakoemulsification system for cataract surgery*

Phanacōl Cough syrup OTC *decongestant; antitussive; expectorant; analgesic; antipyretic* [phenylpropanolamine HCl; dextromethorphan hydrobromide; guaifenesin; acetaminophen]

Phanadex Cough syrup OTC *antitussive; expectorant; antihistamine; decongestant* [dextromethorphan hydrobromide; guaifenesin; phenylpropanolamine HCl; pyrilamine maleate]

Phanatuss Cough syrup OTC *antitussive; expectorant; demulcent* [dextromethorphan hydrobromide; guaifenesin; potassium citrate; citric acid]

phanchinone [see: phanquinone; phanquone]

phanquinone INN [also: phanquone]

phanquone BAN [also: phanquinone]

pharmaceutical glaze [see: glaze, pharmaceutical]

Pharmadine ointment, perineal wash, skin cleanser, solution, swabs, swab sticks, spray, surgical scrub, surgical scrub sponge/brush, whirlpool solution OTC *broad-spectrum antimicrobial* [povidone-iodine]

Pharmaflur; Pharmaflur df; Pharmaflur 1.1 chewable tablets ℞ *dental caries preventative* [sodium fluoride]

Pharmalgen subcu or IM injection ℞ *venom sensitivity testing; allergenic hyposensitization therapy* [extracts of honeybee, yellow jacket, yellow hornet, white-faced hornet, mixed vespid & wasp venom]

Phazyme 125 softgels OTC *antiflatulent* [simethicone]

Phazyme 95 tablets OTC *antiflatulent* [simethicone]

Phazyme tablets, drops OTC *antiflatulent* [simethicone]

Phazyme-PB tablets (discontinued 1991) ℞ *digestive enzymes; antiflatulent; sedative* [amylase; protease; lipase; simethicone; phenobarbital]

phebutazine [see: febuverine]
phebutyrazine [see: febuverine]
phemfilcon A USAN *hydrophilic contact lens material*
phenacaine INN [also: phenacaine HCl]
phenacaine HCl USP [also: phenacaine]
PhenaCal capsules (discontinued 1993) OTC *dietary supplement* [multiple amino acids, vitamins & minerals]
phenacemide USP, INN *anticonvulsant*
phenacetin USP, INN (*withdrawn from market*)
phenacon [see: fenaclon]
phenactropinium chloride INN, BAN
phenacyl 4-morpholineacetate [see: mobecarb]
***N*-phenacylhomatropinium chloride** [see: phenactropinium chloride]
phenacylpivalate [see: pibecarb]

phenadoxone INN, BAN
phenaglycodol INN
Phenahist-TR sustained-release tablets ℞ *decongestant; antihistamine; anticholinergic* [phenylpropanolamine HCl; phenylephrine HCl; chlorpheniramine maleate; hyoscyamine sulfate; atropine sulfate; scopolamine hydrobromide]
phenamazoline INN
phenamazoline HCl [see: phenamazoline]
Phenameth DM syrup ℞ *antihistamine; antitussive* [promethazine HCl; dextromethorphan hydrobromide]
Phenameth tablets ℞ *antihistamine; motion sickness; sleep aid; antiemetic; sedative* [promethazine HCl]
phenampromide INN
Phenapap Sinus Headache & Congestion tablets OTC *decongestant; antihistamine; analgesic* [pseudoephedrine HCl; chlorpheniramine maleate; acetaminophen]
Phenaphen caplets OTC *analgesic; antipyretic* [acetaminophen]
Phenaphen with Codeine No. 2, No. 3 & No. 4 capsules ℞ *narcotic analgesic* [codeine phosphate; acetaminophen]
Phenaphen-650 with Codeine tablets ℞ *narcotic analgesic* [codeine phosphate; acetaminophen]
phenaphthazine
phenarbutal [see: phetharbital]
phenarsone sulfoxylate INN
Phenaseptic mouthwash/gargle (discontinued 1991) OTC *oral antiseptic* [phenol; sodium phenolate; menthol; thymol]
Phenate T.D. timed-release tablets ℞ *decongestant; antihistamine; analgesic* [phenylpropanolamine HCl; chlorpheniramine maleate; acetaminophen]
Phenazine 25; Phenazine 50 injection ℞ *antihistamine; motion sickness;*

sleep aid; antiemetic; sedative [promethazine HCl]
phenazocine INN
phenazocine hydrobromide [see: phenazocine]
Phenazodine tablets ℞ *urinary analgesic* [phenazopyridine HCl]
phenazone INN, BAN *analgesic* [also: antipyrine]
phenazopyridine INN, BAN *urinary tract analgesic* [also: phenazopyridine HCl]
phenazopyridine HCl USAN, USP *urinary tract analgesic* [also: phenazopyridine]
phenbenicillin BAN [also: fenbenicillin]
phenbutazone sodium glycerate USAN *anti-inflammatory*
phenbutrazate BAN [also: fenbutrazate]
phencarbamide USAN *anticholinergic* [also: fencarbamide]
Phencen-50 injection ℞ *sedative; antihistamine* [promethazine HCl]
Phenchlor SHA sustained-release tablets ℞ *decongestant; antihistamine; anticholinergic* [phenylpropanolamine HCl; phenylephrine HCl; chlorpheniramine maleate; hyoscyamine sulfate; atropine sulfate; scopolamine hydrobromide]
phencyclidine INN *anesthetic* [also: phencyclidine HCl]
phencyclidine HCl USAN *anesthetic* [also: phencyclidine]
phendimetrazine INN *anorexiant* [also: phendimetrazine tartrate]
phendimetrazine tartrate USP *anorexiant; CNS stimulant* [also: phendimetrazine]
Phendry; Phendry Children's Allergy Medicine elixir OTC *antihistamine* [diphenhydramine HCl]
phenelzine INN *antidepressant: MAO inhibitor* [also: phenelzine sulfate]
phenelzine sulfate USP *antidepressant* [also: phenelzine]

phenemal [see: phenobarbital]
Phenerbel-S tablets ℞ *analgesic specific for migraine; sedative* [phenobarbital; ergotamine tartrate; belladonna alkaloids]
Phenergan Fortis syrup ℞ *antihistamine; motion sickness; sleep aid; antiemetic; sedative* [promethazine HCl]
Phenergan Plain syrup ℞ *antihistamine; motion sickness; sleep aid; antiemetic; sedative* [promethazine HCl]
Phenergan tablets, suppositories, injection ℞ *antihistamine; motion sickness; sleep aid; antiemetic; sedative* [promethazine HCl]
Phenergan VC syrup ℞ *decongestant; antihistamine* [phenylephrine HCl; promethazine HCl; alcohol]
Phenergan VC with Codeine syrup ℞ *decongestant; antihistamine; antitussive* [phenylephrine HCl; promethazine HCl; codeine phosphate; alcohol]
Phenergan with Codeine syrup ℞ *antihistamine; antitussive* [promethazine HCl; codeine phosphate]
Phenergan with Dextromethorphan syrup ℞ *antihistamine; antitussive* [promethazine HCl; dextromethorphan hydrobromide; alcohol]
Phenergan-D tablets ℞ *antihistamine; decongestant* [promethazine HCl; pseudoephedrine HCl]
pheneridine INN
phenethanol [see: phenylethyl alcohol]
phenethazine [see: fenethazine]
phenethicillin potassium USP [also: pheneticillin]
phenethyl alcohol BAN *antimicrobial agent* [also: phenylethyl alcohol]
***N*-phenethylanthranilic acid** [see: enfenamic acid]
phenethylazocine bromide [see: phenazocine hydrobromide]
phenethylhydrazine sulfate [see: phenelzine sulfate]

pheneticillin INN [also: phenethicillin potassium]
pheneticillin potassium [see: phenethicillin potassium]
Phenetron Compound sugar-coated tablets OTC *antihistamine; analgesic* [chlorpheniramine maleate; aspirin; caffeine]
Phenetron tablets, syrup ℞ *antihistamine; antitussive* [chlorpheniramine maleate]
phenetsal [see: acetaminosalol]
pheneturide INN, BAN
phenformin INN, BAN *hypoglycemic agent* [also: phenformin HCl]
phenformin HCl USP *hypoglycemic agent (removed from market in 1977 by FDA, now available as an investigational drug)* [also: phenformin]
phenglutarimide INN, BAN
Phenhist DH w/Codeine liquid ℞ *decongestant; antihistamine; antitussive* [pseudoephedrine HCl; chlorpheniramine maleate; codeine phosphate; alcohol]
Phenhist Expectorant liquid ℞ *decongestant; antitussive; expectorant* [pseudoephedrine HCl; codeine phosphate; guaifenesin; alcohol]
phenicarbazide INN
phenidiemal [see: phetharbital]
phenindamine INN *antihistamine* [also: phenindamine tartrate]
phenindamine tartrate USAN *antihistamine* [also: phenindamine]
phenindione USP, INN *anticoagulant*
pheniodol sodium INN [also: iodoalphionic acid]
pheniprazine INN, BAN
pheniprazine HCl [see: pheniprazine]
pheniramine INN [also: pheniramine maleate]
pheniramine maleate USAN [also: pheniramine]
phenisonone hydrobromide
Phenistix reagent strips OTC *in vitro diagnostic aid for phenylketonuria*

phenmetraline HCl [see: phenmetrazine HCl]
phenmetrazine INN *anorexiant* [also: phenmetrazine HCl]
phenmetrazine HCl USP *anorexiant; CNS stimulant* [also: phenmetrazine]
phenobamate [see: febarbamate]
phenobarbital USP, INN *anticonvulsant; hypnotic; sedative*
phenobarbital sodium USP, INN *anticonvulsant; hypnotic; sedative*
phenobarbitone [see: phenobarbital]
phenobutiodil INN
phenododecinium bromide [see: domiphen bromide]
Phenoject-50 injection ℞ *antihistamine; motion sickness; sleep aid; antiemetic; sedative* [promethazine HCl]
phenol USP *topical antiseptic/antipruritic; local anesthetic; preservative*
phenol, liquefied USP *topical antipruritic*
phenol, sodium salt [see: phenolate sodium]
phenol red [see: phenolsulfonphthalein]
phenolate sodium USAN *disinfectant*
Phenolated Calamine lotion OTC *topical poison ivy treatment* [calamine; zinc oxide; phenol]
Phenolax wafers OTC *laxative* [phenolphthalein]
phenolphthalein USP, INN *stimulant laxative*
phenolphthalein, white [see: phenolphthalein]
phenolphthalein, yellow USP *stimulant laxative*
phenolsulfonphthalein USP
phenolsulphonate sodium USP
phenomorphan INN, BAN
phenomycilline [see: penicillin V]
phenoperidine INN, BAN
phenopryldiasulfone sodium [see: solasulfone]
phenosulfophthalein [see: phenolsulfonphthalein]
phenothiazine NF, INN *antipsychotic*

phenothrin INN, BAN
phenoxazoline HCl [see: fenoxazoline HCl]
Phenoxine tablets OTC *diet aid* [phenylpropanolamine HCl]
phenoxybenzamine INN *antihypertensive* [also: phenoxybenzamine HCl]
phenoxybenzamine HCl USP *antihypertensive; pheochromocytomic agent* [also: phenoxybenzamine]
phenoxymethylpenicillin INN *bactericidal antibiotic* [also: penicillin V]
phenoxypropazine BAN [also: fenoxypropazine]
phenoxypropylpenicillin [see: propicillin]
phenozolone [see: fenozolone]
phenprobamate INN, BAN
phenprocoumon USAN, USP, INN *anticoagulant*
phenprocumone [see: phenprocoumon]
phenpromethadrine [see: phenpromethamine]
phenpromethamine INN
phenpropamine citrate [see: alverine citrate]
phensuximide USP, INN, BAN *anticonvulsant*
phentermine USAN, INN *anorexiant*
phentermine HCl USP *anorexiant; CNS stimulant*
phenthiazine [see: phenothiazine]
phentolamine INN *antihypertensive; pheochromocytomic agent* [also: phentolamine HCl]
phentolamine HCl USP [also: phentolamine]
phentolamine mesylate USP *antiadrenergic; antihypertensive; pheochromocytomic agent*
phentolamine methanesulfonate [now: phentolamine mesylate]
Phentrol; Phentrol 2; Phentrol 4; Phentrol 5 tablets ℞ *anorexiant* [phentermine HCl]
phentydrone

Phenurone tablets ℞ *anticonvulsant* [phenacemide]
phenyl aminosalicylate USAN *antibacterial; tuberculostatic* [also: fenamisal]
phenyl salicylate NF *analgesic; not generally regarded as safe and effective as an antidiarrheal*
phenylalanine (L-phenylalanine) USAN, USP, INN *essential amino acid; symbols: Phe, F*
L-phenylalanine mustard (L-PAM) [see: melphalan]
phenylalanine mustard (PAM) [see: melphalan]
phenylazo diamino pyridine HCl [see: phenazopyridine HCl]
phenylbenzyl atropine [see: xenytropium bromide]
phenylbutazone USP, INN *antirheumatic; anti-inflammatory; antipyretic; analgesic*
phenylbutyrate sodium (*orphan: sickling disorders; S-S, S-C and S-thalassemia hemoglobinopathy*)
2-phenylbutyrylurea [see: pheneturide]
phenylcarbinol [see: benzyl alcohol]
phenylcinchoninic acid [now: cinchophen]
α-phenyl-p-cresol carbamate [see: diphenan]
2-phenylcyclopentylamine HCl [see: cypenamine HCl]
phenyldimazone [see: normethadone]
Phenyldrine timed-release tablets OTC *diet aid* [phenylpropanolamine HCl]
phenylephrine (PE) INN, BAN *nasal decongestant; ocular vasoconstrictor; vasopressor for shock* [also: phenylephrine HCl]
phenylephrine bitartrate *bronchodilator; vasoconstrictor*
phenylephrine HCl USP *nasal decongestant; ocular vasoconstrictor; vasopressor for shock* [also: phenylephrine]

phenylephrine tannate
phenylethanol [see: phenylethyl alcohol]
phenylethyl alcohol USP *antimicrobial agent; preservative* [also: phenethyl alcohol]
phenylethylmalonylurea [see: phenobarbital]
Phenylfenesin L.A. long-acting tablets ℞ *decongestant; expectorant* [phenylpropanolamine HCl; guaifenesin]
Phenyl-Free liquid OTC *special diet for infants with phenylketonuria (PKU)*
Phenylgesic tablets OTC *antihistamine; analgesic* [phenyltoloxamine citrate; acetaminophen]
phenylindanedione [see: phenindione]
phenylmercuric acetate NF *antimicrobial agent; preservative*
phenylmercuric borate INN
phenylmercuric chloride NF
phenylmercuric nitrate NF *antimicrobial agent; preservative; topical antiseptic*
phenylone [see: antipyrine]
phenylpropanolamine (PPA) INN, BAN *vasoconstrictor; nasal decongestant; nonprescription diet aid* [also: phenylpropanolamine HCl]
phenylpropanolamine HCl USP *vasoconstrictor; nasal decongestant; nonprescription diet aid* [also: phenylpropanolamine]
phenylpropanolamine polistirex USAN *adrenergic; vasoconstrictor*
1-phenylsemicarbazide [see: phenicarbazide]
phenylthilone [see: phenythilone]
phenyltoloxamine INN
phenyltoloxamine citrate *antihistamine*
Phenylzin eye drops OTC *topical ocular decongestant; astringent; antiseptic* [phenylephrine HCl; zinc sulfate]
phenyracillin INN

phenyramidol HCl USAN *analgesic; skeletal muscle relaxant* [also: fenyramidol]
phenythilone INN
phenytoin USAN, USP, INN, BAN *anticonvulsant*
phenytoin redox [see: redox-phenytoin]
phenytoin sodium USP *anticonvulsant*
Phenzine tablets (discontinued 1991) ℞ *anorexiant* [phendimetrazine tartrate]
Pherazine DM syrup ℞ *antihistamine; antitussive* [promethazine HCl; dextromethorphan; alcohol]
Pherazine syrup ℞ *antihistamine* [promethazine HCl]
Pherazine VC syrup ℞ *antihistamine; decongestant* [promethazine HCl; phenylephrine HCl; alcohol]
Pherazine VC with Codeine syrup ℞ *decongestant; antihistamine; antitussive* [phenylephrine HCl; promethazine HCl; codeine phosphate; alcohol]
Pherazine with Codeine syrup ℞ *antihistamine; antitussive* [promethazine HCl; codeine phosphate; alcohol]
Pheryl E 400 tablets OTC *vitamin supplement* [vitamin E]
phetharbital INN
phezathion [see: fezatione]
Phicon cream OTC *topical anesthetic; emollient* [pramoxine HCl; vitamins A & E]
Phicon F cream OTC *topical anesthetic; antifungal* [pramoxine HCl; undecylenic acid]
Phillips' LaxCaps capsules OTC *laxative; stool softener* [docusate sodium; phenolphthalein]
Phillips' Milk of Magnesia liquid OTC *laxative* [magnesium hydroxide]
pHiso Scrub sponge (discontinued 1991) ℞ *antiseptic; germicidal* [hexachlorophene]

pHisoAc BP cream (discontinued 1992) OTC *topical keratolytic for acne* [benzoyl peroxide]

pHisoDan shampoo (discontinued 1991) OTC *antiseborrheic; keratolytic* [sulfur; sodium salicylate]

pHisoDerm Gentle Cleansing Bar OTC *therapeutic skin cleanser*

pHisoDerm liquid OTC *soap-free cleanser*

pHisoHex liquid ℞ *bacteriostatic skin cleanser* [hexachlorophene]

phloropropiophenone [see: flopropione]

pholcodine INN

pholedrine INN, BAN

pholescutol [see: folescutol]

PhosChol 565; PhosChol 900 softgels, liquid concentrate OTC *neurotransmitter; lipotropic* [phosphatidylcholine]

phoscolic acid [see: foscolic acid]

Phos-Ex 125 capsules OTC *calcium supplement* [calcium acetate]

Phos-Ex 62.5 Mini-Tabs; Phos-Ex 167; Phos-Ex 250 tablets OTC *calcium supplement* [calcium acetate]

Phos-Flur oral rinse ℞ *dental caries preventative* [acidulated phosphate fluoride]

PhosLo tablets ℞ *(orphan: hyperphosphatemia in end-stage renal failure)* [calcium acetate]

pHos-pHaid E.C. enteric-coated tablets ℞ *urinary acidifier* [ammonium biphosphate; sodium biphosphate; sodium acid pyrophosphate]

pHos-pHaid tablets ℞ *urinary acidifier* [ammonium biphosphate; sodium biphosphate; sodium acid pyrophosphate]

Phosphaljel oral suspension OTC *no longer labeled for use as an antacid* [aluminum phosphate gel]

phosphate salt of tricyclic nucleoside [now: triciribine phosphate]

phosphatidylcholine (PC) [see: lecithin]

phosphinic acid [see: hypophosphorous acid]

2,2′-phosphinicodilactic acid (PDLA) [see: foscolic acid]

Phosphocol P32 intracavitary instillation, interstitial injection ℞ *radiopharmaceutical antineoplastic* [chromic phosphate P 32]

phosphocysteamine *(orphan: cystinosis)*

Phospholine Iodide powder for eye drops ℞ *antiglaucoma agent; irreversible cholinesterase inhibitor miotic* [echothiophate iodide]

phosphonoformic acid [see: foscarnet sodium]

phosphorated carbohydrate solution (fructose, dextrose & orthophosphoric acid) *antinauseant; antiemetic*

phosphoric acid NF *solvent; acidifying agent*

phosphoric acid, aluminum salt [see: aluminum phosphate]

phosphoric acid, calcium salt [see: calcium phosphate, dibasic]

phosphoric acid, chromium salt [see: chromic phosphate Cr 51 & P 32]

phosphoric acid, diammonium salt [see: ammonium phosphate]

phosphoric acid, dipotassium salt [see: potassium phosphate, dibasic]

phosphoric acid, disodium salt heptahydrate [see: sodium phosphate, dibasic]

phosphoric acid, disodium salt hydrate [see: sodium phosphate, dibasic]

phosphoric acid, magnesium salt [see: magnesium phosphate]

phosphoric acid, monopotassium salt [see: potassium phosphate, monobasic]

phosphoric acid, monosodium salt dihydrate [see: sodium phosphate, monobasic]

phosphoric acid, monosodium salt monohydrate [see: sodium phosphate, monobasic]
phosphorofluoridic acid, disodium salt [see: sodium monofluorophosphate]
phosphorus *element (P)*
Phospho-Soda [see: Fleet Phospho-Soda]
phosphothiamine [see: monophosphothiamine]
Photofrin *(orphan: bladder carcinoma; esophgeal carcinoma)* [dihematoporphyrin ethers]
Photoplex lotion OTC *broad-spectrum sunscreen* [avobenzone; padimate O]
phoxim INN, BAN
Phrenilin Forte capsules ℞ *analgesic; antipyretic; sedative* [acetaminophen; caffeine; butalbital]
Phrenilin tablets ℞ *analgesic; antipyretic; sedative* [acetaminophen; caffeine; butalbital]
PHRT (procarbazine, hydroxyurea, radiotherapy) *chemotherapy protocol*
phthalofyne USAN *veterinary anthelmintic* [also: ftalofyne]
phthalylsulfacetamide NF
phthalylsulfamethizole INN
phthalylsulfathiazole USP, INN
phylcardin [see: aminophylline]
phyllindon [see: aminophylline]
Phyllocontin controlled-release tablets ℞ *bronchodilator* [aminophylline]
phylloquinone [see: phytonadione]
Phylorinol liquid OTC *minor topical anesthetic; antiseptic; astringent; oral deodorant* [phenol; boric acid; strong iodine solution; chlorophyllin copper complex]
physiological irrigating solution *for general irrigating, washing and rinsing; not for injection*
Physiolyte liquid ℞ *sterile irrigant* [physiological irrigating solution]
PhysioSol liquid ℞ *sterile irrigant* [physiological irrigating solution]

physostigmine USP, BAN *antiglaucoma agent; reversible cholinesterase inhibitor miotic*
physostigmine salicylate USP *ophthalmic cholinergic; (orphan: Friedreich's and other ataxias)*
physostigmine sulfate USP *ophthalmic cholinergic*
phytate persodium USAN *pharmaceutic aid*
phytate sodium USAN *calcium-chelating agent*
phytic acid [see: fytic acid]
phytomenadione INN, BAN *vitamin K$_1$; prothrombogenic* [also: phytonadione]
phytonadiol sodium diphosphate INN
phytonadione USP *vitamin K$_1$; prothrombogenic* [also: phytomenadione]
PIA (Platinol, ifosfamide, Adriamycin) *chemotherapy protocol*
pibecarb INN
piberaline INN
picafibrate INN
picartamide INN
picenadol INN *analgesic* [also: picenadol HCl]
picenadol HCl USAN *analgesic* [also: picenadol]
picilorex INN
piclonidine INN
piclopastine INN
picloxydine INN, BAN
picobenzide INN
picodralazine INN
picolamine INN
piconol INN
picoperine INN
picoprazole INN
picotrin INN *keratolytic* [also: picotrin diolamine]
picotrin diolamine USAN *keratolytic* [also: picotrin]
picric acid [see: trinitrophenol]
picrotoxin NF
picumast INN, BAN

picumeterol INN, BAN *bronchodilator* [also: picumeterol fumarate]
picumeterol fumarate USAN *bronchodilator* [also: picumeterol]
pidolacetamol INN
pidolic acid INN
pifarnine USAN, INN *gastric antiulcerative*
pifenate INN, BAN
pifexole INN
piflutixol INN
pifoxime INN
piketoprofen INN
Pilagan eye drops ℞ *antiglaucoma agent; direct-acting miotic* [pilocarpine nitrate]
pildralazine INN
Pilocar eye drops ℞ *antiglaucoma agent; direct-acting miotic* [pilocarpine HCl]
pilocarpine USP, BAN *antiglaucoma agent; ophthalmic cholinergic*
pilocarpine HCl USP *ophthalmic cholinergic; antiglaucoma miotic; (orphan: xerostomia; keratoconjunctivitis sicca)*
pilocarpine nitrate USP *ophthalmic cholinergic; antiglaucoma agent; miotic*
Pilopine HS ophthalmic gel ℞ *antiglaucoma agent; direct-acting miotic* [pilocarpine HCl]
Piloptic-½; Piloptic-1; Piloptic-2; Piloptic-3; Piloptic-4; Piloptic-6 eye drops ℞ *antiglaucoma agent; direct-acting miotic* [pilocarpine HCl]
Pilopto-Carpine eye drops ℞ *antiglaucoma agent; direct-acting miotic* [pilocarpine HCl]
Pilostat eye drops ℞ *antiglaucoma agent; direct-acting miotic* [pilocarpine HCl]
Pima syrup ℞ *expectorant* [potassium iodide]
pimeclone INN
pimefylline INN
pimelautide INN
pimetacin INN
pimethixene INN

pimetine INN *antihyperlipoproteinemic* [also: pimetine HCl]
pimetine HCl USAN *antihyperlipoproteinemic* [also: pimetine]
pimetixene [see: pimethixene]
pimetremide INN
pimeverine [see: pimetremide]
piminodine INN [also: piminodine esylate]
piminodine esylate NF [also: piminodine]
piminodine ethanesulfonate [see: piminodine esylate]
pimobendan USAN, INN *cardiotonic*
pimonidazole INN, BAN
pimozide USAN, USP, INN *antipsychotic; suppresses symptoms of Tourette syndrome*
pinacidil USAN, INN *antihypertensive*
pinadoline USAN, INN *analgesic*
pinafide INN
pinaverium bromide INN
pinazepam INN
pincainide INN
Pindac ℞ *investigational antihypertensive* [pinacidil]
pindolol USAN, USP, INN, BAN *vasodilator; antiadrenergic (β-receptor)*
pine needle oil NF
pine tar USP
Pink Bismuth liquid OTC *antidiarrheal* [bismuth subsalicylate]
pinolcaine INN
pinoxepin INN *antipsychotic* [also: pinoxepin HCl]
pinoxepin HCl USAN *antipsychotic* [also: pinoxepin]
Pin-Rid soft gel capsules, liquid OTC *anthelmintic* [pyrantel pamoate]
Pin-X liquid OTC *anthelmintic* [pyrantel pamoate]
pioglitazone INN *antidiabetic* [also: pioglitazone HCl]
pioglitazone HCl USAN *antidiabetic* [also: pioglitazone]
pipacycline INN
pipamazine INN

pipamperone USAN, INN *antipsychotic*
pipaneperone [see: pipamperone]
pipazetate INN *antitussive* [also: pipazethate]
pipazethate USAN *antitussive* [also: pipazetate]
pipebuzone INN
pipecuronium bromide USAN, INN, BAN *muscle relaxant; neuromuscular blocker*
pipemidic acid INN
pipenzolate bromide INN
pipenzolate methylbromide [see: pipenzolate bromide]
pipenzolone bromide [see: pipenzolate bromide]
pipequaline INN
piperacetazine USAN, USP, INN *antipsychotic*
piperacillin INN, BAN *antibacterial* [also: piperacillin sodium]
piperacillin sodium USAN, USP *bactericidal antibiotic* [also: piperacillin]
piperamide INN *anthelmintic* [also: piperamide maleate]
piperamide maleate USAN *anthelmintic* [also: piperamide]
piperamine [see: bamipine]
piperazine USP *anthelmintic*
piperazine calcium edetate INN *anthelmintic* [also: piperazine edetate calcium]
piperazine citrate USP *anthelmintic*
piperazine citrate hydrate [see: piperazine citrate]
piperazine edetate calcium USAN *anthelmintic* [also: piperazine calcium edetate]
piperazine estrone sulfate [now: estropipate]
piperazine hexahydrate [see: piperazine citrate]
piperazine phosphate
piperazine phosphate monohydrate [see: piperazine phosphate]

piperazine theophylline ethanoate [see: acefylline piperazine]
piperidine phosphate
piperidolate INN [also: piperidolate HCl]
piperidolate HCl USP [also: piperidolate]
piperilate [see: pipethanate]
piperine USP
piperocaine INN [also: piperocaine HCl]
piperocaine HCl USP [also: piperocaine]
piperonyl butoxide *pediculicide*
piperoxan INN
piperphenidol HCl
piperylone INN
pipethanate INN
pipobroman USAN, USP, INN *antineoplastic*
pipoctanone INN
pipofezine INN
piposulfan USAN, INN *antineoplastic*
pipotiazine INN *antipsychotic* [also: pipotiazine palmitate]
pipotiazine palmitate USAN *antipsychotic* [also: pipotiazine]
pipoxizine INN
pipoxolan INN *muscle relaxant* [also: pipoxolan HCl]
pipoxolan HCl USAN *muscle relaxant* [also: pipoxolan]
Pipracil powder for IV or IM injection, ADD-vantage vials ℞ *extended-spectrum penicillin-type antibiotic* [piperacillin sodium]
pipradimadol INN
pipradrol INN [also: pipradrol HCl]
pipradrol HCl NF [also: pipradrol]
pipramadol INN
pipratecol INN
piprinhydrinate INN, BAN
piprocurarium iodide INN
piprofurol INN
piprozolin USAN, INN *choleretic*
piquindone INN *antipsychotic* [also: piquindone HCl]

piquindone HCl USAN *antipsychotic* [also: piquindone]
piquizil INN *bronchodilator* [also: piquizil HCl]
piquizil HCl USAN *bronchodilator* [also: piquizil]
piracetam USAN, INN, BAN *cognition adjuvant; (orphan: myoclonus)*
pirandamine INN *antidepressant* [also: pirandamine HCl]
pirandamine HCl USAN *antidepressant* [also: pirandamine]
pirarubicin INN
piraxelate INN
pirazmonam INN *antimicrobial* [also: pirazmonam sodium]
pirazmonam sodium USAN *antimicrobial* [also: pirazmonam]
pirazofurin INN *antineoplastic* [also: pyrazofurin]
pirazolac USAN, INN, BAN *antirheumatic*
pirbenicillin INN *antibacterial* [also: pirbenicillin sodium]
pirbenicillin sodium USAN *antibacterial* [also: pirbenicillin]
pirbuterol INN *bronchodilator* [also: pirbuterol acetate]
pirbuterol acetate USAN *bronchodilator* [also: pirbuterol]
pirbuterol HCl USAN *bronchodilator*
pirdonium bromide INN
pirenoxine INN
pirenperone USAN, INN, BAN *tranquilizer*
pirenzepine INN, BAN *antiulcerative* [also: pirenzepine HCl]
pirenzepine HCl USAN *antiulcerative* [also: pirenzepine]
pirepolol INN
piretanide USAN, INN *diuretic*
pirfenidone USAN, INN *analgesic; anti-inflammatory; antipyretic*
piribedil INN
piribenzyl methylsulfate [see: bevonium metilsulfate]
piridicillin INN *antibacterial* [also: piridicillin sodium]
piridicillin sodium USAN *antibacterial* [also: piridicillin]
piridocaine INN
piridocaine HCl [see: piridocaine]
piridoxilate INN, BAN
piridronate sodium USAN *calcium regulator*
piridronic acid INN
pirifibrate INN
pirinidazole INN
pirinitramide [see: piritramide]
pirinixic acid INN
pirinixil INN
piriprost USAN *antiasthmatic*
piriprost potassium USAN *antiasthmatic*
piriqualone INN
pirisudanol INN
piritramide INN, BAN
piritrexim INN *antiproliferative agent* [also: piritrexim isethionate]
piritrexim isethionate USAN *antiproliferative; (orphan: Pneumocystis carinii; Mycobacterium avium complex; Toxoplasma gondii)* [also: piritrexim]
pirlimycin HCl USAN *antibacterial*
pirlindole INN
pirmagrel USAN, INN *thromboxane synthetase inhibitor*
pirmenol INN *antiarrhythmic* [also: pirmenol HCl]
pirmenol HCl USAN *antiarrhythmic* [also: pirmenol]
pirnabin INN *antiglaucoma agent* [also: pirnabine]
pirnabine USAN *antiglaucoma agent* [also: pirnabin]
piroctone USAN, INN *antiseborrheic*
piroctone olamine USAN *antiseborrheic*
pirogliride INN *antidiabetic* [also: pirogliride tartrate]
pirogliride tartrate USAN *antidiabetic* [also: pirogliride]
piroheptine INN
pirolate USAN, INN *antiasthmatic*

pirolazamide USAN, INN *antiarrhythmic*
piromidic acid INN
piroxantrone INN *antineoplastic* [also: piroxantrone HCl]
piroxantrone HCl USAN *antineoplastic* [also: piroxantrone]
piroxicam USAN, USP, INN, BAN *antiarthritic; nonsteroidal anti-inflammatory drug (NSAID); analgesic; antiarthritic*
piroxicam cinnamate USAN *anti-inflammatory*
piroxicam olamine USAN *analgesic; anti-inflammatory*
piroxicillin INN
piroximone USAN, INN, BAN *cardiotonic*
pirozadil INN
pirprofen USAN, INN, BAN *anti-inflammatory*
pirquinozol USAN, INN *antiallergic*
pirralkonium bromide INN
pirroksan [now: proroxan HCl]
pirtenidine INN
pitenodil INN
Pitocin IV, IM injection ℞ *induction of labor; postpartum bleeding; incomplete abortion* [oxytocin]
pitofenone INN
Pitressin IM or subcu injection, intranasal cotton pledgets ℞ *diabetes insipidus; abdominal distention* [vasopressin]
Pitressin Tannate IM injection (discontinued 1991) ℞ *diabetes insipidus; abdominal distention* [vasopressin tannate]
pituitary, anterior
pituitary, posterior USP *antidiuretic hormone*
Pituitrin (S) IM injection (discontinued 1991) ℞ *postoperative ileus; surgical hemostasis; enuresis* [posterior pituitary]
pituxate INN
pivampicillin INN *antibacterial* [also: pivampicillin HCl]

pivampicillin HCl USAN *antibacterial* [also: pivampicillin]
pivampicillin pamoate USAN *antibacterial*
pivampicillin probenate USAN *antibacterial*
pivenfrine INN
pivmecillinam INN, BAN *antibacterial* [also: amdinocillin pivoxil]
pivopril USAN *antihypertensive*
pivoxazepam INN
pivsulbactam BAN *β-lactamase inhibitor; penicillin/cephalosporin synergist* [also: sulbactam pivoxil]
pix pini [see: pine tar]
PIXY321 ℞ *investigational agent for chemotherapy-related neutropenia and thrombocytopenia* [granulocyte macrophage colony-stimulating factor]
Pixykine ℞ *investigational second-generation colony stimulating factor*
pizotifen INN, BAN *anabolic; antidepressant; serotonin inhibitor (migraine specific)* [also: pizotyline]
pizotyline USAN *anabolic; antidepressant; serotonin inhibitor (migraine specific)* [also: pizotifen]
placebo *no medicinal value* [also: obecalp]
Placidyl capsules ℞ *hypnotic* [ethchlorvynol]
plafibride INN
plague vaccine USP *active bacterin for plague (Yersinia pestis)*
planadalin [see: carbromal]
plantago seed USP *laxative*
plantain seed [see: plantago seed]
Plaquenil Sulfate tablets ℞ *antimalarial; antirheumatic* [hydroxychloroquine sulfate]
Plasbumin-5; Plasbumin-25 IV infusion ℞ *blood volume expander; shock; burns; hypoproteinemia* [human albumin]
plasma, antihemophilic human USP
plasma concentrate factor IX [see: factor IX complex]

Plasma Plex IV infusion ℞ *blood volume support; protein replenisher* [plasma protein fraction]
plasma protein fraction USP *blood volume supporter*
plasma protein fraction, human [now: plasma protein fraction]
plasma thromboplastin component (PTC) [see: factor IX]
Plasma-Lyte A pH 7.4; Plasma-Lyte R; Plasma-Lyte 56; Plasma-Lyte 148 IV infusion ℞ *intravenous electrolyte therapy* [combined electrolyte solution]
Plasma-Lyte M (R; 56; 148) and 5% Dextrose IV infusion ℞ *intravenous nutritional/electrolyte therapy* [combined electrolyte solution; dextrose]
Plasmanate IV infusion ℞ *blood volume expander; shock due to burns, trauma and surgery* [plasma protein fraction]
Plasmatein 5% IV infusion ℞ *antihemophilic* [plasma protein fraction]
plasmin BAN [also: fibrinolysin, human]
Plateau Caps (trademarked form) *controlled-release capsules*
platelet cofactor II [see: factor IX]
platelet concentrate USP *platelet replenisher*
platelet-derived growth factor *investigational vulnerary*
Platinol powder for IV injection ℞ *antineoplastic* [cisplatin]
Platinol-AQ IV injection ℞ *antineoplastic* [cisplatin]
platinum *element (Pt)*
***cis*-platinum** [now: cisplatin]
***cis*-platinum II** [now: cisplatin]
platinum diamminodichloride [see: cisplatin]
plaunotol INN
plauracin USAN, INN *veterinary growth stimulant*
Plegine tablets ℞ *anorexiant* [phendimetrazine tartrate]

Plegisol solution ℞ *cardioplegic solution* [calcium chloride; magnesium chloride; potassium chloride; sodium chloride]
Plendil extended-release tablets ℞ *antihypertensive* [felodipine]
pleuromulin INN
Pliagel solution OTC *contact lens surfactant cleaning solution*
plicamycin USAN, USP, INN *antineoplastic*
plomestane USAN *antineoplastic; aromatase inhibitor*
plutonium *element (Pu)*
PMB 200; PMB 400 tablets ℞ *estrogen deficiency; menopausal symptoms* [conjugated estrogens; meprobamate]
PMMA (polymethylmethacrylate) [q.v.]
P-MVAC (Platinol, methotrexate, vinblastine, Adriamycin, carboplatin) *chemotherapy protocol*
pneumococcal vaccine, polyvalent *active bacterin for pneumococcal pneumonia*
Pneumopent ℞ *(orphan: Pneumocystis carinii pneumonia)* [pentamidine isethionate]
Pneumovax 23 subcu or IM injection ℞ *pneumonia vaccine* [pneumococcal vaccine, polyvalent]
Pnu-Imune 23 subcu or IM injection ℞ *pneumonia vaccine* [pneumococcal vaccine, polyvalent]
POC (procarbazine, Oncovin, CCNU) *chemotherapy protocol*
POCA (prednisone, Oncovin, cytarabine, Adriamycin) *chemotherapy protocol*
POCC (procarbazine, Oncovin, cyclophosphamide, CCNU) *chemotherapy protocol*
Pod-Ben-25 liquid ℞ *topical keratolytic* [podophyllum resin; benzoin]
podilfen INN
Podoben liquid (discontinued 1991) ℞ *topical keratolytic* [podophyllum resin; benzoin]

Podocon-25 liquid ℞ *topical keratolytic* [podophyllum resin; benzoin]
podofilox USAN *antimitotic* [also: podophyllotoxin]
Podofin liquid ℞ *topical keratolytic* [podophyllum resin; benzoin]
podophyllin [see: podophyllum resin]
podophyllotoxin BAN *antimitotic* [also: podofilox]
podophyllum USP *pharmaceutic necessity*
podophyllum resin USP *caustic*
Point-Two oral rinse ℞ *topical dental caries preventative* [sodium fluoride]
Poison Antidote Kit OTC *emergency poison treatment* [syrup of ipecac; charcoal suspension]
poison ivy extract, alum precipitated USAN *ivy poisoning counteractant*
poison oak extract USAN *antiallergic*
Poison Oak-N-Ivy Armor lotion OTC *topical poison ivy treatment*
polacrilin USAN, INN *pharmaceutic aid*
polacrilin potassium USAN, NF *tablet disintegrant*
Poladex timed-release tablets ℞ *antihistamine* [dexchlorpheniramine maleate]
Polaramine Expectorant liquid ℞ *decongestant; antihistamine; expectorant* [pseudoephedrine sulfate; dexchlorpheniramine maleate; guaifenesin; alcohol]
Polaramine tablets, Repetabs (repeat-action tablets), syrup ℞ *antihistamine* [dexchlorpheniramine maleate]
Polargen timed-release tablets (discontinued 1991) ℞ *antihistamine* [dexchlorpheniramine maleate]
poldine methylsulfate USAN, USP *anticholinergic* [also: poldine metilsulfate]
poldine metilsulfate INN *anticholinergic* [also: poldine methylsulfate]
policapram USAN, INN *tablet binder*
policresulen INN

polidexide sulfate INN
polidocanol
polifeprosan INN *pharmaceutic aid* [also: polifeprosan 20]
polifeprosan 20 USAN *pharmaceutic aid* [also: polifeprosan]
poligeenan USAN, INN *dispersing agent*
poliglecaprone 25 USAN *absorbable surgical suture material*
poliglecaprone 90 USAN *absorbable surgical suture coating*
poliglusam USAN *antihemorrhagic*
polignate sodium USAN *pepsin enzyme inhibitor*
polihexanide INN [also: polyhexanide]
poliomyelitis vaccine [now: poliovirus vaccine, inactivated]
Poliovax subcu injection (discontinued 1993) ℞ *poliomyelitis vaccine* [poliovirus vaccine, inactivated]
poliovirus vaccine, inactivated (IPV) USP *active immunizing agent for poliomyelitis*
poliovirus vaccine, live oral USP *active immunizing agent for poliomyelitis*
polipropene 25 USAN *tablet excipient*
polisaponin INN
politef INN *prosthetic aid* [also: polytef]
Polocaine injection ℞ *injectable local anesthetic* [mepivacaine HCl]
polonium *element (Po)*
Poloris Dental Poultice OTC *topical oral anesthetic* [benzocaine; capsicum]
poloxalene USAN, INN, BAN *surfactant*
poloxamer USAN, NF, INN, BAN *ointment and suppository base; tablet binder*
poloxamer 124 USAN *surfactant; emulsifier; solubilizer; stabilizer*
poloxamer 188 USAN *surfactant; emulsifier; solubilizer; (orphan: sickle cell crisis; severe burns)*
poloxamer 237 USAN *surfactant; emulsifier; solubilizer; stabilizer*

poloxamer 331 (orphan: toxoplasmosis of AIDS)
poloxamer 338 USAN surfactant; emulsifier; solubilizer; stabilizer
poloxamer 407 USAN surfactant; emulsifier; solubilizer; stabilizer
poly I: poly C12U investigational antiviral/immunomodulator; (orphan: AIDS; renal cell carcinoma)
polyamine resin [see: polyamine-methylene resin]
polyamine-methylene resin
polyanhydroglucose [see: dextran]
polyanhydroglucuronic acid [see: dextran]
polybenzarsol INN
polybutester USAN surgical suture material
polybutilate USAN surgical suture coating
polycarbokane [see: polycarbophil]
polycarbophil USP, INN, BAN bulk laxative
Polycillin capsules, powder for oral suspension, pediatric drops ℞ penicillin-type antibiotic [ampicillin trihydrate]
Polycillin-N powder for IV or IM injection ℞ penicillin-type antibiotic [ampicillin sodium]
Polycillin-PRB powder for oral suspension ℞ antibiotic for Neisseria gonorrhoeae [ampicillin trihydrate; probenecid]
Polycitra syrup ℞ urinary alkalinizing agent [potassium citrate; sodium citrate; citric acid]
Polycitra-K solution, crystals ℞ urinary alkalizing agent; (orphan: dissolution of uric acid and cysteine calculi) [potassium citrate; citric acid]
Polycitra-LC solution ℞ urinary alkalizing agent; (orphan: dissolution of urinary stones) [potassium citrate; sodium citrate; citric acid]
Polycose liquid, powder OTC carbohydrate caloric supplement [glucose polymers]

polydextrose USAN food additive
Polydine ointment, scrub, solution OTC broad-spectrum antimicrobial [povidone-iodine]
polydioxanone USAN absorbable surgical suture material
polyelectrolyte 211 [see: sodium alginate]
polyestradiol phosphate INN, BAN antineoplastic; estrogen
polyetadene INN antacid [also: polyethadene]
polyethadene USAN antacid [also: polyetadene]
polyethylene excipient NF stiffening agent
polyethylene glycol (PEG) NF ointment and suppository base; solvent
polyethylene glycol n [n refers to the molecular weight: 300, 400, 1000, etc.]
polyethylene glycol n dioleate [n refers to the molecular weight: 300, 400, 1000, etc.]
polyethylene glycol 8 monostearate [see: polyoxyl 8 stearate]
polyethylene glycol 1000 monocetyl ether [see: cetomacrogol 1000]
polyethylene glycol 1540 NF
polyethylene glycol 4000 USP [also: macrogol 4000]
polyethylene glycol 6000 USP
polyethylene glycol-electrolyte solution (PEG-ES) pre-procedure bowel evacuant [contains PEG 3350]
polyethylene glycol monoleyl ether [see: polyoxyl 10 oleyl ether]
polyethylene glycol monomethyl ether NF excipient
polyethylene glycol monostearate [see: polyoxyl 40 & 50 stearate]
polyethylene oxide NF suspending and viscosity agent; tablet binder
polyferose USAN hematinic
Polyflex tablets (discontinued 1991) ℞ skeletal muscle relaxant; analgesic [chlorzoxazone; acetaminophen]

Polygam powder for IV infusion ℞ *passive immunizing agent* [immune globulin]
polygeline INN, BAN
polyglactin 370 USAN *absorbable surgical suture coating*
polyglactin 910 USAN *absorbable surgical suture material*
polyglycolic acid USAN, INN *surgical suture material*
polyglyconate USAN, BAN *absorbable surgical suture material*
polyhexanide BAN [also: polihexanide]
Poly-Histine CS syrup ℞ *decongestant; antihistamine; antitussive* [phenylpropanolamine HCl; brompheniramine maleate; codeine phosphate]
Poly-Histine DM syrup ℞ *decongestant; antihistamine; antitussive* [phenylpropanolamine HCl; brompheniramine maleate; dextromethorphan hydrobromide]
Poly-Histine elixir ℞ *antihistamine* [pheniramine maleate; pyrilamine maleate; phenyltoloxamine citrate]
Poly-Histine-D Ped Caps sustained-release capsules ℞ *pediatric decongestant and antihistamine* [phenylpropanolamine HCl; phenyltoloxamine citrate; pyrilamine maleate; pheniramine maleate]
Poly-Histine-D sustained-release capsules, elixir ℞ *decongestant; antihistamine* [phenylpropanolamine HCl; phenyltoloxamine citrate; pyrilamine maleate; pheniramine maleate]
polyloxyl 8 stearate USAN *surfactant*
polymacon USAN *hydrophilic contact lens material*
polymanoacetate [now: acemannan]
polymeric oxygen [see: oxygen, polymeric]
polymetaphosphate P 32 USAN *radioactive agent*
polymethylmethacrylate (PMMA) *rigid hydrophobic polymer used for hard contact lenses*

polymixin E [see: colistin sulfate]
polymonine
Polymox capsules, powder for oral suspension, pediatric drops ℞ *penicillin-type antibiotic* [amoxicillin trihydrate]
polymyxin BAN *bactericidal antibiotic* [also: polymyxin B sulfate; polymyxin B]
polymyxin B INN *bactericidal antibiotic* [also: polymyxin B sulfate; polymyxin]
polymyxin B sulfate USP *bactericidal antibiotic* [also: polymyxin B; polymyxin]
polymyxin B$_1$ [see: polymyxin B]
polymyxin B$_2$ [see: polymyxin B]
polymyxin B$_3$ [see: polymyxin B]
polymyxin E [see: colistin sulfate]
polynoxylin INN, BAN
polyoxyethylene 20 sorbitan monolaurate [see: polysorbate 20]
polyoxyethylene 20 sorbitan monooleate [see: polysorbate 80]
polyoxyethylene 20 sorbitan monopalmitate [see: polysorbate 40]
polyoxyethylene 20 sorbitan monostearate [see: polysorbate 60]
polyoxyethylene 20 sorbitan trioleate [see: polysorbate 85]
polyoxyethylene 20 sorbitan tristearate [see: polysorbate 65]
polyoxyethylene 50 stearate [now: polyoxyl 50 stearate]
polyoxyethylene glycol 1000 monocetyl ether [see: cetomacrogol 1000]
polyoxyethylene nonyl phenol *surfactant/wetting agent*
polyoxyl 10 oleyl ether NF *surfactant*
polyoxyl 20 cetostearyl ether NF *surfactant*
polyoxyl 35 castor oil NF *emulsifying agent; surfactant*
polyoxyl 40 hydrogenated castor oil NF *emulsifying agent; surfactant*

polyoxyl 40 stearate USAN, NF *surfactant*
polyoxyl 50 stearate NF *surfactant; emulsifying agent*
polyoxypropylene 15 stearyl ether USAN *solvent*
polyphosphoric acid, sodium salt [see: sodium polyphosphate]
Poly-Pred eye drop suspension ℞ *topical ophthalmic corticosteroidal anti-inflammatory; antibiotic* [prednisolone acetate; neomycin sulfate]
polypropylene glycol NF
polyribonucleotide [see: poly I: poly C12U]
polysaccharide-iron complex *hematinic*
Polysorb Hydrate cream OTC *moisturizer; emollient*
polysorbate 20 USAN, NF, INN *surfactant/wetting agent*
polysorbate 40 USAN, NF, INN *surfactant*
polysorbate 60 USAN, NF, INN *surfactant*
polysorbate 65 USAN, INN *surfactant*
polysorbate 80 USAN, NF, INN *surfactant/wetting agent; viscosity-increasing agent*
polysorbate 85 USAN, INN *surfactant*
Polysporin aerosol spray (discontinued 1993) OTC *topical/ophthalmic antibiotic* [polymyxin B sulfate; bacitracin zinc]
Polysporin ointment, powder, ophthalmic ointment OTC *topical/ophthalmic antibiotic* [polymyxin B sulfate; bacitracin zinc]
Polytabs-F chewable tablets ℞ *pediatric vitamin supplement and dental caries preventative* [multiple vitamins; fluoride; folic acid]
Polytar Bath oil OTC *antipsoriatic; antiseborrheic; antipruritic; emollient* [coal tar]

Polytar shampoo, soap OTC *antiseborrheic; antipsoriatic; antipruritic; antibacterial* [coal tar, pine tar, & juniper tar solution]
polytef USAN *prosthetic aid* [also: politef]
polytetrafluoroethylene (PTFE) [see: polytef]
polythiazide USAN, USP, INN *diuretic; antihypertensive*
Polytrim eye drops ℞ *ophthalmic antibiotic* [polymyxin B sulfate; trimethoprim]
polyurethane foam USAN *internal bone splint*
polyvalent Crotaline antivenin [see: antivenin (Crotalidae) polyvalent]
polyvalent gas gangrene antitoxin [see: gas gangrene antitoxin, pentavalent]
polyvidone INN *dispersing, suspending and viscosity-increasing agent* [also: povidone]
Poly-Vi-Flor chewable tablets, drops ℞ *pediatric vitamin supplement and dental caries preventative* [multiple vitamins; sodium fluoride; folic acid]
Poly-Vi-Flor with Iron chewable tablets, drops ℞ *pediatric vitamin/iron supplement and dental caries preventative* [multiple vitamins & minerals; sodium fluoride; iron; folic acid]
polyvinyl acetate phthalate NF *coating agent*
polyvinyl alcohol (PVA) USP *viscosity-increasing agent*
polyvinylpyrrolidone [now: povidone]
Poly-Vi-Sol chewable tablets OTC *vitamin supplement* [multiple vitamins; folic acid]
Poly-Vi-Sol drops OTC *vitamin supplement* [multiple vitamins]
Poly-Vitamin drops OTC *vitamin supplement* [multiple vitamins]
Polyvitamin Drops with Iron and Fluoride ℞ *pediatric vitamin/iron supplement and dental caries preventa-*

tive [multiple vitamins; iron; fluoride]

Polyvitamin Fluoride chewable tablets, drops ℞ *pediatric vitamin supplement and dental caries preventative* [multiple vitamins; fluoride; folic acid]

Polyvitamin Fluoride with Iron chewable tablets ℞ *pediatric vitamin/iron supplement and dental caries preventative* [multiple vitamins & minerals; fluoride; iron; folic acid]

Polyvitamin with Fluoride chewable tablets, drops ℞ *pediatric vitamin supplement and dental caries preventative* [multiple vitamins; fluoride; folic acid]

Poly-Vitamin with Iron drops OTC *vitamin/iron supplement* [multiple vitamins; iron]

Polyvitamins with Fluoride and Iron chewable tablets ℞ *pediatric vitamin/iron supplement and dental caries preventative* [multiple vitamins; fluoride; iron; folic acid]

Polyvite with Fluoride drops (discontinued 1993) ℞ *pediatric vitamin deficiency and dental caries prevention* [multiple vitamins; fluoride]

POMP (prednisone, Oncovin, methotrexate, Purinethol) *chemotherapy protocol*

ponalrestat USAN, INN, BAN *aldose reductase inhibitor*

Pondimin tablets ℞ *anorexiant* [fenfluramine HCl]

ponfibrate INN

Ponstel capsules ℞ *nonsteroidal anti-inflammatory drug (NSAID); analgesic; for primary dysmenorrhea* [mefenamic acid]

Pontocaine cream OTC *topical local anesthetic* [tetracaine HCl]

Pontocaine Eye ointment ℞ *topical ocular anesthetic* [tetracaine]

Pontocaine HCl eye drops ℞ *topical ocular anesthetic* [tetracaine HCl]

Pontocaine HCl solution ℞ *nose/throat anesthetic to abolish laryngeal and esophageal reflex* [tetracaine HCl; chlorobutanol]

Pontocaine HCl spinal injection, powder for reconstitution ℞ *injectable local anesthetic* [tetracaine HCl]

Pontocaine ointment OTC *topical local anesthetic* [tetracaine]

Po-Pon-S sugar-coated tablets OTC *vitamin/mineral supplement* [multiple vitamins & minerals]

Porcelana cream OTC *hyperpigmentation bleaching agent* [hydroquinone]

Porcelana with Sunscreen cream OTC *hyperpigmentation bleaching agent; sunscreen* [hydroquinone; padimate O]

porfimer sodium USAN, INN *antineoplastic*

porfiromycin USAN, INN *antibacterial; antineoplastic*

porofocon A USAN *hydrophobic contact lens material*

porofocon B USAN *hydrophobic contact lens material*

Portagen powder OTC *nutritional and fat supplement*

porton asparaginase [see: erwinia L-asparaginase]

posatirelin INN

posedrine [see: benzchlorpropamide]

poskine INN, BAN

posterior pituitary [see: pituitary, posterior]

Posterisan anorectal ointment, suppositories (discontinued 1991) OTC *antibacterial; antiseptic* [sterilized coli-vaccine; liquefied phenol]

Posture tablets OTC *calcium supplement* [calcium phosphate, tribasic]

Posture-D film-coated tablets OTC *dietary supplement* [calcium phosphate, tribasic; vitamin D]

Potaba tablets, capsules, Envules (powder for reconstitution), powder ℞ *treatment of scleroderma and other*

skin diseases [potassium para-aminobenzoate]
Potable Aqua tablets OTC *emergency disinfectant for drinking water* [tetraglycine hydroperiodide]
Potachlor 10%; Potachlor 20% liquid (discontinued 1992) ℞ *potassium supplement* [potassium chloride]
Potage powder (discontinued 1991) ℞ *potassium supplement* [potassium chloride]
Potasalan liquid ℞ *potassium supplement* [potassium chloride; alcohol]
potash, sulfurated USP *source of sulfides*
potassic saline, lactated NF
Potassine liquid (discontinued 1991) ℞ *potassium supplement* [potassium chloride]
potassium *element (K)*
potassium acetate USP *electrolyte replenisher*
potassium acid phosphate *urinary acidifier*
potassium alpha-phenoxyethyl penicillin [see: phenethicillin potassium]
potassium alum [see: alum, potassium]
potassium aspartate & magnesium aspartate USAN *nutrient*
potassium benzoate NF *preservative*
potassium benzyl penicillin [see: penicillin G potassium]
potassium bitartrate USAN
potassium borate *pH buffer*
potassium carbonate USP *alkalizing agent*
potassium chloride (KCl) USP *electrolyte replenisher*
potassium chloride K 42 USAN *radioactive agent*
potassium citrate USP *alkalizer; electrolyte replacement; (orphan: nephrolithiasis; hypocitraturia)*
potassium citrate & citric acid *(orphan: dissolution of uric acid and cysteine calculi)*

Potassium Cl enteric-coated tablets (discontinued 1992) ℞ *potassium supplement* [potassium chloride]
potassium clavulanate & amoxicillin [see: amoxicillin]
potassium clavulanate & ticarcillin [see: ticarcillin disodium]
potassium dichloroisocyanurate [see: troclosene potassium]
potassium glucaldrate USAN, INN *antacid*
potassium gluconate USP *electrolyte replenisher*
potassium guaiacolsulfonate USP *expectorant* [also: sulfogaiacol]
potassium hydroxide (KOH) NF *alkalizing agent*
potassium hydroxymethoxybenzenesulfonate hemihydrate [see: potassium guaiacolsulfonate]
potassium iodide USP *antifungal; expectorant; iodine supplement*
potassium mercuric iodide NF
potassium metabisulfite NF *antioxidant*
potassium metaphosphate NF *buffering agent*
potassium nitrate *tooth desensitizer*
potassium nitrazepate INN
potassium para-aminobenzoate (PAB)
potassium penicillin G [see: penicillin G potassium]
potassium perchlorate *adjunct in radioimaging*
potassium permanganate USP *topical anti-infective*
potassium phosphate, dibasic USP *calcium regulator; phosphorus replacement; pH buffer*
potassium phosphate, monobasic NF *pH buffer; phosphorus replacement*
potassium sodium tartrate USP *laxative*
potassium sorbate NF *antimicrobial agent*
potassium tetraborate *pH buffer*
potassium thiocyanate NF

potasssium bicarbonate USP *pH buffer; electrolyte replacement*

Povadyne ointment, scrub, solution, swabsticks, wipes, whirlpool concentrate (discontinued 1992) OTC *broad-spectrum antimicrobial* [povidone-iodine]

Povidine ointment, scrub, solution OTC *broad-spectrum antimicrobial* [povidone-iodine]

povidone USAN, USP *dispersing, suspending and viscosity-increasing agent* [also: polyvidone]

povidone I 125 USAN *radioactive agent*

povidone I 131 USAN *radioactive agent*

povidone-iodine USP, BAN *broad-spectrum antimicrobial*

powdered cellulose [see: cellulose, powdered]

powdered ipecac [see: ipecac, powdered]

powdered opium [see: opium, powdered]

PPA (phenylpropanolamine) [q.v.]

PPA/Guaifenesin tablets (discontinued 1992) ℞ *decongestant; expectorant* [phenylpropanolamine HCl; guaifenesin]

PPD (purified protein derivative [of tuberculin]) [see: tuberculin]

PPG-15 stearyl ether [now: polyoxypropylene 15 stearyl ether]

PPI-002 (*orphan: malignant mesothelioma*)

PR-122 (redox-phenytoin) (*orphan: emergency rescue status epilepticus*)

PR-225 (redox-acyclovir) (*orphan: herpes simplex encephalitis in AIDS*)

PR-239 (redox penicillin Q) (*orphan: AIDS-associated neurosyphilis*)

PR-320 (molecusol-carbamazepine) (*orphan: emergency rescue status epilepticus*)

practolol USAN, INN *antiadrenergic* (β-receptor)

Pragmatar ointment (discontinued 1991) OTC *topical antipsoriatic; antiseborrheic; keratolytic; antifungal* [cetyl-alcohol-coal tar distillate; precipitated sulfur; salicylic acid]

prajmalium bitartrate INN, BAN

pralidoxime chloride USAN, USP *cholinesterase reactivator*

pralidoxime iodide USAN, INN *cholinesterase reactivator*

pralidoxime mesylate USAN *cholinesterase reactivator*

PrameGel liquid OTC *topical local anesthetic; antiseptic* [pramoxine HCl; menthol]

Pramet FA controlled-release Filmtabs (film-coated tablets) ℞ *prenatal vitamin/calcium/iron supplement* [multiple vitamins; calcium; iron; folic acid]

Pramilet FA Filmtabs (film-coated tablets) ℞ *prenatal vitamin/mineral/calcium/iron supplement* [multiple vitamins & minerals; calcium; iron; folic acid]

pramipexole INN *investigational dopaminergic for Parkinson's disease and schizophrenia*

pramiracetam INN *cognition adjuvant* [also: pramiracetam HCl]

pramiracetam HCl USAN *cognition adjuvant* [also: pramiracetam]

pramiracetam sulfate USAN *cognition adjuvant*; (*orphan: adjunct to electroconvulsive therapy*)

pramiverine INN, BAN

pramocaine INN *topical anesthetic* [also: pramoxine HCl; pramoxine]

pramocaine HCl [see: pramoxine HCl]

Pramosone cream, lotion, ointment ℞ *topical corticosteroid; local anesthetic* [hydrocortisone acetate; pramoxine]

pramoxine BAN *topical anesthetic* [also: pramoxine HCl; pramocaine]

pramoxine HCl USP *topical anesthetic* [also: pramocaine; pramoxine]

prampine INN, BAN
pranolium chloride USAN, INN *antiarrhythmic*
pranoprofen INN
pranosal INN
praseodymium *element (Pr)*
prasterone INN
Pravachol tablets ℞ *cholesterol-lowering antihyperlipidemic* [pravastatin sodium]
pravadoline INN *analgesic* [also: pravadoline maleate]
pravadoline maleate USAN *analgesic* [also: pravadoline]
pravastatin INN, BAN *antihyperlipoproteinemic* [also: pravastatin sodium]
pravastatin sodium USAN *antihyperlipoproteinemic* [also: pravastatin]
Prax lotion, cream OTC *topical local anesthetic* [pramoxine HCl]
praxadine INN
prazepam USAN, USP, INN *sedative*
prazepine INN
praziquantel USAN, USP, INN, BAN *anthelmintic; (orphan: neurocysticercosis)*
prazitone INN, BAN
prazocillin INN
prazosin INN *antihypertensive;* $_1$*-adrenergic blocker* [also: prazosin HCl]
prazosin HCl USAN, USP *antihypertensive* [also: prazosin]
Pre-Attain liquid OTC *oral nutritional supplement*
Precef powder for IV or IM injection, StrapKap vials (discontinued 1993) ℞ *cephalosporin-type antibiotic* [ceforanide]
precipitated calcium carbonate [see: calcium carbonate, precipitated]
precipitated chalk [see: calcium carbonate]
precipitated sulfur [see: sulfur, precipitated]
Precision High Nitrogen Diet; Precision Isotonic Diet; Precision LR Diet powder OTC *oral nutritional supplement*

preclamol INN
Pred Mild Ophthalmic; Pred Forte eye drop suspension ℞ *ophthalmic topical corticosteroidal anti-inflammatory* [prednisolone acetate]
Predaject-50 IM injection ℞ *glucocorticoids* [prednisolone acetate]
Predalone 50 IM injection ℞ *glucocorticoids* [prednisolone acetate]
Predalone T.B.A. intra-articular, intralesional, or soft tissue injection ℞ *glucocorticoids* [prednisolone tebutate]
Predamide eye drop suspension (discontinued 1992) ℞ *topical ophthalmic corticosteroidal anti-inflammatory; bacteriostatic* [prednisolone acetate; sodium sulfacetamide]
Predcor-25; Predcor-50 IM injection ℞ *glucocorticoids* [prednisolone acetate]
Predforte eye drop suspension ℞ *ophthalmic topical corticosteroid anti-inflammatory agent* [prednisolone acetate]
Pred-G eye drop suspension ℞ *topical ophthalmic corticosteroidal anti-inflammatory; antibiotic* [prednisolone acetate; gentamicin sulfate]
Pred-G ophthalmic ointment ℞ *topical ophthalmic corticosteroidal anti-inflammatory; antibiotic* [prednisolone acetate; gentamicin sulfate; chlorobutanol]
Predicort-50 IM injection (discontinued 1991) ℞ *glucocorticoids* [prednisolone acetate]
prednazate USAN, INN *anti-inflammatory*
prednazoline INN
prednicarbate USAN, INN *glucocorticoid*
Prednicen-M tablets ℞ *corticosteroid* [prednisone]
prednimustine USAN, INN *antineoplastic; (orphan: malignant non-Hodgkin's lymphomas)*

Prednisol TBA intra-articular, intralesional, or soft tissue injection ℞ *glucocorticoids* [prednisolone tebutate]
prednisolamate INN, BAN
prednisolone USP, INN *glucocorticoid*
prednisolone acetate USP, BAN *glucocorticoid; ophthalmic anti-inflammatory*
prednisolone hemisuccinate USP *glucocorticoid*
prednisolone sodium phosphate USP *glucocorticoid; ophthalmic anti-inflammatory*
prednisolone sodium succinate USP *glucocorticoid*
prednisolone steaglate INN, BAN
prednisolone tebutate USP *glucocorticoid*
prednisone USP, INN *glucocorticoid*
prednival USAN *glucocorticoid*
prednylidene INN, BAN
Predsulfair eye drop suspension, ophthalmic ointment ℞ *topical ophthalmic corticosteroidal anti-inflammatory; bacteriostatic* [prednisolone acetate; sodium sulfacetamide]
prefenamate INN
Prefill (dosage form) *prefilled applicator*
Preflex for Sensitive Eyes solution OTC *contact lens surfactant cleaning solution*
Prefrin Liquifilm eye drops OTC *topical ocular decongestant; local anesthetic* [phenylephrine HCl; antipyrine]
Prefrin-A eye drops ℞ *topical ocular decongestant/antihistamine; local anesthetic* [phenylephrine HCl; pyrilamine maleate; antipyrine]
pregelatinized starch [see: starch, pregelatinized]
Pregestimil liquid, powder OTC *hypoallergenic infant food* [protein hydrolysate formula]
pregneninolone [see: ethisterone]

pregnenolone INN *non-hormonal sterol derivative* [also: pregnenolone succinate]
pregnenolone succinate USAN *non-hormonal sterol derivative* [also: pregnenolone]
Pregnopsia II test kit (discontinued 1991) ℞ *in vitro diagnostic aid for urine pregnancy test*
Pregnosis test kit ℞ *in vitro diagnostic aid for urine pregnancy test*
Pregnosticon Dri-Dot test kit (discontinued 1991) ℞ *in vitro diagnostic aid for urine pregnancy test*
Pregnyl powder for injection ℞ *hormone for prepubertal cryptorchidism and hypogonadism* [chorionic gonadotropin]
Pre-H Cal tablets ℞ *vitamin/calcium/iron supplement* [multiple vitamins; calcium; iron; folic acid]
Prehist D sustained-release capsules ℞ *decongestant; antihistamine; anticholinergic* [phenylephrine HCl; chlorpheniramine maleate; methscopolamine nitrate]
Prehist sustained-release capsules ℞ *decongestant; antihistamine* [phenylephrine HCl; chlorpheniramine maleate]
Prelone syrup ℞ *glucocorticoids* [prednisolone]
Prelu-2 timed-release capsules ℞ *anorexiant* [phendimetrazine tartrate]
Preludin sustained-release tablets (discontinued 1992) ℞ *anorexiant* [phenmetrazine HCl]
Premarin Intravenous ℞ *estrogen deficiency; inoperable prostatic and breast cancer* [conjugated estrogens]
Premarin tablets, vaginal cream ℞ *estrogen deficiency; inoperable prostatic and breast cancer* [conjugated estrogens]
Premarin with Methyltestosterone tablets ℞ *estrogen/androgen for menopausal vasomotor symptoms* [conjugated estrogens; methyltestosterone]

Premarin/MPA ℞ *investigational osteoporosis treatment* [conjugated estrogens; medroxyprogesterone acetate]

premazepam INN, BAN

Prēmsyn PMS caplets OTC *analgesic; antipyretic; diuretic; antihistaminic sleep aid* [acetaminophen; pamabrom; pyrilamine maleate]

Prēmsyn PMS capsules (discontinued 1992) OTC *analgesic; antipyretic; diuretic; antihistaminic sleep aid* [acetaminophen; pamabrom; pyrilamine maleate]

prenalterol INN, BAN *adrenergic* [also: prenalterol HCl]

prenalterol HCl USAN *adrenergic* [also: prenalterol]

Prenatal 1/1 tablets ℞ *vitamin/mineral supplement* [multiple vitamins & minerals]

Pre-Natal cellulose-coated caplets OTC *vitamin/mineral supplement for pregnant and lactating women* [multiple vitamins & minerals]

Prenatal FA tablets ℞ *prenatal vitamin/mineral supplement* [multiple vitamins & minerals]

Prenatal One film-coated tablets ℞ *vitamin/calcium/iron supplement* [multiple vitamins; calcium; iron; folic acid]

Prenatal Plus Improved tablets ℞ *vitamin/calcium/iron supplement* [multiple vitamins; calcium; iron; folic acid]

Prenatal Rx tablets ℞ *vitamin/calcium/iron supplement* [multiple vitamins; calcium; iron; folic acid; biotin]

Prenatal with Folic Acid tablets OTC *vitamin/calcium/iron supplement* [multiple vitamins; calcium; iron; folic acid]

Prenatal-1 + Iron tablets ℞ *vitamin/calcium/iron supplement* [multiple vitamins; calcium; iron; folic acid]

Prenatal-S tablets OTC *vitamin/calcium/iron supplement* [multiple vitamins; calcium; iron; folic acid]

Prenate 90 film-coated delayed-release tablets ℞ *vitamin/calcium/iron supplement* [multiple vitamins; calcium; iron; folic acid]

Prenavite tablets OTC *vitamin/calcium/iron supplement* [multiple vitamins; calcium; iron; folic acid]

prenisteine INN

prenoverine INN

prenoxdiazine INN

prenylamine USAN, INN *coronary vasodilator*

Preparation H anorectal ointment, suppositories OTC *antifungal; antiseptic* [live yeast cell derivative; phenylmercuric nitrate; shark liver oil]

Preparation H Cleansing anorectal pads (discontinued 1992) OTC *astringent; antiseptic; antifungal* [witch hazel; alcohol; glycerin; methylparaben]

Preparation H Cleansing tissues OTC *moisturizer and cleanser for external rectal/vaginal areas*

Preparation H cream OTC *antifungal; antiseptic* [live yeast cell derivative; shark liver oil]

prepared chalk [see: calcium carbonate]

Prepcat suspension ℞ *GI contrast radiopaque agent* [barium sulfate; sorbitol]

Pre-Pen solution for dermal scratch test ℞ *penicillin hypersensitivity assessment* [benzylpenicilloyl polylysine]

Pre-Pen/MDM solution for dermal scratch test ℞ *(orphan: penicillin hypersensitivity assessment)* [benzylpenicillin]

Prepidil gel ℞ *prostaglandin for cervical ripening at term* [dinoprostone]

Presalin tablets OTC *analgesic; antipyretic; anti-inflammatory* [acetaminophen; aspirin; salicylamide; aluminum hydroxide]

pretamazium iodide INN, BAN

prethcamide

prethrombin [see: prothrombin complex, activated]

pretiadil INN

Pretts Diet-Aid chewable tablets OTC *diet aid* [sodium carboxymethylcellulose; sodium bicarbonate]

Pretz Irrigating solution OTC *for postoperative irrigation* [sodium chloride (saline); glycerin; eriodictyon]

Pretz Moisturizing nose drops OTC *nasal moisturizer* [sodium chloride (saline); glycerin; eriodictyon]

Pretz solution OTC *nasal moisturizer* [sodium chloride (saline)]

Pretz-D nasal spray OTC *nasal decongestant and moisturizer* [ephedrine sulfate; glycerin; saline; eriodictyon]

PretzPak ointment OTC *antimicrobial postoperative nasal pack* [benzyl alcohol; urea; eriodictyon; allantoin]

Prevacid ℞ *investigational antiulcerative*

PreviDent Plus topical gel (for professional application) ℞ *dental caries preventative* [sodium fluoride]

PreviDent topical gel (for self-application) ℞ *dental caries preventative* [sodium fluoride]

pribecaine INN

pridefine INN *antidepressant* [also: pridefine HCl]

pridefine HCl USAN *antidepressant* [also: pridefine]

prideperone INN

pridinol INN

prifelone USAN, INN *dermatologic anti-inflammatory*

prifinium bromide INN

prifuroline INN

prilocaine INN *local anesthetic* [also: prilocaine HCl]

prilocaine HCl USAN, USP *local anesthetic* [also: prilocaine]

Prilosec sustained-release capsules ℞ *duodenal ulcer treatment; antisecretory for erosive esophagitis* [omeprazole]

primachine phosphate [see: primaquine phosphate]

Primacor IV infusion ℞ *vasodilator for congestive heart failure* [milrinone lactate]

Primaderm ointment (discontinued 1992) OTC *moisturizer; emollient; astringent; antiseptic* [cod liver oil concentrate; zinc oxide]

Primaderm-B anorectal ointment OTC *topical anesthetic; astringent* [benzocaine; zinc oxide; cod liver oil]

primaperone INN

primaquine INN *antimalarial* [also: primaquine phosphate]

primaquine phosphate USP *cure for malaria; prevention of malarial relapse* [also: primaquine]

Primatene M Formula tablets (discontinued 1991) OTC *antiasthmatic* [theophylline monohydrate; ephedrine HCl; pyrilamine maleate]

Primatene Mist inhalation aerosol OTC *bronchodilator for bronchial asthma* [epinephrine]

Primatene Mist Suspension inhalation aerosol OTC *bronchodilator for bronchial asthma* [epinephrine bitartrate]

Primatene P Formula tablets (discontinued 1991) OTC *antiasthmatic* [theophylline monohydrate; ephedrine HCl]

Primatene tablets OTC *antiasthmatic; bronchodilator; decongestant* [theophylline; ephedrine HCl]

Primatuss Cough Mixture 4 liquid OTC *antihistamine; antitussive* [dextromethorphan hydrobromide; chlorpheniramine maleate; alcohol]

Primatuss Cough Mixture 4D liquid OTC *decongestant; antitussive; expectorant* [pseudoephedrine HCl; dextromethorphan hydrobromide; guaifenesin; alcohol]

Primaxin powder for IV or IM injection, ADD-vantage vials ℞ *thienamycin-type antibiotic* [imipenem; cilastatin sodium]

primidolol USAN, INN *antihypertensive; antianginal; antiarrhythmic*

primidone USP, INN, BAN *anticonvulsant*

primycin INN

Principen '125'; Principen '250' powder for oral suspension ℞ *penicillin-type antibiotic* [ampicillin trihydrate]

Principen '250'; Principen '500' capsules ℞ *penicillin-type antibiotic* [ampicillin trihydrate]

Principen with Probenecid capsules ℞ *antibiotic for Neisseria gonorrhoeae* [ampicillin trihydrate; probenecid]

Prinivil tablets ℞ *antihypertensive; angiotensin-converting enzyme inhibitor* [lisinopril]

prinodolol [see: pindolol]

prinomide INN *antirheumatic* [also: prinomide tromethamine]

prinomide tromethamine USAN *antirheumatic* [also: prinomide]

prinoxodan USAN, INN *cardiotonic*

Prinzide 12.5; Prinzide 25 tablets ℞ *antihypertensive; angiotensin-converting enzyme inhibitor; diuretic* [hydrochlorothiazide; lisinopril]

Priscoline HCl IV injection ℞ *antihypertensive* [tolazoline HCl]

pristinamycin INN, BAN

Privine nasal spray, nose drops OTC *nasal decongestant* [naphazoline HCl]

prizidilol INN, BAN *antihypertensive* [also: prizidilol HCl]

prizidilol HCl USAN *antihypertensive* [also: prizidilol]

Pro-50 injection ℞ *antihistamine; motion sickness; sleep aid; antiemetic; sedative* [promethazine HCl]

proadifen INN *non-specific synergist* [also: proadifen HCl]

proadifen HCl USAN *non-specific synergist* [also: proadifen]

Pro-Air ℞ *investigational antiasthmatic* [procaterol]

Proaqua tablets (discontinued 1991) ℞ *diuretic; antihypertensive* [benzthiazide]

Probalan tablets ℞ *uricosuric for gout* [probenecid]

Probampacin powder for oral suspension ℞ *antibiotic for Neisseria gonorrhoeae* [ampicillin trihydrate; probenecid]

Pro-Banthīne tablets ℞ *peptic ulcer treatment adjunct; antispasmodic; antisecretory* [propantheline bromide]

probarbital sodium NF, INN

Probax oral gel OTC *relief from minor oral irritations* [propolis]

Probec-T tablets OTC *vitamin supplement* [multiple B vitamins; vitamin C]

Proben-C tablets ℞ *uricosuric for gout* [probenecid; colchicine]

probenecid USP, INN, BAN *uricosuric*

Probeta ℞ *investigational antihypertensive (β-blocker)* [bisoprolol]

probicromil calcium USAN *prophylactic antiallergic* [also: ambicromil]

probucol USAN, USP, INN *antihyperlipoproteinemic*

procainamide INN *antiarrhythmic* [also: procainamide HCl]

procainamide HCl USP *antiarrhythmic* [also: procainamide]

procaine INN [also: procaine borate]

procaine borate NF [also: procaine]

procaine HCl USP *local anesthetic*

procaine penicillin BAN *bactericidal antibiotic* [also: penicillin G procaine]

ProcalAmine IV infusion ℞ *peripheral parenteral nutrition* [multiple essential & nonessential amino acids; electrolytes]

Pro-Cal-Sof capsules OTC *stool softener* [docusate calcium]

Procamide SR sustained-release tablets (discontinued 1991) ℞ *antiarrhythmic* [procainamide HCl]
Procan SR sustained-release tablets ℞ *antiarrhythmic* [procainamide HCl]
procarbazine INN *antineoplastic* [also: procarbazine HCl]
procarbazine HCl USAN, USP *antineoplastic* [also: procarbazine]
Procardia capsules ℞ *antianginal* [nifedipine]
Procardia XL film-coated sustained-release tablets ℞ *antianginal; antihypertensive* [nifedipine]
procaterol INN, BAN *bronchodilator* [also: procaterol HCl]
procaterol HCl USAN *bronchodilator* [also: procaterol]
prochlorperazine USP, INN *antiemetic; antipsychotic; antidopaminergic*
prochlorperazine edisylate USP *antiemetic; antipsychotic*
prochlorperazine ethanedisulfonate [see: prochlorperazine edisylate]
prochlorperazine maleate USP *antiemetic; antipsychotic*
procinolol INN
procinonide USAN, INN *adrenocortical steroid*
proclonol USAN, INN *anthelmintic; antifungal*
procodazole INN
proconvertin [see: factor VII]
Procrit IV or subcu injection ℞ *(orphan: anemia of end-stage renal disease, prematurity or HIV)* [epoetin alfa; human albumin]
Proctacain ointment OTC *hemorrhoidal relief*
Proctocort anorectal cream ℞ *topical corticosteroidal anti-inflammatory* [hydrocortisone]
ProctoCream-HC cream ℞ *topical corticosteroid; local anesthetic* [hydrocortisone acetate; pramoxine HCl]
ProctoFoam anorectal aerosol foam OTC *topical anesthetic* [pramoxine HCl]

Proctofoam-HC anorectal aerosol foam ℞ *topical corticosteroid; local anesthetic* [hydrocortisone acetate; pramoxine HCl]
Pro-Cute lotion OTC *moisturizer; emollient*
procyclidine INN *antiparkinsonian; skeletal muscle relaxant; anticholinergic* [also: procyclidine HCl]
procyclidine HCl USP *antiparkinsonian; skeletal muscle relaxant; anticholinergic* [also: procyclidine]
procymate INN
Procysteine ℞ *investigational immunomodulator for AIDS* [oxothiazolidine carboxylate]
prodeconium bromide INN
Pro-Depo IM injection ℞ *progestin; amenorrhea; functional uterine bleeding* [hydroxyprogesterone caproate]
Proderm Topical dressing OTC *dressing for decubitus ulcers* [castor oil; balsam Peru]
prodilidine INN *analgesic* [also: prodilidine HCl]
prodilidine HCl USAN *analgesic* [also: prodilidine]
prodipine INN
prodolic acid USAN, INN *anti-inflammatory*
profadol INN *analgesic* [also: profadol HCl]
profadol HCl USAN *analgesic* [also: profadol]
Profasi HP powder for IM injection ℞ *hormone for prepubertal cryptorchidism and hypogonadism* [chorionic gonadotropin]
Profenal Drop-Tainers (eye drops) ℞ *ocular nonsteroidal anti-inflammatory; intraoperative miosis inhibitor* [suprofen]
profenamine INN *antiparkinsonian* [also: ethopropazine HCl; ethopropazine]
profenamine HCl [see: ethopropazine HCl]

Proferdex IV or IM injection (discontinued 1991) ℞ *antianemic* [iron dextran]
profexalone INN
Profiber liquid OTC *oral nutritional supplement*
Profilate HP; Profilate OSD IV injection ℞ *hemostatic* [antihemophilic factor VIII:C]
Profilnine Heat-Treated IV suspension ℞ *hemostatic* [factor IX complex]
proflavine INN [also: proflavine dihydrochloride]
proflavine dihydrochloride NF [also: proflavine]
proflavine sulfate NF
proflazepam INN
ProFree/GP Weekly Enzymatic Cleaner tablets OTC *contact lens cleaning solution*
progabide USAN, INN *anticonvulsant; muscle relaxant*
Pro-gesic liquid OTC *topical analgesic* [trolamine salicylate]
Progestaject IM injection (discontinued 1991) ℞ *progestin; amenorrhea; functional uterine bleeding* [progesterone]
Progestasert IUD ℞ *intrauterine contraceptive* [progesterone]
progesterone USP, INN *progestin; intrauterine contraceptive*
proglumetacin INN
proglumide USAN, INN *anticholinergic*
Proglycem capsules, oral suspension ℞ *glucose-elevating agent* [diazoxide]
proguanil INN, BAN [also: chloroguanide HCl]
proguanil HCl [see: chloroguanide HCl]
ProHance injection ℞ *contrast media for magnetic imaging* [gadoteridol]
proheptazine INN
ProHIBiT IM injection ℞ *Haemophilus influenzae type b (HIB) vaccine* [Hemophilus b conjugate vaccine]

proinsulin human USAN *antidiabetic*
Prokine powder for IV infusion ℞ *myeloid reconstitution after autologous bone marrow transplant* [sargramostim]
Prolamine capsules (discontinued 1992) OTC *diet aid* [phenylpropanolamine HCl]
Prolastin IV injection ℞ *(orphan: alpha$_1$ proteinase inhibitor deficiency)* [alpha$_1$-proteinase inhibitor]
Proleukin powder for IV infusion ℞ *antineoplastic for renal cell carcinoma; (orphan: renal cell carcinoma; immunodeficiency diseases)* [aldesleukin]
Proleukin-PEG ℞ *investigational immune enhancer for AIDS*
proligestone INN
proline (L-proline) USAN, USP, INN *nonessential amino acid; symbols:* Pro, P
prolintane INN *antidepressant* [also: prolintane HCl]
prolintane HCl USAN *antidepressant* [also: prolintane]
Prolixin Decanoate subcu or IM injection, Unimatic (prefilled) syringe ℞ *antipsychotic* [fluphenazine decanoate]
Prolixin Enanthate subcu or IM injection ℞ *antipsychotic* [fluphenazine enanthate]
Prolixin tablets, elixir, oral concentrate, IM injection ℞ *antipsychotic* [fluphenazine HCl]
Proloid tablets (discontinued 1992) ℞ *hypothyroidism; thyroid cancer* [thyroglobulin]
prolonium iodide INN
Proloprim tablets ℞ *anti-infective; antibacterial* [trimethoprim]
ProMACE (prednisone, methotrexate, Adriamycin, cyclophosphamide, etoposide) *chemotherapy protocol*
promazine INN *antipsychotic* [also: promazine HCl]

promazine HCl USP *antipsychotic* [also: promazine]
Promega Pearles (softgels) OTC *dietary supplement* [omega-3 fatty acids; multiple vitamins & minerals]
promegestone INN
promelase INN
promestriene INN
Prometa syrup ℞ *bronchodilator* [metaproterenol sulfate]
Prometh syrup ℞ *antihistamine* [promethazine HCl; alcohol]
Prometh VC liquid ℞ *decongestant; antihistamine* [promethazine HCl; phenylephrine HCl; alcohol]
Prometh VC Plain liquid ℞ *decongestant; antihistamine* [phenylephrine HCl; promethazine HCl; alcohol]
Prometh VC with Codeine syrup ℞ *decongestant; antihistamine; antitussive* [codeine phosphate; promethazine HCl; phenylephrine HCl; alcohol]
Prometh with Codeine syrup ℞ *antihistamine; antitussive* [codeine phosphate; promethazine HCl; alcohol]
Prometh with Dextromethorphan syrup ℞ *antihistamine; antitussive* [promethazine HCl; dextromethorphan hydrobromide; alcohol]
Prometh-50 injection ℞ *antihistamine; motion sickness; sleep aid; antiemetic; sedative* [promethazine HCl]
promethazine INN *antiemetic; antihistamine; antidopaminergic; motion sickness relief* [also: promethazine HCl]
Promethazine DC Plain syrup ℞ *decongestant; antihistamine* [promethazine HCl; phenylephrine HCl; alcohol]
Promethazine DM syrup ℞ *antihistamine; antitussive* [promethazine HCl; dextromethorphan hydrobromide]
promethazine HCl USP *antiemetic; antihistamine; antidopaminergic* [also: promethazine]
promethazine teoclate INN

Promethazine VC syrup ℞ *decongestant; antihistamine* [promethazine HCl; phenylephrine HCl; alcohol]
Promethazine VC with Codeine syrup ℞ *decongestant; antihistamine; antitussive* [promethazine HCl; phenylephrine HCl; codeine phosphate; alcohol]
promethestrol [see: methestrol]
promethium *element (Pm)*
Promine capsules ℞ *antiarrhythmic* [procainamide HCl]
Promise with Fluoride toothpaste (discontinued 1991) OTC *tooth desensitizer; dental caries prophylaxis* [potassium nitrate; sodium monofluorophosphate]
Promit IV injection ℞ *hapten for prophylaxis of dextran-induced anaphylactic reactions* [dextran 1]
ProMod powder OTC *oral protein supplement* [D-whey protein concentrate; soy lecithin]
promolate INN
promoxolane INN
prompt insulin zinc [see: insulin zinc, prompt]
Pronemia Hematinic capsules ℞ *hematinic* [ferrous fumarate; vitamins B$_{12}$ & C; intrinsic factor concentrate; folic acid]
Pronestyl capsules, tablets, IV or IM injection ℞ *antiarrhythmic* [procainamide HCl]
Pronestyl-SR sustained-release tablets ℞ *antiarrhythmic* [procainamide HCl]
pronetalol INN [also: pronethalol]
pronethalol BAN [also: pronetalol]
Pronto shampoo + creme rinse OTC *pediculicide* [pyrethrins; piperonyl butoxide]
Pronto-Gel (discontinued 1992) OTC *counterirritant* [methyl salicylate; methyl nicotinate; camphor; menthol; isopropanol]
Propa P.H. liquid soap (discontinued 1992) OTC *topical keratolytic for acne* [benzoyl peroxide]

Propa P.H. with Aloe cleansing pads OTC *topical acne treatment* [salicylic acid; aloe extract]
Propa P.H. with Aloe cream (discontinued 1993) OTC *topical acne treatment* [salicylic acid; aloe extract]
Propa P.H. with Aloe stick (discontinued 1992) OTC *topical acne treatment* [salicylic acid; aloe extract]
Propac powder OTC *oral protein supplement* [whey protein; lactose]
Propacet 100 film-coated tablets ℞ *narcotic analgesic* [propoxyphene napsylate; acetaminophen]
propacetamol INN
propafenone INN, BAN *antiarrhythmic* [also: propafenone HCl]
propafenone HCl USAN *antiarrhythmic* [also: propafenone]
Propagest tablets OTC *nasal decongestant; diet aid* [phenylpropanolamine HCl]
propamidine INN, BAN
propamidine isethionate (orphan: Acanthamoeba keratitis)
propaminodiphen [see: pramiverine]
propane NF *aerosol propellant*
1,2-propanediol [see: propylene glycol]
propanidid USAN, INN *intravenous anesthetic*
propanocaine INN
propanoic acid, sodium salt hydrate [see: sodium propionate]
2-propanol [see: isopropyl alcohol]
2-propanone [see: acetone]
propantheline bromide USP, INN *peptic ulcer adjunct*
proparacaine HCl USP *topical ophthalmic anesthetic* [also: proxymetacaine]
propatyl nitrate USAN *coronary vasodilator* [also: propatylnitrate]
propatylnitrate INN *coronary vasodilator* [also: propatyl nitrate]
propazolamide INN
1-propene homopolymer [see: polipropene 25]

propenidazole INN
propentofylline INN
***p*-propenylanisole** [see: anethole]
propenzolate HCl USAN *anticholinergic* [also: oxyclipine]
propericiazine [see: periciazine]
properidine INN, BAN
propetamide INN
propetandrol INN
prophenamine HCl [see: ethopropazine HCl]
Prophyllin ointment, powder OTC *topical antifungal; vulnerary; wound deodorant* [sodium propionate; chlorophyll derivatives]
propicillin INN, BAN
propikacin USAN, INN *antibacterial*
Propine eye drops ℞ *antiglaucoma agent* [dipivefrin HCl]
propinetidine INN
propiodal [see: prolonium iodide]
propiolactone (β-propiolactone) USAN, INN *disinfectant*
propiomazine USAN, INN *preanesthetic sedative*
propiomazine HCl USP *sedative; analgesic adjunct*
propionic acid NF *antimicrobial; acidifying agent*
propionyl erythromycin lauryl sulfate [see: erythromycin estolate]
propipocaine INN
propiram INN *analgesic* [also: propiram fumarate]
propiram fumarate USAN *analgesic* [also: propiram]
propisergide INN
propitocaine HCl [now: prilocaine HCl]
propiverine INN
propizepine INN
Proplex SX-T IV (discontinued 1991) ℞ *factor IX deficiency; correct anticoagulant-induced hemorrhage* [factor IX complex, human]
Proplex T IV infusion ℞ *factor IX deficiency; control bleeding in factor VII*

deficiency [factor IX complex, human]
propofol USAN, INN, BAN *general anesthetic*
propoxate INN
propoxycaine INN *local anesthetic* [also: propoxycaine HCl]
propoxycaine HCl USP *local anesthetic* [also: propoxycaine]
propoxyphene HCl USAN, USP *narcotic analgesic* [also: dextropropoxyphene HCl]
propoxyphene napsylate USAN, USP *narcotic analgesic*
propranolol INN, BAN *antiarrhythmic; migraine preventative; antiadrenergic (β-receptor)* [also: propranolol HCl]
propranolol HCl USAN, USP *antiarrhythmic; migraine preventative; antiadrenergic (β-receptor)* [also: propranolol]
Propulsid ℞ *investigational treatment for gastroesophageal reflux*
propyl p-aminobenzoate [see: risocaine]
propyl docetrizoate INN, BAN
propyl gallate NF *antioxidant*
propyl p-hydroxybenzoate [see: propylparaben]
propyl p-hydroxybenzoate, sodium salt [see: propylparaben sodium]
***N*-propylajmalinium tartrate** [see: prajmalinum bitartrate]
propylene carbonate NF *gelling agent*
propylene glycol USP *humectant; solvent; suspending and viscosity-increasing agent*
propylene glycol alginate NF *suspending agent; viscosity-increasing agent*
propylene glycol diacetate NF *solvent*
propylene glycol ether of methylcellulose [see: hydroxypropyl methylcellulose]
propylene glycol monostearate NF *emulsifying agent*

propylhexedrine USP, INN, BAN *vasoconstrictor; nasal decongestant*
propyliodone USP, INN *radiopaque medium*
propylorvinol [see: etorphine]
propylparaben USAN, NF *antifungal agent; preservative*
propylparaben sodium USAN, NF *antimicrobial preservative*
2-propylpentanoic acid [see: valproic acid]
propylthiouracil (PTU) USP, INN *thyroid inhibitor*
2-propylvaleramide [see: valpromide]
propylvaleric acid [see: valproic acid]
propyperone INN
propyphenazone INN, BAN
propyromazine bromide INN
proquamezine BAN [also: aminopromazine]
proquazone USAN, INN *anti-inflammatory*
proquinolate USAN, INN *coccidiostat for poultry*
prorenoate potassium USAN, INN *aldosterone antagonist*
Prorex-25; Prorex-50 injection ℞ *antihistamine; motion sickness; sleep aid; antiemetic; sedative* [promethazine HCl]
proroxan INN *antiadrenergic (α-receptor)* [also: proroxan HCl]
proroxan HCl USAN *antiadrenergic (α-receptor)* [also: proroxan]
Proscar film-coated tablets ℞ *androgen hormone inhibitor for benign prostatic hyperplasia* [finasteride]
proscillaridin USAN, INN *cardiotonic*
proscillaridin A [see: proscillaridin]
Prosed tablets (discontinued 1991) ℞ *urinary anti-infective; analgesic; antispasmodic; acidifier* [methenamine; phenyl salicylate; atropine sulfate; methylene blue; hyoscyamine; benzoic acid]
Prosed/DS tablets ℞ *urinary anti-infective; antiseptic; analgesic; antispasmodic* [methenamine; phenyl salicyl-

ate; methylene blue; benzoic acid; atropine sulfate; hyoscyamine sulfate]
ProSobee liquid, Nursette (prefilled disposable bottle) OTC *hypoallergenic infant food* [soy protein formula]
Pro-Sof capsules, syrup (discontinued 1992) OTC *stool softener* [docusate sodium]
Pro-Sof Plus capsules OTC *laxative; stool softener* [docusate sodium; casanthranol]
ProSom tablets ℞ *sedative; hypnotic* [estazolam]
prospidium chloride INN
prostacyclin [now: epoprostenol]
prostaglandin E₁ (PGE₁) [now: alprostadil]
prostaglandin E₂ (PGE₂) [see: dinoprostone]
prostaglandin F₂ (PGF₂) [see: dinoprost]
prostaglandin I₂ (PGI₂) [now: epoprostenol]
prostaglandin X (PGX) [now: epoprostenol]
prostalene USAN, INN *prostaglandin*
Prostaphlin capsules, powder for oral solution, powder for IV or IM injection ℞ *bactericidal antibiotic (penicillinase-resistant penicillin)* [oxacillin sodium]
ProStep transdermal patch ℞ *smoking deterrent; nicotine withdrawal aid* [nicotine]
Prostigmin subcu or IM injection ℞ *postsurgical cholinergic bladder muscle stimulant* [neostigmine methylsylfate]
Prostigmin tablets ℞ *myasthenia gravis treatment; antidote for neuromuscular blockers* [neostigmine bromide]
Prostin E2 vaginal suppository ℞ *abortifacient* [dinoprostone]
Prostin F2 alpha IM injection (discontinued 1991) ℞ *abortion; postpartum uterine bleeding* [dinoprost tromethamine]
Prostin VR Pediatric IV injection ℞ *vasodilator; platelet aggregate inhibitor* [alprostadil]
Prostin/15 M (name changed to Hemabate in 1990)
prosulpride INN
prosultiamine INN
Protac troches OTC *topical anesthetic; oral antiseptic* [benzocaine; cetylpyridinium chloride]
protactinium *element (Pa)*
protamine sulfate USP, INN *antidote to heparin* [also: protamine sulphate]
protamine sulphate BAN *antidote to heparin* [also: protamine sulfate]
Protamine Zinc Iletin I subcu injection (discontinued 1992) OTC *antidiabetic* [protamine zinc insulin (beef-pork)]
Protamine Zinc Iletin II (beef) subcu injection (discontinued 1992) OTC *antidiabetic* [protamine zinc insulin]
Protamine Zinc Iletin II (pork) subcu injection (discontinued 1992) OTC *antidiabetic* [protamine zinc insulin]
protamine zinc insulin (PZI) INN *antidiabetic* [also: insulin, protamine zinc]
protargin, mild [see: silver protein, mild]
protease inhibitor *investigational antiviral for AIDS*
ProTech First Aid Stick liquid OTC *topical antiseptic; analgesic* [povidone-iodine; lidocaine]
Protectol Medicated powder OTC *topical antifungal* [calcium undecylenate]
Protegra OTC *investigational antioxidant vitamin/mineral supplement*
Protein C ℞ *investigational anticoagulant*
protein C concentrate *(orphan: protein C deficiency)*
protein hydrolysate USP *fluid and nutrient replenisher*

α₁-**proteinase inhibitor** [see: alpha₁-proteinase inhibitor]
Protenate IV infusion ℞ *blood volume expander; shock due to burns, trauma and surgery* [plasma protein fraction]
proterguride INN
Prothazine Plain syrup ℞ *antihistamine; motion sickness; sleep aid; antiemetic; sedative* [promethazine HCl]
Prothazine subcu or IM injection ℞ *antihistamine; motion sickness; sleep aid; antiemetic; sedative* [promethazine HCl]
protheobromine INN
Prothiaden ℞ *investigational antidepressant* [dothiepin HCl]
prothionamide BAN [also: protionamide]
prothipendyl INN
prothipendyl HCl [see: prothipendyl]
prothixene INN
prothrombin complex, activated BAN
Protilase capsules containing enteric-coated spheres ℞ *digestive enzymes* [pancrelipase]
protiofate INN
protionamide INN [also: prothionamide]
protirelin USAN, INN, BAN *prothyrotropin; (orphan status withdrawn 1993)*
protizinic acid INN
protokylol HCl
Protopam Chloride emergency kit, hospital package ℞ *antidote for organophosphate and anticholinesterase chemicals* [pralidoxime chloride]
Protostat tablets ℞ *antibiotic; antiprotozoal; amebicide* [metronidazole]
protoveratrine A
Protox ℞ *(orphan: toxoplasmosis of AIDS)* [poloxamer 331]
protriptyline INN *antidepressant* [also: protriptyline HCl]
protriptyline HCl USAN, USP *tricyclic antidepressant* [also: protriptyline]

Protropin powder for IM or subcu injection ℞ *growth hormone (orphan: growth failure; Turner syndrome)* [somatrem]
Protropin II ℞ *(orphan: growth failure; Turner syndrome; anovulation; severe burns)* [somatropin]
prourokinase [see: saruplase]
Provatene soft gel perles OTC *to reduce photosensitivity reaction* [beta-carotene]
Proventil inhalation aerosol ℞ *bronchodilator* [albuterol]
Proventil tablets, syrup, solution for inhalation, Repetabs (extended-release tablets) ℞ *bronchodilator* [albuterol sulfate]
Provera tablets ℞ *progestin; secondary amenorrhea; functional uterine bleeding* [medroxyprogesterone acetate]
Provir ℞ *investigational antiviral for respiratory viruses*
provitamin A [see: beta carotene]
Provocholine powder for reconstitution for inhalation ℞ *in vivo pulmonary function test challenge* [methacholine chloride]
proxazole USAN, INN *smooth muscle relaxant; analgesic; anti-inflammatory*
proxazole citrate USAN *smooth muscle relaxant; analgesic; anti-inflammatory*
proxibarbal INN
proxibutene INN
proxicromil USAN, INN *antiallergic*
proxifezone INN
Proxigel OTC *topical oral anti-inflammatory/anti-infective for braces* [carbamide peroxide]
proxorphan INN *analgesic; antitussive* [also: proxorphan tartrate]
proxorphan tartrate USAN *analgesic; antitussive* [also: proxorphan]
Proxy 65 tablets ℞ *analgesic* [propoxyphene HCl; acetaminophen]
proxymetacaine INN *topical ophthalmic anesthetic* [also: proparacaine HCl]

proxymetacaine HCl [see: proparacaine HCl]
proxyphylline INN, BAN
Prozac Pulvules (capsules), liquid ℞ *antidepressant* [fluoxetine HCl]
prozapine INN
Prozine-50 IM injection ℞ *antipsychotic* [promazine HCl]
Prulet tablets OTC *laxative* [white phenolphthalein]
Pseudo liquid OTC *nasal decongestant* [pseudoephedrine HCl]
Pseudo-Car DM syrup ℞ *decongestant; antihistamine; antitussive* [pseudoephedrine HCl; carbinoxamine maleate; dextromethorphan hydrobromide; alcohol]
Pseudo-Chlor sustained-release capsules ℞ *decongestant; antihistamine* [pseudoephedrine HCl; chlorpheniramine maleate]
pseudoephedrine INN, BAN *vasoconstrictor; nasal decongestant* [also: pseudoephedrine HCl]
pseudoephedrine HCl USAN, USP *vasoconstrictor; nasal decongestant* [also: pseudoephedrine]
pseudoephedrine polistirex USAN *nasal decongestant*
pseudoephedrine sulfate USAN, USP *bronchodilator; nasal decongestant*
Pseudo-gest Plus tablets OTC *decongestant; antihistamine* [pseudoephedrine HCl; chlorpheniramine maleate]
Pseudo-Gest tablets OTC *nasal decongestant* [pseudoephedrine HCl]
Pseudo-Hist (name changed to Vanex Expectorant in 1990)
pseudomonas hyperimmune globulin [see: mucoid exopolysaccharide pseudomonas hyperimmune globulin]
pseudomonic acid [see: mupirocin]
psilocybine INN, BAN

Psorcon ointment ℞ *topical corticosteroidal anti-inflammatory* [diflorasone diacetate]
Psorex shampoo (discontinued 1991) OTC *antipsoriatic; antiseborrheic* [coal tar]
PsoriGel OTC *topical antipsoriatic; antiseborrheic; antiseptic* [coal tar solution; alcohol]
PsoriNail liquid OTC *topical antipsoriatic; antiseborrheic; antiseptic* [coal tar solution; alcohol]
Psorion ℞ *investigational topical anti-inflammatory drug*
psyllium husk USP *bulk laxative*
psyllium hydrocolloid *bulk laxative*
psyllium hydrophilic mucilloid *bulk laxative*
psyllium seed [see: plantago seed]
PTC (plasma thromboplastin component) [see: factor IX]
P.T.E.-4; P.T.E.-5 IV injection ℞ *intravenous nutritional therapy* [multiple trace elements (metals)]
pteroyldiglutamic acid (PDGA)
pteroylglutamic acid (PGA) [see: folic acid]
PTFE (polytetrafluoroethylene) [see: polytef]
PTU (propylthiouracil) [q.v.]
Pulmocare liquid OTC *oral nutritional supplement for pulmonary problems*
pulmonary surfactant replacement (orphan: infant respiratory distress syndrome)
Pulmozyme ℞ *investigational treatment for cystic fibrosis* [DNase]
pulse VAC (vincristine, Adriamycin, cyclophosphamide) *chemotherapy protocol* [also: VAC]
Pulvules (trademarked form) *capsules*
pumice USP *dental abrasive*
pumitepa INN
Puralube ophthalmic ointment OTC *ocular moisturizer/lubricant*
Pure Sept Disinfecting solution (discontinued 1992) OTC *contact lens disinfectant*

Pure Sept Murine Saline Solution
(discontinued 1993) OTC *contact lens rinse*
Purge liquid OTC *laxative* [castor oil]
purified cotton [see: cotton, purified]
purified protein derivative (PPD) of tuberculin [see: tuberculin]
purified rayon [see: rayon, purified]
purified siliceous earth [see: siliceous earth, purified]
purified water [see: water, purified]
Purinethol tablets ℞ *antineoplastic for multiple leukemias* [mercaptopurine]
Purisol 4 solution (discontinued 1992) OTC *contact lens rinsing and storage solution* [saline solution]
puromycin USAN, INN *antineoplastic; antiprotozoal (Trypanosoma)*
puromycin HCl USAN *antineoplastic; antiprotozoal (Trypanosoma)*
Purpose Dry Skin cream OTC *moisturizer; emollient*
Purpose Soap bar (discontinued 1992) OTC *therapeutic skin cleanser*
PVA (polyvinyl alcohol) [q.v.]
PVB (Platinol, vinblastine, bleomycin) *chemotherapy protocol*
PVDA (prednisone, vincristine, daunorubicin, asparaginase) *chemotherapy protocol*
PVP (Platinol, VP-16) *chemotherapy protocol*
P-V-Tussin syrup ℞ *decongestant; antihistamine; antitussive; expectorant* [phenylephrine HCl; pyrilamine maleate; phenindamine tartrate; chlorpheniramine maleate; hydrocodone bitartrate; ammonium chloride; alcohol]
P-V-Tussin tablets ℞ *antihistamine; antitussive; expectorant* [phenindamine tartrate; hydrocodone bitartrate; guaifenesin]
Pyocidin-Otic ear drops ℞ *topical corticosteroidal anti-inflammatory; antibiotic* [hydrocortisone; polymyxin B sulfate]
pyrabrom USAN *antihistamine*

pyradone [see: aminopyrine]
pyrantel INN *anthelmintic* [also: pyrantel pamoate]
pyrantel pamoate USAN, USP *anthelmintic* [also: pyrantel]
pyrantel tartrate USAN *anthelmintic*
pyrathiazine HCl [see: parathiazine]
pyrazinamide USP, INN, BAN *bactericidal; primary tuberculostatic*
pyrazinecarboxamide [see: pyrazinamide]
pyrazofurin USAN *antineoplastic* [also: pirazofurin]
pyrazoline [see: antipyrine]
pyrbenzindole [see: benzindopyrine HCl]
pyrbuterol HCl [see: pirbuterol HCl]
pyrethrins
pyribenzamine (PBZ) [see: tripelennamine]
pyricarbate INN
pyridarone INN
Pyridiate tablets ℞ *urinary analgesic* [phenazopyridine HCl]
2-pyridine aldoxime methylchloride (2-PAM) [see: pralidoxime chloride]
3-pyridinecarboxamide [see: niacinamide]
3-pyridinecarboxylic acid [see: niacin]
4-pyridinecarboxylic acid hydrazide [see: isoniazid]
3-pyridinecarboxylic acid methyl ester [see: methyl nicotinate]
3-pyridinemethanol [see: nicotinyl alcohol]
2-pyridinemethanol [see: piconol]
3-pyridinemethanol tartrate [see: nicotinyl tartrate]
Pyridium Plus tablets ℞ *urinary analgesic; antispasmodic; sedative* [phenazopyridine HCl; hyoscyamine hydrobromide; butabarbital]
Pyridium tablets ℞ *urinary analgesic* [phenazopyridine HCl]
pyridofylline INN

pyridostigmine bromide USP, INN *cholinergic; anticholinesterase muscle stimulant*
pyridoxal [see: pyridoxine HCl]
pyridoxamine [see: pyridoxine HCl]
pyridoxine INN *vitamin B_6; enzyme cofactor* [also: pyridoxine HCl]
pyridoxine HCl USP *vitamin B_6; enzyme cofactor* [also: pyridoxine]
β-pyridylcarbinol [see: nicotinyl alcohol]
pyridylmethanol *me+* [see: nicotinyl alcohol]
pyrilamine maleate USP *anticholinergic; antihistamine; sleep aid* [also: mepyramine]
pyrilamine tannate
pyrimethamine USP, INN *malaria suppression and transmission control*
pyrimitate INN, BAN
Pyrinex Pediculicide shampoo OTC *pediculicide* [pyrethrins; piperonyl butoxide; deodorized kerosene]
pyrinoline USAN, INN *antiarrhythmic*
Pyrinyl liquid OTC *pediculicide* [pyrethrins; piperonyl butoxide; deodorized kerosene]
Pyrinyl II liquid OTC *pediculicide* [pyrethrins; piperonyl butoxide]
Pyrinyl Plus shampoo OTC *pediculicide* [pyrethrins; piperonyl butoxide]
pyrithen [see: chlorothen citrate]
pyrithione sodium USAN *topical antimicrobial*
pyrithione zinc USAN, INN, BAN *antibacterial; antifungal; antiseborrheic*
pyrithyldione INN
pyritidium bromide INN
pyritinol INN, BAN

pyrodifenium bromide [see: prifinium bromide]
pyrogallic acid [see: pyrogallol]
pyrogallol NF
pyrophendane INN
pyrophenindane [see: pyrophendane]
pyrovalerone INN *CNS stimulant* [also: pyrovalerone HCl]
pyrovalerone HCl USAN *CNS stimulant* [also: pyrovalerone]
pyroxamine INN *antihistamine* [also: pyroxamine maleate]
pyroxamine maleate USAN *antihistamine* [also: pyroxamine]
pyroxylin USP, INN *pharmaceutic necessity for collodion*
pyrrobutamine phosphate USP
pyrrocaine USAN, INN *local anesthetic*
pyrrocaine HCl NF
pyrrolifene INN *analgesic* [also: pyrroliphene HCl]
pyrrolifene HCl [see: pyrroliphene HCl]
pyrroliphene HCl USAN *analgesic* [also: pyrrolifene]
pyrrolnitrin USAN, INN *antifungal*
pyrroxane [now: proroxan HCl]
Pyrroxate capsules OTC *decongestant; antihistamine; analgesic* [phenylpropanolamine HCl; chlorpheniramine maleate; acetaminophen]
pyrvinium chloride INN
pyrvinium embonate [see: pyrvinium pamoate]
pyrvinium pamoate USP *anthelmintic* [also: viprynium embonate]
pytamine INN
PZI (protamine zinc insulin) [q.v.]

Q

Q.B. liquid ℞ *antiasthmatic; bronchodilator; expectorant* [theophylline; guaifenesin]

Q-Pam tablets ℞ *skeletal muscle relaxant* [diazepam]

quadazocine INN, BAN *opioid antagonist* [also: quadazocine mesylate]

quadazocine mesylate USAN *opioid antagonist* [also: quadazocine]

Quadra-Hist ER syrup ℞ *decongestant; antihistamine* [phenylpropanolamine HCl; phenylephrine HCl; phenyltoloxamine citrate; chlorpheniramine maleate]

Quadra-Hist extended-release tablets ℞ *decongestant; antihistamine* [phenylpropanolamine HCl; phenylephrine HCl; phenyltoloxamine citrate; chlorpheniramine maleate]

Quadrinal tablets ℞ *antiasthmatic; bronchodilator; decongestant; expectorant; sedative* [theophylline; ephedrine HCl; potassium iodide; phenobarbital]

quadrosilan INN

Quarzan capsules ℞ *anticholinergic; peptic ulcer treatment* [clidinium bromide]

quatacaine INN

quazepam USAN, INN *sedative; hypnotic*

quazinone USAN, INN *cardiotonic*

quazodine USAN, INN *cardiotonic; bronchodilator*

quazolast USAN, INN *antiasthmatic; mediator release inhibitor*

Quelan liquid ℞ *bronchodilator; expectorant* [theophylline; guaifenesin]

Quelicin IV or IM injection ℞ *neuromuscular blocker* [succinylcholine chloride]

Quelidrine Cough syrup OTC *antihistamine; antitussive* [dextromethorphan hydrobromide; chlorpheniramine maleate; ephedrine HCl; phenylephrine HCl; ammonium chloride; ipecac; alcohol]

Queltuss tablets OTC *antitussive; expectorant* [dextromethorphan hydrobromide; guaifenesin]

Quercetin tablets OTC *dietary supplement* [eucalyptus bioflavonoids]

Questran; Questran Light powder for oral suspension ℞ *cholesterol-lowering antihyperlipidemic* [cholestyramine resin]

Quibron liquid (discontinued 1992) ℞ *antiasthmatic; bronchodilator; expectorant* [theophylline; guaifenesin]

Quibron Plus capsules (discontinued 1992) ℞ *antiasthmatic; bronchodilator; decongestant; expectorant; sedative* [theophylline; ephedrine HCl; guaifenesin; butabarbital]

Quibron Plus elixir ℞ *antiasthmatic; bronchodilator; decongestant; expectorant; sedative* [theophylline; ephedrine HCl; guaifenesin; butabarbital]

Quibron; Quibron-300 capsules ℞ *antiasthmatic; bronchodilator; expectorant* [theophylline; guaifenesin]

Quibron-T Dividose (multiple-scored tablets) ℞ *bronchodilator* [theophylline]

Quibron-T/SR sustained-release Dividose (multiple-scored tablets) ℞ *bronchodilator* [theophylline]

Quick Pep tablets OTC *CNS stimulant; analeptic* [caffeine]

Quiess IM injection ℞ *anxiolytic* [hydroxyzine HCl]

Quiet World tablets (discontinued 1992) OTC *antihistaminic sleep aid; analgesic* [pyrilamine maleate; acetaminophen; aspirin]

quifenadine INN

Quik-Sept System solution (discontinued 1991) OTC *three-step contact lens disinfectant*

quillifoline INN

quinacainol INN

quinacillin INN, BAN
quinacrine HCl USP *anthelmintic; antimalarial* [also: mepacrine]
Quinaglute Dura-Tabs (sustained-release tablets) ℞ *antiarrhythmic* [quinidine gluconate]
Quinalan sustained-release tablets ℞ *antiarrhythmic* [quinidine gluconate]
quinalbarbitone sodium BAN *hypnotic; sedative* [also: secobarbital sodium]
quinaldine blue USAN *obstetric diagnostic aid*
quinambicide [see: clioquinol]
Quinamm tablets ℞ *prevention and treatment of nocturnal leg cramps* [quinine sulfate]
quinapril INN, BAN *antihypertensive; angiotensin-converting enzyme (ACE) inhibitor* [also: quinapril HCl]
quinapril HCl USAN *antihypertensive; angiotensin-converting enzyme (ACE) inhibitor* [also: quinapril]
quinaprilat USAN, INN *antihypertensive; angiotensin-converting enzyme (ACE) inhibitor*
Quinatime sustained-release tablets (discontinued 1992) ℞ *antiarrhythmic* [quinidine gluconate]
quinazosin INN *antihypertensive* [also: quinazosin HCl]
quinazosin HCl USAN *antihypertensive* [also: quinazosin]
quinbolone USAN, INN *anabolic*
quincarbate INN
quindecamine INN *antibacterial* [also: quindecamine acetate]
quindecamine acetate USAN *antibacterial* [also: quindecamine]
quindonium bromide USAN, INN *antiarrhythmic*
quindoxin INN, BAN
quinelorane INN *antihypertensive; antiparkinsonian* [also: quinelorane HCl]
quinelorane HCl USAN *antihypertensive; antiparkinsonian* [also: quinelorane]

quinestradol INN, BAN
quinestrol USAN, USP, INN, BAN *estrogen*
quinetalate INN *smooth muscle relaxant* [also: quinetolate]
quinethazone USP, INN *diuretic; antihypertensive*
quinetolate USAN *smooth muscle relaxant* [also: quinetalate]
quinezamide INN
quinfamide USAN, INN *antiamebic*
quingestanol INN *progestin* [also: quingestanol acetate]
quingestanol acetate USAN *progestin* [also: quingestanol]
quingestrone USAN, INN *progestin*
Quinidex Extentabs (extended-release tablets) ℞ *antiarrhythmic* [quinidine sulfate]
quinidine NF, BAN *antiarrhythmic*
quinidine gluconate USP *antiarrhythmic*
quinidine polygalacturonate *antiarrhythmic*
quinidine sulfate USP *antiarrhythmic*
quinine NF, BAN
quinine ascorbate USAN *smoking deterrent*
quinine biascorbate [now: quinine ascorbate]
quinine bisulfate NF
quinine dihydrochloride NF *investigational anti-infective for pernicious malaria*
quinine ethylcarbonate NF
quinine glycerophosphate NF
quinine HCl NF
quinine hydrobromide NF
quinine hypophosphite NF
quinine monohydrobromide [see: quinine hydrobromide]
quinine monohydrochloride [see: quinine HCl]
quinine monosalicylate [see: quinine salicylate]
quinine phosphate NF
quinine phosphinate [see: quinine hypophosphite]

quinine salicylate NF
quinine sulfate USP *antimalarial schizonticide*
quinine sulfate dihydrate [see: quinine sulfate]
quinine tannate USP
quinisocaine INN [also: dimethisoquin HCl; dimethisoquin]
quinocide INN
8-quinolinol [see: oxyquinoline]
8-quinolinol benzoate [see: benzoxiquine]
Quinora tablets ℞ *antiarrhythmic* [quinidine sulfate]
quinoxyl [see: chiniofon]
quinpirole INN *antihypertensive* [also: quinpirole HCl]
quinpirole HCl USAN *antihypertensive* [also: quinpirole]
quinprenaline INN *bronchodilator* [also: quinterenol sulfate]
quinprenaline sulfate [see: quinterenol sulfate]
Quin-Release sustained-release tablets ℞ *antiarrhythmic* [quinidine gluconate]

Quinsana Plus powder OTC *topical antifungal* [tolnaftate]
Quintabs tablets OTC *vitamin supplement* [multiple vitamins; folic acid]
Quintabs-M tablets OTC *vitamin/mineral/iron supplement* [multiple vitamins & minerals; iron; folic acid]
quinterenol sulfate USAN *bronchodilator* [also: quinprenaline]
quintiofos INN, BAN
3-quinuclidinol benzoate [see: benzoclidine]
quinuclium bromide USAN, INN *antihypertensive*
quinupramine INN
quipazine INN *antidepressant; oxytocic* [also: quipazine maleate]
quipazine maleate USAN *antidepressant; oxytocic* [also: quipazine]
Quiphile tablets ℞ *prevention and treatment of nocturnal leg cramps* [quinine sulfate]
quisultazine INN
quisultidine [see: quisultazine]
Q-Vel tablets, soft caplets OTC *prevention and treatment of nocturnal leg cramps* [quinine sulfate]

R

R A Lotion OTC *topical acne treatment* [resorcinol; calamine; sodium borate]
R & C shampoo OTC *pediculicide* [pyrethrins; piperonyl butoxide]
R & D Calcium Carbonate/600 *(orphan: hyperphosphatemia of end-stage renal disease)* [calcium carbonate]
r-VIII SQ ℞ *investigational antihemophilic* [recombinant factor VIII]
rabies immune globulin (RIG) USP *passive immunizing agent*
rabies vaccine USP *active immunizing agent*

rabies vaccine, HDCV (human diploid cell vaccine) [see: rabies vaccine]
racefemine INN
racefenicol INN *antibacterial* [also: racephenicol]
racemethadol [see: dimepheptanol]
racemethionine USAN *urinary acidifier* [also: methionine (DL- form)]
racemethorphan INN, BAN
racemetirosine INN
racemic amphetamine phosphate
racemic amphetamine sulfate [see: amphetamine sulfate]

racemic calcium pantothenate [see: calcium pantothenate, racemic]
racemoramide INN, BAN
racemorphan INN
racephedrine HCl USAN
racephenicol USAN *antibacterial* [also: racefenicol]
racepinefrine INN *bronchodilator* [also: racepinephrine]
racepinephrine USP *bronchodilator* [also: racepinefrine]
racepinephrine HCl USP *bronchodilator*
Racet cream (discontinued 1991) ℞ *topical corticosteroid; antifungal; antibacterial* [hydrocortisone; clioquinol]
raclopride INN, BAN
ractopamine INN *veterinary growth stimulant* [also: ractopamine HCl]
ractopamine HCl USAN *veterinary growth stimulant* [also: ractopamine]
radio-chromated serum albumin [see: albumin, chromated]
radio-iodinated I 125 serum albumin [see: albumin, iodinated]
radio-iodinated I 131 serum albumin [see: albumin, iodinated]
radiomerisoprol ¹⁹⁷Hg [see: merisoprol Hg 197]
radioselenomethionine ⁷⁵Se [see: selenomethionine Se 75]
radiotolpovidone I 131 INN *hypoalbuminemia test; radioactive agent* [also: tolpovidone I 131]
radium *element (Ra)*
radon *element (Rn)*
rafoxanide USAN, INN *anthelmintic*
Ragus tablets OTC *dietary supplement* [multiple vitamins, minerals & amino acids]
ralitoline USAN, INN *anticonvulsant*
raloxifene INN *antiestrogen* [also: raloxifene HCl]
raloxifene HCl USAN *antiestrogen* [also: raloxifene]
rambufaside [see: meproscillarin]
ramciclane INN
ramifenazone INN

ramipril USAN, INN, BAN *antihypertensive; angiotensin-converting enzyme inhibitor*
ramiprilat INN
ramixotidine INN
ramnodigin INN
ramoplanin INN
RAMP Urine hCG Assay test kit ℞ *in vitro diagnostic aid for urine pregnancy test*
Ramses Extra condom OTC *spermicidal/barrier contraceptive* [nonoxynol 9]
Ramses vaginal jelly OTC *spermicidal contraceptive* [nonoxynol 9]
ranimustine INN
ranimycin USAN, INN *antibacterial*
ranitidine USAN, INN, BAN *treatment of GI ulcers; histamine H_2 antagonist*
ranitidine HCl USP *treatment of GI ulcers; histamine H_2 antagonist*
ranolazine INN *antianginal* [also: ranolazine HCl]
ranolazine HCl USAN *antianginal* [also: ranolazine]
RapidTest Strep throat swab test kit ℞ *in vitro diagnostic test for streptococci*
raspberry [syrup] USP
rathyronine INN
rattlesnake antivenin [see: antivenin (Crotalidae) polyvalent]
Raudixin tablets ℞ *antihypertensive; antipsychotic* [rauwolfia serpentina (whole root)]
Rauverid tablets ℞ *antihypertensive; antipsychotic* [rauwolfia serpentina (whole root)]
Rauwiloid tablets (discontinued 1991) ℞ *hypertension* [alseroxylon]
rauwolfia serpentina USP *antihypertensive*
Rauzide tablets ℞ *antihypertensive* [bendroflumethiazide; rauwolfia serpentina]
Ravocaine & Novocaine with Levophed injection ℞ *injectable local*

anesthetic for dental procedures [proproxycaine HCl; procaine; norepinephrine]

Ravocaine & Novocaine with Neo-Cobefrin injection ℞ *injectable local anesthetic for dental procedures* [proproxycaine HCl; procaine; levonordefrin]

rayon, purified USAN, USP *surgical aid*

razinodil INN

razobazam INN

razoxane INN, BAN

[86]Rb [see: rubidium chloride Rb 86]

rCD4 (recombinant soluble human CD4) [see: CD4, recombinant soluble human]

RCF liquid concentrate OTC *total or supplementary infant feeding* [soy protein formula]

Reabilan; Reabilan HN liquid OTC *oral nutritional supplement*

Reactine ℞ *investigational antiallergic* [cetirizine]

reactrol [see: clemizole HCl]

Rea-Lo cream, lotion (discontinued 1992) OTC *moisturizer; emollient; keratolytic* [urea]

rebamipide INN

reboxetine INN

recainam INN, BAN *antiarrhythmic* [also: recainam HCl]

recainam HCl USAN *antiarrhythmic* [also: recainam]

recainam tosylate USAN *antiarrhythmic*

recanescin [see: deserpidine]

Receptin (*orphan: AIDS*) [CD4, recombinant soluble human]

reclazepam USAN, INN *sedative*

Reclomide tablets ℞ *antidopaminergic; antiemetic for chemotherapy; peristaltic* [metoclopramide monohydrochloride monohydrate]

Recombigen HIV-1 LA Test OTC *in vitro diagnostic aid for HIV-1 antibody*

recombinant alpha$_1$ antitrypsin [see: alpha$_1$ antitrypsin, recombinant]

recombinant antihemophilic factor [see: antihemophilic factor, recombinant]

recombinant factor VIIa [see: factor VIIa, recombinant]

recombinant factor VIII [see: antihemophilic factor, recombinant]

recombinant human CD4 immunoglobulin G [CD4 immunoglobulin G, recombinant human]

recombinant human deoxyribonuclease (rhDNase) [see: deoxyribonuclease, recombinant human]

recombinant human erythropoietin [see: erythropoietin, recombinant human]

recombinant human growth hormone [see: human growth hormone, recombinant]

recombinant human interferon beta [see: interferon beta, recombinant human]

recombinant human superoxide dismutase (SOD) [see: superoxide dismutase, recombinant human]

recombinant interferon alfa-2a [see: interferon alfa-2a, recombinant]

recombinant interferon alfa-2b [see: interferon alfa-2b, recombinant]

recombinant interferon beta [see: interferon beta, recombinant]

recombinant interleukin-2 [see: interleukin-2, recombinant]

recombinant methionyl granulocyte CSF [see: methionyl granulocyte CSF, recombinant]

recombinant methionyl human granulocyte CSF [see: methionyl human granulocyte CSF, recombinant]

recombinant soluble human CD4 (rCD4) [see: CD4, recombinant soluble human]

recombinant tissue plasminogen activator (rtPA; rt-PA) [see: alteplase]

Recombinate powder for injection ℞ *coagulant* [antihemophilic factor, recombinant]

Recombivax HB IM injection, dialysis formulation ℞ *hepatitis B vaccine* [hepatitis B virus vaccine, recombinant]

Rectacort rectal suppositories ℞ *topical corticosteroidal anti-inflammatory; antipruritic* [hydrocortisone acetate; zinc oxide; bismuth salts]

Rectagene II suppositories OTC *temporary relief of hemorrhoidal symptoms* [bismuth subgallate; bismuth resorcin; benzyl benzoate; peruvian balsam; zinc oxide]

Rectagene Medicated Rectal Balm ointment OTC *temporary relief of hemorrhoidal symptoms* [skin respiratory factor; phenyl mercuric nitrate]

Rectal Medicone ointment, suppositories OTC *topical anesthetic; antiseptic; astringent; counterirritant* [benzocaine; hydroxyquinoline sulfate; zinc oxide; menthol]

Rectolax suppositories OTC *laxative* [bisacodyl]

red blood cells [see: blood cells, red]

red ferric oxide [see: ferric oxide, red]

red veterinarian petrolatum (RVP) [see: petrolatum]

Redi Vial (trademarked form) *dual-compartment vial*

Redisol injection (discontinued 1991) ℞ *antianemic; vitamin supplement* [cyanocobalamin]

redox-acyclovir (orphan: *herpes simplex encephalitis in AIDS*)

redox-penicillin G (orphan: *AIDS-associated neurosyphilis*)

redox-phenytoin (orphan: *emergency rescue of grand mal status epilepticus*)

Reducin (orphan: *nonoperative management of cutaneous fistulas of the GI tract*) [somatostatin]

Redutemp tablets OTC *analgesic; antipyretic* [acetaminophen]

Reese's Pinworm liquid OTC *anthelmintic* [pyrantel pamoate]

Refresh eye drops OTC *ocular moisturizer/lubricant*

Refresh P.M. ophthalmic ointment OTC *ocular moisturizer/lubricant*

Regaine ℞ *investigational baldness remedy*

Regitine IV or IM injection ℞ *antihypertensive for pheochromocytoma* [phentolamine mesylate]

Reglan syrup, IV infusion, tablets ℞ *antidopaminergic; antiemetic for chemotherapy; peristaltic* [metoclopramide monohydrochloride monohydrate]

Regonol IM or IV injection ℞ *anticholinesterase muscle stimulant; muscle relaxant reversal* [pyridostigmine bromide]

regramostim USAN *biological response modifier; bone marrow stimulant*

Regroton tablets ℞ *antihypertensive* [chlorthalidone; reserpine]

Regulace capsules OTC *laxative; stool softener* [docusate sodium; casanthranol]

Regular Iletin I subcu injection OTC *antidiabetic* [insulin (beef-pork)]

Regular Iletin II (beef) subcu injection OTC *antidiabetic* [insulin]

Regular Iletin II (pork) subcu injection OTC *antidiabetic* [insulin]

Regular Iletin II U-500 (concentrated) subcu or IM injection ℞ *antidiabetic* [insulin (pork)]

Regular Insulin injection OTC *antidiabetic* [insulin (pork)]

Regular Purified Pork Insulin injection OTC *antidiabetic* [insulin (pork)]

Regulax SS capsules OTC *stool softener* [docusate sodium]

Reguloid powder OTC *bulk laxative* [psyllium hydrophilic mucilloid]

Regutol tablets OTC *stool softener* [docusate sodium]

Rehydralyte oral solution OTC *electrolyte replacement* [sodium, potassium, and chloride electrolytes]

Rela sugar-coated tablets ℞ *skeletal muscle relaxant* [carisoprodol]

Relafen film-coated tablets ℞ *antiarthritic; nonsteroidal anti-inflammatory drug (NSAID)* [namubetone]

Relaxadon tablets ℞ *anticholinergic; sedative* [atropine sulfate; scopolamine hydrobromide; hyoscyamine hydrobromide; phenobarbital]

relaxin

Relaxin ℞ *investigational agent to facilitate childbirth*

Release-Tabs (dosage form) *timed-release tablets*

Relefact TRH IV injection ℞ *in vivo thyroid function test* [protirelin]

Relief eye drops OTC *topical ocular decongestant; topical anesthetic* [phenylephrine HCl; antipyrine]

relomycin USAN, INN *antibacterial*

remacemide HCl USAN *neuroprotective anticonvulsant*

Remcol Cold capsules OTC *decongestant; antihistamine; analgesic* [phenylpropanolamine HCl; chlorpheniramine maleate; acetaminophen]

Remcol-C capsules OTC *antihistamine; antitussive; analgesic* [chlorpheniramine maleate; dextromethorphan hydrobromide; acetaminophen]

remifentanil HCl USAN *analgesic*

remoxipride USAN, INN, BAN *antipsychotic*

Remular-S tablets ℞ *muscle relaxant* [chlorzoxazone]

Renacidin Irrigation solution ℞ *(orphan: renal and bladder calculi)* [citric acid; glucono-delta-lactone; magnesium carbonate]

Renacidin powder for solution ℞ *bladder and catheter irrigant for calcifications* [citric acid; d-gluconic acid lactone; magnesium hydroxycarbonate]

RenAmin IV infusion ℞ *nutritional therapy for renal failure* [multiple essential & nonessential amino acids; electrolytes]

renanolone INN

Renese tablets ℞ *diuretic; antihypertensive* [polythiazide]

Renese-R tablets ℞ *antihypertensive* [polythiazide; reserpine]

Renografin-76 injection ℞ *parenteral radiopaque agent* [diatrizoate meglumine; diatrizoate sodium]

Reno-M-30; Reno-M-60; Reno-M-Dip intracavitary instillation ℞ *urologic radiopaque agent* [diatrizoate meglumine]

Renoquid tablets ℞ *broad-spectrum bacteriostatic* [sulfacytine]

Renova ℞ *investigational therapy for photodamage* [tretinoin]

Renovist; Renovist II injection ℞ *parenteral radiopaque agent* [diatrizoate meglumine; diatrizoate sodium]

Renovue-Dip; Renovue-65 injection ℞ *parenteral renal radiopaque agent* [iodamide meglumine]

Rentamine liquid ℞ *decongestant; antitussive; antihistamine* [carbetapentane tannate; chlorpheniramine tannate; ephedrine tannate; phenylephrine tannate]

Rentamine Pediatric oral suspension ℞ *pediatric decongestant, antitussive and antihistamine* [carbetapentane tannate; chlorpheniramine tannate; ephedrine tannate; phenylephrine tannate]

rentiapril INN

ReNu Effervescent Enzymatic Cleaner; ReNu Thermal Enzymatic Cleaner tablets OTC *contact lens enzymatic cleaner*

ReNu Multi-Action solution OTC *contact lens disinfectant*

ReNu Saline solution OTC *contact lens rinsing and storage solution* [preserved saline solution]

renytoline INN *anti-inflammatory* [also: paranyline HCl]
renytoline HCl [see: paranyline HCl; renytoline]
renzapride INN, BAN
Repan tablets, capsules ℞ *sedative; analgesic* [butalbital; acetaminophen; caffeine]
Repetabs (trademarked form) *repeat-action tablets*
repirinast USAN, INN *antiallergic; antiasthmatic*
Replena (name changed to Suplena in 1992)
Replens gel OTC *vaginal lubricant*
Replete liquid OTC *oral nutritional supplement*
Replistatin ℞ *investigational postsurgery coagulation restorer (heparin reversal)*
rEPO (recombinant erythropoietin) [see: epoetin alfa; epoetin beta]
Reposans-10 capsules ℞ *anxiolytic* [chlordiazepoxide HCl]
repository corticotropin [see: corticotropin, repository]
Rep-Pred 40; Rep-Pred 80 injection ℞ *corticosteroid* [methylprednisolone acetate]
repromicin USAN, INN *antibacterial*
reproterol INN, BAN *bronchodilator* [also: reproterol HCl]
reproterol HCl USAN *bronchodilator* [also: reproterol]
Resaid sustained-release capsules ℞ *decongestant; antihistamine* [phenylpropanolamine HCl; chlorpheniramine maleate]
Rescaps-D S.R. prolonged-release capsules ℞ *decongestant; antitussive* [pseudoephedrine HCl; codeine phosphate]
rescimetol INN
rescinnamine NF, INN, BAN *antihypertensive; rauwolfia derivative*
Rescon capsules ℞ *antihistamine; decongestant* [chlorpheniramine maleate; pseudoephedrine HCl]

Rescon liquid OTC *decongestant; antihistamine* [phenylpropanolamine HCl; chlorpheniramine maleate]
Rescon-DM liquid OTC *antihistamine; decongestant; antitussive* [chlorpheniramine maleate; pseudoephedrine HCl; dextromethorphan hydrobromide]
Rescon-ED; Rescon Jr. controlled-release capsules ℞ *antihistamine; decongestant* [chlorpheniramine maleate; pseudoephedrine HCl]
Rescon-GG liquid ℞ *decongestant; expectorant* [phenylephrine HCl; guaifenesin]
Resectisol solution ℞ *genitourinary irrigant* [mannitol]
reserpine USP, INN *antihypertensive; rauwolfia derivative*
resibufogenin [see: bufogenin]
Resinol ointment OTC *topical poison ivy treatment* [calamine; zinc oxide; resorcinol]
Resol oral solution OTC *electrolyte replacement* [sodium, potassium, chloride, calcium, magnesium, and phosphate electrolytes]
Resolve/GP Daily Cleaner liquid OTC *contact lens cleaning solution*
resorantel INN
resorcin [see: resorcinol]
resorcin acetate [see: resorcinol monoacetate]
resorcin brown NF
resorcinol USP *keratolytic; antifungal*
resorcinol monoacetate USP *antiseborrheic; keratolytic*
Resource; Resource Plus liquid OTC *oral nutritional supplement*
Respaire-60 SR; Respaire-120 SR prolonged-action capsules ℞ *decongestant; expectorant* [pseudoephedrine HCl; guaifenesin]
Respbid sustained-release tablets ℞ *bronchodilator* [theophylline]
Respihaler (trademarked form) *oral inhalation aerosol*

Respinol-G film-coated tablets ℞ *decongestant; expectorant* [phenylpropanolamine HCl; phenylephrine HCl; guaifenesin]

Respiracult-Strep culture test ℞ *in vitro diagnostic test for streptococci*

Respiralex test kit ℞ *in vitro diagnostic test for streptococci*

respiratory syncytial virus immune globulin, human *(orphan: respiratory syncytial virus)*

Respirgard II (trademarked delivery system) *nebulizer*

Respivir ℞ *investigational preventative for respiratory syncytial viral infections*

Respond tablets OTC *dietary supplement* [multiple vitamins; levoglutamide; bovine brain concentrate]

Resporal sustained-release tablets OTC *decongestant; antihistamine* [pseudoephedrine sulfate; dexbrompheniramine maleate]

Res-Q powder OTC *universal antidote* [activated charcoal; magnesium hydroxide; tannic acid]

Restoril capsules ℞ *sedative; hypnotic* [temazepam]

retelliptine INN

Reticulex Pulvules (discontinued 1991) ℞ *antianemic* [iron & ammonium citrates; intrinsic factor; multiple B vitamins]

Reticulogen; Reticulogen Fortified IM injection (discontinued 1991) ℞ *antianemic; vitamin supplement* [vitamins B_1 & B_{12}]

Retin-A cream, gel, liquid ℞ *topical keratolytic for acne* [tretinoin]

13-*cis*-retinoic acid [see: isotretinoin]

retinoic acid (all-*trans*-retinoic acid) [see: tretinoin]

retinoic acid, 9-C15 *(orphan: acute promyelocytic leukemia)*

retinol INN, BAN *vitamin A_1*

Retinol cream OTC *moisturizer; emollient* [vitamin A]

Retrovir capsules, syrup, IV injection ℞ *antiviral for AIDS and AIDS-related complex (orphan)* [zidovudine]

revenast INN

Reversol IV or IM injection ℞ *myasthenia gravis treatment; antidote to curare-type overdose* [edrophonium chloride]

Rēv-Eyes powder for eye drops ℞ *iatrogenic mydriasis treatment; miotic* [dapiprazole HCl]

revospirone INN, BAN

Rexigen Forte sustained-release capsules ℞ *anorexiant* [phendimetrazine tartrate]

Rexolate IM injection ℞ *analgesic; antipyretic; anti-inflammatory; antirheumatic* [sodium thiosalicylate]

Rezamid lotion OTC *topical acne treatment* [sulfur; resorcinol]

Rezine table ℞ *anxiolytic* [hydroxyzine HCl]

Rezipas *(orphan: ulcerative colitis)* [aminosalicylic acid]

RG 12986 ℞ *investigational antithrombotic* [recombinant human von Willebrand factor]

RG 83894 *investigational antiviral for AIDS* [also: HIV vaccine]

R-Gen elixir ℞ *expectorant* [iodinated glycerol]

R-gene 10 IV injection ℞ *pituitary (growth hormone) function test* [arginine HCl]

rGM-CSF (granulocyte macrophage-colony stimulating factor) [q.v.]

rhamnus purshiana [see: cascara sagrada]

rhDNase (recombinant human deoxyribonuclease) [see: deoxyribonuclease, recombinant human]

Rheaban tablets OTC *antidiarrheal; GI adsorbent* [activated attapulgite; pectin]

rhenium *element (Re)*

Rheomacrodex IV infusion ℞ *plasma-volume expander* [dextran 40]

RheothRx Copolymer *(orphan: sickle cell crisis; severe burns)* [poloxamer 188]

rheotran (45) [see: dextran 45]

Rhesonativ IM injection ℞ *obstetric Rh factor immunity suppressant* [Rh₀(D) immune globulin]

rhetinic acid [see: enoxolone]

Rheumanosticon Dri-Dot slide test (discontinued 1991) OTC *in vitro diagnostic aid for rheumatoid factor in the blood*

Rheumatex test kit OTC *in vitro diagnostic aid for rheumatoid factor in the blood*

Rheumaton test kit OTC *in vitro diagnostic aid for rheumatoid factor in the blood*

Rheumatrex Dose Pack (tablets) ℞ *antirheumatic; antipsoriatic; antineoplastic for leukemia* [methotrexate sodium]

Rheumatrex test kit OTC *in vitro diagnostic aid for rheumatoid factor in the blood*

Rhinall nasal spray, nose drops OTC *nasal decongestant* [phenylephrine HCl]

Rhinall-10 solution (discontinued 1992) OTC *nasal decongestant* [phenylephrine HCl]

Rhinatate tablets ℞ *decongestant; antihistamine* [phenylephrine tannate; chlorpheniramine tannate; pyrilamine tannate]

Rhindecon timed-release capsules ℞ *nasal decongestant; diet aid* [phenylpropanolamine HCl]

Rhinocaps capsules OTC *decongestant* [phenylpropanolamine HCl; acetaminophen; aspirin]

Rhinogesic tablets OTC *decongestant; antihistamine; analgesic* [phenylephrine HCl; chlorpheniramine maleate; acetaminophen; salicylamide]

Rhinolar sustained-release capsules ℞ *decongestant; antihistamine; anticholinergic* [phenylpropanolamine HCl; chlorpheniramine maleate; methscopolamine nitrate]

Rhinolar-EX; Rhinolar-EX 12 sustained-release capsules ℞ *decongestant; antihistamine* [phenylpropanolamine HCl; chlorpheniramine malelate]

Rhinosyn; Rhinosyn-PD liquid OTC *decongestant; antihistamine* [pseudoephedrine HCl; chlorpheniramine maleate; alcohol]

Rhinosyn-DM liquid OTC *decongestant; antihistamine; antitussive* [pseudoephedrine HCl; chlorpheniramine maleate; dextromethorphan hydrobromide; alcohol]

Rhinosyn-DMX liquid OTC *antitussive; expectorant* [dextromethorphan hydrobromide; guaifenesin; alcohol]

Rhinosyn-X liquid OTC *decongestant; antitussive; expectorant* [pseudoephedrine HCl; dextromethorphan hydrobromide; guaifenesin; alcohol]

Rh₀(D) immune globulin USP *passive immunizing agent*

Rh₀(D) immune human globulin [now: Rh₀(D) immune globulin]

rhodine [see: aspirin]

rhodium *element (Rh)*

RhoGAM IM injection ℞ *obstetric Rh factor immunity suppressant* [Rh₀(D) immune globulin]

Rhuli cream, spray OTC *topical poison ivy treatment* [benzocaine; calamine; camphor]

Rhuli gel OTC *topical poison ivy treatment* [benzyl alcohol; menthol; camphor]

Rhulicaine solution (discontinued 1991) OTC *topical local anesthetic* [benzocaine; triclosan; menthol; alcohol; isopropyl alcohol]

Rhus Tox Antigen injection (discontinued 1991) ℞ *poison ivy treatment* [poison ivy extract]

Rhythmin sustained-release tablets ℞ *antiarrhythmic* [procainamide HCl]

ribaminol USAN, INN *memory adjuvant*

ribavirin USP, INN *antiviral; (orphan: hemorrhagic fever with renal syndrome)* [also: tribavirin]

riboflavin USP, INN *vitamin B_2; vitamin G; enzyme cofactor*

riboflavin 5′-phosphate sodium USP *vitamin*

riboflavine [see: riboflavin]

riboprine USAN, INN *antineoplastic*

ribostamycin INN, BAN

riboxamide [see: tiazofurin]

ricainide [see: indecainide HCl]

Ricelyte oral solution OTC *electrolyte replacement* [sodium, potassium, and chloride electrolytes]

ricin (blocked) conjugated murine monoclonal antibody (anti-B4) *(orphan: B-cell leukemia and lymphoma; ex vivo treatment of autologous bone marrow in leukemia)*

ricin (blocked) conjugated murine monoclonal antibody (anti-MY9) *(orphan: myeloid leukemia; ex vivo treatment of autologous bone marrow in leukemia)*

ricin (blocked) conjugated murine monoclonal antibody (N901) *(orphan: small cell lung cancer)*

RID liquid OTC *pediculicide* [pyrethrins; piperonyl butoxide; petroleum distillate]

Rid-A-Pain drops OTC *topical anesthetic; oral antiseptic; astringent* [benzocaine; cetalkonium chloride; hamamelis water]

Rid-A-Pain gel OTC *topical oral anesthetic* [benzocaine]

Rid-A-Pain ointment (discontinued 1992) OTC *counterirritant* [methyl salicylate; methyl nicotinate; menthol; camphor]

Rid-A-Pain with Codeine tablets ℞ *narcotic analgesic* [codeine phosphate; acetaminophen; aspirin; caffeine; salicylamide]

Ridaura capsules ℞ *antirheumatic* [auranofin]

ridazolol INN

RIDD (recombinant interleukin-2, dacarbazine, DDP) *chemotherapy protocol*

ridogrel USAN, INN, BAN *thromboxane synthetase inhibitor*

rifabutin INN *investigational antiviral; (orphan: Mycobacterium avium complex disease; AIDS)*

Rifadin capsules, powder for IV injection ℞ *tuberculostatic; (orphan: IV where oral use is not feasible)* [rifampin]

Rifamate capsules ℞ *tuberculostatic* [rifampin; isoniazid]

rifametane USAN, INN *antibacterial*

rifamexil USAN *antibacterial*

rifamide USAN, INN *antibacterial*

rifampicin INN, BAN *antibacterial* [also: rifampin]

rifampin USAN, USP *antibacterial; (orphan: tuberculosis)* [also: rifampicin]

rifampin, isoniazid & pyrazinamide *(orphan: short-course treatment of tuberculosis)*

rifamycin INN, BAN

rifamycin diethylamide [see: rifamide]

rifamycin M-14 [see: rifamide]

rifapentine USAN, INN, BAN *antibacterial*

Rifater *(orphan: short course treatment of tuberculosis)* [rifampin; isoniazid; pyrazinamide]

rifaxidin [see: rifaximin]

rifaximin INN

rIFN-A (recombinant interferon alfa) [see: interferon alfa-2a, recombinant]

rIFN-α2 (recombinant interferon alfa-2) [see: interferon alfa-2b, recombinant]

R-IFN-beta *(orphan: metastatic renal cell carcinoma)* [interferon beta, recombinant]

rIFN-beta (recombinant interferon beta) [see: interferon beta, recombinant]
rifomycin [see: rifamycin]
RIG (rabies immune globulin) [q.v.]
rilapine INN
rilmazafone INN
rilmenidine INN
rilopirox INN
rilozarone INN
riluzole INN
Rimactane capsules ℞ *tuberculostatic* [rifampin]
Rimactane/INH Dual Pack (two-product package) ℞ *tuberculostatic* [rifampin (2 capsules); isoniazid (1 tablet)]
Rimadyl ℞ *investigational nonsteroidal anti-inflammatory drug (NSAID); analgesic; antipyretic* [carprofen]
rimantadine INN *antiviral* [also: rimantadine HCl]
rimantadine HCl USAN *antiviral* [also: rimantadine]
rimazolium metilsulfate INN
rimcazole INN *antipsychotic* [also: rimcazole HCl]
rimcazole HCl USAN *antipsychotic* [also: rimcazole]
rimexolone USAN, INN, BAN *anti-inflammatory*
rimiterol INN *bronchodilator* [also: rimiterol hydrobromide]
rimiterol hydrobromide USAN *bronchodilator* [also: rimiterol]
rimoprogin INN
Rimso-50 solution for bladder instillation ℞ *for symptomatic relief of cystitis* [dimethyl sulfoxide (DMSO)]
Rinade B.I.D. sustained-release capsules ℞ *decongestant; antihistamine* [d-isoephedrine HCl; chlorpheniramine maleate]
Ringer's injection USP *fluid and electrolyte replenisher* [also: compound solution of sodium chloride]
Ringer's injection, lactated USP *fluid and electrolyte replenisher; systemic alkalizer* [also: compound solution of sodium lactate]
Ringer's irrigation USP *irrigation solution*
Ringer's solution [now: Ringer's irrigation]
riodipine INN
Riopan Plus; Riopan Plus 2 chewable tablets, oral suspension OTC *antacid; antiflatulent* [magaldrate; simethicone]
Riopan tablets, chewable tablets, suspension OTC *antacid* [magaldrate]
rioprostil USAN, INN *gastric antisecretory*
ripazepam USAN, INN *minor tranquilizer*
risedronate sodium USAN *calcium regulator*
risocaine USAN, INN *local anesthetic*
risotilide HCl USAN *antiarrhythmic*
Risperdal ℞ *investigational antischizophrenic*
risperidone USAN, INN, BAN *neuroleptic*
ristianol INN, BAN *immunoregulator* [also: ristianol phosphate]
ristianol phosphate USAN *immunoregulator* [also: ristianol]
ristocetin USP, INN, BAN
Ritalin tablets ℞ *for attention deficit disorders; analeptic* [methylphenidate HCl]
Ritalin-SR sustained-release tablets ℞ *for attention deficit disorders; analeptic* [methylphenidate HCl]
ritanserin USAN, INN, BAN *serotonin antagonist*
ritiometan INN
ritodrine USAN, INN *smooth muscle relaxant*
ritodrine HCl USAN, USP *smooth muscle relaxant; uterine relaxant*
ritolukast USAN, INN *antiasthmatic; leukotriene antagonist*
ritropirronium bromide INN
ritrosulfan INN
rizolipase INN

RMP-7 ℞ *investigational drug for AIDS*
RMS suppositories ℞ *analgesic* [morphine sulfate]
Robafen CF liquid OTC *expectorant; decongestant; antitussive* [guaifenesin; phenylpropanolamine HCl; dextromethorphan hydrobromide; alcohol]
Robafen DAC syrup ℞ *decongestant; antitussive; expectorant* [pseudoephedrine HCl; codeine phosphate; guaifenesin; alcohol]
Robafen DM syrup OTC *expectorant; antitussive* [guaifenesin; dextromethorphan hydrobromide; alcohol]
RoBathol Bath Oil OTC *bath emollient*
Robaxin tablets, IV or IM injection ℞ *skeletal muscle relaxant* [methocarbamol]
Robaxin-750 tablets ℞ *skeletal muscle relaxant* [methocarbamol]
Robaxisal tablets ℞ *skeletal muscle relaxant; analgesic* [methocarbamol; aspirin]
robenidine INN *coccidiostat for poultry* [also: robenidine HCl]
robenidine HCl USAN *coccidiostat for poultry* [also: robenidine]
Robicaps (dosage form) *capsules*
Robicillin VK tablets ℞ *bactericidal antibiotic* [penicillin V potassium]
Ro-Bile tablets (discontinued 1991) ℞ *digestive enzymes; laxative; sedative* [pancreatin; lipase; ox bile extract; dehydrocholic acid; belladonna extract; pepsin]
Robimycin Robitabs (enteric-coated tablets) ℞ *macrolide antibiotic* [erythromycin]
Robinul Forte tablets ℞ *anticholinergic; peptic ulcer treatment adjunct; antisecretory* [glycopyrrolate]
Robinul tablets, IV or IM injection ℞ *anticholinergic; peptic ulcer treatment adjunct; antisecretory* [glycopyrrolate]
Robitabs (dosage form) *enteric-coated tablets*

Robitet Robicaps (capsules) ℞ *broad-spectrum antibiotic* [tetracycline HCl]
Robitussin A-C syrup ℞ *antitussive; expectorant* [codeine phosphate; guaifenesin; alcohol]
Robitussin Cough Calmers lozenge OTC *antitussive* [dextromethorphan hydrobromide]
Robitussin Cough & Cold Formula; Robitussin Pediatric Cough & Cold Formula liquid OTC *antitussive; decongestant* [dextromethorphan hydrobromide; pseudoephedrine HCl]
Robitussin Cough Drops lozenge OTC *mild topical anesthetic; antiseptic* [menthol; eucalyptus oil]
Robitussin Night Relief liquid OTC *analgesic; decongestant; antihistamine; antitussive* [acetaminophen; phenylephrine HCl; pyrilamine maleate; dextromethorphan hydrobromide]
Robitussin Pediatric liquid OTC *antitussive* [dextromethorphan hydrobromide]
Robitussin syrup OTC *expectorant* [guaifenesin; alcohol]
Robitussin-CF syrup OTC *expectorant; decongestant; antitussive* [guaifenesin; phenylpropanolamine HCl; dextromethorphan hydrobromide; alcohol]
Robitussin-DAC syrup ℞ *decongestant; antitussive; expectorant* [pseudoephedrine HCl; codeine phosphate; guaifenesin; alcohol]
Robitussin-DM syrup OTC *expectorant; antitussive* [guaifenesin; dextromethorphan hydrobromide]
Robitussin-PE syrup OTC *expectorant; decongestant* [guaifenesin; pseudoephedrine HCl; alcohol]
Robomol-500; Robomol-750 tablets ℞ *skeletal muscle relaxant* [methocarbamol]
Rocaltrol capsules ℞ *treatment of hypocalcemia in dialysis patients; de-*

creases severity of psoriatic lesions [calcitriol]
rocastine INN *antihistamine* [also: rocastine HCl]
rocastine HCl USAN *antihistamine* [also: rocastine]
Rocephin powder for IV or IM injection, ADD-vantage vials ℞ *cephalosporin-type antibiotic* [ceftriaxone sodium]
rochelle salt [see: potassium sodium tartrate]
rociverine INN
Rocky Mountain spotted fever vaccine USP
rodocaine USAN, INN *local anesthetic*
rodorubicin INN
rofelodine INN
Roferon-A subcu or IM injection ℞ *antineoplastic for hairy cell leukemia and Kaposi sarcoma; (orphan: various cancers)* [interferon alfa-2a, recombinant]
roflurane USAN, INN *inhalation anesthetic*
Rogaine topical solution ℞ *hair growth stimulant* [minoxidil]
Rogenic IM injection ℞ *hematinic* [peptonized iron; vitamin B$_{12}$]
Rogenic slow-release tablets OTC *hematinic* [ferrous fumarate; ferrous gluconate; ferrous sulfate; desiccated liver; multiple vitamins]
rogletimide USAN, INN, BAN *antineoplastic; aromatase inhibitor*
rokitamycin INN
Rolaids Antacid chewable tablets OTC *antacid* [dihydroxyaluminum sodium carbonate]
Rolaids Calcium Rich chewable tablets OTC *antacid* [calcium carbonate]
Rolaids Sodium Free chewable tablets OTC *antacid* [magnesium hydroxide; calcium carbonate]
Rolatuss with Hydrocodone liquid ℞ *decongestant; antihistamine; antitussive* [phenylpropanolamine HCl; phenylephrine HCl; pyrilamine maleate; pheniramine maleate; hydrocodone bitartrate]
roletamide USAN, INN *hypnotic*
rolgamidine USAN, INN, BAN *antidiarrheal*
rolicton [see: amisometradine]
rolicyclidine INN
rolicypram BAN *antidepressant* [also: rolicyprine]
rolicyprine USAN, INN *antidepressant* [also: rolicypram]
rolipram USAN, INN *tranquilizer*
rolitetracycline USAN, USP, INN *antibacterial*
rolitetracycline nitrate USAN *antibacterial*
rolodine USAN, INN *skeletal muscle relaxant*
rolziracetam INN, BAN
romazarit USAN, INN, BAN *anti-inflammatory; antirheumatic*
rometin [see: clioquinol]
romifenone INN
romifidine INN
romurtide INN
ronactolol INN
Ronase tablets (discontinued 1991) ℞ *antidiabetic* [tolazamide]
Rondamine-DM pediatric drops ℞ *decongestant; antihistamine; antitussive* [pseudoephedrine HCl; carbinoxamine maleate; dextromethorphan hydrobromide]
Rondec film-coated tablets, syrup, pediatric drops ℞ *antihistamine; decongestant* [carbinoxamine maleate; pseudoephedrine HCl]
Rondec-DM syrup, pediatric drops ℞ *antihistamine; decongestant; antitussive* [carbinoxamine maleate; pseudoephedrine HCl; dextromethorphan hydrobromide]
Rondec-TR timed-release Filmtabs (film-coated tablets) ℞ *antihistamine; decongestant* [carbinoxamine maleate; pseudoephedrine HCl]

Rondomycin capsules (discontinued 1991) ℞ *tetracycline-type antibiotic* [methacycline HCl]
ronidazole USAN, INN *antiprotozoal*
ronifibrate INN
ronipamil INN
ronnel USAN *systemic insecticide* [also: fenclofos; fenchlorphos]
ropinirole INN, BAN
ropitoin INN *antiarrhythmic* [also: ropitoin HCl]
ropitoin HCl USAN *antiarrhythmic* [also: ropitoin]
ropivacaine INN
ropizine USAN, INN *anticonvulsant*
roquinimex INN *investigational immunomodulator for AIDS*
rosamicin [now: rosaramicin]
rosamicin butyrate [now: rosaramicin butyrate]
rosamicin propionate [now: rosaramicin propionate]
rosamicin sodium phosphate [now: rosaramicin sodium phosphate]
rosamicin stearate [now: rosaramicin stearate]
rosaprostol INN
rosaramicin USAN, INN *antibacterial*
rosaramicin butyrate USAN *antibacterial*
rosaramicin propionate USAN *antibacterial*
rosaramicin sodium phosphate USAN *antibacterial*
rosaramicin stearate USAN *antibacterial*
rose bengal *corneal injury and pathology diagnostic aid*
rose bengal sodium (^{131}I) INN *hepatic function test; radioactive agent* [also: rose bengal sodium I 131]
rose bengal sodium I 125 USAN *radioactive agent*
rose bengal sodium I 131 USAN, USP *hepatic function test; radioactive agent* [also: rose bengal sodium (^{131}I)]
rose oil NF *perfume*

rose petal aqueous infusion *ocular emollient*
rose water, stronger NF *perfume*
rose water ointment USP *emollient; ointment base*
Rosets ophthalmic strips OTC *corneal disclosing agent* [rose bengal]
rosin USP
rosoxacin USAN, INN *antibacterial* [also: acrosoxacin]
Ross SLD powder for oral solution OTC *oral nutritional supplement for patients on clear liquid diets*
rosterolone INN
Rotacaps (trademarked form) *encapsulated powder for inhalation*
Rotalex test kit OTC *in vitro diagnostic aid for fecal rotavirus*
rotamicillin INN
rotoxamine USAN, INN *antihistamine*
rotoxamine tartrate NF
rotraxate INN
Rovamycine (*orphan: cryptosporidiosis in immunodeficiency*) [spiramycin]
Rowasa rectal suspension enema, suppositories ℞ *treatment of active ulcerative colitis, proctosigmoiditis and proctitis* [mesalamine]
roxadimate USAN, INN *sunscreen*
Roxanol; Roxanol 100; Roxanol Rescudose; Roxanol UD oral solution ℞ *narcotic analgesic* [morphine sulfate]
Roxanol SR sustained-release tablets ℞ *narcotic analgesic* [morphine sulfate]
Roxanol suppositories ℞ *narcotic analgesic* [morphine sulfate]
roxarsone USAN, INN *antibacterial*
roxatidine INN, BAN *antiulcerative* [also: roxatidine acetate HCl]
roxatidine acetate HCl USAN *antiulcerative* [also: roxatidine]
Roxiam ℞ *investigational antipsychotic* [remoxipride]
roxibolone INN

Roxicet 5/500 caplets ℞ *narcotic analgesic* [oxycodone HCl; acetaminophen]
Roxicet tablets, oral solution ℞ *narcotic analgesic* [oxycodone HCl; acetaminophen]
Roxicodone tablets, oral solution, Intensol (concentrated oral solution) ℞ *narcotic analgesic* [oxycodone HCl]
Roxilox capsules ℞ *narcotic analgesic* [oxycodone HCl; acetaminophen]
roxindole INN
Roxiprin tablets ℞ *narcotic analgesic* [oxycodone HCl; oxycodone terephthalate; aspirin]
roxithromycin USAN, INN *antibacterial*
roxolonium metilsulfate INN
roxoperone INN
R-Tannamine tablets, pediatric oral suspension ℞ *decongestant; antihistamine* [phenylephrine tannate; chlorpheniramine tannate; pyrilamine tannate]
R-Tannate pediatric oral suspension, tablets ℞ *decongestant; antihistamine* [phenylephrine tannate; chlorpheniramine tannate; pyrilamine tannate]
rtPA; rt-PA (recombinant tissue plasminogen activator) [see: alteplase]
Rubacell II OTC *in vitro diagnostic aid for rubella virus antibody*
Rubazyme OTC *in vitro diagnostic aid for rubella virus antibody*
rubbing alcohol [see: alcohol, rubbing]
rubbing isopropyl alcohol [see: isopropyl alcohol, rubbing]
rubella & mumps virus vaccine, live *active immunizing agent for rubella and mumps*
rubella virus vaccine, live USP *active immunizing agent for rubella*
Rubesol-1000 injection ℞ *vitamin supplement* [cyanocobalamin]

Rubex powder for IV injection ℞ *antineoplastic antibiotic* [doxorubicin HCl]
rubidium *element (Rb)*
rubidium chloride Rb 86 USAN *radioactive agent*
Rubramin PC injection ℞ *antianemic; vitamin supplement* [cyanocobalamin]
Rufen film-coated tablets ℞ *nonsteroidal anti-inflammatory drug (NSAID); antiarthritic; analgesic* [ibuprofen]
rufloxacin INN
rufocromomycin INN, BAN *antineoplastic* [also: streptonigrin]
Ru-lets 500 film-coated tablets OTC *vitamin supplement* [multiple vitamins]
Ru-lets M 500 film-coated tablets OTC *vitamin/mineral supplement* [multiple vitamins & minerals]
Rulox #1; Rulox #2 chewable tablets OTC *antacid* [aluminum hydroxide; magnesium hydroxide]
Rulox oral suspension OTC *antacid; antiflatulent* [aluminum hydroxide; magnesium hydroxide; simethicone]
Rum-K liquid ℞ *potassium supplement* [potassium chloride]
rutamycin USAN, INN *antifungal*
ruthenium *element (Ru)*
rutin NF [also: rutoside]
rutoside INN [also: rutin]
Ru-Tuss liquid OTC *decongestant; antihistamine* [phenylephrine HCl; chlorpheniramine maleate; alcohol]
Ru-Tuss sustained-release tablets ℞ *decongestant; antihistamine; anticholinergic* [phenylpropanolamine HCl; phenylephrine HCl; chlorpheniramine maleate; hyoscyamine sulfate; atropine sulfate; scopolamine hydrobromide]
Ru-Tuss II slow-release capsules ℞ *decongestant; antihistamine* [phenylpropanolamine HCl; chlorpheniramine maleate]

Ru-Tuss DE film-coated prolonged-action tablets ℞ *decongestant; expectorant* [pseudoephedrine HCl; guaifenesin]

Ru-Tuss Expectorant liquid OTC *decongestant; antitussive; expectorant* [pseudoephedrine HCl; dextromethorphan hydrobromide; guaifenesin; alcohol]

Ru-Tuss with Hydrocodone liquid ℞ *decongestant; antihistamine; antitussive* [phenylpropanolamine HCl; phenylephrine HCl; pyrilamine maleate; pheniramine maleate; hydrocodone bitartrate]

ruvazone INN

Ru-Vert-M film-coated tablets ℞ *anticholinergic; antivertigo agent; motion sickness preventative* [meclizine]

RVP (red veterinarian petrolatum) [see: petrolatum]

℞Pak (trademarked form) *prescription package*

Rymed capsules ℞ *decongestant; expectorant* [pseudoephedrine HCl; guaifenesin]

Rymed liquid OTC *decongestant; expectorant* [pseudoephedrine HCl; guaifenesin; alcohol]

Rymed-TR long-acting caplets ℞ *decongestant; expectorant* [phenylpropanolamine HCl; guaifenesin]

Ryna liquid OTC *decongestant; antihistamine* [pseudoephedrine HCl; chlorpheniramine maleate]

Ryna-C liquid ℞ *decongestant; antihistamine; antitussive* [pseudoephedrine HCl; chlorpheniramine maleate; codeine phosphate]

Ryna-CX liquid ℞ *decongestant; antitussive; expectorant* [pseudoephedrine HCl; codeine phosphate; guaifenesin]

Rynatan tablets, pediatric oral suspension ℞ *decongestant; antihistamine* [phenylephrine tannate; chlorpheniramine tannate; pyrilamine tannate]

Rynatan-S pediatric suspension ℞ *decongestant; antihistamine* [phenylephrine tannate; chlorpheniramine tannate; pyrilamine tannate]

Rynatuss tablets, pediatric suspension ℞ *decongestant; antihistamine; antitussive* [phenylephrine tannate; ephedrine tannate; chlorpheniramine tannate; carbetapentane tannate]

Rythmol film-coated tablets ℞ *antiarrhythmic* [propafenone HCl]

S

S-2 solution for inhalation OTC *bronchodilator for bronchial asthma* [racepinephrine]

^{35}S [see: sodium sulfate S 35]

SA (salicylic acid) [q.v.]

SA (serum albumin) [see: albumin, human]

Saave + capsules (discontinued 1993) OTC *dietary supplement* [multiple amino acids, vitamins & minerals]

sabeluzole USAN, INN, BAN *anticonvulsant; antihypoxic*

S-A-C tablets OTC *analgesic; antipyretic; anti-inflammatory* [acetaminophen; salicylamide; caffeine]

saccharin NF *flavoring agent*

saccharin calcium USP *non-nutritive sweetener*

saccharin sodium USP *non-nutritive sweetener*

safflower oil USP *oleaginous vehicle; essential fatty acid supplement*

safrole USP

Saizen ℞ *(orphan: growth failure; Turner syndrome; anovulation; severe burns)* [somatropin]
SalAc liquid OTC *topical acne cleanser* [salicylic acid]
salacetamide INN
salacetin [see: aspirin]
Salacid 25%; Salacid 60% ointment ℞ *topical keratolytic* [salicylic acid]
Sal-Acid plaster ℞ *topical keratolytic* [salicylic acid]
Salactic Film liquid ℞ *topical keratolytic* [salicylic acid; lactic acid]
salafibrate INN
Salagen ℞ *investigational treatment for radiation-induced xerostomia* [pilocarpine]
salantel USAN, INN *veterinary anthelmintic*
Salatin capsules (discontinued 1991) OTC *analgesic; antipyretic; anti-inflammatory* [acetaminophen; aspirin; caffeine]
Salazide; Salazide-Demi tablets ℞ *antihypertensive* [hydroflumethiazide; reserpine]
salazodine INN
salazosulfadimidine INN [also: salazosulphadimidine]
salazosulfamide INN
salazosulfapyridine [see: sulfasalazine]
salazosulfathiazole INN
salazosulphadimidine BAN [also: salazosulfadimidine]
salbutamol INN, BAN *bronchodilator* [also: albuterol]
salcatonin BAN
salcetogen [see: aspirin]
salcolex USAN, INN *analgesic; anti-inflammatory; antipyretic*
Sal-Dex liquid (discontinued 1991) OTC *topical antifungal; keratolytic; antiseptic* [undecylenic acid; salicylic acid; isopropyl alcohol]
Sal-Dex-Boro liquid (discontinued 1991) ℞ *topical astringent; antiseptic; keratolytic* [tannic acid; boric acid; salicylic acid; isopropyl alcohol]

saletamide INN *analgesic* [also: salethamide maleate]
saletamide maleate [see: salethamide maleate]
salethamide maleate USAN *analgesic* [also: saletamide]
saletin [see: aspirin]
Saleto tablets OTC *analgesic; antipyretic; anti-inflammatory* [acetaminophen; aspirin; salicylamide; caffeine]
Saleto-200 tablets OTC *nonsteroidal anti-inflammatory drug (NSAID); antiarthritic; analgesic* [ibuprofen]
Saleto-400; Saleto-600; Saleto-800 tablets ℞ *nonsteroidal anti-inflammatory drug (NSAID); antiarthritic; analgesic* [ibuprofen]
Saleto-D capsules OTC *decongestant* [phenylpropanolamine HCl; acetaminophen; salicylamide; caffeine]
Salflex film-coated tablets OTC *analgesic; antipyretic; anti-inflammatory; antirheumatic* [salsalate]
salfluverine INN
salicain [now: salicyl alcohol]
salicin USP
salicyl alcohol USAN *local anesthetic*
salicylamide USP *analgesic*
salicylanilide NF
salicylate meglumine USAN *antirheumatic; analgesic*
salicylazosulfapyridine [now: sulfasalazine]
salicylic acid (SA) USP *keratolytic; antiseborrheic; antipsoriatic*
salicylic acid, bimolecular ester [see: salsalate]
salicylic acid acetate [see: aspirin]
Salicylic Acid and Sulfur Soap bar OTC *medicated cleanser for acne* [salicylic acid; precipitated sulfur]
salicylic acid dihydrogen phosphate [see: fosfosal]
Salicylic Acid Soap bar OTC *medicated cleanser for acne* [salicylic acid]
salicylsalicylic acid [see: salsalate]
Saligel Acne gel OTC *topical acne treatment* [salicylic acid; alcohol]

Saligel gel OTC *keratolytic for acne* [salicylic acid]
saligenin [now: salicyl alcohol]
saligenol [now: salicyl alcohol]
salinazid INN, BAN
saline, lactated potassic [see: potassic saline, lactated]
saline solution (SS) [also: normal saline]
SalineX nasal mist, nose drops OTC *nasal moisturizer* [sodium chloride (saline)]
saliniazid [see: salinazid]
salinomycin INN, BAN
Saliv-Aid liquid OTC *oral lubricant*
Salivart oral spray OTC *saliva substitute*
salmaterol [see: salmeterol]
salmefamol INN, BAN
salmeterol USAN, INN, BAN *bronchodilator*
salmeterol xinafoate USAN *adrenergic; bronchodilator*
salmisteine INN
salmon calcitonin [see: salcatonin]
salmotin [see: adicillin]
Salocol tablets OTC *analgesic; antipyretic; anti-inflammatory* [acetaminophen; aspirin; salicylamide; caffeine]
Sal-Oil-T hair dressing ℞ *antipsoriatic; antiseborrheic; keratolytic* [coal tar; salicylic acid]
salol [see: phenyl salicylate]
Salonil ointment (discontinued 1992) ℞ *topical keratolytic* [salicylic acid]
Salphenyl capsules OTC *decongestant; antihistamine; analgesic* [phenylephrine HCl; chlorpheniramine maleate; acetaminophen; salicylamide]
Sal-Plant gel ℞ *topical keratolytic* [salicylic acid; lactic acid]
salprotoside INN
salsalate USAN, USP, INN, BAN *analgesic; antipyretic; anti-inflammatory; antirheumatic*
Salsitab film-coated tablets ℞ *analgesic; antipyretic; anti-inflammatory; antirheumatic* [salsalate]

Saluron tablets ℞ *diuretic; antihypertensive* [hydroflumethiazide]
Salutensin; Salutensin-Demi tablets ℞ *antihypertensive* [hydroflumethiazide; reserpine]
saluzide [see: opiniazide]
salvarsan [see: arsphenamine]
salverine INN
samarium *element (Sm)*
San Cura ointment (discontinued 1991) OTC *topical local anesthetic; antifungal; keratolytic; antiseptic* [benzocaine; chlorobutanol; chlorothymol; benzoic acid; salicylic acid; benzyl alcohol]
Sanchia Silicone cream OTC *skin protectant* [silicone; lanolin]
sancycline USAN, INN *antibacterial*
Sandimmune ℞ *investigational agent for psoriasis and atopic dermatitis*
Sandimmune ophthalmic ointment ℞ *(orphan: keratoplasty graft rejection; corneal melting syndrome)* [cyclosporine]
Sandimmune soft gelatin capsules, oral solution, IV injection ℞ *immunosuppressant for organ transplantation* [cyclosporine]
Sandoglobulin powder for IV infusion ℞ *passive immunizing agent* [immune globulin]
Sandostatin IV injection ℞ *carcinoid tumors; vasoactive intestinal peptide tumors (VIPomas)* [octreotide acetate]
Sani-Supp suppositories OTC *hyperosmolar laxative* [glycerin]
Sanitube ointment OTC *venereal prophylactic* [calomel; benzoxiquine; trolamine]
Sanorex tablets ℞ *anorexiant; (orphan: Duchenne's muscular dystrophy)* [mazindol]
Sansert tablets ℞ *agent for migraine and vascular headaches* [methysergide maleate]
santonin NF
Santyl ointment ℞ *topical enzyme for biochemical debridement* [collagenase]

saperconazole USAN, INN, BAN *antifungal*
sapropterin INN
sarafloxacin INN, BAN *anti-infective; DNA gyrase inhibitor* [also: sarafloxacin HCl]
sarafloxacin HCl USAN *anti-infective; DNA gyrase inhibitor* [also: sarafloxacin]
saralasin INN *antihypertensive* [also: saralasin acetate]
saralasin acetate USAN *antihypertensive* [also: saralasin]
Saratoga ointment OTC *astringent; antiseptic; wound protectant* [zinc oxide; boric acid; eucalyptol]
sarcolysin INN
L-sarcolysin [see: melphalan]
sargramostim USAN *antineutropenic; (orphan: neutropenia in bone marrow transplant; graft failure)*
Sarisol No. 2 tablets ℞ *sedative; hypnotic* [butabarbital sodium]
sarmazenil INN
sarmoxicillin USAN, INN *antibacterial*
Sarna Anti-Itch foam, lotion OTC *counterirritant* [camphor; menthol]
saroten [see: amitriptyline]
sarpicillin USAN, INN *antibacterial*
saruplase INN
Sastid (AL) Scrub cream OTC *abrasive cleanser for acne* [aluminum oxide; precipitated sulfur; salicylic acid]
Sastid cream, bar soap OTC *keratolytic for acne* [precipitated sulfur; salicylic acid]
Sastid Plain Therapeutic Shampoo & Acne Wash OTC *topical acne cleanser* [sulfur; salicylic acid]
saterinone INN
satranidazole INN
Satric tablets (discontinued 1991) ℞ *bactericidal antibiotic* [metronidazole]
savoxepin INN
S.B.P. tablets (discontinued 1991) ℞ *sedative; hypnotic* [secobarbital sodium; butabarbital sodium; phenobarbital]
SC (succinylcholine) [see: succinylcholine chloride]
SCA proteins (single-chain antigen-binding proteins) *investigational class of antineoplastics*
Scabene lotion, shampoo ℞ *scabicide; pediculicide* [lindane]
Scadan scalp lotion OTC *antiseptic; antiseborrheic* [myristyltrimethylammonium bromide; stearyl dimethyl benzyl ammonium chloride]
scandium *element (Sc)*
scarlet fever streptococcus toxin
scarlet red NF *promotes wound healing*
Scarlet Red Ointment Dressings medication-impregnated gauze ℞ *wound dressings* [scarlet red; lanolin; olive oil; petrolatum]
sCD4-PE40 *investigational antiviral for AIDS*
Schamberg lotion OTC *antiseptic; astringent; antifungal; counterirritant* [zinc oxide; menthol; phenol]
Schick test [see: diphtheria toxin for Schick test]
Schick test control USP *dermal reactivity indicator*
Sclavo Test-PPD single-use intradermal puncture test device ℞ *tuberculosis skin test* [tuberculin purified protein derivative]
Sclerex tablets OTC *vitamin/mineral supplement* [multiple vitamins & minerals]
Scleromate IV injection ℞ *sclerosing agent for varicose veins* [morrhuate sodium]
Sclerosol ℞ *(orphan: scleroderma)* [dimethyl sulfoxide (DMSO)]
Scooby-Doo Children's Chewable Plus Iron tablets (discontinued 1992) OTC *vitamin/iron supplement* [multiple vitamins; iron; folic acid]
Scooby-Doo Children's Chewable Tablets (discontinued 1992) OTC

vitamin supplement [multiple vitamins; folic acid]
Scooby-Doo Children's Complete Formula chewable tablets (discontinued 1992) OTC *vitamin/mineral/iron supplement* [multiple vitamins & minerals; iron; folic acid; biotin]
Scooter Rabbit chewable tablets OTC *vitamin/mineral supplement* [multiple vitamins & minerals; bioflavonoids]
scopafungin USAN *antibacterial; antifungal*
Scope mouthwash OTC *oral antiseptic* [cetylpyridinium chloride; domiphen bromide]
scopolamine *transdermal motion sickness preventative*
scopolamine hydrobromide USP *GI antispasmodic; anticholinergic; motion sickness preventative; cycloplegic; mydriatic* [also: hyoscine hydrobromide]
scopolamine methyl nitrate [see: methscopolamine nitrate]
scopolamine methylbromide [see: methscopolamine bromide]
Scorbex/12 injection (discontinued 1992) ℞ *vitamin therapy* [multiple B vitamins; vitamin C]
Scott's Emulsion OTC *vitamin supplement* [vitamins A & D]
Scot-Tussin Allergy liquid OTC *antihistamine* [diphenhydramine HCl]
Scot-Tussin DM 2 syrup (discontinued 1992) OTC *antitussive; expectorant* [dextromethorphan hydrobromide; guaifenesin; alcohol]
Scot-Tussin DM Cough Chasers lozenges OTC *antitussive* [dextromethorphan hydrobromide]
Scot-Tussin DM liquid OTC *antitussive; antihistamine* [dextromethorphan hydrobromide; chlorpheniramine maleate]
Scot-Tussin Expectorant sugar-free liquid OTC *expectorant* [guaifenesin; alcohol]

Scot-Tussin Original 5-Action Cold Formula syrup, sugar-free liquid OTC *decongestant; antihistamine; analgesic* [phenylephrine HCl; pheniramine maleate; sodium citrate; sodium salicylate; caffeine citrate]
sCR1 ℞ *investigational complement inhibitor for severe burns* [soluble complement receptor 1]
Scrip Zinc capsules (discontinued 1991) OTC *zinc supplement* [zinc sulfate]
Scriptene ℞ *investigational antiviral for AIDS* [AZT-P-ddI (drug code—generic not yet approved)]
scuroforme [see: butyl aminobenzoate]
SD (streptodornase) [q.v.]
SDZ MSL-109 (orphan: *cytomegalovirus of organ transplants; cytomegalovirus retinitis of AIDS*)
[75]Se [see: selenomethionine Se 75]
Sea Mist nasal spray OTC *nasal moisturizer* [sodium chloride (saline)]
Seale's Lotion Modified OTC *topical acne treatment* [sulfur; zinc oxide; bentonite; sodium borate; acetone]
Sea-Omega 30; Sea-Omega 50 softgels OTC *dietary supplement* [omega-3 fatty acids; vitamin E]
Sebacide Cleanser liquid OTC *topical acne cleanser*
Seba-Nil Cleansing Mask suspension (discontinued 1991) OTC *abrasive cleanser for acne; astringent* [sulfated castor oil; titanium dioxide]
Seba-Nil Liquid Cleanser OTC *topical acne cleanser* [alcohol; acetone]
Sebaquin shampoo OTC *antiseborrheic; antimicrobial* [iodoquinol]
Sebasorb liquid OTC *topical acne treatment* [sulfur; salicylic acid; attapulgite]
Sebex shampoo OTC *antiseborrheic; keratolytic* [sulfur; salicylic acid]
Sebex-T shampoo OTC *antiseborrheic; antipsoriatic; keratolytic* [sulfur; salicylic acid; coal tar]

Sebizon lotion ℞ *bacteriostatic; antiseborrheic* [sulfacetamide sodium]
Sebucare hair lotion OTC *antiseborrheic; keratolytic* [salicylic acid; alcohol]
Sebulex shampoo, cream, liquid OTC *antiseborrheic; keratolytic* [sulfur; salicylic acid]
Sebulex with Conditioners shampoo OTC *antiseborrheic; keratolytic* [sulfur; salicylic acid]
Sebulon shampoo OTC *antiseborrheic; antibacterial; antifungal* [pyrithione zinc]
Sebutone cream shampoo, liquid shampoo OTC *antiseborrheic; antipsoriatic; keratolytic* [coal tar; sulfur; salicylic acid]
secalciferol USAN, BAN *calcium regulator*
secbutabarbital sodium INN *sedative* [also: butabarbital sodium]
secbutobarbitone BAN *hypnotic; sedative* [also: butabarbital]
seclazone USAN, INN *anti-inflammatory; uricosuric*
secnidazole INN, BAN
secobarbital USP, INN *hypnotic; sedative*
secobarbital sodium USP *hypnotic; sedative* [also: quinalbarbitone sodium]
Seconal Sodium IV, IM or rectal injection (discontinued 1992) ℞ *sedative; hypnotic* [secobarbital sodium]
Seconal Sodium Pulvules (capsules) ℞ *sedative; hypnotic* [secobarbital sodium]
secoverine INN
Secran liquid OTC *vitamin supplement* [vitamins B_1, B_3 & B_{12}; alcohol]
Secran Prenatal tablets ℞ *vitamin/calcium/iron supplement* [multiple vitamins; calcium; iron; folic acid]
Secran/Fe elixir (discontinued 1991) OTC *antianemic* [ferric pyrophosphate; vitamins B_1, B_3 & B_{12}]

secretin INN, BAN *pancreatic function diagnostic aid*
Secretin Ferring powder for IV injection ℞ *in vivo pancreatic function test* [secretin]
Secretin-Kabi (name changed to Secretin Ferring in 1990)
Sectral capsules ℞ *antihypertensive; antiarrhythmic; β-blocker* [acebutolol HCl]
Secule (trademarked form) *single-dose powder for injection*
securinine INN
sedaform [see: chlorobutanol]
Sedapap caplet ℞ *analgesic; antipyretic; sedative* [acetaminophen; caffeine; butalbital]
sedatine [see: antipyrine]
sedecamycin USAN, INN *veterinary antibacterial*
sedeval [see: barbital]
seganserin INN, BAN
seglitide INN *antidiabetic* [also: seglitide acetate]
seglitide acetate USAN *antidiabetic* [also: seglitide]
Seldane tablets ℞ *antihistamine* [terfenadine]
Seldane-D sustained-release tablets ℞ *antihistamine; decongestant* [terfenadine; pseudoephedrine HCl]
Selecor tablets ℞ *antihypertensive* [celiprolol HCl]
selegiline INN, BAN *antiparkinsonian*
selegiline HCl (*orphan*: Parkinson's disease)
selenious acid USP *dietary selenium supplement*
selenium *element* (Se)
selenium dioxide, monohydrated [see: selenious acid]
selenium sulfide USP *antifungal; antiseborrheic*
selenomethionine (^{75}Se) INN *pancreas function test; radioactive agent* [also: selenomethionine Se 75]
selenomethionine Se 75 USAN, USP *pancreas function test; radioac-*

tive agent [also: selenomethionine (^{75}Se)]

Sele-Pak IV injection ℞ *intravenous nutritional therapy* [selenious acid]

Selepen IV injection ℞ *intravenous nutritional therapy* [selenious acid]

Selestoject IV, IM injection ℞ *glucocorticoids* [betamethasone sodium phosphate]

Seloken ZOC (foreign name for U.S. product Toprol XL)

selprazine INN

Selsun Blue lotion/shampoo OTC *antiseborrheic* [selenium sulfide]

Selsun lotion/shampoo ℞ *antiseborrheic; antifungal* [selenium sulfide]

sematilide INN *antiarrhythmic* [also: sematilide HCl]

sematilide HCl USAN *antiarrhythmic* [also: sematilide]

semduramicin USAN, INN *coccidiostat*

semduramicin sodium USAN *coccidiostat*

Semets troches (discontinued 1991) OTC *topical anesthetic; oral antiseptic* [benzocaine; cetylpyridinium chloride]

Semicid vaginal suppositories OTC *spermicidal contraceptive* [nonoxynol 9]

Semilente Iletin I subcu injection OTC *antidiabetic* [insulin zinc (beef-pork)]

Semilente Insulin suspension for injection OTC *antidiabetic* [prompt insulin zinc (beef)]

semisodium valproate BAN *anticonvulsant* [also: divalproex sodium; valproate semisodium]

semustine USAN, INN *antineoplastic*

Senexon tablets OTC *laxative* [senna concentrate]

Senilezol elixir ℞ *vitamin/iron supplement* [multiple B vitamins; ferric pyrophosphate]

senna USP *stimulant laxative*

Senna-Gen tablets OTC *laxative* [senna concentrate]

sennosides USP *stimulant laxative*

Senokot; Senokotxtra tablets, granules, suppositories, syrup OTC *laxative* [senna concentrate]

Senokot-S tablets OTC *laxative; stool softener* [docusate sodium; senna concentrate]

Senolax tablets OTC *laxative* [senna concentrate]

Sensitive Eyes Daily Cleaner; Sensitive Eyes Saline/Cleaning Solution solution OTC *contact lens surfactant cleaning solution*

Sensitive Eyes Drops OTC *contact lens rewetting solution*

Sensitive Eyes Saline solution OTC *contact lens rinsing and storage solution* [preserved saline solution]

Sensodyne, Mint toothpaste OTC *tooth desensitizer* [potassium nitrate]

Sensodyne, Original toothpaste OTC *tooth desensitizer* [strontium chloride hexahydrate]

Sensodyne-F toothpaste (discontinued 1991) OTC *tooth desensitizer; dental caries prophylaxis* [potassium nitrate; sodium monofluorophosphate]

Sensorcaine injection ℞ *local anesthetic* [bupivacaine HCl]

Sensorcaine Spinal spinal injection ℞ *anesthetic; obstetric nerve block* [bupivacaine HCl; dextrose]

Sensorcaine with Epinephrine 1:200,000 injection ℞ *local anesthetic* [bupivacaine HCl; epinephrine]

Sensorcaine with Epinephrine injection ℞ *injectable local anesthetic* [bupivacaine HCl; epinephrine]

sepazonium chloride USAN, INN *topical anti-infective*

seperidol HCl USAN *antipsychotic* [also: clofluperol]

Sepo throat lozenges OTC *oral anesthetic; demulcent* [benzocaine; sugar]

Sepp Antiseptic tincture applicators (discontinued 1991) OTC *broad-spectrum antimicrobial* [iodine]

seproxetine HCl USAN *antidepressant*

Septa ointment OTC *topical antibiotic* [polymyxin B sulfate; neomycin sulfate; bacitracin]

Septi-Soft solution ℞ *antiseptic; disinfectant* [triclosan]

Septisol foam ℞ *bacteriostatic skin cleanser* [hexachlorophene; alcohol]

Septisol solution ℞ *antiseptic; disinfectant* [triclosan]

septomonab [see: nebacumab]

Septopal polymethyl methacrylate (PMMA) beads on surgical wire *(orphan: osteomyelitis)* [gentamicin]

Septra DS double strength tablets ℞ *anti-infective; antibacterial* [trimethoprim; sulfamethoxazole]

Septra tablets, oral suspension, IV infusion ℞ *anti-infective; antibacterial* [trimethoprim; sulfamethoxazole]

Sequels (trademarked form) *sustained-release capsules*

sequifenadine INN

seractide INN *adrenocorticotropic hormone* [also: seractide acetate]

seractide acetate USAN *adrenocorticotropic hormone* [also: seractide]

Ser-A-Gen tablets ℞ *antihypertensive* [hydrochlorothiazide; reserpine; hydralazine HCl]

Seralazide tablets (discontinued 1992) ℞ *antihypertensive* [hydrochlorothiazide; reserpine; hydralazine HCl]

Ser-Ap-Es tablets ℞ *antihypertensive* [hydrochlorothiazide; reserpine; hydralazine HCl]

Serax capsules, tablets ℞ *anxiolytic* [oxazepam]

serazapine HCl USAN *anxiolytic*

Sereine solution OTC *contact lens cleaning and soaking solution*

Sereine solution OTC *contact lens wetting/soaking solution*

Serentil tablets, oral concentrate, IM injection ℞ *antipsychotic* [mesoridazine besylate]

Serevent ℞ *investigational beta agonist for bronchial asthma and bronchospasm* [salmeterol]

serfibrate INN

sergolexole INN *antimigraine* [also: sergolexole maleate]

sergolexole maleate USAN *antimigraine* [also: sergolexole]

serine (L-serine) USAN, USP, INN *nonessential amino acid; symbols: Ser, S*

L-serine diazoacetate [see: azaserine]

sermetacin USAN, INN *anti-inflammatory*

sermorelin INN, BAN *growth hormone deficiency diagnosis and treatment* [also: sermorelin acetate]

sermorelin acetate USAN *diagnostic aid; (orphan: growth hormone deficiency; anovulation; AIDS-related weight loss)* [also: sermorelin]

Seromycin Pulvules (capsules) ℞ *tuberculostatic* [cycloserine]

Serophene tablets ℞ *ovulation stimulant* [clomiphene citrate]

Seroxat (European name for U.S. product Paxil)

Serpalan tablets ℞ *antihypertensive; antipsychotic* [reserpine]

Serpasil tablets (discontinued 1992) ℞ *antihypertensive; antipsychotic* [reserpine]

Serpasil-Apresoline #1; Serpasil-Apresoline #2 tablets (discontinued 1992) ℞ *antihypertensive* [reserpine; hydralazine HCl]

Serpasil-Esidrix #1; Serpasil-Esidrex #2 tablets (discontinued 1992) ℞ *antihypertensive* [reserpine; hydrochlorothiazide]

Serpazide tablets ℞ *antihypertensive* [hydrochlorothiazide; reserpine; hydralazine HCl]

serrapeptase INN

Serratia marcescens extract (polyribosomes) *(orphan: primary brain malignancies)*
sertaconazole INN
sertindole INN *investigational schizophrenia treatment*
sertraline INN, BAN *antidepressant* [also: sertraline HCl]
sertraline HCl USAN *antidepressant* [also: sertraline]
serum albumin (SA) [see: albumin, human]
serum albumin, iodinated (^{125}I) human [see: albumin, iodinated I 125 serum]
serum albumin, iodinated (^{131}I) human [see: albumin, iodinated I 131 serum]
serum fibrinogen (SF) [see: fibrinogen, human]
serum globulin (SG) [see: globulin, immune]
serum gonadotrophin [see: gonadotrophin, serum]
serum gonadotropin [see: gonadotrophin, serum]
serum prothrombin conversion accelerator (SPCA) factor [see: factor VII]
Serutan powder, granules OTC *bulk laxative* [psyllium]
sesame oil NF *solvent; oleaginous vehicle*
Sesame Street Complete chewable tablets OTC *vitamin/mineral/calcium/iron supplement* [multiple vitamins and minerals; calcium; iron; folic acid; biotin]
Sesame Street Plus Iron chewable tablets OTC *vitamin/iron supplement* [multiple vitamins; iron; folic acid]
Sesame Street Vitamins and Minerals (name changed to Sesame Street Complete in 1993)
Sesame Street Vitamins chewable tablets (discontinued 1993) OTC *vitamin supplement* [multiple vitamins; folic acid]

Sesame Street with Extra C chewable tablets OTC *vitamin supplement* [multiple vitamins; folic acid]
setastine INN
setazindol INN
setiptiline INN
setoperone USAN, INN *antipsychotic*
Seudotabs tablets OTC *nasal decongestant* [pseudoephedrine HCl]
sevitropium mesilate INN
sevoflurane USAN, INN *inhalation anesthetic*
sevopramide INN
sezolamide HCl USAN *carbonic anhydrase inhibitor*
SF (serum fibrinogen) [see: fibrinogen, human]
SFC lotion OTC *cleanser* [stearyl alcohol]
sfericase INN
SG (serum globulin) [see: globulin, immune]
SG (soluble gelatin) [see: gelatin]
shark liver oil *emollient/protectant*
Sheik Elite condom OTC *spermicidal/barrier contraceptive* [nonoxynol 9]
shellac NF *tablet coating agent*
Shepard's Cream Lotion; Shepard's Skin Cream OTC *moisturizer; emollient*
Shepard's Moisturizing Soap bar (discontinued 1992) OTC *therapeutic skin cleanser*
Shohl solution, modified (sodium citrate & citric acid) *urinary alkalizer; compounding agent*
short chain fatty acids *(orphan: left-sided ulcerative colitis)*
Shur-Clens solution OTC *wound cleanser* [poloxamer 188]
Shur-Seal Gel vaginal jelly OTC *spermicidal contraceptive* [nonoxynol 9]
siagoside INN
Sibelium *(orphan: alternating hemiplegia)* [flunarizine]
Siblin granules OTC *bulk laxative* [blond psyllium seed coatings]

sibutramine INN, BAN *anorexic; antidepressant* [also: sibutramine HCl]
sibutramine HCl USAN *anorexic; antidepressant* [also: sibutramine]
siccanin INN
Sickledex tube test ℞ *in vitro diagnostic aid for hemoglobin S (sickle cell)*
Sigtab tablets OTC *vitamin supplement* [multiple vitamins; folic acid]
siguazodan INN, BAN
SilaClean solution OTC *contact lens cleaning solution*
silafilcon A USAN *hydrophilic contact lens material*
silafocon A USAN *hydrophobic contact lens material*
Silain tablets (discontinued 1991) OTC *antiflatulent* [simethicone]
Silain-Gel gel (discontinued 1991) OTC *antacid; antiflatulent* [aluminum hydroxide; magnesium hydroxide; simethicone]
silandrone USAN, INN *androgen*
Silexin syrup OTC *antitussive; expectorant* [dextromethorphan hydrobromide; guaifenesin]
Silexin tablets OTC *antitussive; oral anesthetic* [dextromethorphan hydrobromide; benzocaine]
silibinin INN
silica, dental-type NF *pharmaceutic aid*
silica gel [now: silicon dioxide]
siliceous earth, purified NF *filtering medium*
silicic acid, magnesium salt [see: magnesium trisilicate]
silicon *element (Si)*
silicon dioxide NF *dispersing and suspending agent*
silicon dioxide, colloidal NF *suspending agent; tablet and capsule diluent*
silicone
Silicone No. 2 ointment OTC *skin protectant* [silicone in petrolatum; hydrophobic starch derivative]
silicristin INN
silidianin INN

silodrate USAN *antacid* [also: simaldrate]
Silphen Cough syrup OTC *antihistamine; antitussive* [diphenhydramine HCl; alcohol]
Silvadene cream ℞ *broad-spectrum bactericidal for adjunctive burn treatment* [silver sulfadiazine]
silver *element (Ag)*
silver nitrate USP *ophthalmic neonatal anti-infective; strong caustic*
silver nitrate, toughened USP *caustic*
silver protein, mild NF *ophthalmic antiseptic; ophthalmic surgical aid*
silver sulfadiazine (SSD) USAN, USP *bactericidal; adjunct to burn therapy*
Simaal Gel; Simaal Gel 2 liquid OTC *antacid; antiflatulent* [aluminum hydroxide; magnesium hydroxide; simethicone]
Simaal; Simaal 2 gel OTC *antacid; antiflatulent* [aluminum hydroxide; magnesium hydroxide; simethicone]
simaldrate INN *antacid* [also: silodrate]
simethicone USAN, USP *antiflatulent*
simetride INN
simfibrate INN
Similac; Similac PM 60/40; Similac with Iron liquid OTC *total or supplementary infant feeding* [whey protein formula]
simple syrup [see: syrup]
Simplet tablets OTC *decongestant; antihistamine; analgesic* [pseudoephedrine HCl; chlorpheniramine maleate; acetaminophen]
Simron Plus capsules OTC *vitamin/iron supplement* [multiple vitamins; ferrous gluconate; folic acid]
Simron soft gelatin capsules OTC *hematinic* [ferrous gluconate]
simtrazene USAN, INN *antineoplastic*
simvastatin USAN, INN, BAN *antihyperlipidemic*
Sinapils tablets OTC *decongestant; antihistamine; analgesic* [phenylpropa-

nolamine HCl; chlorpheniramine maleate; acetaminophen; caffeine]

Sinarest, 12 Hour nasal spray OTC *nasal decongestant* [oxymetazoline HCl]

Sinarest No Drowsiness tablets OTC *decongestant; analgesic* [pseudoephedrine HCl; acetaminophen]

Sinarest tablets OTC *decongestant; antihistamine; analgesic* [phenylpropanolamine HCl; chlorpheniramine maleate; acetaminophen]

sincalide USAN, INN *choleretic*

Sine-Aid caplets, tablets OTC *decongestant; analgesic* [pseudoephedrine HCl; acetaminophen]

sinefungin USAN, INN *antifungal*

Sinemet 10/100; Sinemet 25/100; Sinemet 25/250 tablets ℞ *antiparkinsonian* [carbidopa; levodopa]

Sinemet CR sustained-release tablets ℞ *antiparkinsonian* [carbidopa; levodopa]

Sine-Off Allergy/Sinus caplets OTC *decongestant; antihistamine; analgesic* [pseudoephedrine HCl; chlorpheniramine maleate; acetaminophen]

Sine-Off No Drowsiness Formula caplets OTC *decongestant; analgesic* [pseudoephedrine HCl; acetaminophen]

Sine-Off Sinus Medicine tablets OTC *decongestant; antihistamine; analgesic* [phenylpropanolamine HCl; chlorpheniramine maleate; aspirin]

Sinequan capsules, oral concentrate ℞ *anxiolytic; antidepressant* [doxepin HCl]

Sinex Long-Acting nasal spray OTC *nasal decongestant* [oxymetazoline HCl]

Sinex nasal spray OTC *nasal decongestant* [phenylephrine HCl]

single-chain antigen-binding proteins (SCA proteins) *investigational class of antineoplastics*

Singlet Tablets for Adults OTC *decongestant; antihistamine; analgesic* [pseudoephedrine HCl; chlorpheniramine maleate; acetaminophen]

Sinografin intracavitary instillation ℞ *radiopaque agent* [diatrizoate meglumine; iodipamide meglumine]

sintropium bromide INN

Sinubid sustained-release tablets ℞ *decongestant; antihistamine; analgesic* [phenylpropanolamine HCl; phenyltoloxamine citrate; acetaminophen]

Sinufed Timecelles (sustained-release capsules) ℞ *decongestant; expectorant* [pseudoephedrine HCl; guaifenesin]

Sinulin tablets OTC *decongestant; antihistamine; analgesic* [phenylpropanolamine HCl; chlorpheniramine maleate; acetaminophen]

Sinumist-SR sustained-release Capsulets (capsule-shaped tablet) ℞ *expectorant* [guaifenesin]

Sinupan controlled-release capsules ℞ *decongestant; expectorant* [phenylephrine HCl; guaifenesin]

Sinus Relief tablets OTC *decongestant; analgesic* [pseudoephedrine HCl; acetaminophen]

Sinusol-B subcu or IM injection ℞ *anthistamine; anaphylaxis* [brompheniramine maleate]

SinuStat capsules OTC *decongestant* [pseudoephedrine HCl]

Sinustop Pro capsules OTC *nasal decongestant* [pseudoephedrine HCl]

Sinutab, Allergy Formula sustained-release tablets (discontinued 1992) OTC *decongestant; antihistamine* [pseudoephedrine sulfate; dexbrompheniramine maleate]

Sinutab caplets, tablets OTC *decongestant; antihistamine; analgesic* [pseudoephedrine HCl; chlorpheniramine maleate; acetaminophen]

Sinutab Without Drowsiness tablets, caplets OTC *decongestant; analgesic* [pseudoephedrine HCl; acetaminophen]

Sinutrex tablets OTC *analgesic; decongestant; antihistamine* [acetaminophen; chlorpheniramine maleate; pseudoephedrine HCl]

SinuVent long-acting tablets ℞ *decongestant; expectorant* [phenylpropanolamine; guaifenesin]

SIS solution (discontinued 1991) OTC *ocular presurgical germicidal cleanser*

sisomicin USAN, INN *antibacterial* [also: sissomicin]

sisomicin sulfate USAN, USP *antibacterial*

sissomicin BAN *antibacterial* [also: sisomicin]

sitalidone INN

sitofibrate INN

sitogluside USAN, INN *antiprostatic hypertrophy*

sitosterols NF

Sitzmarks capsules ℞ *GI contrast radiopaque agent* [radiopaque polyvinyl chloride]

sizofiran INN

SK (streptokinase) [q.v.]

Skeeter Stik liquid OTC *topical local anesthetic; counterirritant; antifungal* [lidocaine; phenol; isopropyl alcohol]

Skelaxin tablets ℞ *skeletal muscle relaxant* [metaxalone]

Skelex capsules (discontinued 1991) ℞ *skeletal muscle relaxant; analgesic* [chlorzoxazone; acetaminophen]

SKF 105657 *investigational treatment for benign prostatic hyperplasia*

SK&F 110679 (*orphan: growth failure due to lack of endogenous growth hormone*)

skin respiratory factor (SRF) *claimed to promote wound healing*

Skin Shield liquid OTC *skin protectant; topical local anesthetic* [dyclonine HCl; benzethonium chloride]

SK-Quinidine Sulfate tablets (discontinued 1991) ℞ *antiarrhythmic* [quinidine sulfate]

SL (sodium lactate) [q.v.]

SLC solution (discontinued 1992) OTC *contact lens cleaning solution*

Sleep-Eze 3 tablets OTC *antihistaminic sleep aid* [diphenhydramine HCl]

Sleepinal capsules OTC *antihistaminic sleep aid* [diphenhydramine HCl]

Slim-Mint gum OTC *decrease taste perception of sweetness* [benzocaine]

Sloan's Liniment (discontinued 1992) OTC *counterirritant* [methyl salicylate; oil of camphor; capsicum oleoresin; turpentine oil; oil of pine]

Slo-bid Gyrocaps (extended-release capsules) ℞ *antiasthmatic; bronchodilator* [theophylline]

Slocaps (trademarked form) *sustained-release capsules*

Slo-Niacin controlled-release tablets OTC *nutritional supplement* [niacin]

Slo-phyllin GG capsules, syrup ℞ *antiasthmatic; bronchodilator; expectorant* [theophylline; guaifenesin]

Slo-phyllin tablets, syrup, Gyrocaps (extended-release capsules) ℞ *antiasthmatic; bronchodilator* [theophylline]

Slo-Salt slow-release tablets (discontinued 1993) OTC *sodium chloride replacement; dehydration preventative* [sodium chloride]

Slo-Salt-K slow-release tablets OTC *sodium chloride/potassium replacement; dehydration preventative* [sodium chloride; potassium chloride]

Slow Fe slow-release tablets OTC *hematinic* [ferrous sulfate, dried]

Slow-K controlled-release tablets ℞ *potassium supplement* [potassium chloride]

Slow-Mag delayed-release enteric-coated tablets OTC *magnesium supplement* [magnesium chloride]

Slow-Mag delayed-release tablets OTC *magnesium supplement* [magnesium chloride]

Slow-Mag tablets OTC *magnesium supplement* [magnesium chloride]

SLT hair lotion OTC *antiseborrheic; antipsoriatic; keratolytic; antiseptic* [coal tar; salicylic acid; lactic acid; benzalkonium chloride; alcohol]

Slyn-LL sustained-release capsules (discontinued 1993) ℞ *anorexiant* [phendimetrazine tartrate]

SMA Iron Fortified; SMA Lo-Iron; SMA with Whey liquid OTC *total or supplementary infant feeding* [whey protein formula]

smallpox vaccine USP *active immunizing agent*

SMF (streptozocin, mitomycin, fluorouracil) *chemotherapy protocol*

SMX; SMZ (sulfamethoxazole) [q.v.]

SN (streptonigrin) [q.v.]

snakebite antivenin [see: antivenin, Crotalidae & Micrurus fulvius]

Snaplets-D granules OTC *pediatric decongestant and antihistamine* [phenylpropanolamine HCl; chlorpheniramine maleate]

Snaplets-DM granules OTC *pediatric decongestant and antitussive* [phenylpropanolamine HCl; dextromethorphan hydrobromide]

Snaplets-EX granules OTC *pediatric decongestant and expectorant* [phenylpropanolamine HCl; guaifenesin]

Snaplets-Multi granules OTC *pediatric decongestant, antihistamine and antitussive* [phenylpropanolamine HCl; chlorpheniramine maleate; dextromethorphan hydrobromide]

SnapTabs (trademarked form) *scored tablets*

Sno Strips ophthalmic strips OTC *Schirmer tear flow test*

Soaclens solution OTC *contact lens wetting/soaking solution*

Soakare solution (discontinued 1992) OTC *contact lens storage/soaking solution*

soap, green USP *detergent*

SOD (superoxide dismutase) [see: orgotein]

soda lime NF *carbon dioxide absorbent*

Soda Mint tablets OTC *antacid* [sodium bicarbonate]

sodium *element (Na)*

sodium acetate USP *dialysis aid; electrolyte replenisher; pH buffer*

sodium acetate trihydrate [see: sodium acetate]

sodium acetrizoate INN [also: acetrizoate sodium]

sodium acetylsalicylate *analgesic*

sodium acid phosphate *urinary acidifier*

sodium acid pyrophosphate *urinary acidifier*

sodium alginate NF *suspending agent*

sodium amidotrizoate INN *radiopaque medium* [also: diatrizoate sodium; sodium diatrizoate]

sodium aminobenzoate [see: aminobenzoate sodium]

sodium amylopectin sulfate [see: sodium amylosulfate]

sodium amylosulfate USAN *enzyme inhibitor*

sodium anoxynaphthonate BAN *blood volume and cardiac output test* [also: anazolene sodium]

sodium antimony gluconate [see: sodium stibogluconate]

sodium antimonylgluconate BAN

sodium apolate INN, BAN *anticoagulant* [also: lyapolate sodium]

sodium arsenate, exsiccated NF

sodium arsenate As 74 USAN *radioactive agent*

sodium ascorbate USP, INN *vitamin C; antiscorbutic*

sodium aurothiomalate INN *antirheumatic* [also: gold sodium thiomalate]

sodium aurotiosulfate INN [also: gold sodium thiosulfate]

sodium azodisalicylate [now: olsalazine sodium]

sodium benzoate USAN, NF *antihyperammonemic; antifungal agent; preservative*

sodium benzyl penicillin [see: penicillin G sodium]
sodium bicarbonate USP *electrolyte replenisher; systemic alkalizer; antacid*
sodium biphosphate *urinary acidifier; pH buffer*
sodium bisulfite NF *antioxidant*
sodium bitionolate INN *topical antiinfective* [also: bithionolate sodium]
sodium borate NF *alkalizing agent; antipruritic*
sodium borocaptate (^{10}B) INN *antineoplastic; radioactive agent* [also: borocaptate sodium B 10]
sodium cacodylate NF
sodium calcium edetate INN *metal-chelating agent* [also: edetate calcium disodium; sodium calciumedetate]
sodium calciumedetate BAN *metal-chelating agent* [also: edetate calcium disodium; sodium calcium edetate]
sodium caprylate *antifungal*
sodium carbonate NF *alkalizing agent*
sodium chloride (NaCl) USP *ophthalmic hypertonic; electrolyte replacement; abortifacient*
0.45% sodium chloride (½ normal saline; ½ NS) *electrolyte replacement*
0.9% sodium chloride (normal saline; NS) *electrolyte replacement* [also: saline solution]
sodium chloride, compound solution of INN *fluid and electrolyte replenisher* [also: Ringer's injection]
sodium chloride Na 22 USAN *radioactive agent*
sodium chromate (^{51}Cr) INN *blood volume test; radioactive agent* [also: sodium chromate Cr 51]
sodium chromate Cr 51 USAN *blood volume test; radioactive agent* [also: sodium chromate (^{51}Cr)]
sodium citrate USP *systemic alkalizer; pH buffer*
sodium colistin methanesulfonate [see: colistimethate sodium]
sodium cyclamate NF, INN

sodium cyclohexanesulfamate [see: sodium cyclamate]
sodium dehydroacetate NF *antimicrobial preservative*
sodium dehydrocholate INN [also: dehydrocholate sodium]
sodium denyl [see: phenytoin sodium]
sodium diatrizoate BAN *radiopaque medium* [also: diatrizoate sodium; sodium amidotrizoate]
sodium dibunate INN, BAN
sodium dicloroacetate (*orphan: lactic acidosis; homozygous hypercholesterolemia*)
sodium diethyldithiocarbamate [see: ditiocarb sodium]
sodium diiodomethanesulfonate [see: dimethiodal sodium]
sodium dioctyl sulfosuccinate INN *stool softener; surfactant* [also: docusate sodium]
sodium diphenylhydantoin [see: phenytoin sodium]
sodium diprotrizoate INN, BAN [also: diprotrizoate sodium]
Sodium Edecrin powder for IV injection ℞ *loop diuretic* [ethacrynate sodium]
sodium edetate [see: edetate sodium]
sodium etasulfate INN *detergent* [also: sodium ethasulfate]
sodium ethasulfate USAN *detergent* [also: sodium etasulfate]
sodium feredetate INN [also: sodium ironedetate]
sodium fluoride USP *dental caries preventative*
sodium fluoride F 18 USP
sodium fluoride & phosphoric acid USP *dental caries prophylactic*
sodium formaldehyde sulfoxylate NF *preservative*
sodium gammahydroxyburate [see: sodium oxybate]
sodium gentisate INN
sodium glucaspaldrate INN, BAN

sodium gluconate USP *electrolyte replenisher*
sodium glucosulfone USP
sodium glutamate
sodium glycerophosphate NF
sodium glycocholate [see: bile salts]
sodium gualenate INN
sodium hyaluronate [see: hyaluronate sodium]
sodium hydroxide NF *alkalizing agent*
sodium hydroxybenzenesulfonate [see: phenolsulphonate sodium]
sodium 4-hydroxybutyrate [see: sodium oxybate]
sodium hypochlorite USP *disinfectant; bleach; used for utensils and equipment*
sodium hypochlorite, diluted NF
sodium hypophosphite NF
sodium iodide USP *dietary iodine supplement*
sodium iodide (^{125}I) INN *thyroid function test; radioactive agent* [also: sodium iodide I 125]
sodium iodide I 123 USP *thyroid function test; radioactive agent*
sodium iodide I 125 USAN, USP *thyroid function test; radioactive agent* [also: sodium iodide (^{125}I)]
sodium iodide I 131 USAN, USP *antineoplastic; thyroid function test; radioactive agent*
sodium iodohippurate (^{131}I) INN *renal function test; radioactive agent* [also: iodohippurate sodium I 131]
sodium iodomethanesulfonate [see: methiodal sodium]
sodium iopodate INN, BAN *radiopaque medium* [also: ipodate sodium]
sodium iotalamate (^{125}I) INN *radioactive agent* [also: iothalamate sodium I 125]
sodium iotalamate (^{131}I) INN *radioactive agent* [also: iothalamate sodium I 131]
sodium iothalamate BAN *radiopaque medium* [also: iothalamate sodium]
sodium ioxaglate BAN *radiopaque medium* [also: ioxaglate sodium]
sodium ironedetate BAN [also: sodium feredetate]
sodium lactate (SL) USP *electrolyte replenisher*
sodium lactate, compound solution of INN *electrolyte and fluid replenisher; systemic alkalizer* [also: Ringer's injection, lactated]
sodium lauryl sulfate NF *surfactant/wetting agent*
sodium lignosulfonate [see: polignate sodium]
sodium metabisulfite NF *antioxidant*
sodium metrizoate INN *radiopaque medium* [also: metrizoate sodium]
sodium monododecyl sulfate [see: sodium lauryl sulfate]
sodium monofluorophosphate USP *dental caries prophylactic*
sodium morrhuate INN *sclerosing agent* [also: morrhuate sodium]
sodium nitrite USP *antidote to cyanide poisoning*
sodium nitroferricyanide [see: sodium nitroprusside]
sodium nitroferricyanide dihydrate [see: sodium nitroprusside]
sodium nitroprusside USP *emergency antihypertensive*
sodium noramidopyrine methanesulfonate [see: dipyrone]
sodium oxybate USAN *adjunct to anesthesia; (orphan status withdrawn 1993)*
sodium oxychlorosene [see: oxychlorosene sodium]
sodium paratoluenesulfan chloramide [see: chloramine-T]
Sodium P.A.S. tablets ℞ *tuberculostatic* [aminosalicylate sodium]
sodium penicillin G [see: penicillin G sodium]
sodium pentosan polysulphate *(orphan: interstitial cystitis)*
sodium perborate *topical antiseptic/germicidal*

sodium perborate monohydrate USAN

sodium pertechnetate Tc 99m USAN, USP *radioactive agent*

sodium phenolate [see: phenolate sodium]

sodium phenylacetate USAN *antihyperammonemic*

sodium phosphate (^{32}P) INN *antineoplastic; antipolycythemic; neoplasm test* [also: sodium phosphate P 32]

sodium phosphate, dibasic USP *saline laxative; phosphorus replacement; pH buffer*

sodium phosphate, monobasic USP *phosphorus replacement; pH buffer*

sodium phosphate P 32 USAN, USP *antineoplastic; antipolycythemic; neoplasm test* [also: sodium phosphate (^{32}P)]

sodium picofosfate INN

sodium picosulfate INN

sodium polyphosphate USAN *pharmaceutic aid*

sodium polystyrene sulfonate USP *potassium-removing ion-exchange resin*

sodium propionate NF *preservative; antifungal*

sodium propionate hydrate [see: sodium propionate]

sodium 2-propylvalerate [see: valproate sodium]

sodium psylliate NF

sodium pyrophosphate USAN *pharmaceutic aid*

sodium radiochromate [see: sodium chromate Cr 51]

sodium rhodanate [see: thiocyanate sodium]

sodium salicylate (SS) USP *analgesic; antipyretic; anti-inflammatory; antirheumatic*

sodium starch glycolate NF *tablet excipient*

sodium stearate NF *emulsifying and stiffening agent*

sodium stearyl fumarate NF *tablet and capsule lubricant*

sodium stibocaptate INN [also: stibocaptate]

sodium stibogluconate INN, BAN *investigational anti-infective for leishmaniasis*

Sodium Sulamyd eye drops, ophthalmic ointment ℞ *ophthalmic bacteriostatic* [sodium sulfacetamide]

sodium sulfacetamide [see: sulfacetamide sodium]

sodium sulfate USP *calcium regulator*

sodium sulfate S 35 USAN *radioactive agent*

sodium sulfocyanate [see: thiocyanate sodium]

sodium taurocholate [see: bile salts]

sodium tetradecyl (STD) sulfate INN *sclerosing agent; (orphan: bleeding esophageal varices)*

sodium thiomalate, gold [see: gold sodium thiomalate]

sodium thiosalicylate *analgesic; antipyretic; anti-inflammatory; antirheumatic*

sodium thiosulfate USP *antidote to cyanide poisoning; antiseptic; antifungal*

sodium thiosulfate, gold [see: gold sodium thiosulfate]

sodium timerfonate INN *topical anti-infective* [also: thimerfonate sodium]

sodium trimetaphosphate USAN *pharmaceutic aid*

sodium tyropanoate INN *cholecystographic radiopaque medium* [also: tyropanoate sodium]

sodium valproate [see: valproate sodium]

Sodol Compound tablets ℞ *skeletal muscle relaxant; analgesic* [carisoprodol; aspirin]

Sodol tablets ℞ *skeletal muscle relaxant* [carisoprodol]

sofalcone INN

Sofarin tablets ℞ *anticoagulant* [warfarin sodium]

Sofenol 5 lotion OTC *moisturizer; emollient*

Sof/Pro-Clean; Sof/Pro-Clean (s.a.) solution OTC *contact lens surfactant cleaning solution*

Soft Mate Comfort Drops (discontinued 1991) OTC *contact lens rewetting solution*

Soft Mate Comfort Drops for Sensitive Eyes OTC *contact lens rewetting solution*

Soft Mate Consept solution OTC *two-step contact lens disinfectant*

Soft Mate Daily Cleaning for Sensitive Eyes solution OTC *contact lens surfactant cleaning solution*

Soft Mate Enzyme Plus Cleaner tablets OTC *contact lens enzymatic cleaner* [subtilisin]

Soft Mate Hands Off Daily Cleaner solution (discontinued 1992) OTC *contact lens surfactant cleaning solution*

Soft Mate Lens Drops (discontinued 1992) OTC *contact lens rewetting solution*

Soft Mate Protein Remover solution OTC *contact lens surfactant cleaning solution*

Soft Mate Saline for Sensitive Eyes solution (discontinued 1992) OTC *contact lens rinsing and storage solution* [preserved saline solution]

Soft Mate Saline Preservative-Free solution (discontinued 1992) OTC *contact lens rinsing and storage solution* [saline solution]

Soft Mate solution OTC *contact lens disinfectant*

Soft 'N Soothe cream (discontinued 1991) OTC *topical local anesthetic* [benzocaine; menthol]

Soft Rinse 135; Soft Rinse 250 tablets OTC *contact lens rinsing and storage solution* [sodium chloride for normal saline solution]

Softabs (trademarked form) *chewable tablets*

softgels (dosage form) *soft gelatin capsules*

Soft-Stress capsules OTC *vitamin/mineral/calcium/iron supplement* [multiple vitamins & minerals; calcium; iron; folic acid; biotin]

sol particle immunoassay (SPIA) *detects hCG in urine for pregnancy testing*

solapsone BAN [also: solasulfone]

Solaquin cream OTC *hyperpigmentation bleaching agent; sunscreen* [hydroquinone; ethyl dihydroxypropyl PABA; dioxybenzone; oxybenzone]

Solaquin Forte cream, gel ℞ *hyperpigmentation bleaching agent; sunscreen* [hydroquinone; ethyl dihydroxypropyl PABA; dioxybenzone; oxybenzone]

Solarcaine aerosol spray, lotion OTC *topical local anesthetic; antiseptic* [benzocaine; triclosan]

Solarcaine cream OTC *topical local anesthetic* [lidocaine]

solasulfone INN [also: solapsone]

Solatene capsules ℞ *to reduce photosensitivity reaction* [beta-carotene]

Solfoton tablets, capsules ℞ *barbiturate sedative; hypnotic* [phenobarbital]

Solganal IM injection ℞ *antirheumatic* [aurothioglucose]

solpecainol INN

Soltice Quick-Rub OTC *counterirritant* [methyl salicylate; camphor; menthol; eucalyptus oil]

soluble ferric pyrophosphate [see: ferric pyrophosphate, soluble]

soluble gelatin (SG) [see: gelatin]

Soluble T4 (*orphan: AIDS*) [CD4, human truncated 369 AA polypeptide]

Solu-Cortef powder for IV or IM injection ℞ *glucocorticoids* [hydrocortisone sodium succinate]

Solu-Medrol powder for IV or IM injection ℞ *glucocorticoids* [methylprednisolone sodium succinate]

Solumol OTC *ointment base*

Solurex intra-articular, intralesional, soft tissue, or IM injection ℞ *gluco-*

corticoids [dexamethasone sodium phosphate]

Solurex LA intralesional, intra-articular, soft tissue, or IM injection ℞ *glucocorticoids* [dexamethasone acetate]

Soluspan (trademarked form) *injectable suspension*

Soluvite C.T. chewable tablets ℞ *pediatric vitamin supplement and dental caries preventative* [multiple vitamins; fluoride; folic acid]

Soluvite-F drops ℞ *pediatric vitamin supplement and dental caries preventative* [vitamins A, C & D; fluoride]

Solvent-G OTC *liquid base*

Solvet (trademarked form) *soluble tablet*

solypertine INN *antiadrenergic* [also: solypertine tartrate]

solypertine tartrate USAN *antiadrenergic* [also: solypertine]

Soma Compound tablets ℞ *skeletal muscle relaxant; analgesic* [carisoprodol; aspirin]

Soma Compound with Codeine tablets ℞ *skeletal muscle relaxant; analgesic* [carisoprodol; aspirin; codeine phosphate]

Soma tablets ℞ *skeletal muscle relaxant* [carisoprodol]

Somagard (*orphan: central precocious puberty*) [deslorelin]

somagrebove USAN *veterinary galactopoietic agent*

somalapor USAN, INN, BAN *porcine growth hormone*

somantadine INN *antiviral* [also: somantadine HCl]

somantadine HCl USAN *antiviral* [also: somantadine]

somatorelin INN *growth hormone-releasing factor (GH-RF)*

somatostatin (SS) INN, BAN *growth hormone-release inhibiting factor; (orphan: GI fistulas)*

somatotropin, human [see: somatropin]

Somatrel ℞ (*orphan: diagnostic aid for pituitary release of growth hormone*) [NG-29 (drug code–generic name not yet approved)]

somatrem USAN, INN, BAN *human growth hormone; (orphan: Turner syndrome; growth delay)*

somatropin USAN, INN, BAN *human growth hormone; (orphan: Turner syndrome; growth delay; severe burns; anovulation)*

somavubove USAN, INN *veterinary galactopoietic agent*

somenopor USAN *porcine growth hormone*

sometribove USAN, INN, BAN *veterinary growth stimulant*

sometripor USAN, INN, BAN *veterinary growth stimulant*

somfasepor USAN *veterinary growth stimulant*

somidobove USAN, INN *synthetic bovine growth hormone*

Sominex 2 Pain Relief tablets OTC *antihistaminic sleep aid; analgesic* [diphenhydramine HCl; acetaminophen]

Sominex 2 tablets OTC *antihistaminic sleep aid* [diphenhydramine HCl]

Sominex caplets OTC *antihistaminic sleep aid* [diphenhydramine HCl]

Soothaderm lotion OTC *topical anesthetic; topical antihistamine; emollient* [pyrilamine maleate; benzocaine; zinc oxide]

Soothe eye drops OTC *topical ocular decongestant* [tetrahydrozoline HCl]

Soothers Throat Drops lozenges OTC *topical antipruritic/counterirritant; mild local anesthetic* [menthol]

sopecainol [see: solpecainol]

sopitazine INN

Soprodol tablets ℞ *skeletal muscle relaxant* [carisoprodol]

sopromidine INN

Sopronol ointment, powder (discontinued 1991) OTC *topical antifungal*

[sodium propionate; sodium caprylate; zinc caprylate]
Sopronol solution (discontinued 1991) OTC *topical antifungal* [sodium propionate; sodium caprylate]
Soquette solution (discontinued 1992) OTC *contact lens storage/soaking solution*
soquinolol INN
sorbic acid NF *antimicrobial agent; preservative*
Sorbi-Care solution OTC *contact lens aid*
sorbide nitrate [see: isosorbide dinitrate]
sorbimacrogol laurate 300 [see: polysorbate 20]
sorbimacrogol oleate 300 [see: polysorbate 80]
sorbimacrogol palmitate 300 [see: polysorbate 40]
sorbimacrogol stearate [see: polysorbate 60]
sorbimacrogol tristearate 300 [see: polysorbate 65]
sorbinicate INN
sorbinil USAN, INN, BAN *aldose reductase enzyme inhibitor*
sorbitan laurate INN *surfactant* [also: sorbitan monolaurate]
sorbitan monolaurate USAN, NF *surfactant* [also: sorbitan laurate]
sorbitan monooleate USAN, NF *surfactant* [also: sorbitan oleate]
sorbitan monopalmitate USAN, NF *surfactant* [also: sorbitan palmitate]
sorbitan monostearate USAN, NF *surfactant* [also: sorbitan stearate]
sorbitan oleate INN *surfactant* [also: sorbitan monooleate]
sorbitan palmitate INN *surfactant* [also: sorbitan monopalmitate]
sorbitan sesquioleate USAN, INN *surfactant*
sorbitan stearate INN *surfactant* [also: sorbitan monostearate]
sorbitan trioleate USAN, INN *surfactant*

sorbitan tristearate USAN, INN *surfactant*
Sorbi-Tinic-F liquid ℞ *vitamin supplement* [multiple B vitamins; lysine HCl]
sorbitol NF *flavoring agent; tablet excipient; urologic irrigant*
sorbitol (solution) USP *flavoring agent; tablet excipient*
Sorbitrate SA sustained-action tablets ℞ *antianginal* [isosorbide dinitrate]
Sorbitrate tablets, sublingual tablets, chewable tablets ℞ *antianginal* [isosorbide dinitrate]
Sorbsan pads, wound packing ℞ *wound dressing* [calcium alginate fiber]
Soretts lozenges (discontinued 1993) OTC *topical anesthetic; antipruritic/counterirritant* [benzocaine; menthol]
sornidipine INN
SOSS-10 eye drops ℞ *ophthalmic bacteriostatic* [sodium sulfacetamide]
sotalol INN, BAN *antiadrenergic (β-receptor)* [also: sotalol HCl]
sotalol HCl USAN *antiadrenergic (β-receptor); (orphan: ventricular arrhythmias)* [also: sotalol]
soterenol INN *adrenergic; bronchodilator* [also: soterenol HCl]
soterenol HCl USAN *adrenergic; bronchodilator* [also: soterenol]
Sotradecol IV injection, Dosette (unit-of-use injection) ℞ *sclerosing agent; (orphan: bleeding esophageal varices)* [sodium tetradecyl sulfate]
Soyacal 10%; Soyacal 20% IV infusion (discontinued 1991) ℞ *nutritional therapy* [intravenous fat emulsion]
Soyalac; I-Soyalac liquid OTC *hypoallergenic infant food* [soybean protein formula]
soybean oil USP *pharmaceutic necessity*
S/P Cola oral liquid ℞ *glucose tolerance test beverage* [glucose]
spaglumic acid INN

Span C tablets OTC *dietary supplement* [vitamin C; citrus & rose hips bioflavonoids]

Spancap No. 1 sustained-release capsules ℞ *CNS stimulant* [dextroamphetamine sulfate]

Spancaps (dosage form) *timed-release capsules*

Span-FF controlled-release capsules OTC *hematinic* [ferrous fumarate]

Spansule (trademarked form) *sustained-release capsules*

sparfloxacin USAN, INN, BAN *antibacterial*

sparfosate sodium USAN *antineoplastic* [also: sparfosic acid]

sparfosic acid INN *antineoplastic* [also: sparfosate sodium]

Sparine tablets, Tubex (cartridge-needle unit for IM injection) ℞ *antipsychotic* [promazine HCl]

Sparkles effervescent granules OTC *antacid; aid in endoscopic examination* [sodium bicarbonate]

sparsomycin USAN, INN *antineoplastic*

sparteine INN *oxytocic* [also: sparteine sulfate]

sparteine sulfate USAN *oxytocic* [also: sparteine]

Spartus + Iron tablets (discontinued 1991) OTC *antianemic* [ferrous fumarate; multiple vitamins]

Spaslin tablets (discontinued 1991) ℞ *anticholinergic; sedative* [atropine sulfate; scopolamine hydrobromide; hyoscyamine hydrobromide; phenobarbital]

Spasmoject IM injection ℞ *gastrointestinal antispasmodic* [dicyclomine HCl]

Spasmolin capsules, tablets ℞ *anticholinergic; sedative* [atropine sulfate; scopolamine hydrobromide; hyoscyamine hydrobromide; phenobarbital]

Spasmophen tablets, elixir ℞ *anticholinergic; sedative* [atropine sulfate; scopolamine hydrobromide; hyoscyamine hydrobromide; phenobarbital]

Spasquid elixir ℞ *anticholinergic; sedative* [atropine sulfate; scopolamine hydrobromide; hyoscyamine hydrobromide; phenobarbital]

Spastosed chewable tablets OTC *antacid* [calcium carbonate; magnesium carbonate]

SPCA (serum prothrombin conversion accelerator) factor [see: factor VII]

spearmint NF

spearmint oil NF

Specifid ℞ *investigational antineoplastic for non-Hodgkin's and AIDS-related lymphomas* [monoclonal antibodies]

Spec-T Sore Throat Anesthetic lozenges OTC *topical anesthetic* [benzocaine]

Spec-T Sore Throat/Decongestant lozenges OTC *decongestant; topical anesthetic* [phenylpropanolamine HCl; phenylephrine HCl; benzocaine]

Spec-T; Spec-T Sore Throat/Cough Suppressant lozenges OTC *topical anesthetic; antitussive* [benzocaine; dextromethorphan hydrobromide]

Spectazole cream ℞ *topical antifungal* [econazole nitrate]

spectinomycin INN *bactericidal antibiotic* [also: spectinomycin HCl]

spectinomycin HCl USAN, USP *bactericidal antibiotic* [also: spectinomycin]

Spectrobid film-coated tablets, powder for oral suspension ℞ *penicillin-type antibiotic* [bacampicillin HCl]

Spectrocin ointment (discontinued 1991) OTC *topical antibiotic* [neomycin sulfate; gramicidin]

Spectrocin Plus ointment OTC *topical antibiotic; local anesthetic* [neomycin sulfate; polymyxin B sulfate; bacitracin; lidocaine]

Spectro-Jel liquid OTC *soap-free cleanser*

spenbolic [see: methandriol]
spermaceti, synthetic [see: cetyl esters wax]
Sperti ointment (discontinued 1992) OTC *treatment for burns, scalds, cuts and abrasions* [live yeast cell derivative; shark liver oil; phenylmercuric nitrate]
Spherulin intradermal injection ℞ *diagnostic aid for coccidioidomycosis* [coccidioidin]
SPIA (sol particle immunoassay) [q.v.]
spiclamine INN
spiclomazine INN
spider bite antivenin [see: antivenin (Latrodectus mactans)]
Spider-Man Children's Chewable Vitamin Tablets (discontinued 1993) OTC *vitamin supplement* [multiple vitamins; folic acid]
spiperone USAN, INN *antipsychotic*
spiradoline INN *analgesic* [also: spiradoline mesylate]
spiradoline mesylate USAN *analgesic* [also: spiradoline]
spiramide INN
spiramycin USAN, INN, BAN *antibacterial; (orphan: cryptosporidiosis in immunodeficiency)*
spirapril INN, BAN *angiotensin-converting enzyme (ACE) inhibitor* [also: spirapril HCl]
spirapril HCl USAN *angiotensin-converting enzyme (ACE) inhibitor* [also: spirapril]
spiraprilat USAN, INN *angiotensin-converting enzyme (ACE) inhibitor*
spirazine INN
spirazine HCl [see: spirazine]
spirendolol INN
spirgetine INN
spirilene INN, BAN
spirit of nitrous ether [see: ethyl nitrite]
spirobarbital sodium
spirofylline INN

spirogermanium INN, BAN *antineoplastic* [also: spirogermanium HCl]
spirogermanium HCl USAN *antineoplastic* [also: spirogermanium]
spirohydantoin mustard [now: spiromustine]
spiromustine USAN, INN *antineoplastic*
Spironazide tablets ℞ *diuretic* [spironolactone; hydrochlorothiazide]
spironolactone USP, INN *potassium-sparing diuretic; aldosterone antagonist*
spiroplatin USAN, INN, BAN *antineoplastic*
spirorenone INN
spirotriazine HCl [see: spirazine]
spiroxamide [see: spiroxatrine]
spiroxasone USAN, INN *diuretic*
spiroxatrine INN
spiroxepin INN
Spirozide tablets ℞ *diuretic* [spironolactone; hydrochlorothiazide]
spizofurone INN
SPL (staphage lysate) [q.v.]
SPL-Serologic types I and III solution for subcu injection, nasal aerosol, nasal drop, oral, or topical irrigation ℞ *staphylococcal or polymicrobial vaccine* [staphage lysate (Staphylococcus aureus; Staphylococcus bacteriophage plaque-forming units)]
Sporanox capsules ℞ *systemic antifungal* [itraconazole]
Sports Spray OTC *counterirritant; topical antiseptic* [methyl salicylate; menthol; camphor; alcohol]
Sportscreme cream OTC *topical analgesic* [trolamine salicylate]
Sportscreme gel OTC *topical analgesic; counterirritant* [trolamine; menthol]
Sprinkle Caps (trademarked form) *powder*
SPS oral suspension ℞ *potassium-removing agent for hyperkalemia* [sodium polystyrene sulfonate]

S-P-T "liquid" capsules ℞ *hypothyroidism; thyroid cancer* [pork thyroid, desiccated]

squalane NF *oleaginous vehicle*

⁸⁵Sr [see: strontium chloride Sr 85]

⁸⁵Sr [see: strontium nitrate Sr 85]

⁸⁵Sr [see: strontium Sr 85]

SRC Expectorant liquid ℞ *decongestant; antitussive; expectorant* [pseudoephedrine HCl; hydrocodone bitartrate; guaifenesin; alcohol]

SRF (skin respiratory factor) [q.v.]

SS (saline solution)

SS (sodium salicylate) [q.v.]

SS (somatostatin) [q.v.]

SSD (silver sulfadiazine) [q.v.]

SSD; SSD AF cream ℞ *broad-spectrum bactericidal for adjunctive burn treatment* [silver sulfadiazine]

SSKI oral solution ℞ *expectorant* [potassium iodide]

S.T. 37 solution OTC *topical antiseptic* [hexylresorcinol]

S-T Cort cream (discontinued 1992) ℞ *topical corticosteroid* [hydrocortisone]

S-T Cort lotion ℞ *topical corticosteroid* [hydrocortisone]

S-T Forte liquid ℞ *antitussive; antihistamine* [hydrocodone bitartrate; chlorpheniramine maleate]

S-T Forte syrup (discontinued 1992) ℞ *antitussive; decongestant; antihistamine; expectorant* [hydrocodone bitartrate; phenylephrine HCl; phenylpropanolamine HCl; pheniramine maleate; guaifenesin]

St. Joseph Anti-Diarrheal for Children liquid OTC *antidiarrheal; GI adsorbent* [attapulgite]

St. Joseph Aspirin-Free Cold Tablets for Children chewable tablets OTC *decongestant* [phenylpropanolamine HCl; acetaminophen]

St. Joseph Aspirin-Free Fever Reducer for Children liquid OTC *analgesic; antipyretic* [acetaminophen]

St. Joseph Aspirin-Free for Children chewable tablets OTC *analgesic; antipyretic* [acetaminophen]

St. Joseph Aspirin-Free Infant Drops OTC *analgesic; antipyretic* [acetaminophen]

St. Joseph Complete Nighttime Cold Relief, Aspirin Free liquid OTC *pediatric decongestant, antihistamine, antitussive and analgesic* [pseudoephedrine HCl; chlorpheniramine maleate; dextromethorphan hydrobromide; acetaminophen]

St. Joseph Cough Suppressant syrup OTC *antitussive* [dextromethorphan hydrobromide]

St. Joseph Measured Dose solution (discontinued 1992) OTC *nasal decongestant* [phenylephrine HCl]

ST1-RTA immunotoxin (SR 44163) (*orphan: graft vs. host disease; B-chronic lymphocytic leukemia*)

stable factor [see: factor VII]

Stadol IV or IM injection ℞ *narcotic agonist-antagonist analgesic* [butorphanol tartrate]

Stadol NS nasal spray ℞ *narcotic agonist-antagonist analgesic* [butorphanol tartrate]

Stagesic capsules ℞ *narcotic analgesic* [hydrocodone bitartrate; acetaminophen]

Stahist sustained-release tablets ℞ *decongestant; antihistamine; bronchodilator; GI antispasmodic* [phenylpropanolamine HCl; phenylephrine HCl; chlorpheniramine maleate; hyoscyamine sulfate; atropine sulfate; scopolamine hydrobromide]

stallimycin INN *antibacterial* [also: stallimycin HCl]

stallimycin HCl USAN *antibacterial* [also: stallimycin]

Stamoist E sustained-release tablets ℞ *decongestant; expectorant* [pseudoephedrine HCl; guaifenesin]

Stamoist LA film-coated sustained-release tablets ℞ *decongestant; expecto-*

rant [phenylpropanolamine HCl; guaifenesin]

standard VAC *chemotherapy protocol* [see: VAC standard (under VAC)]

stannous chloride USAN *pharmaceutic aid*

stannous fluoride USP *dental caries prophylactic*

stannous pyrophosphate USAN *skeletal imaging aid*

stannous sulfur colloid USAN *bone, liver and spleen imaging aid*

stanolone BAN [also: androstanolone]

stanozolol USAN, USP, INN, BAN *androgen; anabolic steroid*

staphage lysate (SPL) *active bacterin for staphylococcal infections*

Staphage Lysate (SPL) liquid (nasal, oral, injection, topical) ℞ *staphylococcal vaccine (bacterin); immunomodulator* [bacterial antigen made from Staphylococcus]

Staphcillin powder for IV or IM injection ℞ *bactericidal antibiotic (penicillinase-resistant penicillin)* [methicillin sodium]

starch NF *dusting powder; pharmaceutic aid*

starch, pregelatinized NF *tablet excipient*

starch, topical USP *dusting powder*

starch carboxymethyl ether, sodium salt [see: sodium starch glycolate]

starch glycerite NF

starch 2-hydroxyethyl ether [see: hetastarch; pentastarch]

Star-Optic Eye Wash OTC *extraocular irrigating solution* [balanced saline solution]

Star-Otic ear drops OTC *antibacterial/antifungal* [acetic acid; aluminum acetate; boric acid]

Staticin topical solution ℞ *topical antibiotic for acne vulgaris* [erythromycin]

Statobex tablets (discontinued 1991) ℞ *anorexiant* [phendimetrazine tartrate]

statolon USAN *antiviral* [also: vistatolon]

Stat-One gel OTC *topical antiseptic* [hydrogen peroxide]

Stat-One gel OTC *topical antiseptic* [isopropyl alcohol]

Stat-Pak (trademarked form) *single-use dispensing package*

Statrol Drop-Tainers (eye drops), ophthalmic ointment ℞ *ophthalmic antibiotic* [polymyxin B sulfate; neomycin sulfate]

Statuss Expectorant liquid ℞ *decongestant; antihistamine; antitussive; expectorant* [phenylephrine HCl; chlorpheniramine maleate; codeine phosphate; ammonium chloride; alcohol]

Statuss Green liquid ℞ *decongestant; antihistamine; antitussive; expectorant* [phenylpropanolamine HCl; phenylephrine HCl; pheniramine maleate; pyrilamine maleate; hydrocodone bitartrate; alcohol]

stavudine USAN, INN *antiviral*

Stay Trim gum, mints OTC *diet aid* [phenylpropanolamine HCl]

Stay-Brite solution OTC *contact lens cleaning solution*

Stay-Wet 3 solution OTC *contact lens wetting/rewetting solution*

STD (sodium tetradecyl sulfate) [q.v.]

STEAM (streptonigrin, thioguanine, cyclophosphamide, actinomycin, mitomycin) *chemotherapy protocol*

stearethate 40 [see: polyoxyl 40 stearate]

stearic acid NF *emulsion adjunct; tablet and capsule lubricant*

stearyl alcohol NF *emulsion adjunct*

stearyl dimethyl benzyl ammonium chloride

stearylsulfamide INN

steffimycin USAN, INN *antibacterial; antiviral*

Stelazine film-coated tablets, oral concentrate, IM injection ℞ *antianxiety; antipsychotic* [trifluoperazine HCl]
stem cell factor *investigational agent for blood-related disorders*
stenbolone INN *anabolic* [also: stenbolone acetate]
stenbolone acetate USAN *anabolic* [also: stenbolone]
Step 2 creme rinse OTC *for use following a pediculicide shampoo to remove lice eggs from hair*
stepronin INN
Sterapred; Sterapred DS tablets, Unipak (dispensing pack) ℞ *glucocorticoids* [prednisone]
stercuronium iodide INN
Sterecyt *(orphan: malignant non-Hodgkin's lymphomas)* [prednimustine]
Steri-Dose (trademarked delivery system) *unit-dose disposable syringes*
Sterile Lens Lubricant solution OTC *contact lens rewetting solution*
SteriNail solution OTC *topical antifungal* [undecylenic acid; tolnaftate]
Steri-Vial (trademarked form) *ampules*
stevaladil INN
stibamine glucoside INN, BAN
stibocaptate BAN [also: sodium stibocaptate]
stibophen NF
stibosamine INN
stilbamidine isethionate [see: stilbamidine isetionate]
stilbamidine isetionate INN
stilbazium iodide USAN, INN *anthelmintic*
stilbestroform [see: diethylstilbestrol]
stilbestrol [see: diethylstilbestrol]
stilbestronate [see: diethylstilbestrol dipropionate]
stilboestroform [see: diethylstilbestrol]
stilboestrol BAN *estrogen* [also: diethylstilbestrol]
stilboestrol DP [see: diethylstilbestrol dipropionate]

Stilnoct; Stilnox (European name for U.S. product Ambien)
stilonium iodide USAN, INN *antispasmodic*
Stilphostrol tablets, IV injection ℞ *antineoplastic for prostatic carcinoma* [diethylstilbestrol diphosphate]
stilronate [see: diethylstilbestrol dipropionate]
Stimurub cream (discontinued 1992) OTC *topical anesthetic; counterirritant; anti-inflammatory; vasodilator* [methyl salicylate; menthol; capsicum oleoresin]
Sting Relief lotion, concentrate (discontinued 1991) OTC *topical anesthetic; antipruritic; antibacterial* [benzocaine; camphor; chloroxylenol]
Sting-Eze concentrate OTC *topical antihistamine; antipruritic; anesthetic; bacteriostatic* [diphenhydramine HCl; camphor; phenol; benzocaine; eucalyptol]
Stinging Insect Antigen No. 108 subcu or IM injection ℞ *venom sensitivity testing; allergenic hyposensitization therapy* [bumblebee, honeybee, wasp, hornet & yellow jacket antigen extracts]
Sting-Kill swabs OTC *topical local anesthetic* [benzocaine; menthol]
stirimazole INN, BAN
stiripentol USAN, INN *anticonvulsant*
stirocainide INN
stirofos USAN *veterinary insecticide*
Stoko Gard cream OTC *topical protection from the effects of poison ivy*
Stop gel ℞ *topical dental caries preventative* [stannous fluoride]
storax USP
Storzolamide tablets (discontinued 1992) ℞ *anticonvulsant; diuretic* [acetazolamide]
Stoxil eye drops, ophthalmic ointment (discontinued 1992) ℞ *ophthalmic antiviral* [idoxuridine]
Sto-Zyme enteric-coated tablets (discontinued 1991) OTC *digestive en-*

zymes [pancreatic enzyme concentrate; ox bile extract; cellulase; pepsin]

StrapKap (dosage form) *piggyback vials*

Streptase powder for IV or intracoronary infusion ℞ *thrombolytic enzyme; lysis of thrombi; catheter clearance* [streptokinase]

streptococcus immune globulin, group B *(orphan: neonatal group B streptococcal infection)*

streptodornase (SD) INN, BAN

streptoduocin USP

streptokinase (SK) INN *thrombolytic enzyme*

streptomycin INN, BAN *aminoglycoside bactericidal antibiotic; primary tuberculostatic* [also: streptomycin sulfate]

streptomycin sulfate USP *aminoglycoside bactericidal antibiotic; primary tuberculostatic* [also: streptomycin]

Streptonase-B tube test ℞ *in vitro diagnostic test for streptococci*

streptoniazid INN *antibacterial* [also: streptonicozid]

streptonicozid USAN *antibacterial* [also: streptoniazid]

streptonigrin (SN) USAN *antineoplastic* [also: rufocromomycin]

Strepto-Sec slide test (discontinued 1991) ℞ *in vitro diagnostic test for streptococci*

streptovarycin INN

streptozocin USAN, INN *antineoplastic*

streptozotocin [see: streptozocin]

Stress 600 with Zinc tablets OTC *vitamin/zinc supplement* [multiple vitamins; zinc; folic acid; biotin]

Stress "1000" tablets (discontinued 1993) OTC *vitamin supplement* [multiple vitamins]

Stress B Complex tablets OTC *vitamin/mineral supplement* [multiple vitamins; zinc; folic acid; biotin]

Stress B Complex with Vitamin C timed-release tablets OTC *vitamin/mineral supplement* [multiple B vitamins; vitamin C; zinc]

Stress B with C tablets OTC *vitamin supplement* [multiple B vitamins; vitamin C; folic acid; biotin]

Stress Formula 500 Plus Iron tablets (discontinued 1993) OTC *vitamin/iron supplement* [multiple B vitamins; vitamins C & E; ferrous fumarate; folic acid; biotin]

Stress Formula 500 Plus Zinc tablets (discontinued 1993) OTC *vitamin/zinc supplement* [multiple vitamins; zinc; folic acid; biotin]

Stress Formula 500 tablets (discontinued 1993) OTC *vitamin supplement* [multiple vitamins; biotin; folic acid]

Stress Formula 600 plus Iron tablets OTC *antianemic* [ferrous fumarate, dried; vitamins E & C; multiple B vitamins; folic acid]

Stress Formula 600 plus Zinc tablets (discontinued 1993) OTC *vitamin/mineral supplement* [multiple vitamins & minerals; folic acid; biotin]

Stress Formula 600 tablets OTC *vitamin supplement* [multiple vitamins; folic acid; biotin]

Stress Formula "605" tablets OTC *vitamin supplement* [multiple vitamins; folic acid; biotin]

Stress Formula "605" with Iron tablets OTC *vitamin/iron supplement* [multiple vitamins; iron; biotin; folic acid]

Stress Formula "605" with Zinc tablets OTC *vitamin/mineral supplement* [multiple vitamins & minerals; biotin; folic acid]

Stress Formula Vitamin capsules, tablets OTC *vitamin supplement* [multiple vitamins; folic acid; biotin]

Stress Formula with Iron film-coated tablets OTC *vitamin/iron supplement* [multiple B vitamins; vitamins C & E; ferrous fumarate; folic acid; biotin]

Stress-Bee capsules (discontinued 1991) OTC *vitamin supplement* [multiple B vitamins; vitamin C]
Stresscaps capsules OTC *vitamin supplement* [multiple B vitamins; vitamin C]
StressForm "605" with Iron tablets OTC *hematinic* [multiple vitamins; iron; folic acid; biotin]
Stresstabs 600 Advanced Formula (name changed to Stresstabs Advanced Formula in 1991)
Stresstabs 600 with Iron tablets OTC *antianemic* [ferrous fumarate, dried; vitamins E & C; multiple B vitamins; folic acid]
Stresstabs Advanced Formula tablets OTC *vitamin supplement* [multiple vitamins; folic acid; biotin]
Stresstabs + Iron film-coated tablets OTC *vitamin/iron supplement* [multiple B vitamins; vitamins C & E; ferrous fumarate; folic acid; biotin]
Stresstabs + Zinc film-coated tablets OTC *vitamin/mineral supplement* [multiple vitamins & minerals; biotin; folic acid]
Stresstein powder OTC *oral nutritional supplement for metabolic stress, trauma and sepsis*
Stri-Dex pads OTC *topical acne cleanser* [salicylic acid; alcohol; citric acid]
strinoline INN
strong ammonia solution [see: ammonia solution, strong]
Strong Iodine solution, tincture ℞ *thyroid-blocking therapy; topical antimicrobial* [iodine; potassium iodide]
stronger rose water [see: rose water, stronger]
strontium *element (Sr)*
strontium chloride Sr 85 USAN *radioactive agent*
strontium nitrate Sr 85 USAN *radioactive agent*
strontium salicylate NF
strontium Sr 85 USP

Strovite Plus caplets ℞ *geriatric vitamin/mineral therapy* [multiple vitamins & minerals; folic acid; biotin]
Strovite tablets ℞ *vitamin supplement* [multiple B vitamins; vitamin C; folic acid]
strychnine NF
strychnine glycerophosphate NF
strychnine nitrate NF
strychnine phosphate NF
strychnine sulfate NF
strychnine valerate NF
Stuart Formula tablets OTC *vitamin/mineral/iron supplement* [multiple vitamins & minerals; iron; folic acid]
Stuart Prenatal tablets OTC *vitamin/calcium/iron supplement* [multiple vitamins; calcium; iron; folic acid]
Stuartinic film-coated tablets OTC *hematinic* [ferrous fumarate; multiple B vitamins; ascorbic acid; sodium ascorbate]
Stuartnatal 1 + 1 tablets ℞ *vitamin/calcium/iron supplement* [multiple vitamins; calcium; iron; folic acid]
stugeron [see: cinnarizine]
stutgin [see: cinnarizine]
Stye ophthalmic ointment OTC *stye treatment* [boric acid; yellow mercuric oxide; zinc sulfate]
Stypto-Caine solution OTC *to stop bleeding of minor cuts* [aluminum chloride; tetracaine HCl; oxyquinoline sulfate]
styramate INN
styronate resins
subathizone INN
subendazole INN
Sublimaze IV or IM injection ℞ *narcotic analgesic; anesthetic* [fentanyl citrate]
sublimed sulfur [see: sulfur, sublimed]
Sublingual B Total drops OTC *vitamin supplement* [multiple B vitamins; vitamin C]
substance F [see: demecolcine]
Suby's G solution; Suby's solution G (citric acid, magnesium oxide,

sodium carbonate) *urologic irrigant to dissolve phosphatic calculi*

succimer USAN, INN, BAN *metal-chelating agent; (orphan: lead and mercury poisoning; cysteine kidney stones)*

succinchlorimide NF

succinylcholine chloride USP *neuromuscular blocker; muscle relaxant* [also: suxamethonium chloride]

succinyldapsone [see: succisulfone]

succinylsulfathiazole USP

succisulfone INN

Succus Cineraria Maritima ophthalmic ointment ℞ *treatment for optic opacity caused by cataract* [aqueous/glycerin solution of senecio compositae, hamamelis water & boric acid]

suclofenide INN, BAN

Sucostrin IV or IM injection ℞ *neuromuscular blocker* [succinylcholine chloride]

sucralfate USAN, INN, BAN *treatment of gastric ulcers; (orphan: oral ulcerations)*

sucralose BAN

sucralox INN, BAN

Sucrets Children's Formula Sore Throat; Vapor Lemon Sucrets lozenges OTC *topical antipruritic/counterirritant; mild local anesthetic* [dyclonine HCl]

Sucrets Cough Control lozenge OTC *antitussive* [dextromethorphan hydrobromide]

Sucrets lozenges, mouthwash/gargle, throat spray OTC *topical antipruritic/counterirritant; mild local anesthetic* [dyclonine HCl]

Sucrets Sore Throat Lozenges OTC *oral antiseptic* [hexylresorcinol]

sucrose NF *flavoring agent; tablet excipient*

sucrose octaacetate NF *alcohol denaturant*

sucrosofate potassium USAN *antiulcerative*

Sudafed, Children's liquid OTC *nasal decongestant* [pseudoephedrine HCl]

Sudafed 12 Hour Caplets extended-release tablets OTC *nasal decongestant* [pseudoephedrine HCl]

Sudafed 12 Hour timed-release capsules (discontinued 1991) OTC *nasal decongestant* [pseudoephedrine HCl]

Sudafed Cough syrup OTC *decongestant; antitussive; expectorant* [pseudoephedrine HCl; dextromethorphan hydrobromide; guaifenesin; alcohol]

Sudafed Plus tablets, liquid OTC *decongestant; antihistamine* [pseudoephedrine HCl; chlorpheniramine maleate]

Sudafed Severe Cold Formula tablets OTC *decongestant; antitussive; analgesic; antipyretic* [pseudoephedrine HCl; dextromethorphan hydrobromide; acetaminophen]

Sudafed Sinus tablets, caplets OTC *decongestant; analgesic* [pseudoephedrine HCl; acetaminophen]

Sudafed tablets OTC *nasal decongestant* [pseudoephedrine HCl]

sudexanox INN

sudismase INN

sudoxicam USAN, INN *anti-inflammatory*

Sudrin tablets (discontinued 1992) OTC *nasal decongestant* [pseudoephedrine HCl]

Sufenta IV injection ℞ *narcotic analgesic; anesthetic* [sufentanil citrate]

sufentanil USAN, INN, BAN *analgesic*

sufentanil citrate USAN *narcotic analgesic*

sufosfamide INN

sufotidine USAN, INN, BAN *antagonist to histamine H_2 receptors*

sugar, compressible NF *flavoring agent; tablet excipient*

sugar, confectioner's NF *flavoring agent; tablet excipient*

sugar, invert (50% dextrose & 50% fructose) USP *fluid and nutrient replenisher; caloric replacement*
sugar spheres NF *solid carrier vehicle*
Sulamyd [see: Sodium Sulamyd]
sulazepam USAN, INN *minor tranquilizer*
sulbactam INN, BAN
sulbactam benzathine USAN *β-lactamase inhibitor; penicillin/cephalosporin synergist*
sulbactam pivoxil USAN *β-lactamase inhibitor; penicillin/cephalosporin synergist* [also: pivsulbactam]
sulbactam sodium USAN, USP *β-lactamase inhibitor; penicillin/cephalosporin synergist*
sulbenicillin INN
sulbenox USAN, INN *veterinary growth stimulant*
sulbentine INN
sulbutiamine INN
sulclamide INN
sulconazole INN, BAN *antifungal* [also: sulconazole nitrate]
sulconazole nitrate USAN, USP *antifungal* [also: sulconazole]
Suldiazo film-coated tablets ℞ *urinary anti-infective; urinary analgesic* [sulfisoxazole; phenazopyridine HCl]
sulergine [see: disulergine]
Sulf-10 eye drops ℞ *ophthalmic bacteriostatic* [sodium sulfacetamide]
sulfabenz USAN, INN *antibacterial; coccidiostat for poultry*
sulfabenzamide USAN, USP, INN *bacteriostatic antibiotic*
sulfabromomethazine sodium NF
sulfacarbamide INN [also: sulphaurea]
sulfacecole INN
sulfacetamide USP, INN *bacteriostatic antibiotic*
sulfacetamide sodium USP *bacteriostatic antibiotic*
Sulfacet-R lotion ℞ *topical acne treatment* [sulfacetamide sodium; precipitated sulfur]

sulfachlorpyridazine INN
sulfachrysoidine INN
sulfacitine INN *antibacterial* [also: sulfacytine]
sulfaclomide INN
sulfaclorazole INN
sulfaclozine INN
sulfacombin [see: sulfadiazine]
sulfacytine USAN *broad-spectrum bacteriostatic* [also: sulfacitine]
sulfadiasulfone sodium INN *antibacterial; leprostatic* [also: acetosulfone sodium]
sulfadiazine USP, INN *broad-spectrum bacteriostatic*
sulfadiazine silver [see: silver sulfadiazine]
sulfadiazine sodium USP, INN *antibacterial* [also: sulphadiazine sodium]
sulfadicramide INN
sulfadicrolamide [see: sulfadicramide]
sulfadimethoxine NF [also: sulphadimethoxine]
sulfadimidine INN, BAN *antibacterial* [also: sulfamethazine]
sulfadoxine USAN, USP *bacteriostatic; antimalarial adjunct*
sulfaethidole NF, INN [also: sulphaethidole]
sulfafurazole INN *antibacterial* [also: sulfisoxazole; sulphafurazole]
sulfaguanidine NF, INN
sulfaguanole INN
Sulfa-Gyn vaginal cream (discontinued 1992) ℞ *bacteriostatic* [sulfathiazole; sulfacetamide; sulfabenzamide; urea]
Sulfair 15 eye drops (discontinued 1992) ℞ *ophthalmic bacteriostatic* [sodium sulfacetamide]
sulfaisodimidine [see: sulfisomidine]
Sulfalax Calcium capsules OTC *stool softener* [docusate calcium]
sulfalene USAN, INN *antibacterial* [also: sulfametopyrazine]
sulfaloxic acid INN [also: sulphaloxic acid]
sulfamazone INN

sulfamerazine USP, INN *broad-spectrum bacteriostatic*
sulfamerazine sodium NF, INN
sulfameter USAN *antibacterial* [also: sulfametoxydiazine; sulfamethoxydiazine]
sulfamethazine USP *broad-spectrum bacteriostatic* [also: sulfadimidine]
sulfamethizole USP, INN *antibacterial* [also: sulphamethizole]
Sulfamethoprim IV infusion ℞ *anti-infective; antibacterial* [trimethoprim; sulfamethoxazole]
sulfamethoxazole (SMX; SMZ) USAN, USP, INN *broad-spectrum bacteriostatic* [also: sulphamethoxazole]
sulfamethoxydiazine BAN *antibacterial* [also: sulfameter; sulfametoxydiazine]
sulfamethoxypyridazine USP, INN [also: sulphamethoxypyridazine]
sulfamethoxypyridazine acetyl
sulfametin [see: sulfameter]
sulfametomidine INN
sulfametopyrazine BAN *antibacterial* [also: sulfalene]
sulfametoxydiazine INN *antibacterial* [also: sulfameter; sulfamethoxydiazine]
sulfametrole INN, BAN
Sulfamide eye drop suspension ℞ *topical ophthalmic corticosteroidal anti-inflammatory; bacteriostatic* [prednisolone acetate; sodium sulfacetamide]
sulfamidothiodiazol [see: glybuzole]
sulfamonomethoxine USAN, INN, BAN *antibacterial*
sulfamoxole USAN, INN *antibacterial* [also: sulphamoxole]
***p*-sulfamoylbenzoic acid** [see: carzenide]
4′-sulfamoylsuccinanilic acid [see: sulfasuccinamide]
Sulfamylon cream, solution ℞ *broad-spectrum bacteriostatic; (orphan: meshed autograft loss in burns)* [mafenide acetate]

sulfanilamide NF, INN *bacteriostatic antibiotic*
sulfanilanilide [see: sulfabenz]
sulfanilate zinc USAN *antibacterial*
***N*-sulfanilylacetamide** [see: sulfacetamide]
***N*-sulfanilylacetamide monosodium salt monohydrate** [see: sulfacetamide sodium]
***N-p*-sulfanilylphenylglycine sodium** [see: acediasulfone sodium]
***N*-sulfanilylstearamide** [see: stearylsulfamide]
4′-sulfanilylsuccinanilic acid [see: succisulfone]
sulfanilylurea [see: sulfacarbamide]
sulfanitran USAN, INN, BAN *antibacterial; coccidiostat for poultry*
sulfaperin INN
sulfaphenazole INN [also: sulphaphenazole]
sulfaphthalylthiazol [see: phthalylsulfathiazole]
sulfaproxyline INN [also: sulphaproxyline]
sulfapyrazole INN, BAN *antibacterial* [also: sulfazamet]
sulfapyridine USP, INN *dermatitis herpetiformis suppressant (orphan)* [also: sulphapyridine]
sulfapyridine sodium NF
sulfaquinoxaline INN, BAN
sulfarsphenamine NF, INN
sulfasalazine USAN, USP, INN *broad-spectrum bacteriostatic*
sulfasomizole USAN, INN *antibacterial* [also: sulphasomizole]
sulfastearyl [see: stearylsulfamide]
sulfasuccinamide INN
sulfasymazine INN
sulfathiazole USP, INN *bacteriostatic antibiotic* [also: sulphathiazole]
sulfathiazole sodium NF
sulfathiocarbamide [see: sulfathiourea]
sulfathiourea INN
sulfatolamide INN

Sulfatrim; Sulfatrim D/S oral suspension, pediatric suspension, tablets ℞ *anti-infective; antibacterial* [sulfamethoxazole; trimethoprim]
Sulfa-Trip vaginal cream ℞ *bacteriostatic* [sulfathiazole; sulfacetamide; sulfabenzamide; urea]
sulfatroxazole INN
sulfatrozole INN
sulfazamet USAN *antibacterial* [also: sulfapyrazole]
sulfinalol INN *antihypertensive* [also: sulfinalol HCl]
sulfinalol HCl USAN *antihypertensive* [also: sulfinalol]
sulfinpyrazone USP, INN *uricosuric* [also: sulphinpyrazone]
sulfiram INN [also: monosulfiram]
sulfisomidine [also: sulphasomidine]
sulfisoxazole USP *broad-spectrum bacteriostatic* [also: sulfafurazole; sulphafurazole]
sulfisoxazole acetyl USP *broad-spectrum bacteriostatic*
sulfisoxazole diolamine USAN, USP *broad-spectrum bacteriostatic*
Sulfoam shampoo OTC *antiseborrheic; keratolytic* [salicylic acid]
sulfobenzylpenicillin [see: sulbenicillin]
sulfobromophthalein sodium USP *hepatic function test*
sulfobromphthalein sodium [see: sulfobromophthalein sodium]
sulfogaiacol INN *expectorant* [also: potassium guaiacolsulfonate]
Sulfoil liquid OTC *soap-free cleanser*
sulfomyxin USAN, INN *antibacterial* [also: sulphomyxin sodium]
sulfonal [see: sulfonmethane]
sulfonated hydrogenated castor oil [see: hydroxystearin sulfate]
sulfonethylmethane NF
sulfonmethane NF
sulfonterol INN *bronchodilator* [also: sulfonterol HCl]
sulfonterol HCl USAN *bronchodilator* [also: sulfonterol]

Sulforcin lotion OTC *topical acne treatment* [sulfur; resorcinol; alcohol]
sulforidazine INN
sulfosalicylic acid
sulfoxone sodium USP *antibacterial; leprostatic* [also: aldesulfone sodium]
Sulfoxyl Regular; Sulfoxyl Strong lotion ℞ *keratolytic for acne* [benzoyl peroxide; precipitated sulfur]
sulfur *element (S)* [see: sulfur, precipitated; sulfur, sublimed]
sulfur, precipitated USP *scabicide; topical antibacterial; topical exfoliant*
sulfur, sublimed USP *scabicide; topical antibacterial; topical exfoliant*
sulfur dioxide NF *antioxidant*
Sulfur Soap bar OTC *medicated cleanser for acne* [precipitated sulfur]
sulfurated lime solution [see: lime, sulfurated]
sulfurated potash [see: potash, sulfurated]
sulfuric acid NF *acidifying agent*
sulfuric acid, calcium salt [see: calcium sulfate]
sulfuric acid, copper salt pentahydrate [see: cupric sulfate]
sulfuric acid, disodium salt decahydrate [see: sodium sulfate]
sulfuric acid, magnesium salt [see: magnesium sulfate]
sulfuric acid, manganese salt [see: manganese sulfate]
sulfuric acid, zinc salt hydrate [see: zinc sulfate]
sulfurous acid, monosodium salt [see: sodium bisulfite]
sulglicotide INN [also: sulglycotide]
sulglycotide BAN [also: sulglicotide]
sulicrinat INN
sulindac USAN, USP, INN, BAN *antiarthritic; nonsteroidal anti-inflammatory drug (NSAID); analgesic*
sulisatin INN
sulisobenzone USAN, INN *ultraviolet screen*
sulmarin USAN, INN *hemostatic*
sulmazole INN

sulmepride INN
sulnidazole USAN, INN *antiprotozoal (Trichomonas)*
sulocarbilate INN
suloctidil USAN, INN, BAN *peripheral vasodilator*
sulodexide INN
sulofenur USAN, INN *antineoplastic*
sulosemide INN
sulotroban USAN, INN, BAN *treatment for glomerulonephritis*
suloxifen INN *bronchodilator* [also: suloxifen oxalate]
suloxifen oxalate USAN *bronchodilator* [also: suloxifen]
sulphabutin [see: busulfan]
sulphadiazine sodium BAN *antibacterial* [also: sulfadiazine sodium]
sulphadimethoxine BAN [also: sulfadimethoxine]
sulphaethidole BAN [also: sulfaethidole]
sulphafurazole BAN *antibacterial* [also: sulfisoxazole; sulfafurazole]
sulphaloxic acid BAN [also: sulfaloxic acid]
sulphamethizole BAN *antibacterial* [also: sulfamethizole]
sulphamethoxazole BAN *antibacterial* [also: sulfamethoxazole]
sulphamethoxypyridazine BAN [also: sulfamethoxypyridazine]
sulphamoxole BAN *antibacterial* [also: sulfamoxole]
sulphan blue BAN *lymphangiography aid* [also: isosulfan blue]
sulphaphenazole BAN [also: sulfaphenazole]
sulphaproxyline BAN [also: sulfaproxyline]
sulphapyridine BAN *dermatitis herpetiformis suppressant* [also: sulfapyridine]
sulphasomidine BAN [also: sulfisomidine]
sulphasomizole BAN *antibacterial* [also: sulfasomizole]
sulphathiazole BAN *antibacterial* [also: sulfathiazole]
sulphaurea BAN [also: sulfacarbamide]
sulphinpyrazone BAN *uricosuric* [also: sulfinpyrazone]
sulphocarbolate sodium [see: phenolsulphonate sodium]
Sulpho-Lac Acne Medication solution OTC *antibacterial; exfoliant* [sulfur; zinc sulfate]
Sulpho-Lac soap OTC *antibacterial; exfoliant* [sulfur]
sulphomyxin sodium BAN *antibacterial* [also: sulfomyxin]
sulphonal [see: sulfonmethane]
Sulphrin eye drop suspension ℞ *topical ophthalmic corticosteroidal anti-inflammatory; bacteriostatic* [prednisolone acetate; sodium sulfacetamide]
sulpiride USAN, INN *antidepressant*
Sulpred eye drop suspension ℞ *topical ophthalmic corticosteroidal anti-inflammatory; bacteriostatic* [prednisolone acetate; sodium sulfacetamide]
sulprosal INN
sulprostone USAN, INN *prostaglandin*
sultamicillin USAN, INN, BAN *antibacterial*
Sulten-10 eye drops (discontinued 1992) ℞ *ophthalmic bacteriostatic* [sodium sulfacetamide]
sulthiame USAN *anticonvulsant* [also: sultiame]
sultiame INN *anticonvulsant* [also: sulthiame]
sultopride INN
sultosilic acid INN
Sultrin Triple Sulfa vaginal tablets, vaginal cream ℞ *bacteriostatic* [sulfathiazole; sulfacetamide; sulfabenzamide; urea]
sultroponium INN
sulukast USAN, INN *antiasthmatic; leukotriene antagonist*
sulverapride INN

Sumacal powder OTC *carbohydrate caloric supplement* [glucose polymers]
sumacetamol INN, BAN
sumarotene USAN, INN *keratolytic*
sumatriptan INN, BAN *antimigraine* [also: sumatriptan succinate]
sumatriptan succinate USAN *antimigraine* [also: sumatriptan]
sumetizide INN
Summer's Eve Disposable Douche solution OTC *vaginal cleansing and deodorizing; acidity modifier* [sodium citrate; citric acid]
Summer's Eve Disposable Douche solution OTC *vaginal cleansing and deodorizing; acidity modifier* [vinegar (acetic acid)]
Summer's Eve Medicated Disposable Douche solution OTC *antiseptic/germicidal; vaginal cleansing and deodorizing* [povidone-iodine]
Summer's Eve Post-Menstrual Disposable Douche solution OTC *vaginal cleansing and deodorizing*
Summer's Eve vaginal suppositories (discontinued 1991) OTC *counterirritant* [potassium sorbate; sodium metabisulfite]
Sumycin '250'; Sumycin '500' capsules, tablets ℞ *broad-spectrum antibiotic* [tetracycline HCl]
Sumycin syrup ℞ *broad-spectrum antibiotic* [tetracycline HCl]
sunagrel INN
suncillin INN *antibacterial* [also: suncillin sodium]
suncillin sodium USAN *antibacterial* [also: suncillin]
Sunkist Children's Multivitamins chewable tablets OTC *dietary supplement* [multiple vitamins]
Sunkist Vitamin C chewable tablets, caplets OTC *vitamin supplement* [ascorbic acid]
Sunshine chewable tablets (discontinued 1992) OTC *dietary supplement* [multiple vitamins & minerals; iron; folic acid; biotin]

Supac tablets OTC *analgesic; antipyretic; anti-inflammatory* [acetaminophen; aspirin; caffeine; calcium gluconate]
Super CalciCaps M-Z tablets OTC *dietary supplement* [vitamins A & D; multiple minerals]
Super CalciCaps tablets OTC *dietary supplement* [dibasic calcium phosphate; calcium gluconate; calcium carbonate; vitamin D]
Super Calcium '1200' softgels OTC *dietary supplement* [calcium; vitamin D]
Super Citro Cee sustained-release tablets OTC *dietary supplement* [ascorbic acid; lemon & rose hips bioflavonoids; rutin]
Super Complex C-500 Caplets OTC *dietary supplement* [ascorbic acid; various bioflavonoids; citrus hesperidin; rutin]
Super D Perles (capsules) OTC *vitamin supplement* [vitamins A & D]
Super Hi Potency tablets OTC *vitamin/mineral supplement* [multiple vitamins & minerals]
Super Omega-3 soft capsules OTC *dietary supplement* [eicosapentaenoic acid; docosahexaenoic acid; alpha-linolenic acid]
Super Quints-50 tablets OTC *vitamin supplement* [multiple B vitamins; folic acid; biotin]
Super-1-Daily; Vegetarian Super-1-Daily cellulose-coated caplets OTC *vitamin/mineral supplement* [multiple vitamins & minerals; betaine HCl]
Super-75 cellulose-coated caplets OTC *vitamin/mineral supplement* [multiple vitamins & minerals; bioflavonoids; betaine HCl]
Superchar powder, liquid (discontinued 1991) OTC *adsorbent poisoning antidote* [activated charcoal]
SuperEPA 1200; SuperEPA 2000 softgels OTC *dietary supplement* [omega-3 fatty acids; vitamin E]

Superfed liquid OTC *decongestant* [pseudoephedrine HCl]
superoxide dismutase (SOD) [see: orgotein]
superoxide dismutase, recombinant human (SOD) (*orphan: prevent reperfusion injury to donor organ tissue; neonatal bronchopulmonary dysplasia*)
Superplex-T tablets OTC *vitamin supplement* [multiple B vitamins; vitamin C]
supidimide INN
Suplena liquid OTC *oral nutritional supplement for renal failure*
Suppap-120; Suppap-325; Suppap-650 suppositories OTC *analgesic; antipyretic* [acetaminophen]
Supprelin subcu injection ℞ *gonadotropin-releasing hormone for central precocious puberty (orphan)* [histrelin acetate]
Suppress lozenges OTC *antitussive* [dextromethorphan hydrobromide]
Supprettes (trademarked form) *suppositories*
Suprane liquid for vaporization ℞ *inhalation general anesthetic* [desflurane]
Suprax film-coated tablets, powder for oral suspension ℞ *cephalosporin-type antibiotic* [cefixime]
suproclone USAN, INN *sedative*
suprofen USAN, INN, BAN *ocular nonsteroidal anti-inflammatory drug (NSAID); antimiotic*
suramin sodium USP, BAN *investigational anti-infective for trypanosomiasis and onchocerciasis*
Surbex 750 with Iron Filmtabs (film-coated tablets) OTC *vitamin/iron supplement* [multiple B vitamins; ferrous sulfate; vitamins C & E; folic acid]
Surbex 750 with Zinc Filmtabs (film-coated tablets) OTC *vitamin/zinc supplement* [multiple vitamins; zinc sulfate; folic acid]

Surbex Filmtabs (film-coated tablets) OTC *vitamin supplement* [multiple B vitamins]
Surbex-T; Surbex with C Filmtabs (film-coated tablets) OTC *vitamin supplement* [multiple B vitamins; vitamin C]
Surbu-Gen-T film-coated tablets OTC *vitamin supplement* [multiple B vitamins; vitamin C]
SureCell Chlamydia Test kit OTC *in vitro diagnostic aid for Chlamydia trachomatis*
SureCell hCG-Urine Test kit ℞ *in vitro diagnostic aid for urine pregnancy test*
SureCell Herpes (HSV) Test kit OTC *in vitro diagnostic aid for herpes simplex virus in lesions*
SureCell Strep A Test kit ℞ *in vitro diagnostic aid for streptococci*
SureLac chewable tablets OTC *digestive aid for lactose intolerance* [lactase enzyme]
surface active extract of saline lavage of bovine lungs (*orphan: respiratory failure in premature infants*)
surfactant, human amniotic fluid derived (*orphan: neonatal respiratory distress syndrome*)
surfactant TA [see: beractant]
surfactant TA, modified bovine lung surfactant extract (*orphan: neonatal respiratory distress syndrome*) [see: beractant]
Surfadil cream, lotion (discontinued 1991) OTC *topical antihistamine* [diphenhydramine HCl; alcohol]
Surfak Liquigels (capsules) OTC *stool softener* [docusate calcium]
surfilcon A USAN *hydrophilic contact lens material*
Surfol Post-Immersion Bath Oil OTC *bath emollient*
surfomer USAN, INN *hypolipidemic*
Surgel vaginal gel OTC *lubricant for gynecologic procedures*
surgibone USAN *internal bone splint*

surgical catgut [see: suture, absorbable surgical]
surgical gut [see: suture, absorbable surgical]
Surgicel strips ℞ *topical hemostatic aid in surgical hemostasis* [oxidized cellulose]
Surgi-Sep scrub (discontinued 1991) OTC *broad-spectrum antimicrobial* [povidone-iodine]
suricainide INN *antiarrhythmic* [also: suricainide maleate]
suricainide maleate USAN, INN *antiarrhythmic* [also: suricainide]
suriclone INN, BAN
Surital IV ℞ *general anesthetic* [thiamylal sodium]
Surmontil capsules ℞ *tricyclic antidepressant* [trimipramine maleate]
suronacrine INN *cholinesterase inhibitor* [also: suronacrine maleate]
suronacrine maleate USAN *cholinesterase inhibitor* [also: suronacrine]
Survanta suspension for intratracheal instillation ℞ *pulmonary surfactant; (orphan: neonatal respiratory distress syndrome)* [beractant]
Susano tablets, elixir ℞ *anticholinergic; sedative* [phenobarbital; atropine sulfate; scopolamine hydrobromide; hyoscyamine hydrobromide]
Sus-Phrine subcu injection ℞ *bronchodilator for bronchial asthma, bronchospasm and COPD; vasopressor used in shock* [epinephrine]
Sust-A 10,000; Sust-A 25,000 sustained-release tablets OTC *vitamin supplement* [vitamin A palmitate]
Sustacal HC liquid OTC *high-calorie nutritional supplement*
Sustacal liquid, powder, pudding OTC *total enteral nutrition; nutritional supplement*
Sustacal with Fiber liquid OTC *nutritional supplement*
Sustagen powder OTC *nutritional supplement*

Sustaire timed-release tablets ℞ *bronchodilator* [theophylline]
sutilains USAN, USP, INN, BAN *topical proteolytic enzymes for necrotic tissue debridement*
sutoprofen [see: suprofen]
suture, absorbable surgical USP *surgical aid*
suture, nonabsorbable surgical USP *surgical aid*
suxamethone [see: succinylcholine chloride]
suxamethonium chloride INN, BAN *neuromuscular blocking agent* [also: succinylcholine chloride]
suxemerid INN *antitussive* [also: suxemerid sulfate]
suxemerid sulfate USAN *antitussive* [also: suxemerid]
suxethonium chloride INN
suxibuzone INN
sweet birch oil [see: methyl salicylate]
sweet orange peel tincture [see: orange peel tincture, sweet]
sweet spirit of nitre [see: ethyl nitrite]
Swim-Ear ear drops OTC *antiseptic* [isopropyl alcohol]
SWS solution (discontinued 1992) OTC *contact lens wetting/soaking solution*
Syllact powder OTC *bulk laxative* [psyllium seed husks]
Syllamalt powder OTC *laxative* [malt soup extract; psyllium seed husks]
Symadine capsules ℞ *antiviral* [amantadine HCl]
symclosene USAN, INN *topical anti-infective*
symetine INN *antiamebic* [also: symetine HCl]
symetine HCl USAN *antiamebic* [also: symetine]
Symmetrel capsules, syrup ℞ *antiviral; antiparkinsonian agent* [amantadine HCl]
Synacort cream ℞ *topical corticosteroid* [hydrocortisone]

Synalar cream, ointment, topical solution ℞ *topical corticosteroid* [fluocinolone acetonide]

Synalar-HP cream ℞ *topical corticosteroid* [fluocinolone acetonide]

Synalgos capsules (discontinued 1991) OTC *analgesic; antipyretic; anti-inflammatory* [aspirin; caffeine]

Synalgos-DC capsules ℞ *narcotic analgesic* [dihydrocodeine bitartrate; aspirin; caffeine]

Synapton ℞ *investigational cholinesterase inhibitor for Alzheimer's disease*

Synarel nasal spray ℞ *gonadotropin-releasing hormone for endometriosis and central precocious puberty (orphan)* [nafarelin acetate]

Synemol cream ℞ *topical corticosteroid* [fluocinolone acetonide]

synestrin [see: diethylstilbestrol]

Synkayvite tablets, subcu, IM or IV injection (discontinued 1992) ℞ *coagulant; for vitamin K deficiency or hypoprothrombinemia* [menadiol sodium diphosphate]

synnematin B [see: adicillin]

Synophylate-GG syrup ℞ *antiasthmatic; bronchodilator; expectorant* [theophylline sodium glycinate; guaifenesin]

Synthaloids throat lozenges OTC *oral antiseptic; topical anesthetic* [Calpuridin (q.v.); benzocaine]

synthestrin [see: diethylstilbestrol]

synthetic lung surfactant [see: colfosceril palmitate]

synthetic paraffin [see: paraffin, synthetic]

synthetic spermaceti [now: cetyl esters wax]

synthoestrin [see: diethylstilbestrol]

Synthroid tablets, powder for injection ℞ *hypothyroidism; myxedema coma; TSH suppression in thyroid cancer* [levothyroxine sodium]

Syntocinon IV, IM injection ℞ *induction of labor; postpartum bleeding; incomplete abortion* [oxytocin]

Syntocinon nasal spray ℞ *initial milk let-down* [oxytocin]

synvinolin [now: simvastatin]

Synvisc ℞ *investigational antiarthritic* [hylan fluid-gel mixture]

Syprine capsules ℞ *chelating agent for copper; (orphan: Wilson's disease)* [trientine HCl]

syrosingopine NF, INN, BAN

syrup NF *flavoring agent*

syrupus cerasi [see: cherry juice]

Syrvite liquid OTC *vitamin supplement* [multiple vitamins]

Sytobex injection ℞ *antianemic; vitamin supplement* [cyanocobalamin]

T

T-2 protocol (dactinomycin, doxorubicin, vincristine, cyclophosphamide, radiation) *chemotherapy protocol*

T₃ (liothyronine sodium) [q.v.]

T₄ (levothyroxine sodium) [q.v.]

T4, recombinant soluble human *investigational antiviral for AIDS*

T4 endonuclease V, liposome encapsulated *(orphan: prevent cutaneous neoplasms in xeroderma pigmentosum)*

T4N5 *(orphan: prevent cutaneous neoplasms in xeroderma pigmentosum)* [T4 endonuclease V, liposome encapsulated]

T-88 ℞ *investigational treatment for gram-negative sepsis* [monoclonal antibodies]

Tab-A-Vite + Iron tablets OTC *vitamin/iron supplement* [multiple vitamins; iron; folic acid]

Tab-A-Vite tablets OTC *vitamin supplement* [multiple vitamins; folic acid]

tabilautide INN

Tabron Filmseals (film-coated tablets) ℞ *hematinic* [ferrous fumarate; vitamins C & E; multiple B vitamins; folic acid]

Tabules (dosage form) *tablets*

Tac suspension ℞ *topical corticosteroid* [triamcinolone acetonide]

Tac-3 IM, intra-articular, intrabursal, intradermal injection ℞ *glucocorticoids* [triamcinolone acetonide]

Tac-40 suspension ℞ *topical corticosteroid* [triamcinolone acetonide]

Tacaryl chewable tablets ℞ *antihistamine* [methdilazine HCl]

Tacaryl HCl syrup, tablets ℞ *antihistamine* [methdilazine HCl]

Tace capsules ℞ *hormone for estrogen replacement therapy or inoperable prostatic carcinoma* [chlorotrianisene]

taclamine INN *minor tranquilizer* [also: taclamine HCl]

taclamine HCl USAN *minor tranquilizer* [also: taclamine]

tacrine INN, BAN *cognition adjuvant* [also: tacrine HCl]

tacrine HCl USAN *cognition adjuvant* [also: tacrine]

TAD (thioguanine, ara-C, daunorubicin) *chemotherapy protocol*

Tagamet film-coated tablets (status change from ℞ to OTC pending) *gastric and duodenal ulcer treatment; for gastric hypersecretory conditions* [cimetidine]

Tagamet liquid, IV or IM injection ℞ *gastric and duodenal ulcer treatment; for gastric hypersecretory conditions* [cimetidine HCl]

taglutimide INN

Talacen caplets ℞ *narcotic agonist-antagonist analgesic; antipyretic* [pentazocine HCl; acetaminophen]

talampicillin INN *antibacterial* [also: talampicillin HCl]

talampicillin HCl USAN *antibacterial* [also: talampicillin]

talastine INN

talbutal USP, INN *sedative; hypnotic*

talc USP *dusting powder; tablet and capsule lubricant*

taleranol USAN, INN *gonadotropin enzyme inhibitor*

talinolol INN

talipexole INN

talisomycin USAN, INN *antineoplastic*

tallysomycin A [now: talisomycin]

talmetacin USAN, INN *analgesic; anti-inflammatory; antipyretic*

talmetoprim INN

talniflumate USAN, INN *anti-inflammatory; analgesic*

Taloin ointment (discontinued 1992) OTC *topical diaper rash treatment* [methylbenzethonium chloride; zinc oxide; calamine; eucalyptol]

talopram INN *catecholamine potentiator* [also: talopram HCl]

talopram HCl USAN *catecholamine potentiator* [also: talopram]

talosalate USAN, INN *analgesic; anti-inflammatory*

taloximine INN, BAN

talsupram INN

taltibride [see: metibride]

taltrimide INN

taludipine [see: teludipine]

taludipine HCl *(previously used USAN)* [see: teludipine HCl]

Talwin Compound caplets ℞ *narcotic agonist-antagonist analgesic; antipyretic* [pentazocine HCl; aspirin]

Talwin IV, subcu or IM injection ℞ *narcotic agonist-antagonist analgesic* [pentazocine lactate]

Talwin NX tablets ℞ *narcotic agonist-antagonist analgesic* [pentazocine HCl; naloxone HCl]
Tambocor tablets ℞ *antiarrhythmic* [flecainide acetate]
tameridone USAN, INN, BAN *veterinary sedative*
tameticillin INN
tametraline INN *antidepressant* [also: tametraline HCl]
tametraline HCl USAN *antidepressant* [also: tametraline]
Tamine S.R. sustained-release tablets ℞ *decongestant; antihistamine* [phenylpropanolamine HCl; phenylephrine HCl; brompheniramine maleate]
tamitinol INN
tamoxifen INN *antiestrogen* [also: tamoxifen citrate]
tamoxifen citrate USAN, USP *antineoplastic; antiestrogen* [also: tamoxifen]
tampramine INN *antidepressant* [also: tampramine fumarate]
tampramine fumarate USAN *antidepressant* [also: tampramine]
Tanac liquid, stick, roll-on liquid OTC *topical anesthetic; oral antiseptic; astringent* [benzocaine; benzalkonium chloride; tannic acid]
tandamine INN *antidepressant* [also: tandamine HCl]
tandamine HCl USAN *antidepressant* [also: tandamine]
tandospirone INN *anxiolytic* [also: tandospirone citrate]
tandospirone citrate USAN *anxiolytic* [also: tandospirone]
taniplon INN
tannic acid USP *astringent; topical mucosal protectant*
tannic acid acetate [see: acetyltannic acid]
tannin [see: tannic acid]
tannyl acetate [see: acetyltannic acid]
Tanoral tablets ℞ *decongestant; antihistamine* [phenylephrine tannate; chlorpheniramine tannate; pyrilamine tannate]
tantalum *element (Ta)*
Tao capsules ℞ *macrolide antibiotic* [troleandomycin]
taoryi edisylate [see: caramiphen edisylate]
Tapanol tablets OTC *analgesic; antipyretic* [acetaminophen]
Tapazole tablets ℞ *antithyroid agent* [methimazole]
tape, adhesive USP *surgical aid*
taprostene INN
tar [see: coal tar]
Tarabine PFS injection ℞ *antineoplastic* [cytarabine]
Taractan IM injection ℞ *antipsychotic* [clorprothixene HCl]
Taractan oral concentrate ℞ *antipsychotic* [clorprothixene lactate]
Taractan tablets ℞ *antipsychotic* [clorprothixene]
Taraphilic Ointment OTC *topical antipsoriatic; antiseborrheic* [coal tar]
Targocid ℞ *investigational glycopeptide antibiotic* [teicoplanin]
Tarlene hair lotion OTC *antiseborrheic; antipsoriatic; keratolytic* [salicylic acid; coal tar]
Tarsum shampoo OTC *antipsoriatic; antiseborrheic; keratolytic* [coal tar; salicylic acid]
tartar emetic [see: antimony potassium tartrate]
tartaric acid NF *buffering agent*
tasuldine INN
TAT antagonist *investigational antiviral for AIDS*
T-Athlete cream, powder, aerosol powder, solution OTC *antifungal* [tolnaftate]
taurine INN
taurocholate sodium [see: sodium taurocholate]
taurolidine INN, BAN
tauromustine INN
tauroselcholic acid INN, BAN
taurultam INN, BAN

Tavist tablets, syrup ℞ *antihistamine* [clemastine fumarate]
Tavist-1 tablets OTC *antihistamine* [clemastine fumarate]
Tavist-D sustained-release tablets OTC *decongestant; antihistamine* [phenylpropanolamine HCl; clemastine fumarate]
Taxol IV infusion ℞ *antineoplastic for metastatic carcinoma of the ovary* [paclitaxel]
Taxotere *investigational antineoplastic for metastatic carcinoma of the ovary* [semisynthetic analog to paclitaxel]
tazadolene INN *analgesic* [also: tazadolene succinate]
tazadolene succinate USAN *analgesic* [also: tazadolene]
tazanolast INN
tazasubrate INN, BAN
tazeprofen INN
Tazicef powder for IV or IM injection ℞ *cephalosporin-type antibiotic* [ceftazidime]
Tazidime powder for IV or IM injection, ADD-vantage vials, Faspaks ℞ *cephalosporin-type antibiotic* [ceftazidime]
tazifylline INN *antihistamine* [also: tazifylline HCl]
tazifylline HCl USAN *antihistamine* [also: tazifylline]
taziprinone INN
tazobactam USAN, INN, BAN β-*lactamase inhibitor*
tazobactam sodium USAN β-*lactamase inhibitor*
tazolol INN *cardiotonic* [also: tazolol HCl]
tazolol HCl USAN *cardiotonic* [also: tazolol]
TBZ (thiabendazole) [q.v.]
3TC ℞ *investigational antiviral for AIDS*
^{99m}**Tc** [see: macrosalb (^{99m}Tc)]
^{99m}**Tc** [see: sodium pertechnetate Tc 99m]
^{99m}**Tc** [see: technetium Tc 99m albumin]
^{99m}**Tc** [see: technetium Tc 99m albumin aggregated]
^{99m}**Tc** [see: technetium Tc 99m albumin colloid]
^{99m}**Tc** [see: technetium Tc 99m albumin microaggregated]
^{99m}**Tc** [see: technetium Tc 99m antimony trisulfide colloid]
^{99m}**Tc** [see: technetium Tc 99m disofenin]
^{99m}**Tc** [see: technetium Tc 99m etidronate]
^{99m}**Tc** [see: technetium Tc 99m exametazine]
^{99m}**Tc** [see: technetium Tc 99m ferpentetate]
^{99m}**Tc** [see: technetium Tc 99m gluceptate]
^{99m}**Tc** [see: technetium Tc 99m lidofenin]
^{99m}**Tc** [see: technetium Tc 99m mebrofenin]
^{99m}**Tc** [see: technetium Tc 99m medronate]
^{99m}**Tc** [see: technetium Tc 99m medronate disodium]
^{99m}**Tc** [see: technetium Tc 99m mertiatide]
^{99m}**Tc** [see: technetium Tc 99m oxidronate]
^{99m}**Tc** [see: technetium Tc 99m pentetate]
^{99m}**Tc** [see: technetium Tc 99m (pyro- & trimeta-) phosphates]
^{99m}**Tc** [see: technetium Tc 99m pyrophosphate]
^{99m}**Tc** [see: technetium Tc 99m red blood cells]
^{99m}**Tc** [see: technetium Tc 99m sestamibi]
^{99m}**Tc** [see: technetium Tc 99m succimer]
^{99m}**Tc** [see: technetium Tc 99m sulfur colloid]
^{99m}**Tc** [see: technetium Tc 99m teboroxime]
^{99m}**Tc** [see: technetium Tc 99m tiatide]

T-Caine lozenges (discontinued 1993) OTC *topical anesthetic* [benzocaine]
TCC (trichlorocarbanilide) [see: triclocarban]
TD; Td (tetanus & diphtheria [toxoids]) [q.v.]
T-Dry Jr. sustained-release capsules (discontinued 1992) ℞ *decongestant; antihistamine* [pseudoephedrine HCl; chlorpheniramine maleate]
T-Dry sustained-release capsules OTC *decongestant; antihistamine* [pseudoephedrine HCl; chlorpheniramine maleate]
TEAB (tetraethylammonium bromide) [see: tetrylammonium bromide]
teaberry oil [see: methyl salicylate]
TEAC (tetraethylammonium chloride) [q.v.]
TearGard eye drops OTC *ocular moisturizer/lubricant*
Teargen eye drops OTC *ocular moisturizer/lubricant*
Tearisol eye drops OTC *ocular moisturizer/lubricant*
Tears Naturale; Tears Naturale II Drop-Tainers (eye drops) OTC *ocular moisturizer/lubricant*
Tears Plus eye drops OTC *ocular moisturizer/lubricant*
Tears Renewed eye drops, ophthalmic ointment OTC *ocular moisturizer/lubricant*
Tears Renewed ophthalmic solution OTC *artificial tears* [dextran 70; methylcellulose]
Tebamide suppositories ℞ *anticholinergic; antiemetic* [trimethobenzamide HCl]
tebatizole INN
tebethion [see: thioacetazone; thiacetazone]
tebufelone USAN, INN *analgesic; anti-inflammatory*
tebuquine USAN, INN *antimalarial*
TEC (thiotepa, etoposide, carboplatin) *chemotherapy protocol*

T.E.C. IV injection (discontinued 1992) ℞ *intravenous nutritional therapy* [multiple trace elements (metals)]
teceleukin USAN, INN, BAN *immunostimulant; (orphan: renal cell cancer; malignant melanoma)*
technetium *element (Tc)*
technetium (^{99m}Tc) labeled macroaggregated human albumin [see: macrosalb (^{99m}Tc)]
technetium Tc 99m albumin USP *radioactive agent*
technetium Tc 99m albumin aggregated USAN, USP *radioactive diagnostic aid for lung imaging*
technetium Tc 99m albumin colloid USAN *radioactive agent*
technetium Tc 99m albumin microaggregated USAN *radioactive agent*
technetium Tc 99m antimelanoma murine monoclonal antibody *(orphan: diagnostic aid for metastases of malignant melanoma)*
technetium Tc 99m antimony trisulfide colloid USAN *radioactive agent*
technetium Tc 99m bicisate USAN, INN, BAN *radioactive diagnostic aid for brain imaging*
technetium Tc 99m disofenin USP *radioactive diagnostic aid for hepatobiliary function testing*
technetium Tc 99m etidronate USP *radioactive agent*
technetium Tc 99m exametazine USAN *radioactive agent*
technetium Tc 99m ferpentetate USP *radioactive agent*
technetium Tc 99m gluceptate USP *radioactive agent*
technetium Tc 99m iron ascorbate pentetic acid complex [now: technetium Tc 99m ferpentetate]
technetium Tc 99m lidofenin USAN, USP *radioactive agent*

technetium Tc 99m mebrofenin USAN *radioactive agent*

technetium Tc 99m medronate USP *radioactive diagnostic aid for skeletal imaging*

technetium Tc 99m medronate disodium USAN *radioactive agent*

technetium Tc 99m mertiatide USAN *radioactive diagnostic aid for renal function testing*

technetium Tc 99m murine monoclonal antibody IgG$_2$a to B cell (*orphan: diagnostic aid for B-cell leukemia and lymphoma*)

technetium Tc 99m murine monoclonal antibody to human alpha-fetoprotein (AFP) (*orphan: diagnostic aid for AFP-producing tumors; hepatoblastoma*)

technetium Tc 99m murine monoclonal antibody to human chorionic gonadotropin (hCG) (*orphan: diagnostic aid for hCG-producing tumors*)

technetium Tc 99m oxidronate USP *radioactive diagnostic aid for skeletal imaging*

technetium Tc 99m pentetate USP *radioactive agent*

technetium Tc 99m pentetate calcium USAN *radioactive agent*

technetium Tc 99m pentetate sodium [now: technetium Tc 99m pentetate]

technetium Tc 99m (pyro- & trimeta-) phosphates USP *radioactive agent*

technetium Tc 99m pyrophosphate USP *radioactive agent*

technetium Tc 99m red blood cells USAN *radioactive agent*

technetium Tc 99m sestamibi USAN, INN, BAN *radioactive/radiopaque diagnostic aid for cardiac perfusion imaging*

technetium Tc 99m siboroxime USAN, INN *radioactive diagnostic aid for brain imaging*

technetium Tc 99m sodium gluceptate [now: technetium Tc 99m gluceptate]

technetium Tc 99m succimer USP *diagnostic aid for renal function testing*

technetium Tc 99m sulfur colloid (TSC) USAN, USP *radioactive agent*

technetium Tc 99m teboroxime USAN, INN *radioactive/radiopaque diagnostic aid for cardiac perfusion imaging*

technetium Tc 99m tiatide BAN

teclothiazide INN, BAN

teclozan USAN, INN *antiamebic*

Tecnu Poison Oak-N-Ivy liquid OTC *topical poison ivy treatment* [deodorized mineral spirits]

tedisamil INN

Tedral SA sustained-action tablets ℞ *antiasthmatic; bronchodilator; decongestant; sedative* [theophylline; ephedrine HCl; phenobarbital]

Tedral tablets, suspension OTC *antiasthmatic; bronchodilator; decongestant; sedative* [theophylline; ephedrine HCl; phenobarbital]

Tedrigen tablets OTC *antiasthmatic; bronchodilator; decongestant; sedative* [theophylline; ephedrine HCl; phenobarbital]

tefazoline INN

tefenperate INN

tefludazine INN

teflurane USAN, INN *inhalation anesthetic*

teflutixol INN

Tega Caine solution OTC *topical local anesthetic* [benzocaine; urea; parachlormetaxylenol]

Tega D & E, SR sustained-release tablets (discontinued 1992) ℞ *decongestant; expectorant* [phenylpropanolamine HCl; guaifenesin]

Tega-Atric elixir (discontinued 1993) OTC *vitamin/mineral supplement* [multiple B vitamins & minerals]

Tega-Atric M elixir OTC *vitamin/ mineral supplement* [multiple B vitamins & minerals]

Tega-Cort; Tega-Cort Forte lotion ℞ *topical corticosteroid* [hydrocortisone]

tegafur USAN, INN, BAN *antineoplastic*

Tega-Otic ear drops ℞ *topical corticosteroid; antibacterial/antifungal; anesthetic* [hydrocortisone; pramoxine; chloroxylenol; acetic acid]

Tega-Tussin syrup (discontinued 1992) ℞ *decongestant; antihistamine; antitussive* [phenylephrine HCl; chlorpheniramine maleate; hydrocodone bitartrate]

Tega-Vert capsules OTC *antinauseant; antiemetic; antivertigo; motion sickness preventative* [dimenhydrinate]

Tegison capsules ℞ *systemic antipsoriatic* [etretinate]

Tegopen capsules, powder for oral solution ℞ *bactericidal antibiotic (penicillinase-resistant penicillin)* [cloxacillin sodium]

Tegretol chewable tablets, tablets, oral suspension ℞ *anticonvulsant* [carbamazepine]

Tegrin for Psoriasis cream, lotion, soap OTC *topical antipsoriatic; antiseborrheic; antiseptic* [coal tar solution; alcohol]

Tegrin Medicated cream, lotion (name changed to Tegrin for Psoriasis in 1992)

Tegrin Medicated cream shampoo (discontinued 1991) OTC *antiseborrheic; antipsoriatic; antipruritic; antibacterial* [coal tar]

Tegrin Medicated Extra Conditioning shampoo OTC *antiseborrheic; antipsoriatic; antipruritic; antibacterial* [coal tar]

Tegrin Medicated gel shampoo, lotion shampoo OTC *antiseborrheic; antipsoriatic; antipruritic; antibacterial* [coal tar]

Tegrin-HC ointment OTC *topical corticosteroid* [hydrocortisone]

T.E.H. tablets ℞ *antiasthmatic; bronchodilator; decongestant; anxiolytic* [theophylline; ephedrine sulfate; hydroxyzine HCl]

teholamine [see: aminophylline]

TEIB (triethyleneiminobenzoquinone) [see: triaziquone]

teicoplanin USAN, INN, BAN *glycopeptide antibacterial antibiotic*

Teladar cream ℞ *topical corticosteroid* [betamethasone dipropionate]

Teldrin timed-release capsules OTC *antihistamine* [chlorpheniramine maleate]

Telechlor timed-release capsules ℞ *antihistamine* [chlorpheniramine maleate]

Tel-E-Dose (trademarked form) *unit dose package*

Tel-E-Ject (trademarked form) *prefilled disposable syringe*

teleleukin (*orphan:* metastatic renal cell carcinoma)

telenzepine INN

Telepaque tablets ℞ *oral cholecystographic radiopaque agent* [iopanoic acid]

Teline; Teline-500 capsules ℞ *broad-spectrum antibiotic* [tetracycline HCl]

tellurium *element (Te)*

teludipine INN, BAN *antihypertensive; calcium channel antagonist* [also: teludipine HCl]

teludipine HCl USAN *antihypertensive; calcium channel antagonist* [also: teludipine] [USAN previously used: taludipine HCl]

temafloxacin INN, BAN *antibacterial; microbial DNA topoisomerase inhibitor* [also: temafloxacin HCl]

temafloxacin HCl USAN *antibacterial; microbial DNA topoisomerase inhibitor* [also: temafloxacin]

Temaril tablets, syrup, Spansules (sustained-release capsules) ℞ *antipruritic* [trimeprazine tartrate]

temarotene INN
tematropium methylsulfate USAN *anticholinergic* [also: tematropium metilsulfate]
tematropium metilsulfate INN *anticholinergic* [also: tematropium methylsulfate]
temazepam USAN, INN *minor tranquilizer; hypnotic*
Tembids (trademarked form) *controlled-release capsules and tablets*
temefos USAN, INN *veterinary ectoparasiticide*
temelastine USAN, INN, BAN *antihistamine*
temocillin USAN, INN, BAN *antibacterial*
temodox USAN, INN *veterinary growth stimulant*
Temovate ointment, cream, scalp application ℞ *topical corticosteroidal anti-inflammatory* [clobetasol propionate]
temozolomide INN, BAN
TEMP (tamoxifen, etoposide, mitoxantrone, Platinol) *chemotherapy protocol*
Tempo chewable tablets (discontinued 1992) OTC *antacid; antiflatulent* [aluminum hydroxide; magnesium hydroxide; calcium carbonate; simethicone]
Tempra drops, syrup, chewable tablets OTC *analgesic; antipyretic* [acetaminophen]
Tempules (trademarked form) *timed-release capsules*
temurtide USAN, INN, BAN *vaccine adjuvant*
10 Benzagel; 5 Benzagel gel ℞ *keratolytic for acne* [benzoyl peroxide]
10% LMD IV ℞ *plasma volume expander; shock due to hemorrhage, burns, surgery* [dextran 40]
tenamfetamine INN
Tencet capsules ℞ *analgesic; antipyretic; sedative* [acetaminophen; caffeine; butalbital]

Tencon capsules ℞ *analgesic* [butalbital; acetaminophen]
tendamistat INN
Tenex tablets ℞ *antihypertensive* [guanfacine HCl]
tenidap USAN, INN *anti-inflammatory for osteoarthritis and rheumatoid arthritis*
tenidap sodium USAN *anti-inflammatory for osteoarthritis and rheumatoid arthritis*
tenilapine INN
teniloxazine INN
tenilsetam INN
teniposide USAN, INN, BAN *antineoplastic; (orphan: refractory childhood acute lymphocytic leukemia)*
Ten-K controlled-release tablets ℞ *potassium supplement* [potassium chloride]
tenocyclidine INN
Tenol-Plus tablets OTC *analgesic; antipyretic; anti-inflammatory* [acetaminophen; aspirin; caffeine]
tenonitrozole INN
Tenoretic 50; Tenoretic 100 tablets ℞ *antihypertensive* [chlorthalidone; atenolol]
Tenormin tablets, IV injection ℞ *antianginal; antihypertensive; β-blocker* [atenolol]
tenoxicam USAN, INN, BAN *anti-inflammatory*
Tensilon IV or IM injection ℞ *myasthenia gravis treatment; antidote to curare-type overdose* [edrophonium chloride]
Ten-tab (trademarked form) *sustained-release tablets*
Tenuate tablets, Dosepan (controlled-release tablets) ℞ *anorexiant* [diethylpropion HCl]
tenylidone INN
teopranitol INN
teoprolol INN
T.E.P. tablets OTC *antiasthmatic; bronchodilator; decongestant; sedative*

[theophylline; ephedrine HCl; phenobarbital]
Tepanil tablets, Ten-tab (sustained-release tablets) ℞ *anorexiant* [diethylpropion HCl]
tepirindole INN
tepoxalin USAN, INN *antipsoriatic*
teprenone INN
teprotide USAN, INN *angiotensin-converting enzyme (ACE) inhibitor*
Terazol 3 vaginal suppositories, vaginal cream ℞ *antifungal* [terconazole]
Terazol 7 vaginal cream ℞ *antifungal* [terconazole]
terazosin INN, BAN *antihypertensive;* $_1$-adrenergic blocker [also: terazosin HCl]
terazosin HCl USAN *antihypertensive* [also: terazosin]
terbinafine USAN, INN, BAN *antifungal*
terbium *element (Tb)*
terbucromil INN
terbufibrol INN
terbuficin INN
terbuprol INN
terbutaline INN, BAN *bronchodilator* [also: terbutaline sulfate]
terbutaline sulfate USAN, USP *bronchodilator* [also: terbutaline]
terciprazine INN
terconazole USAN, INN, BAN *antifungal*
terfenadine USAN, USP, INN *antihistamine*
terflavoxate INN
terfluranol INN
terguride INN
teriparatide INN *diagnostic aid for hypocalcemia (orphan)* [also: teriparatide acetate]
teriparatide acetate USAN *diagnostic aid for hypocalcemia* [also: teriparatide]
terizidone INN
terlakiren USAN *antihypertensive; renin inhibitor*

terlipressin INN, BAN *(orphan: bleeding esophageal varices)*
ternidazole INN
terodiline INN, BAN *coronary vasodilator* [also: terodiline HCl]
terodiline HCl USAN *coronary vasodilator; investigational agent for urinary incontinence* [also: terodiline]
terofenamate INN
teroxalene INN *antischistosomal* [also: teroxalene HCl]
teroxalene HCl USAN *antischistosomal* [also: teroxalene]
teroxirone USAN, INN *antineoplastic*
terpin hydrate USP *(disapproved for use as an expectorant in 1991)*
Terpin-Dex elixir (discontinued 1992) OTC *antitussive; expectorant* [dextromethorphan hydrobromide; terpin hydrate]
terpinol [see: terpin hydrate]
Terra-Cortril eye drop suspension ℞ *topical ophthalmic corticosteroidal antiinflammatory; antibiotic* [hydrocortisone acetate; oxytetracycline HCl]
terrafungine [see: oxytetracycline]
Terramycin capsules ℞ *tetracycline-type antibiotic* [oxytetracycline HCl]
Terramycin film-coated tablets ℞ *tetracycline-type antibiotic* [oxytetracycline]
Terramycin IM injection ℞ *tetracycline-type antibiotic* [oxytetracycline; lidocaine]
Terramycin with Polymyxin B ophthalmic ointment ℞ *ophthalmic antibiotic* [oxytetracycline HCl; polymyxin B sulfate]
Terramycin with Polymyxin B Sulfate ointment, powder (discontinued 1991) OTC *topical antibiotic* [oxytetracycline HCl; polymyxin B sulfate]
Terramycin with Polymyxin B vaginal tablets (discontinued 1992) ℞ *topical antibiotic* [oxytetracycline HCl; polymyxin B sulfate]
tertatolol INN, BAN

tertiary amyl alcohol [see: amylene hydrate]
***tert*-pentyl alcohol** [see: amylene hydrate]
Tesamone IM injection ℞ *androgen replacement for delayed puberty or breast cancer* [testosterone]
tesicam USAN, INN *anti-inflammatory*
tesimide USAN, INN *anti-inflammatory*
Teslac tablets ℞ *adjunctive hormonal chemotherapy for breast carcinoma* [testolactone]
TESPA (triethylenethiophosphoramide) [see: thiotepa]
Tessalon Perles (capsules) ℞ *antitussive* [benzonatate]
Tes-Tape reagent strips OTC *in vitro diagnostic aid for urine glucose*
Test-Estro Cypionates IM injection ℞ *estrogen/androgen for menopausal vasomotor symptoms* [estradiol cypionate; testosterone cypionate]
Testex IM injection ℞ *androgen replacement for delayed puberty or breast cancer* [testosterone propionate]
Testoderm transdermal patch ℞ *investigational hormone replacement therapy* [testosterone]
testolactone USAN, USP, INN *antineoplastic; androgen hormone*
Testone LA 100; Testone LA 200 IM injection ℞ *androgen replacement for delayed puberty or breast cancer* [testosterone ethanate]
testosterone USP, INN, BAN *androgen; (orphan: sublingual treatment of growth delay in boys)*
testosterone cyclopentanepropionate [see: testosterone cypionate]
testosterone cyclopentylpropionate [see: testosterone cypionate]
testosterone cypionate USP *parenteral androgen*
testosterone enanthate USP *parenteral androgen*
testosterone heptanoate [see: testosterone enanthate]
testosterone ketolaurate USAN, INN *androgen*
testosterone 3-oxododecanoate [see: testosterone ketolaurate]
testosterone phenylacetate USAN *androgen*
testosterone propionate USP *parenteral androgen; (orphan: vulvar dystrophies)*
TestPack [see: Abbott TestPack]
Testred capsules ℞ *androgen for male hypogonadism, impotence and breast cancer* [methyltestosterone]
Testred Cypionate IM injection ℞ *androgen replacement for delayed puberty or breast cancer* [testosterone cypionate]
Testrin PA IM injection ℞ *androgen replacement for delayed puberty or breast cancer* [testosterone enanthate]
tetanus antitoxin USP *passive immunizing agent*
tetanus & gas gangrene antitoxins NF
tetanus & gas gangrene polyvalent antitoxin [see: tetanus & gas gangrene antitoxins]
tetanus immune globulin USP *passive immunizing agent*
tetanus immune human globulin [now: tetanus immune globulin]
tetanus toxoid USP *active immunizing agent*
tetanus toxoid adsorbed USP *active immunizing agent*
tetiothalein sodium [see: iodophthalein sodium]
tetnicoran [see: nicofurate]
tetrabarbital INN
tetrabenazine INN, BAN
tetracaine USP, INN *topical anesthetic* [also: amethocaine]
tetracaine HCl USP *local anesthetic* [also: amethocaine HCl]

Tetracap capsules ℞ *broad-spectrum antibiotic* [tetracycline HCl]
tetrachloroethylene USP
tetrachloromethane [see: carbon tetrachloride]
Tetraclear eye drops OTC *topical ocular vasoconstrictor* [tetrahydrozoline HCl; sodium borate; boric acid; sodium chloride]
tetracosactide INN *adrenocorticotropic hormone* [also: cosyntropin; tetracosactrin]
tetracosactrin BAN *adrenocorticotropic hormone* [also: cosyntropin; tetracosactide]
tetracycline USP, INN, BAN *bacteriostatic antibiotic; antirickettsial*
tetracycline HCl USP *bacteriostatic antibiotic; antirickettsial*
tetracycline phosphate complex USP, BAN *antibacterial*
Tetracyn; Tetracyn 500 capsules ℞ *antibiotic* [tetracycline HCl]
tetradecanoic acid, methylethyl ester [see: isopropyl myristate]
tetradonium bromide INN
tetraethylammonium bromide (TEAB) [see: tetrylammonium bromide]
tetraethylammonium chloride (TEAC)
tetraethylthiuram disulfide [see: disulfiram]
tetrafilcon A USAN *hydrophilic contact lens material*
tetraglycine hydroperiodide *source of iodine for disinfecting water*
tetrahydroaminoacridine (THA) [see: tacrine HCl]
tetrahydrocannabinol (THC) [see: dronabinol]
tetrahydrozoline BAN *vasoconstrictor; nasal decongestant; topical ocular decongestant* [also: tetrhydrozoline HCl; tetryzoline]
tetrahydrozoline HCl USP *vasoconstrictor; nasal decongestant; topical ocular decongestant* [also: tetryzoline; tetrahydrozoline]
tetraiodophenolphthalein sodium [see: iodophthalein sodium]
Tetralan "250"; Tetralan-500 capsules ℞ *broad-spectrum antibiotic* [tetracycline HCl]
Tetralan syrup ℞ *broad-spectrum antibiotic* [tetracycline HCl]
tetrallobarbital [see: butalbital]
Tetram capsules ℞ *broad-spectrum antibiotic* [tetracycline HCl]
tetramal [see: tetrabarbital]
tetrameprozine [see: aminopromazine]
tetramethrin INN
tetramethylene dimethanesulfonate [see: busulfan]
tetramisole INN *anthelmintic* [also: tetramisole HCl]
tetramisole HCl USAN *anthelmintic* [also: tetramisole]
Tetramune ℞ *investigational pediatric vaccine for diphtheria, pertussis, tetanus and Haemophilus b*
tetranitrol [see: erythrityl tetranitrate]
tetrantoin
tetrasodium ethylenediaminetetraacetate [see: edetate sodium]
tetrasodium pyrophosphate [see: sodium pyrophosphate]
tetrazepam INN
tetrazolast meglumine USAN *antiallergic; antiasthmatic*
tetridamine INN *analgesic; anti-inflammatory* [also: tetrydamine]
tetriprofen INN
tetronasin BAN [also: tetronasin 5930]
tetronasin 5930 INN [also: tetronasin]
tetroquinone USAN, INN *systemic keratolytic*
tetroxoprim USAN, INN *antibacterial*
tetrydamine USAN *analgesic; anti-inflammatory* [also: tetridamine]
tetrylammonium bromide INN

tetryzoline INN *vasoconstrictor; nasal decongestant; topical ocular decongestant* [also: tetrahydrozoline HCl; tetrahydrozoline]
tetryzoline HCl [see: tetrahydrozoline HCl]
Texacort solution ℞ *topical corticosteroid* [hydrocortisone]
texacromil INN
TG (thioguanine) [q.v.]
TG (thyroglobulin) [q.v.]
T/Gel Scalp Solution gel (discontinued 1992) OTC *topical antipsoriatic; antiseborrheic; keratolytic* [coal tar solution; salicylic acid]
T-Gen suppositories ℞ *anticholinergic; antiemetic* [trimethobenzamide HCl]
T-Gesic capsules ℞ *narcotic analgesic* [hydrocodone bitartrate; acetaminophen]
α-TGI (α-triglycidyl isocyanurate) [see: teroxirone]
TH (theophylline) [q.v.]
TH (thyroid hormone) [see: levothyroxine sodium]
THA (tetrahydroaminoacridine) [see: tacrine HCl]
thalidomide USAN, INN, BAN *sedative; hypnotic; (orphan: graft vs. host disease; leprosy)*
Thalitone tablets ℞ *antihypertensive* [chlorthalidone]
thallium *element (Tl)*
thallous chloride Tl 201 USAN, USP *radiopaque medium; radioactive agent*
Tham IV infusion ℞ *corrects systemic acidosis associated with cardiac bypass surgery or cardiac arrest* [tromethamine]
Tham-E powder for IV infusion (discontinued 1992) ℞ *corrects systemic acidosis associated with cardiac bypass surgery or cardiac arrest* [tromethamine]
Thames Lotion OTC *moisturizer*
thaumatin BAN

THC (tetrahydrocannabinol) [see: dronabinol]
THC (thiocarbanidin)
thebacon INN, BAN
Theelin Aqueous IM injection ℞ *estrogen replacement therapy; antineoplastic for prostatic and breast cancer* [estrone]
theine [see: caffeine]
thenalidine INN
thenium closilate INN *veterinary anthelmintic* [also: thenium closylate]
thenium closylate USAN *veterinary anthelmintic* [also: thenium closilate]
thenyldiamine INN
thenylpyramine HCl [see: methapyrilene HCl]
Theo-24 timed-release capsules ℞ *bronchodilator* [theophylline]
Theobid Duracaps (sustained-release capsules) ℞ *bronchodilator* [theophylline]
Theobid Jr. Duracaps (sustained-release capsules) ℞ *bronchodilator* [theophylline]
theobromine NF
theobromine calcium salicylate NF
theobromine sodium acetate NF
theobromine sodium salicylate NF
Theochron extended-release tablets ℞ *bronchodilator* [theophylline]
Theoclear L.A.-130; Theoclear L.A.-260 extended-release capsules ℞ *bronchodilator* [theophylline]
Theoclear-80 oral solution ℞ *bronchodilator* [theophylline]
Theocolate liquid (discontinued 1991) ℞ *antiasthmatic* [theophylline; guaifenesin]
theodrenaline INN, BAN
Theodrine tablets OTC *antiasthmatic; bronchodilator; decongestant; sedative* [theophylline; ephedrine HCl; phenobarbital]
Theo-Dur extended-release tablets ℞ *bronchodilator* [theophylline]

Theo-Dur Sprinkle sustained-release capsules ℞ *bronchodilator* [theophylline]

Theofedral tablets ℞ *antiasthmatic* [theophylline; ephedrine HCl]

theofibrate USAN *antihyperlipoproteinemic* [also: etofylline clofibrate]

Theo-G capsules ℞ *antiasthmatic; bronchodilator; expectorant* [theophylline; guaifenesin]

Theolair tablets, liquid ℞ *antiasthmatic* [theophylline]

Theolair-SR sustained-release tablets ℞ *antiasthmatic* [theophylline]

Theolate liquid ℞ *antiasthmatic; bronchodilator; expectorant* [theophylline; guaifenesin]

Theomax DF syrup ℞ *decongestant; bronchodilator; antihistamine* [ephedrine sulfate; theophylline; hydroxyzine HCl; alcohol]

Theo-Organidin elixir ℞ *antiasthmatic; bronchodilator; expectorant* [theophylline; iodinated glycerol]

theophyldine [see: aminophylline]

theophyllamine [see: aminophylline]

Theophyllin KI elixir ℞ *antiasthmatic; bronchodilator; expectorant* [theophylline; potassium iodide]

theophylline (TH) USP, BAN *bronchodilator*

theophylline aminoisobutanol [see: ambuphylline]

theophylline ethylenediamine [now: aminophylline]

Theophylline Extended-Release tablets ℞ *bronchodilator* [theophylline]

theophylline monohydrate [see: theophylline]

theophylline olamine USP

theophylline sodium acetate NF

theophylline sodium glycinate USP *smooth muscle relaxant*

Theo-R-Gen elixir ℞ *antiasthmatic; bronchodilator; expectorant* [theophylline; iodinated glycerol]

Theo-Sav controlled-release tablets ℞ *bronchodilator* [theophylline]

Theospan-SR timed-release capsules ℞ *bronchodilator* [theophylline]

Theostat 80 syrup ℞ *bronchodilator* [theophylline]

Theotal tablets OTC *antiasthmatic; bronchodilator; decongestant; sedative* [theophylline; ephedrine HCl; phenobarbital]

Theovent timed-release capsules ℞ *bronchodilator* [theophylline]

Theox controlled-release tablets ℞ *antibiotic* [theophylline anhydrous]

Theozine tablets ℞ *bronchodilator; antihistamine; decongestant* [theophylline; hydroxyzine HCl; ephedrine sulfate]

Thera Hematinic tablets OTC *vitamin/iron* [multiple vitamins; ferrous fumarate; folic acid]

Thera Multi-vitamin liquid OTC *vitamin supplement* [multiple vitamins]

Therabid tablets OTC *vitamin supplement* [multiple vitamins]

Therac lotion OTC *topical acne treatment* [sulfur; salicylic acid]

Theracebrin Pulvules (capsules) (discontinued 1991) ℞ *vitamin supplement* [multiple vitamins]

Thera-Combex H P Kapseals (capsules) (discontinued 1992) OTC *vitamin supplement* [multiple B vitamins; vitamin C]

TheraCys freeze-dried suspension for intrevesical injection ℞ *antineoplastic for urinary bladder cancer* [BCG vaccine]

TheraFlu Flu, Cold & Cough Medicine; NightTime TheraFlu powder OTC *decongestant; antihistamine; antitussive; analgesic* [pseudoephedrine HCl; chlorpheniramine maleate; dextromethorphan hydrobromide; acetaminophen]

TheraFlu Flu & Cold Medicine powder OTC *decongestant; antihistamine; analgesic* [pseudoephedrine

HCl; chlorpheniramine maleate; acetaminophen]

Thera-Flur gel drops (for self-application) ℞ *dental caries preventative* [acidulated phosphate fluoride]

Thera-Flur-N gel drops (for self-application) ℞ *dental caries preventative* [sodium fluoride]

Theragenerix tablets OTC *vitamin supplement* [multiple vitamins; folic acid; biotin]

Theragenerix-H tablets OTC *vitamin/iron supplement* [multiple vitamins; ferrous fumarate; folic acid]

Theragenerix-M tablets OTC *vitamin/mineral/iron supplement* [multiple vitamins & minerals; iron; folic acid; biotin]

Thera-Gesic cream OTC *counterirritant* [methyl salicylate; menthol]

Theragran Hematinic tablets ℞ *vitamin/iron supplement* [multiple vitamins; ferrous fumarate; folic acid]

Theragran Jr. Children's Chewable Tablets (discontinued 1991) OTC *vitamin supplement* [multiple vitamins; folic acid]

Theragran Jr. with Extra Vitamin C chewable tablets (discontinued 1991) OTC *vitamin supplement* [multiple vitamins; folic acid]

Theragran Jr. with Iron chewable tablets (discontinued 1992) OTC *vitamin/iron supplement* [multiple vitamins; iron; folic acid]

Theragran liquid OTC *vitamin supplement* [multiple vitamins]

Theragran Stress Formula tablets OTC *vitamin/iron supplement* [ferrous fumarate; vitamins C & E; multiple B vitamins; folic acid; biotin]

Theragran tablets OTC *vitamin supplement* [multiple vitamins; folic acid; biotin]

Theragran-M film-coated tablets OTC *vitamin/mineral/calcium/iron supplement* [multiple vitamins & minerals; calcium; iron; folic acid; biotin]

Thera-Hist powder OTC *decongestant; antihistamine; analgesic* [pseudoephedrine HCl; chlorpheniramine maleate; acetaminophen]

Thera-M tablets OTC *vitamin/mineral/iron supplement* [multiple vitamins & minerals; iron]

Theramill Forte capsules OTC *vitamin replacement therapy* [multiple vitamins & minerals]

Theramine Expectorant liquid OTC *decongestant; expectorant* [phenylpropanolamine HCl; guaifenesin]

Theramycin Z topical solution ℞ *topical antibiotic* [erythromycin; alcohol]

Therapeutic B with C capsules OTC *vitamin supplement* [multiple B vitamins; vitamin C]

Therapeutic Bath lotion, oil OTC *moisturizer; emollient*

Therapeutic Mineral Ice; Therapeutic Mineral Ice Exercise Formula gel OTC *counterirritant* [menthol]

Theraplex T shampoo OTC *antiseborrheic; antipsoriatic; antipruritic; antibacterial* [coal tar]

Theraplex Z shampoo OTC *antiseborrheic; antibacterial; antifungal* [pyrithione zinc]

Theravee Hematinic tablets OTC *vitamin/iron supplement* [multiple vitamins; ferrous fumarate; folic acid]

Theravee tablets OTC *vitamin supplement* [multiple vitamins; folic acid; biotin]

Theravee-M tablets OTC *vitamin/mineral/iron supplement* [multiple vitamins & minerals; iron; folic acid; biotin]

Theravim tablets OTC *vitamin supplement* [multiple vitamins; folic acid; biotin]

Theravim-M tablets OTC *vitamin/mineral/iron supplement* [multiple vitamins & minerals; iron; folic acid; biotin]

Theravir ℞ *investigational anti-HIV drug* [monoclonal antibodies]

Theravite liquid OTC *vitamin supplement* [multiple vitamins]

Theravit-M tablets OTC *vitamin/mineral supplement* [multiple vitamins & minerals]

Theravits tablets OTC *vitamin supplement* [multiple vitamins]

Therems tablets OTC *vitamin supplement* [multiple vitamins; folic acid; biotin]

Therems-M tablets OTC *vitamin/mineral/iron supplement* [multiple vitamins & minerals; iron; biotin]

Therevac-Plus enema OTC *laxative; stool softener* [docusate sodium; benzocaine; soft soap; PEG 400; glycerin]

Therevac-SB enema OTC *laxative; stool softener* [docusate sodium; soft soap; PEG 400; glycerin]

Theri bath oil OTC *emollient* [mineral oil; PEG; 4-dilaurate; lanolin oil; benzophenone-3]

Theri-Care lotion OTC *moisturizer; emollient* [mineral oil; propylene glycol; lanolin; trolamine; alcohol]

Thermazene cream ℞ *broad-spectrum bactericidal for adjunctive burn treatment* [silver sulfadiazine]

ThermoRub ointment, lotion (discontinued 1992) OTC *counterirritant; topical analgesic* [methyl nicotinate; histamine dihydrochloride; salicylamide; dipropylene glycol salicylate; capsicum]

Theroxide lotion, wash ℞ *topical keratolytic for acne* [benzoyl peroxide]

Thex Forte caplets OTC *vitamin supplement* [multiple B vitamins; vitamin C]

thiabendazole (TBZ) USAN, USP *anthelmintic* [also: tiabendazole]

thiabutazide [see: buthiazide]

thiacetarsamide sodium INN

thiacetazone BAN [also: thioacetazone]

Thiacide film-coated tablets ℞ *urinary anti-infective; acidifier* [methenamine mandelate; potassium acid phosphate]

thialbarbital INN [also: thialbarbitone]

thialbarbitone BAN [also: thialbarbital]

thialisobumal sodium [see: buthalital sodium]

thiamazole INN *thyroid inhibitor* [also: methimazole]

thiambutosine INN, BAN

Thiamilate enteric-coated tablets OTC *vitamin supplement* [thiamine HCl]

thiamine INN *vitamin B$_1$; enzyme cofactor* [also: thiamine HCl]

thiamine HCl USP *vitamin B$_1$; enzyme cofactor* [also: thiamine]

thiamine mononitrate USP *vitamin B$_1$; enzyme cofactor*

thiamine propyl disulfide [see: prosultiamine]

thiamiprine USAN *antineoplastic* [also: tiamiprine]

thiamphenicol USAN, INN, BAN *antibacterial*

thiamylal sodium USP *general anesthetic*

thiazesim HCl USAN *antidepressant* [also: tiazesim]

thiazinamium chloride USAN *antiallergic*

thiazinamium metilsulfate INN

4-thiazolidinecarboxylic acid [see: timonacic]

thiazolsulfone [see: thiazosulfone]

thiazosulfone INN

thiazothielite [see: antienite]

thiazothienol [see: antazonite]

thiethylperazine USAN, INN *antiemetic; antidopaminergic*

thiethylperazine malate USP *antiemetic; antipsychotic*

thiethylperazine maleate USAN, USP *antiemetic*
thihexinol methylbromide NF, INN
thimerfonate sodium USAN *topical anti-infective* [also: sodium timerfonate]
thimerosal USP *topical anti-infective; preservative* [also: thiomersal]
thioacetazone INN [also: thiacetazone]
thiocarbanidin (THC)
thiocarlide BAN [also: tiocarlide]
thiocolchicine glycoside [see: thiocolchicoside]
thiocolchicoside INN
thiocyanate sodium NF
thiodiglycol INN
thiodiphenylamine [see: phenothiazine]
thiofuradene INN
6-thioguanine [see: thioguanine]
thioguanine (TG) USAN, USP *antineoplastic* [also: tioguanine]
thiohexallymal [see: thialbarbital]
thiohexamide INN
Thiola tablets ℞ *(orphan: cystine nephrolithiasis in homozygous cystinuria)* [tiopronin]
thiomebumal sodium [see: thiopental sodium]
thiomersal INN, BAN *topical anti-infective; preservative* [also: thimerosal]
thiomesterone BAN [also: tiomesterone]
thiomicid [see: thioacetazone; thiacetazone]
thioparamizone [see: thioacetazone; thiacetazone]
thiopental sodium USP, INN *general anesthetic; anticonvulsant*
thiopentone sodium [see: thiopental sodium]
thiophanate BAN
thiophosphoramide [see: thiotepa]
thiopropazate INN [also: thiopropazate HCl]
thiopropazate HCl NF [also: thiopropazate]

thioproperazine INN, BAN [also: thioproperazine mesylate]
thioproperazine mesylate [also: thioproperazine]
thioproperazine methanesulfonate [see: thioproperazine mesylate]
thioridazine USAN, USP, INN *antipsychotic; sedative*
thioridazine HCl USP *antipsychotic; sedative*
thiosalan USAN *disinfectant* [also: tiosalan]
Thiosulfil Duo-Pak (two-product package) (discontinued 1991) ℞ *urinary anti-infective/bacteriostatic; urinary analgesic* [Thiosulfil Forte (q.v.); Thiosulfil-A Forte (q.v.)]
Thiosulfil Forte tablets ℞ *broad-spectrum bacteriostatic* [sulfamethizole]
Thiosulfil-A; Thiosulfil-A Forte tablets (discontinued 1991) ℞ *urinary anti-infective* [sulfamethizole; phenazopyridine HCl]
thiosulfuric acid, disodium salt pentahydrate [see: sodium thiosulfate]
thiotepa USP, INN *antineoplastic*
thiotetrabarbital INN
thiothixene USAN, USP, BAN *antipsychotic* [also: tiotixene]
thiothixene HCl USAN, USP *antipsychotic*
thiouracil
thiourea *antioxidant*
thioxolone BAN [also: tioxolone]
thiphenamil HCl USAN *smooth muscle relaxant* [also: tifenamil]
thiphencillin potassium USAN *antibacterial* [also: tifencillin]
thiram USAN, INN *antifungal*
Thiuretic tablets ℞ *diuretic; antihypertensive* [hydrochlorothiazide]
Thixo-Flur topical gel (for professional application) ℞ *dental caries preventative* [acidulated phosphate fluoride]
thonzonium bromide USAN, USP *detergent* [also: tonzonium bromide]

thonzylamine HCl USAN, INN
Thorazine tablets, Spansules (capsules), IV, IM, syrup, suppositories ℞ *tranquilizer; antiemetic* [chlorpromazine]
Thorets throat lozenges OTC *oral anesthetic* [benzocaine]
thorium *element (Th)*
thozalinone USAN *antidepressant* [also: tozalinone]
THQ (tetrahydroxybenzoquinone) [see: tetroquinone]
THR (trishydroxyethyl rutin) [see: troxerutin]
Threamine DM syrup OTC *decongestant; antihistamine; antitussive* [phenylpropanolamine HCl; chlorpheniramine maleate; dextromethorphan hydrobromide]
Threamine Expectorant liquid OTC *decongestant; expectorant* [phenylpropanolamine HCl; guaifenesin; alcohol]
3TC ℞ *investigational antiviral for AIDS*
threonine (L-threonine) USAN, USP, INN *essential amino acid; (orphan: spasticity; amyotrophic lateral sclerosis)*; symbols: Thr, T
Threostat *(orphan: familial spastic paraparesis; amyotrophic lateral sclerosis)* [L-threonine]
Throat Discs lozenges OTC *analgesic; counterirritant* [capsicum; peppermint; anise; cubeb; licorice; linseed]
Thrombate III *(orphan: antithrombin III deficiency; thrombosis)* [antithrombin III, human]
thrombin USP, INN *local hemostatic*
Thrombinar powder ℞ *topical hemostatic aid in surgical hemostasis* [thrombin]
thrombinogen (prothrombin)
Thrombogen powder ℞ *topical hemostatic aid in surgical hemostasis* [thrombin]
thromboplastin USP

Thrombostat powder ℞ *topical hemostatic aid in surgical hemostasis* [thrombin]
thulium *element (Tm)*
Thylline tablets ℞ *bronchodilator* [dyphylline]
Thylline-GG tablets ℞ *bronchodilator; expectorant* [dyphylline; guaifenesin]
thymic humoral factor *investigational immunomodulator for AIDS*
thymocartin INN
thymol NF *stabilizer; topical antiseptic*
thymol iodide NF
Thymone ℞ *(orphan: amyotrophic lateral sclerosis)* [protirelin]
thymopentin USAN, INN, BAN *immunoregulator*
thymopoietin 32-36 [now: thymopentin]
thymosin alpha-1 *(orphan: chronic active hepatitis B)*
thymostimulin INN *investigational immunomodulator for AIDS*
thymotrinan INN
thymoxamine BAN [also: moxisylyte]
thymoxamine HCl *(orphan: phenylephrine-induced mydriasis)*
Thypinone IV injection ℞ *in vivo thyroid function test* [protirelin]
Thyrar tablets ℞ *thyroid replacement therapy; hypothyroidism; thyroid cancer* [thyroid (bovine)]
Thyro-Block tablets ℞ *thyroid-blocking therapy* [potassium iodide]
thyrocalcitonin [see: calcitonin]
Thyrogen ℞ *(orphan: diagnostic aid for thyroid cancer)* [thyrotropin]
thyroglobulin (TG) USAN, USP, INN *thyroid hormone*
thyroid USP *thyroid hormone*
thyroid hormone (TH) [see: levothyroxine sodium]
thyroid stimulating hormone (TSH) [see: thyrotropin]
Thyroid Strong tablets ℞ *hypothyroidism; thyroid cancer* [thyroid, desiccated]

Thyrolar-0.25; -0.5; -1; -2; -3 tablets ℞ *thyroid hormone therapy* [liotrix]
thyromedan HCl USAN *thyromimetic* [also: tyromedan]
thyropropic acid INN
thyrotrophic hormone [see: thyrotrophin]
thyrotrophin INN *thyroid stimulating hormone* [also: thyrotropin]
thyrotropin *thyroid stimulating hormone; (orphan: diagnostic aid for thyroid cancer)* [also: thyrotrophin]
thyrotropin-releasing hormone (TRH) [see: protirelin]
thyroxine BAN *thyroid hormone* [also: levothyroxine sodium]
D-thyroxine [see: dextrothyroxine sodium]
L-thyroxine [see: levothyroxine sodium]
thyroxine I 125 USAN *radioactive agent*
thyroxine I 131 USAN *radioactive agent*
Thytropar powder for IM or subcu injection ℞ *thyrotrophic hormone; in vivo thyroid function test* [thyrotropin]
tiabendazole INN *anthelmintic* [also: thiabendazole]
tiacrilast USAN, INN *antiallergic*
tiacrilast sodium USAN *antiallergic*
tiadenol INN
tiafibrate INN
Tiagabine ℞ *investigational anticonvulsant*
tiamenidine USAN, INN *antihypertensive*
tiamenidine HCl USAN *antihypertensive*
tiametonium iodide INN
tiamiprine INN *antineoplastic* [also: thiamiprine]
tiamizide INN *diuretic; antihypertensive* [also: diapamide]
tiamulin USAN, INN *veterinary antibacterial*
tiamulin fumarate USAN *veterinary antibacterial*

tianafac INN
tianeptine INN
tiapamil INN, BAN *antagonist to calcium* [also: tiapamil HCl]
tiapamil HCl USAN *antagonist to calcium* [also: tiapamil]
tiapirinol INN
tiapride INN
tiaprofenic acid INN
tiaprost INN
tiaramide INN, BAN *antiasthmatic* [also: tiaramide HCl]
tiaramide HCl USAN *antiasthmatic* [also: tiaramide]
tiazesim INN *antidepressant* [also: thiazesim HCl]
tiazesim HCl [see: thiazesim HCl]
tiazofurin USAN *antineoplastic* [also: tiazofurine]
tiazofurine INN *antineoplastic* [also: tiazofurin]
tiazuril USAN, INN *coccidiostat for poultry*
tibalosin INN
tibenelast sodium USAN *antiasthmatic; bronchodilator*
tibenzate INN
tibezonium iodide INN
tibolone USAN, INN, BAN *anabolic*
tibric acid USAN, INN *antihyperlipoproteinemic*
tibrofan USAN, INN *disinfectant*
ticabesone INN *glucocorticoid* [also: ticabesone propionate]
ticabesone propionate USAN *glucocorticoid* [also: ticabesone]
Ticar powder for IV or IM injection, ADD-vantage vials ℞ *extended-spectrum penicillin-type antibiotic* [ticarcillin disodium]
ticarbodine USAN, INN *anthelmintic*
ticarcillin INN *antibacterial* [also: ticarcillin disodium]
ticarcillin cresyl sodium USAN *antibacterial*
ticarcillin disodium USAN, USP *bactericidal antibiotic* [also: ticarcillin]

Tice BCG percutaneous injection for TB, intravesical injection for cancer ℞ *tuberculosis immunizing agent; antineoplastic for bladder cancer* [BCG vaccine, Tice strain]

ticlatone USAN, INN *antibacterial; antifungal*

Ticlid film-coated tablets ℞ *platelet aggregation inhibitor for stroke* [ticlopidine HCl]

ticlopidine INN, BAN *platelet aggregation inhibitor* [also: ticlopidine HCl]

ticlopidine HCl USAN *platelet aggregation inhibitor* [also: ticlopidine]

Ticon IM injection ℞ *anticholinergic; antiemetic* [trimethobenzamide HCl]

ticrynafen USAN *diuretic; uricosuric; antihypertensive* [also: tienilic acid]

tidiacic INN

tiemonium iodide INN, BAN

tienilic acid INN *diuretic; uricosuric; antihypertensive* [also: ticrynafen]

tienocarbine INN

tienopramine INN

tienoxolol INN

tifemoxone INN

tifenamil INN *smooth muscle relaxant* [also: thiphenamil HCl]

tifenamil HCl [see: thiphenamil HCl]

tifencillin INN *antibacterial* [also: thiphencillin potassium]

tifencillin potassium [see: thiphencillin potassium]

tiflamizole INN

tiflorex INN

tifluadom INN

tiflucarbine INN

tiformin INN [also: tyformin]

tifurac INN *analgesic* [also: tifurac sodium]

tifurac sodium USAN *analgesic* [also: tifurac]

Tigan capsules, suppositories, IM injection ℞ *antiemetic* [trimethobenzamide HCl]

tigemonam INN *antimicrobial* [also: tigemonam dicholine]

tigemonam dicholine USAN *antimicrobial* [also: tigemonam]

tigestol USAN, INN *progestin*

tigloidine INN, BAN

tiglyl*pseudo*tropine [see: tigloidine]

tiglyltropeine [see: tropigline]

Tiject-20 IM injection (discontinued 1992) ℞ *anticholinergic; antiemetic* [trimethobenzamide HCl]

tilactase INN *digestive enzyme*

Tilad (Spanish name for U.S. product Tilade)

Tilade inhalation aerosol ℞ *bronchodilator for bronchial asthma* [nedocromil sodium]

tilbroquinol INN

tiletamine INN *anesthetic; anticonvulsant* [also: tiletamine HCl]

tiletamine HCl USAN *anesthetic; anticonvulsant* [also: tiletamine]

tilidate HCl BAN *analgesic* [also: tilidine HCl; tilidine]

tilidine INN *analgesic* [also: tilidine HCl; tilidate HCl]

tilidine HCl USAN *analgesic* [also: tilidine; tilidate HCl]

tiliquinol INN

tilisolol INN

tilmicosin USAN, INN, BAN *veterinary antibacterial*

tilomisole USAN, INN *immunoregulator*

tilorone INN *antiviral* [also: tilorone HCl]

tilorone HCl USAN *antiviral* [also: tilorone]

tilozepine INN

tilsuprost INN

Tiludronate ℞ *investigational biphosphonate for Paget's disease and osteoporosis*

tiludronic acid INN

Time-B-50 timed-release caplet OTC *vitamin supplement* [multiple B vitamins]

Time-C; Time-C-1500 timed-release capsules OTC *vitamin supplement* [vitamin C]

Timecaps (trademarked form) *timed-release capsules*

Time-C-Bio timed-release caplet OTC *vitamin supplement* [vitamin C; bioflavonoids]

Timecelles (dosage form) *sustained-release capsules*

timefurone USAN, INN *antiatherosclerotic*

timegadine INN

timelotem INN

Timentin powder for IV injection, ADD-vantage vials ℞ *extended-spectrum penicillin-type antibiotic* [ticarcillin disodium; clavulanate potassium]

timepidium bromide INN

Timespan (trademarked form) *sustained-release tablets*

Timesules (dosage form) *sustained-release capsules*

timiperone INN

timobesone INN *topical adrenocortical steroid* [also: timobesone acetate]

timobesone acetate USAN *topical adrenocortical steroid* [also: timobesone]

timofibrate INN

Timolide 10-25 tablets ℞ *antihypertensive* [timolol maleate; hydrochlorothiazide]

timolol USAN, INN, BAN *antiadrenergic (β-receptor)*

timolol maleate USAN, USP *antiadrenergic (β-receptor); topical antiglaucoma agent; migraine preventative*

timonacic INN

timoprazole INN

Timoptic Ocumeter (eye drops), Ocudose (single-use eye drop dispenser) ℞ *antiglaucoma agent (β-blocker)* [timolol maleate]

Timoptic-XE ℞ *investigational once-daily antiglaucoma formulation* [timolol maleate]

Timunox ℞ *investigational immunomodulator for AIDS* [thymopoentin]

tin *element (Sn)*

tin chloride dihydrate [see: stannous chloride]

tin fluoride [see: stannous fluoride]

tinabinol USAN, INN *antihypertensive*

Tinactin cream, powder, spray powder, spray liquid, solution OTC *topical antifungal* [tolnaftate]

Tinactin for Jock Itch cream, spray powder OTC *topical antifungal* [tolnaftate]

tinazoline INN

TinBen tincture OTC *skin protectant* [benzoin; alcohol]

TinCoBen tincture OTC *skin protectant* [benzoin; aloe; alcohol]

Tincture of Green Soap liquid OTC *antiseptic cleanser* [green soap; alcohol]

Tindal sugar-coated tablets ℞ *antipsychotic* [acetophenazine maleate]

Tine Test OT [see: Tuberculin, Old, Tine Test]

Tine Test PPD single-use intradermal puncture test device ℞ *tuberculosis skin test* [tuberculin purified protein derivative]

Ting cream, powder, spray powder, spray liquid OTC *topical antifungal* [tolnaftate]

tinidazole USAN, INN *antiprotozoal*

tinisulpride INN

tinofedrine INN

tinoridine INN

Tinver lotion ℞ *topical antifungal; keratolytic; antipruritic; anesthetic* [sodium thiosulfate; salicylic acid; menthol; alcohol]

tiocarlide INN [also: thiocarlide]

tioclomarol INN

tioconazole USAN, USP, INN *antifungal*

tioctilate INN

tiodazosin USAN, INN *antihypertensive*

tiodonium chloride USAN, INN *antibacterial*

tiofacic [see: stepronin]

tioguanine INN *antineoplastic* [also: thioguanine]
tiomergine INN
tiomesterone INN [also: thiomesterone]
tioperidone INN *antipsychotic* [also: tioperidone HCl]
tioperidone HCl USAN *antipsychotic* [also: tioperidone]
tiopinac USAN, INN *anti-inflammatory; analgesic; antipyretic*
tiopronin INN *(orphan: cystine nephrolithiasis in homozygous cystinuria)*
tiopropamine INN
tiosalan INN *disinfectant* [also: thiosalan]
tiosinamine [see: allylthiourea]
tiospirone INN *antipsychotic* [also: tiospirone HCl]
tiospirone HCl USAN *antipsychotic* [also: tiospirone]
tiotidine USAN, INN *antagonist to histamine H_2 receptors*
tiotixene INN *antipsychotic* [also: thiothixene]
tioxacin INN
tioxamast INN
tioxaprofen INN
tioxidazole USAN, INN *anthelmintic*
tioxolone INN [also: thioxolone]
tipentosin INN, BAN *antihypertensive* [also: tipentosin HCl]
tipentosin HCl USAN *antihypertensive* [also: tipentosin]
tipepidine INN
tipetropium bromide INN
tipindole INN
tipredane USAN, INN, BAN *topical adrenocortical steroid*
tiprenolol INN *antiadrenergic (β-receptor)* [also: tiprenolol HCl]
tiprenolol HCl USAN *antiadrenergic (β-receptor)* [also: tiprenolol]
tiprinast INN *antiallergic* [also: tiprinast meglumine]
tiprinast meglumine USAN *antiallergic* [also: tiprinast]

tipropidil INN *vasodilator* [also: tipropidil HCl]
tipropidil HCl USAN *vasodilator* [also: tipropidil]
tiprostanide INN, BAN
tiprotimod INN
tiquinamide INN *gastric anticholinergic* [also: tiquinamide HCl]
tiquinamide HCl USAN *gastric anticholinergic* [also: tiquinamide]
tiquizium bromide INN
tirapazamine *investigational cytotoxic antineoplastic to be used in conjunction with radiation therapy*
tiratricol INN *(orphan: thyroid cancer)*
Tirend tablets OTC *CNS stimulant; analeptic* [caffeine]
tirilazad mesylate USAN *lipid peroxidation inhibitor*
tiropramide INN
tisilfocon A USAN *hydrophobic contact lens material*
Tisit Blue liquid OTC *pediculicide* [pyrethrins; piperonyl butoxide; petroleum distillate]
Tisit liquid, shampoo OTC *pediculicide* [pyrethrins; piperonyl butoxide]
tisocromide INN
TiSol solution OTC *anesthetic and antimicrobial throat irrigation* [menthol; benzyl alcohol; saline; eriodictyon; cetylpyridinium chloride; yerba santa]
tisopurine INN
tisoquone INN
tissue factor [see: thromboplastin]
tissue plasminogen activator (tPA; t-PA) [see: alteplase]
Tis-U-Sol solution ℞ *sterile irrigant* [physiologic irrigating solution]
Titan solution OTC *contact lens cleaning solution*
titanium *element (Ti)*
titanium dioxide USP *topical protectant; astringent*
titanium oxide [see: titanium dioxide]
Titracid chewable tablets OTC *antacid* [calcium carbonate; glycine]

Titradose (trademarked form) *tablets*
Titralac chewable tablets OTC *antacid* [calcium carbonate; glycine]
Titralac Plus liquid OTC *antacid; antiflatulent* [calcium carbonate; simethicone]
tivanidazole INN
tivazine [see: piperazine citrate]
tixadil INN
tixanox USAN *antiallergic* [also: tixanoxum]
tixanoxum INN *antiallergic* [also: tixanox]
tixocortol INN *topical anti-inflammatory* [also: tixocortol pivalate]
tixocortol pivalate USAN *topical anti-inflammatory* [also: tixocortol]
tizabrin INN
tizanidine INN, BAN *investigational agent for spasticity of multiple sclerosis*
tizolemide INN
tizoprolic acid INN
T-Koff liquid ℞ *decongestant; antihistamine; antitussive* [phenylpropanolamine HCl; phenylephrine HCl; chlorpheniramine maleate; codeine phosphate]
[201]**Tl** [see: thallous chloride Tl 201]
TLC ABLC ℞ *investigational systemic antifungal* [amphotericin B lipid complex]
TLC C-53 ℞ *investigational cell adhesion antagonist for adult respiratory distress syndrome*
TLC D-99 ℞ *investigational antineoplastic* [liposome-encapsulated doxorubicin]
TMB (trimedoxime bromide) [q.v.]
T-Medic Cold Syrup OTC *decongestant; antihistamine* [phenylpropanolamine HCl; chlorpheniramine maleate]
T-Medic Expectorant syrup OTC *decongestant; expectorant* [phenylpropanolamine HCl; guaifenesin]
TMP (trimethoprim) [q.v.]

TMP-SMZ (trimethoprim & sulfamethoxazole) *antibacterial antibiotics* [q.v.]
TNF (tumor necrosis factor) [q.v.]
TOAP (thioguanine, Oncovin, [cytosine] arabinoside, prednisone) *chemotherapy protocol*
TobraDex eye drop suspension ℞ *topical ophthalmic corticosteroidal anti-inflammatory; antibiotic* [dexamethasone; tobramycin]
TobraDex ophthalmic ointment ℞ *topical ophthalmic corticosteroidal anti-inflammatory; antibiotic* [dexamethasone; tobramycin; chlorobutanol]
tobramycin USAN, USP, INN, BAN *antibacterial antibiotic*
tobramycin sulfate USP *aminoglycoside bactericidal antibiotic*
Tobrex Drop-Tainers (eye drops), ophthalmic ointment ℞ *ophthalmic antibiotic* [tobramycin]
tobuterol INN
tocainide USAN, INN, BAN *antiarrhythmic*
tocainide HCl USP *antiarrhythmic*
tocamphyl USAN, INN *choleretic*
tocofenoxate INN
tocofersolan INN *vitamin E supplement* [also: tocophersolan]
tocofibrate INN
tocopherol, d-alpha [see: vitamin E]
tocopherol, dl-alpha [see: vitamin E]
tocopherols, mixed [see: vitamin E]
tocopherols excipient NF *antioxidant*
tocophersolan USAN *vitamin E supplement; (orphan: cholestatic hepatobiliary disease)* [also: tocofersolan]
tocopheryl acetate, d-alpha [see: vitamin E]
tocopheryl acetate, dl-alpha [see: vitamin E]
tocopheryl acid succinate, d-alpha [see: vitamin E]
tocopheryl acid succinate, dl-alpha [see: vitamin E]

tocopheryl polyethylene glycol succinate (TPGS) [see: tocophersolan]

Today vaginal sponge OTC *spermicidal contraceptive* [nonoxynol 9]

todralazine INN, BAN

tofenacin INN *anticholinergic* [also: tofenacin HCl]

tofenacin HCl USAN *anticholinergic* [also: tofenacin]

tofetridine INN

tofisoline

tofisopam INN

Tofranil film-coated tablets, IM injection ℞ *tricyclic antidepressant; treatment for childhood enuresis* [imipramine HCl]

Tofranil-PM capsules ℞ *tricyclic antidepressant; treatment for childhood enuresis* [imipramine pamoate]

Tolamide tablets (discontinued 1992) ℞ *antidiabetic* [tolazamide]

tolamolol USAN, INN *vasodilator; antiarrhythmic; antiadrenergic (β-receptor)*

tolazamide USAN, USP, INN, BAN *sulfonylurea-type antidiabetic*

tolazoline INN *peripheral vasodilator* [also: tolazoline HCl]

tolazoline HCl USP *antihypertensive; peripheral vasodilator* [also: tolazoline]

tolboxane INN

tolbutamide USP, INN, BAN *sulfonylurea-type antidiabetic*

tolbutamide sodium USP *diagnostic aid for diabetes*

tolciclate USAN, INN *antifungal*

tolclotide [see: disulfamide]

toldimfos INN, BAN

Tolectin 200; Tolectin 600 tablets ℞ *nonsteroidal anti-inflammatory drug (NSAID); antiarthritic; analgesic* [tolmetin sodium]

Tolectin DS capsules ℞ *nonsteroidal anti-inflammatory drug (NSAID); antiarthritic; analgesic* [tolmetin sodium]

Tolectin tablets, capsules ℞ *anti-inflammatory for arthritis* [tolmetin sodium]

Tolerex single-serving packets OTC *enteral maintenance diet* [multiple vitamins & minerals; essential & nonessential amino acids]

tolfamide USAN, INN *urease enzyme inhibitor*

tolfenamic acid INN, BAN

Tolfrinic film-coated tablets ℞ *hematinic* [ferrous fumarate; cyanocobalamin; ascorbic acid]

tolgabide USAN, INN, BAN *anticonvulsant*

tolhexamide [see: glycyclamide]

tolimidone USAN, INN *antiulcerative*

Tolinase tablets ℞ *antidiabetic* [tolazamide]

tolindate USAN, INN *antifungal*

toliodium chloride USAN, INN *veterinary food additive*

toliprolol INN

tolmesoxide INN

tolmetin USAN, INN *nonsteroidal anti-inflammatory drug (NSAID); analgesic*

tolmetin sodium USAN, USP *antiarthritic; nonsteroidal anti-inflammatory drug (NSAID); analgesic*

tolnaftate USAN, USP, INN, BAN *antifungal*

tolnapersine INN

tolnidamine INN

toloconium metilsulfate INN

tolofocon A USAN *hydrophobic contact lens material*

tolonidine INN

tolonium chloride INN

toloxatone INN

toloxichloral [see: toloxychlorinol]

toloxychlorinol INN

tolpadol INN

tolpentamide INN, BAN

tolperisone INN, BAN

tolpiprazole INN, BAN

tolpovidone I 131 USAN *hypoalbuminemia test; radioactive agent* [also: radiotolpovidone I 131]
tolpronine INN, BAN
tolpropamine INN, BAN
tolpyrramide USAN, INN *antidiabetic*
tolquinzole INN
tolrestat USAN, INN, BAN *aldose reductase inhibitor*
toltrazuril USAN, INN, BAN *veterinary coccidiostat*
tolu balsam USP *pharmaceutic aid*
p-**toluenesulfone dichloramine** [see: dichloramine T]
tolufazepam INN
toluidine blue O [see: tolonium chloride]
toluidine blue O chloride [see: tolonium chloride]
Tolu-Sed DM liquid OTC *antitussive; expectorant* [dextromethorphan hydrobromide; guaifenesin; alcohol]
Tolu-Sed liquid (discontinued 1991) ℞ *antitussive; expectorant* [codeine phosphate; guaifenesin; alcohol]
tolycaine INN, BAN
tomclukast USAN, INN *antiasthmatic; leukotriene antagonist*
Tomocat concentrated suspension ℞ *GI contrast radiopaque agent* [barium sulfate; sorbitol]
tomoglumide INN
tomoxetine INN *antidepressant* [also: tomoxetine HCl]
tomoxetine HCl USAN *antidepressant* [also: tomoxetine]
tomoxiprole INN
Tonavite-M liquid OTC *antianemic* [iron ammonium citrate; multiple B vitamins]
tonazocine INN *analgesic* [also: tonazocine mesylate]
tonazocine mesylate USAN *analgesic* [also: tonazocine]
Tonocard film-coated tablets ℞ *antiarrhythmic* [tocainide HCl]

Tonopaque powder for suspension ℞ *GI contrast radiopaque agent* [barium sulfate; sorbitol]
tonzonium bromide INN *detergent* [also: thonzonium bromide]
Topic gel OTC *antipruritic; counterirritant* [benzyl alcohol; camphor; menthol]
topical starch [see: starch, topical]
Topicort LP cream ℞ *topical corticosteroidal anti-inflammatory* [desoximetasone]
Topicort ointment, cream, gel ℞ *topical corticosteroidal anti-inflammatory* [desoximetasone]
Topicycline solution ℞ *topical antibiotic for acne vulgaris* [tetracycline HCl]
topiramate USAN, INN *anticonvulsant*
topotecan INN *antineoplastic; DNA topoisomerase I inhibitor* [also: topotecan HCl]
topotecan HCl USAN *antineoplastic; DNA topoisomerase I inhibitor* [also: topotecan]
toprilidine INN
Toprol XL film-coated extended-release tablets ℞ *antihypertensive; long-term antianginal; β-blocker* [metoprolol succinate]
topterone USAN, INN *antiandrogen*
TOPV (trivalent oral poliovirus vaccine) [see: poliovirus vaccine, live oral]
toquizine USAN, INN *anticholinergic*
Toradol film-coated tablets, Cartrix (prefilled syringes) and Tubex (cartridge-needle unit) for IM injection ℞ *nonsteroidal anti-inflammatory drug (NSAID)* [ketorolac tromethamine]
torasemide INN, BAN *diuretic* [also: torsemide]
torbafylline INN
Torecan IM injection, suppositories, tablets ℞ *antiemetic* [thiethylperazine maleate]

toremifene INN, BAN *antiestrogen; antineoplastic; (orphan: metastatic carcinoma of the breast)* [also: toremifene citrate]

toremifene citrate USAN *antiestrogen; antineoplastic* [also: toremifene]

toripristone INN

Tornalate oral inhalation aerosol, inhalation solution ℞ *bronchodilator* [bitolterol mesylate]

Torofor cream (discontinued 1991) OTC *topical antifungal; antibacterial* [clioquinol]

torsemide USAN *diuretic* [also: torasemide]

tosactide INN [also: octacosactrin]

tosifen USAN, INN *antianginal*

tosufloxacin USAN, INN *antibacterial*

tosulur INN

tosylchloramide sodium INN [also: chloramine-T]

Tota Vite tablets OTC *vitamin/mineral supplement* [multiple vitamins & minerals]

Totacillin capsules, powder for oral suspension ℞ *penicillin-type antibiotic* [ampicillin]

Totacillin-N powder for IV or IM injection ℞ *penicillin-type antibiotic* [ampicillin sodium]

Total Formula; Total Formula-2 tablets OTC *vitamin/mineral/iron supplement* [multiple vitamins & minerals; iron; folic acid; biotin]

Total Formula-3 tablets OTC *vitamin/mineral supplement* [multiple vitamins & minerals; folic acid; biotin]

Total solution OTC *contact lens wetting/soaking solution*

toughened silver nitrate [see: silver nitrate, toughened]

Touro LA long-acting caplets ℞ *decongestant; expectorant* [pseudoephedrine HCl; guaifenesin]

tozalinone INN *antidepressant* [also: thozalinone]

tPA; t-PA (tissue plasminogen activator) [see: alteplase]

T-Panol drops (for infants), oral solution (for children) OTC *analgesic* [acetaminophen]

TPDCV (thioguanine, procarbazine, DCD, CCNU, vincristine) *chemotherapy protocol*

TPGS (tocopheryl polyethylene glycol succinate) [see: tocophersolan]

T-Phyl timed-release tablets ℞ *bronchodilator* [theophylline]

TPI tablets (discontinued 1992) OTC *decongestant; antihistamine; antitussive; analgesic* [pseudoephedrine HCl; chlorpheniramine maleate; dextromethorphan hydrobromide; acetaminophen]

T-P-L troches OTC *oral antibacterial*

TPM Test OTC *in vitro diagnostic aid for toxoplasmosis*

TPN Electrolytes; TPN Electrolytes II; TPN Electrolytes III IV admixture ℞ *intravenous electrolyte therapy* [combined electrolyte solution]

traboxopine INN

Trac Tabs 2X tablets ℞ *urinary anti-infective; analgesic; antispasmodic; acidifier* [methenamine; phenyl salicylate; atropine sulfate; hyoscyamine sulfate; benzoic acid; methylene blue]

tracazolate USAN, INN, BAN *sedative*

Trace Metals Additive in 0.9% NaCl IV injection ℞ *intravenous nutritional therapy* [multiple trace elements (metals)]

Trace-4 IV injection (discontinued 1991) ℞ *intravenous nutritional therapy* [multiple trace elements (metals)]

Tracelyte; Tracelyte II; Tracelyte with Double Electrolytes; Tracelyte II with Double Electrolytes IV admixture ℞ *intravenous nutri-*

tional therapy [multiple trace elements (metals); electrolytes]
Tracer bG reagent strips OTC *in vitro diagnostic aid for blood glucose*
Tracrium IV infusion ℞ *neuromuscular blocker* [atracurium besylate]
tragacanth NF *suspending agent*
Tral Filmtabs (film-coated tablets) (discontinued 1991) ℞ *anticholinergic; peptic ulcer treatment adjunct* [hexocyclium methylsulfate]
tralonide USAN, INN *glucocorticoid*
tramadol INN *analgesic* [also: tramadol HCl]
tramadol HCl USAN *analgesic* [also: tramadol]
tramazoline INN *adrenergic* [also: tramazoline HCl]
tramazoline HCl USAN *adrenergic* [also: tramazoline]
Trancopal caplets ℞ *anxiolytic* [chlormezanone]
Trandate HCT tablets (discontinued 1992) ℞ *antihypertensive* [labetalol HCl; hydrochlorothiazide]
Trandate IV injection, tablets ℞ *antihypertensive; alpha- and beta-adrenergic blocking agent* [labetalol HCl]
trandolapril INN
trandolaprilat INN
tranexamic acid USAN, INN, BAN *systemic hemostatic; (orphan: angioneurotic edema; coagulopathies)*
tranilast USAN, INN *antiasthmatic*
Transact gel (discontinued 1991) OTC *antibacterial; exfoliant* [sulfur; alcohol]
transcainide USAN, INN *antiarrhythmic*
transclomiphene [now: zuclomiphene]
Transderm Scōp transdermal patch ℞ *motion sickness prevention* [scopolamine hydrobromide]
Transderm-Nitro transdermal patch ℞ *antianginal* [nitroglycerin]
Trans-Plantar transdermal patch ℞ *topical keratolytic* [salicylic acid]

***trans*-retinoic acid** [see: tretinoin]
Trans-Ver-Sal transdermal patch ℞ *topical keratolytic* [salicylic acid]
trantelinium bromide INN
Tranxene T-Tabs ("T"-imprinted tablets) ℞ *anxiolytic; minor tranquilizer; anticonvulsant adjunct* [clorazepate dipotassium]
Tranxene-SD; Tranxene-SD Half Strength single-dose tablets ℞ *anxiolytic; minor tranquilizer; anticonvulsant adjunct* [clorazepate dipotassium]
tranylcypromine INN *antidepressant; MAO inhibitor* [also: tranylcypromine sulfate]
tranylcypromine sulfate USP *antidepressant; MAO inhibitor* [also: tranylcypromine]
trapencaine INN
trapidil INN
trapymin [see: trapidil]
TraumaCal liquid OTC *oral nutritional supplement for trauma and severe burns*
Traum-Aid HBC powder OTC *oral nutritional supplement for trauma and sepsis*
Travase ointment ℞ *topical enzyme for biochemical debridement* [sutilains]
Travasol 2.75% in 5% (10%, 25%) Dextrose; Travasol 4.25% in 5% (10%, 25%) Dextrose IV infusion ℞ *total parenteral nutrition; peripheral parenteral nutrition* [multiple essential & nonessential amino acids; dextrose]
Travasol 3.5% (5.5%, 8.5%) with Electrolytes IV infusion ℞ *total parenteral nutrition (all except 3.5%); peripheral parenteral nutrition (all)* [multiple essential & nonessential amino acids & electrolytes]
Travasol 5.5% (8.5%, 10%) IV infusion ℞ *total parenteral nutrition; peripheral parenteral nutrition* [multiple essential & nonessential amino acids]

Travasorb Hepatic powder OTC *oral nutritional supplement for liver disease*
Travasorb HN; Travasorb MCT; Travasorb STD powder OTC *oral nutritional supplement*
Travasorb Renal powder OTC *oral nutritional supplement for renal failure*
5% Travert and Electrolyte No. 2; 10% Travert and Electrolyte No. 2 IV infusion ℞ *intravenous nutritional/electrolyte therapy* [combined electrolyte solution; invert sugar (50% dextrose + 50% fructose)]
Travert IV infusion ℞ *nonelectrolyte fluid and caloric replacement* [invert sugar (50% dextrose + 50% fructose) in water]
traxanox INN
Traypak (trademarked form) *multivial carton*
trazitiline INN
trazium esilate INN
trazodone INN *antidepressant* [also: trazodone HCl]
trazodone HCl USAN *antidepressant; used for panic disorders and aggressive behavior* [also: trazodone]
trazolopride INN
trebenzomine INN *antidepressant* [also: trebenzomine HCl]
trebenzomine HCl USAN *antidepressant* [also: trebenzomine]
trecadrine INN
Trecator-SC tablets ℞ *tuberculostatic* [ethionamide]
trefentanil HCl USAN *analgesic*
treloxinate USAN, INN *antihyperlipoproteinemic*
trenbolone INN, BAN *veterinary anabolic* [also: trenbolone acetate]
trenbolone acetate USAN *veterinary anabolic* [also: trenbolone]
Trendar tablets OTC *nonsteroidal anti-inflammatory drug (NSAID); antiarthritic; analgesic* [ibuprofen]
trengestone INN
trenizine INN

Trental controlled-release tablets ℞ *hemorrheologic agent; improve blood microcirculation* [pentoxifylline]
treosulfan INN, BAN
trepibutone INN
trepipam INN *sedative* [also: trepipam maleate]
trepipam maleate USAN *sedative* [also: trepipam]
trepirium iodide INN
treptilamine INN
trequinsin INN
trestolone INN *antineoplastic; androgen* [also: trestolone acetate]
trestolone acetate USAN *antineoplastic; androgen* [also: trestolone]
tretamine INN, BAN [also: triethylenemelamine]
trethinium tosilate INN
trethocanic acid INN
trethocanoic acid [see: trethocanic acid]
tretinoin USAN, USP, INN, BAN *keratolytic; (orphan: conjunctival and corneal squamous metaplasia; promyelocytic leukemia)*
tretoquinol INN
Trexan tablets ℞ *narcotic antagonist; (orphan: opiate blockage for withdrawal)* [naltrexone HCl]
TRH (thyrotropin-releasing hormone) [see: protirelin]
Tri Vit drops (discontinued 1992) OTC *vitamin supplement* [vitamins A, D & C]
Tri Vit with Fluoride drops ℞ *pediatric vitamin supplement and dental caries preventative* [vitamins A, D & C; fluoride]
triacana ℞ *(orphan: thyroid cancer)* [tiratricol]
Triacet cream ℞ *topical corticosteroid* [triamcinolone acetonide]
triacetin USP, INN *antifungal*
triacetyloleandomycin BAN *macrolide bactericidal antibiotic* [also: troleandomycin]

Triacin syrup OTC *decongestant; antihistamine* [pseudoephedrine HCl; triprolidine HCl]

Triacin-C syrup ℞ *decongestant; antihistamine; antitussive* [codeine phosphate; triprolidine HCl; pseudoephedrine HCl; alcohol]

triaconazole [now: terconazole]

Triad capsules ℞ *sedative; analgesic* [butalbital; acetaminophen; caffeine]

Triafed tablets OTC *decongestant; antihistamine* [pseudoephedrine HCl; triprolidine HCl]

Triafed with Codeine syrup ℞ *antihistamine; decongestant; antitussive* [triprolidine HCl; pseudoephedrine HCl; codeine phosphate]

triafungin USAN, INN *antifungal*

Triam Forte IM injection ℞ *glucocorticoids* [triamcinolone diacetate]

Triam-A IM, intra-articular, intrabursal, intradermal injection ℞ *glucocorticoids* [triamcinolone acetonide]

triamcinolone USP, INN, BAN *glucocorticoid*

triamcinolone acetonide USP *topical corticosteroid; inhalant for asthma*

triamcinolone acetonide sodium phosphate USAN *glucocorticoid*

triamcinolone benetonide INN

triamcinolone diacetate USP *glucocorticoid*

triamcinolone furetonide INN

triamcinolone hexacetonide USAN, USP, INN, BAN *glucocorticoid*

Triaminic Allergy; Triaminic Cold; Triaminic Chewable tablets OTC *decongestant; antihistamine* [phenylpropanolamine HCl; chlorpheniramine maleate]

Triaminic Expectorant DH liquid ℞ *decongestant; antihistamine; antitussive; expectorant* [phenylpropanolamine HCl; pyrilamine maleate; pheniramine maleate; hydrocodone bitartrate; guaifenesin]

Triaminic Expectorant liquid OTC *decongestant; expectorant* [phenylpropanolamine HCl; guaifenesin]

Triaminic Expectorant with Codeine liquid ℞ *decongestant; antitussive; expectorant* [phenylpropanolamine HCl; codeine phosphate; guaifenesin; alcohol]

Triaminic Nite Light liquid OTC *pediatric decongestant, antihistamine and antitussive* [pseudoephedrine HCl; chlorpheniramine maleate; dextromethorphan hydrobromide]

Triaminic oral infant drops ℞ *pediatric decongestant and antihistamine* [phenylpropanolamine HCl; pyrilamine maleate; pheniramine maleate]

Triaminic TR sustained-release tablets ℞ *decongestant; antihistamine* [phenylpropanolamine HCl; pyrilamine maleate; pheniramine maleate]

Triaminic-12 sustained-release tablets OTC *decongestant; antihistamine* [phenylpropanolamine HCl; chlorpheniramine maleate]

Triaminic-DM syrup OTC *decongestant; antitussive* [phenylpropanolamine HCl; dextromethorphan hydrobromide]

Triaminicin (name changed to Triaminicin Cold, Allergy, Sinus in 1993)

Triaminicin Cold, Allergy, Sinus tablets OTC *decongestant; antihistamine; analgesic* [phenylpropanolamine HCl; chlorpheniramine maleate; acetaminophen]

Triaminicol Multi-Symptom Cold tablets OTC *decongestant; antihistamine; antitussive* [phenylpropanolamine HCl; chlorpheniramine maleate; dextromethorphan hydrobromide]

Triaminicol Multi-Symptom Relief liquid OTC *decongestant; antihistamine; antitussive* [phenylpropanolamine HCl; chlorpheniramine maleate; dextromethorphan hydrobromide]

Triamolone 40 IM injection ℞ *glucocorticoids* [triamcinolone diacetate]

Triamonide 40 IM, intra-articular, intrabursal, intradermal injection ℞ *glucocorticoids* [triamcinolone acetonide]

triampyzine INN *anticholinergic* [also: triampyzine sulfate]

triampyzine sulfate USAN *anticholinergic* [also: triampyzine]

triamterene USAN, USP, INN *potassium-sparing diuretic*

trianisestrol [see: chlorotrianisene]

Triaprin capsules ℞ *analgesic; antipyretic; sedative* [acetaminophen; caffeine; butalbital]

Tri-Aqua tablets OTC *diuretic* [caffeine; buchu, uva ursi, zea, & triticum extracts]

Triasyn B capsules, tablets (discontinued 1993) OTC *vitamin supplement* [vitamins B_1, B_2 & B_3]

Triavil 2-10; Triavil 2-25; Triavil 4-10; Triavil 4-25; Triavil 4-50 tablets ℞ *antipsychotic; antidepressant* [perphenazine; amitriptyline HCl]

triaziquone INN, BAN

triazolam USAN, USP, INN *sedative; hypnotic*

Triban; Pediatric Triban suppositories ℞ *anticholinergic; antiemetic* [trimethobenzamide HCl]

Tri-Barbs capsules (discontinued 1993) ℞ *sedative; hypnotic* [phenobarbital; butabarbital sodium; secobarbital sodium]

tribasic calcium phosphate [see: calcium phosphate, tribasic]

tribavirin BAN *antiviral* [also: ribavirin]

tribendilol INN

tribenoside USAN, INN *sclerosing agent*

Tribiotic Plus ointment OTC *topical antibiotic; anesthetic* [polymyxin B sulfate; neomycin sulfate; bacitracin; lidocaine]

tribromoethanol NF

tribromomethane [see: bromoform]

tribromsalan USAN, INN *disinfectant*

Tri-Buffered Aspirin tablets OTC *analgesic; antipyretic; anti-inflammatory* [aspirin; calcium carbonate; magnesium oxide; magnesium carbonate]

tribuzone INN

tricalcium phosphate [see: calcium phosphate, tribasic]

tricetamide USAN *sedative*

Trichinella extract USP

Tri-Chlor liquid ℞ *cauterant; keratolytic* [trichloroacetic acid]

trichlorethoxyphosphamide [see: defosfamide]

Trichlorex tablets ℞ *diuretic; antihypertensive* [trichlormethiazide]

trichlorisobutylalcohol [see: chlorobutanol]

trichlormethiazide USP, INN *diuretic; antihypertensive*

trichlormethine INN [also: trimustine]

trichloroacetic acid USP *strong keratolytic/cauterant*

trichlorocarbanilide (TCC) [see: triclocarban]

trichloroethylene NF, INN

trichlorofluoromethane [see: trichloromonofluoromethane]

trichlorofon [see: metrifonate]

trichloromonofluoromethane NF *aerosol propellant*

trichlorphon [see: metrifonate]

Trichophyton extract *diagnosis and treatment of Trichophyton-induced skin infections*

trichorad [see: acinitrazole]

trichosanthin *investigational antiviral for AIDS*

Trichotine Douche powder OTC *antiseptic/germicidal; vaginal cleanser and deodorizer; acidity modifier* [sodium perborate]

Trichotine Douche solution OTC *antiseptic/germicidal; vaginal cleanser and deodorizer; acidity modifier* [sodium borate]
triciribine INN *antineoplastic* [also: triciribine phosphate]
triciribine phosphate USAN *antineoplastic* [also: triciribine]
triclabendazole INN
triclacetamol INN
triclazate INN
triclobisonium chloride NF, INN
triclocarban USAN, INN *disinfectant*
triclodazol INN
triclofenol piperazine USAN, INN *anthelmintic*
triclofos INN *hypnotic; sedative* [also: triclofos sodium]
triclofos sodium USAN *hypnotic; sedative* [also: triclofos]
triclofylline INN
triclonide USAN, INN *anti-inflammatory*
triclosan USAN, INN, BAN *disinfectant/antiseptic*
Tricodene Cough and Cold liquid ℞ *antihistamine; antitussive* [pyrilamine maleate; codeine phosphate]
Tricodene Forte; Tricodene NN liquid OTC *decongestant; antihistamine; antitussive* [phenylpropanolamine HCl; chlorpheniramine maleate; dextromethorphan hydrobromide]
Tricodene Pediatric liquid OTC *decongestant; antitussive* [phenylpropanolamine HCl; dextromethorphan hydrobromide]
Tricodene Sugar Free liquid OTC *antihistamine; antitussive* [chlorpheniramine maleate; dextromethorphan hydrobromide]
Tricom tablets OTC *decongestant; antihistamine; analgesic* [pseudoephedrine HCl; chlorpheniramine maleate; acetaminophen]
Triconsil chewable tablets (discontinued 1991) OTC *antacid* [aluminum hydroxide; sodium bicarbonate; magnesium trisilicate]
tricosactide INN
Tricosal film-coated tablets ℞ *analgesic; antipyretic; antirheumatic* [choline magnesium trisalicylate]
tricyclamol chloride INN
Triderm cream ℞ *topical corticosteroid* [trimacinolone acetonide]
Tridesilon cream, ointment ℞ *topical corticosteroidal anti-inflammatory* [desonide]
Tridesilon Otic [see: Otic Tridesilon]
Tri-Desogen ℞ *investigational oral contraceptive*
tridihexethyl chloride USP *peptic ulcer adjunct*
tridihexethyl iodide INN
Tridil IV infusion ℞ *antianginal; perioperative antihypertensive; for congestive heart failure with myocardial infarction* [nitroglycerin]
Tridione capsules, Dulcets (chewable tablets), oral solution ℞ *anticonvulsant* [trimethadione]
Tridrate Bowel Evacuant Kit oral solution + 3 tablets + 1 suppository OTC *pre-procedure bowel evacuant* [magnesium citrate (solution); bisacodyl (tablets & suppository)]
trientine INN *chelating agent* [also: trientine HCl; trientine dihydrochloride]
trientine dihydrochloride BAN *chelating agent* [also: trientine HCl; trientine]
trientine HCl USAN, USP *chelating agent; (orphan: Wilson's disease)* [also: trientine; trientine dihydrochloride]
triethanolamine [now: trolamine]
triethyl citrate NF *plasticizer*
triethyleneiminobenzoquinone (TEIB) [see: triaziquone]
triethylenemelamine NF [also: tretamine]
triethylenethiophosphoramide (TSPA; TESPA) [see: thiotepa]

Trifed tablets ℞ *decongestant; antihistamine* [pseudoephedrine HCl; triprolidine HCl]

Trifed-C Cough syrup ℞ *decongestant; antihistamine; antitussive* [pseudoephedrine HCl; triprolidine HCl; codeine phosphate; alcohol]

trifenagrel USAN, INN *antithrombotic*

trifezolac INN

triflocin USAN, INN *diuretic*

triflubazam USAN, INN *minor tranquilizer*

triflumidate USAN, INN *anti-inflammatory*

trifluomeprazine INN, BAN

trifluoperazine INN *antipsychotic; sedative* [also: trifluoperazine HCl]

trifluoperazine HCl USP *antipsychotic; sedative* [also: trifluoperazine]

trifluorothymidine [see: trifluridine]

trifluperidol USAN, INN *antipsychotic*

triflupromazine USP, INN *antiemetic; antipsychotic; antidopaminergic*

triflupromazine HCl USP *antipsychotic; antiemetic*

trifluridine USAN, INN *ophthalmic antiviral*

triflusal INN

Trigesic tablets OTC *analgesic; antipyretic; anti-inflammatory* [acetaminophen; aspirin; caffeine]

trigevolol INN

α-triglycidyl isocyanurate (α-TGI) [see: teroxirone]

TriHemic 600 film-coated tablets ℞ *hematinic* [ferrous fumarate; vitamins B_{12} & C; intrinsic factor concentrate; folic acid]

Trihexy-2; Trihexy-5 tablets ℞ *anticholinergic; antiparkinsonian agent* [trihexyphenidyl HCl]

trihexyphenidyl INN *anticholinergic; antiparkinsonian* [also: trihexyphenidyl HCl; benzhexol]

trihexyphenidyl HCl USP *anticholinergic; antiparkinsonian* [also: trihexyphenidyl; benzhexol]

Tri-Hist Expectorant syrup OTC *decongestant; expectorant* [phenylpropanolamine HCl; guaifenesin]

Tri-Hist syrup OTC *decongestant; antihistamine* [phenylpropanolamine HCl; chlorpheniramine maleate]

Tri-Hydroserpine tablets ℞ *antihypertensive* [hydrochlorothiazide; reserpine; hydralazine HCl]

Tri-Immunol IM injection ℞ *immunization against diphtheria, tetanus and pertussis (DTP)* [diphtheria & tetanus toxoids & pertussis vaccine, adsorbed]

triiodothyronine sodium, levo [see: liothyronine sodium]

Tri-K liquid ℞ *potassium supplement* [potassium acetate; potassium bicarbonate; potassium citrate]

trikates USP *electrolyte replenisher*

Trikates liquid (discontinued 1991) ℞ *potassium supplement* [potassium acetate; potassium bicarbonate; potassium citrate]

Tri-Kort IM, intra-articular, intrabursal, intradermal injection ℞ *glucocorticoids* [triamcinolone acetonide]

Trilafon tablets, oral concentrate, IV or IM injection ℞ *antipsychotic; antidopaminergic; antiemetic* [perphenazine]

triletide INN

Tri-Levlen tablets ℞ *oral contraceptive* [levonorgestrel; ethinyl estradiol]

Trilisate tablets, liquid ℞ *analgesic; antipyretic; anti-inflammatory; antirheumatic* [choline salicylate; magnesium salicylate]

trilithium citrate tetrahydrate [see: lithium citrate]

Trilog IM, intra-articular, intrabursal, intradermal injection ℞ *glucocorticoids* [triamcinolone acetonide]

Trilone IM injection ℞ *glucocorticoids* [triamcinolone diacetate]

trilostane USAN, INN, BAN *adrenocortical suppressant*

Trimazide capsules, suppositories ℞ *anticholinergic; antiemetic* [trimethobenzamide HCl]
trimazosin INN, BAN *antihypertensive* [also: trimazosin HCl]
trimazosin HCl USAN *antihypertensive* [also: trimazosin]
Trimcaps sustained-release capsules (discontinued 1992) ℞ *anorexiant* [phendimetrazine tartrate]
trimebutine INN
trimecaine INN
Trimedine liquid OTC *decongestant; antihistamine; antitussive* [phenylephrine HCl; chlorpheniramine maleate; dextromethorphan hydrobromide]
trimedoxime bromide INN
trimeperidine INN, BAN
trimeprazine tartrate USP *antipruritic; antihistamine* [also: alimemazine]
trimeproprimine [see: trimipramine]
trimetamide INN
trimetaphan camsilate INN *antihypertensive* [also: trimethaphan camsylate; trimetaphan camsylate]
trimetaphan camsylate BAN *antihypertensive* [also: trimethaphan camsylate; trimetaphan camsilate]
trimetazidine INN, BAN
trimethadione USP, INN *anticonvulsant* [also: troxidone]
trimethamide [see: trimetamide]
trimethaphan camphorsulfonate [see: trimethaphan camsylate]
trimethaphan camsylate USP *emergency antihypertensive* [also: trimetaphan camsilate; trimetaphan camsylate]
trimethidinium methosulfate NF, INN
trimethobenzamide INN *antiemetic; anticholinergic* [also: trimethobenzamide HCl]
trimethobenzamide HCl USP *antiemetic; anticholinergic* [also: trimethobenzamide]

trimethoprim (TMP) USAN, USP, INN, BAN *antibacterial antibiotic*
trimethoprim sulfate USAN *antibacterial*
trimethoquinol [see: tretoquinol]
trimethylammonium chloride carbamate [see: bethanechol chloride]
trimethylene [see: cyclopropane]
trimethyltetradecylammonium bromide [see: tetradonium bromide]
trimetozine USAN, INN *sedative*
trimetrexate USAN, INN, BAN *antineoplastic*
trimetrexate glucuronate USAN *antineoplastic; (orphan: Pneumocystis carinii pneumonia of AIDS; multiple cancers)*
trimexiline INN
Triminol Cough syrup OTC *decongestant; antihistamine; antitussive* [phenylpropanolamine HCl; chlorpheniramine maleate; dextromethorphan hydrobromide]
Tri-Minulet ℞ *investigational oral contraceptive* [triphasic gestodene]
trimipramine USAN, INN *antidepressant*
trimipramine maleate USAN *tricyclic antidepressant*
trimolide [see: trimetozine]
trimopam maleate [now: trepipam maleate]
trimoprostil USAN, INN *gastric antisecretory*
Trimo-San vaginal jelly OTC *antibacterial* [oxyquinoline sulfate; boric acid]
Trimox '125'; Trimox '250' powder for oral suspension ℞ *penicillin-type antibiotic* [amoxicillin trihydrate]
Trimox '250'; Trimox '500' capsules ℞ *penicillin-type antibiotic* [amoxicillin trihydrate]
trimoxamine INN *antihypertensive* [also: trimoxamine HCl]
trimoxamine HCl USAN *antihypertensive* [also: trimoxamine]

Trimpex tablets ℞ *anti-infective; antibacterial* [trimethoprim]
Trimstat tablets ℞ *anorexiant* [phendimetrazine tartrate]
Trimtabs tablets (discontinued 1992) ℞ *anorexiant* [phendimetrazine tartrate]
trimustine BAN [also: trichlormethine]
Trimycin ointment (discontinued 1991) OTC *topical antibiotic; antihistamine* [polymyxin B sulfate; neomycin sulfate; bacitracin; diperodon HCl]
Trinalin Repetabs (repeat-action tablets) ℞ *decongestant; antihistamine* [pseudoephedrine sulfate; azatadine maleate]
Trinasal nasal spray ℞ *investigational treatment for allergic rhinitis*
Trind liquid OTC *antihistamine; decongestant* [phenylpropanolamine HCl; chlorpheniramine maleate]
Trind-DM liquid OTC *antitussive; antihistamine; decongestant* [phenylpropanolamine HCl; dextromethorphan hydrobromide; chlorpheniramine maleate; alcohol]
Tri-Nefrin tablets OTC *decongestant; antihistamine* [phenylpropanolamine HCl; chlorpheniramine maleate]
trinitrin [see: nitroglycerin]
trinitrophenol NF
Tri-Norinyl tablets ℞ *oral contraceptive* [norethindrone; ethinyl estradiol]
Trinsicon capsules ℞ *hematinic* [ferrous fumarate; vitamins B_{12} & C; intrinsic factor concentrate; folic acid]
Trinsicon M capsules (discontinued 1992) ℞ *antianemic* [ferrous fumarate; intrinsic factor; vitamins B_{12} & C]
Triofed syrup OTC *decongestant; antihistamine* [triprolidine HCl; pseudoephedrine HCl]
triolein I 125 USAN *radioactive agent*
triolein I 131 USAN *radioactive agent*

Trio-Mycin ointment OTC *topical antibiotic*
trional [see: sulfonethylmethane]
Triostat IV injection ℞ *treatment of myxedema coma or precoma (orphan)* [liothyronine sodium]
Triotann tablets, pediatric oral suspension ℞ *decongestant; antihistamine* [phenylephrine tannate; chlorpheniramine tannate; pyrilamine tannate]
trioxifene INN *antiestrogen* [also: trioxifene mesylate]
trioxifene mesylate USAN *antiestrogen* [also: trioxifene]
trioxsalen USAN, USP *pigmentation agent for vitiligo; antipsoriatic* [also: trioxysalen]
trioxyethylrutin [see: troxerutin]
trioxymethylene [see: paraformaldehyde]
trioxysalen INN *pigmentation agent* [also: trioxsalen]
Tri-Pain tablets OTC *analgesic; antipyretic; anti-inflammatory* [acetaminophen; aspirin; salicylamide; caffeine]
Tripalgen Cold syrup OTC *decongestant; antihistamine* [phenylpropanolamine HCl; chlorpheniramine maleate]
tripamide USAN, INN *antihypertensive; diuretic*
triparanol INN *(withdrawn from market)*
Tripedia IM injection ℞ *immunization against diphtheria, tetanus and pertussis (DTP)* [diphtheria toxoid; tetanus toxoid; pertussis antigens]
tripelennamine INN *antihistamine* [also: tripelennamine citrate]
tripelennamine citrate USP *antihistamine* [also: tripelennamine]
tripelennamine HCl USP *antihistamine*
Triphasil tablets ℞ *oral contraceptive* [levonorgestrel; ethinyl estradiol]
Tri-Phen-Chlor syrup, pediatric syrup, pediatric drops ℞ *decongestant; antihistamine* [phenylpropanol-

amine HCl; phenylephrine HCl; chlorpheniramine maleate; phenyltoloxamine citrate]

Tri-Phen-Chlor T.R. timed-release tablets ℞ *decongestant; antihistamine* [phenylpropanolamine HCl; phenylephrine HCl; chlorpheniramine maleate; phenyltoloxamine citrate]

Triphenyl Expectorant liquid OTC *decongestant; expectorant* [phenylpropanolamine HCl; guaifenesin; alcohol]

Triphenyl syrup OTC *antihistamine; decongestant* [phenylpropanolamine HCl; chlorpheniramine maleate]

Triphenyl T.D. sustained-release tablets (discontinued 1992) ℞ *decongestant; antihistamine* [phenylpropanolamine HCl; pyrilamine maleate; pheniramine maleate]

Triple Antibiotic DP ointment (discontinued 1991) OTC *topical antibiotic; antihistamine* [polymyxin B sulfate; neomycin sulfate; bacitracin; diperodon HCl]

Triple Antibiotic ointment OTC *topical antibiotic* [polymyxin B sulfate; neomycin sulfate; bacitracin]

Triple Antibiotic Ophthalmic ointment ℞ *ophthalmic antibiotic* [polymyxin B sulfate; neomycin sulfate; bacitracin]

Triple Antibiotic with HC ophthalmic ointment ℞ *topical ophthalmic corticosteroidal anti-inflammatory; antibiotic* [hydrocortisone; neomycin sulfate; bacitracin zinc; polymyxin B sulfate]

Triple Paste ointment OTC *topical diaper rash treatment* [zinc oxide; aluminum acetate]

Triple Sulfa No. 2 tablets ℞ *broad-spectrum bacteriostatic* [trisulfapyrimidines]

Triple Sulfa vaginal cream (discontinued 1991) ℞ *broad-spectrum bacteriostatic* [sulfathiazole; sulfacetamide; sulfabenzamide; urea]

Triple Vita Drops (discontinued 1992) OTC *vitamin supplement* [vitamins A, D & C]

Triple Vitamin ADC with Fluoride drops ℞ *pediatric vitamin supplement and dental caries preventative* [vitamins A, D & C; fluoride]

Triple Vitamins with Fluoride chewable tablets ℞ *vitamin supplement; dental caries preventative* [vitamins A, D & C; fluoride]

Triple X Kit liquid + shampoo OTC *pediculicide* [pyrethrins; piperonyl butoxide; petroleum distillate]

Triple-Gen eye drop suspension ℞ *topical ophthalmic corticosteroidal anti-inflammatory; antibiotic* [hydrocortisone; neomycin sulfate; polymyxin B sulfate]

Triple-Vita-Flor drops (discontinued 1993) ℞ *pediatric vitamin supplement and dental caries preventative* [multiple vitamins; fluoride]

Triplevite with Fluoride drops (discontinued 1993) ℞ *pediatric vitamin supplement and dental caries preventative* [multiple vitamins; fluoride]

Tripodrine tablets (discontinued 1992) OTC *decongestant; antihistamine* [pseudoephedrine HCl; triprolidine HCl]

Triposed syrup, tablets OTC *decongestant; antihistamine* [triprolidine HCl; pseudoephedrine HCl]

tripotassium citrate monohydrate [see: potassium citrate]

triprolidine INN *antihistamine* [also: triprolidine HCl]

triprolidine HCl USP *antihistamine* [also: triprolidine]

Triptone long-acting caplets OTC *antinauseant; antiemetic; antivertigo; motion sickness preventative* [dimenhydrinate]

triptorelin USAN, INN *antineoplastic*

triptorelin pamoate *(orphan: ovarian carcinoma)*

trisaccharides A & B (orphan: newborn hemolytic disease; ABO blood incompatibility of organ or bone marrow transplants)
Trisequens ℞ investigational osteoporosis treatment [17-beta-estradiol; norethindrone acetate]
trisodium citrate [see: sodium citrate]
trisodium citrate dihydrate [see: sodium citrate]
trisodium hydrogen ethylenediaminetetraacetate [see: edetate trisodium]
Trisol eye wash OTC *ocular irrigation*
Trisoralen tablets ℞ *taken before exposure to sunlight to enhance repigmentation* [trioxsalen]
Tri-Statin II cream ℞ *topical corticosteroid; antifungal* [triamcinolone acetonide; nystatin]
Tristoject IM injection ℞ *glucocorticoids* [triamcinolone diacetate]
trisulfapyrimidines (a mixture of sulfadiazine, sulfamerazine, and sulfamethazine) USP *broad-spectrum bacteriostatic*
Tritan tablets ℞ *antihistamine; decongestant* [phenylephrine tannate; chlorpheniramine tannate; pyrilamine tannate]
Tritann Pediatric suspension ℞ *pediatric antihistamine and decongestant* [phenylephrine tannate; chlorpheniramine tannate; pyrilamine tannate]
Tri-Tannate Plus Pediatric oral suspension ℞ *pediatric decongestant, antihistamine and antitussive* [phenylephrine tannate; ephedrine tannate; chlorpheniramine tannate; carbetapentane tannate]
Tri-Tannate tablets, pediatric oral suspension ℞ *decongestant; antihistamine* [phenylephrine tannate; chlorpheniramine tannate; pyrilamine tannate]
Tri-Thalmic HC ophthalmic ointment ℞ *topical corticosteroid; antibiotic* [bacitracin zinc; neomycin sulfate; polymyxin B sulfate; hydrocortisone]
Tri-Thalmic ophthalmic ointment, ophthalmic solution ℞ *topical antibiotic* [bacitracin zinc; neomycin sulfate; polymyxin B sulfate]
tritheon [see: acinitrazole]
tritiated water USAN *radioactive agent*
Tri-Tinic capsules ℞ *antianemic* [ferrous fumarate; intrinsic factor; vitamins B_{12} & C; folic acid]
tritiozine INN
tritoqualine INN
Triva Douche powder OTC *antiseptic/germicidal; vaginal cleanser and deodorizer* [oxyquinoline sulfate]
trivalent oral poliovirus vaccine (TOPV) [see: poliovirus vaccine, live oral]
Tri-Vi-Flor chewable tablets, drops ℞ *pediatric vitamin supplement and dental caries preventative* [vitamins A, C & D; sodium fluoride]
Tri-Vi-Flor with Iron drops ℞ *pediatric vitamin/iron supplement and dental caries preventative* [vitamins A, C & D; iron; sodium fluoride]
Tri-Vi-Sol drops OTC *pediatric vitamin supplement* [vitamins A, D & C]
Tri-Vi-Sol with Iron drops OTC *vitamin/iron supplement* [multiple vitamins; iron]
Trivitamin Fluoride chewable tablets, drops ℞ *pediatric vitamin supplement and dental caries preventative* [vitamins A, C & D; fluoride]
Tri-Vitamin Infants' Drops OTC *vitamin supplement* [vitamins A, D & C]
Tri-Vitamin with Fluoride drops ℞ *pediatric vitamin supplement and dental caries preventative* [multiple vitamins; fluoride]
trixolane INN
trizoxime INN
Trizyme (ingredient) OTC *digestive enzymes* [amylolytic, proteolytic &

cellulolytic enzymes (amylase; protease; cellulase)]

Trobicin powder for IM injection ℞ *antibiotic* [spectinomycin HCl]

Trocaine lozenges OTC *topical anesthetic; oral antiseptic; expectorant* [benzocaine; cetylpyridinium chloride; terpin hydrate]

Trocal lozenges OTC *antitussive* [dextromethorphan hydrobromide]

trocimine INN

troclosene potassium USAN, INN *topical anti-infective*

Trofan; Trofan-DS tablets OTC *dietary amino acid supplement* [L-tryptophan]

trofosfamide INN

trolamine NF *alkalizing agent; analgesic*

troleandomycin USAN, USP *macrolide bactericidal antibiotic; (orphan: severe asthma)* [also: triacetyloleandomycin]

trolnitrate INN

trolnitrate phosphate [see: trolnitrate]

tromantadine INN

trometamol INN, BAN *alkalizer for cardiac bypass surgery* [also: tromethamine]

tromethamine USAN, USP *alkalizer for cardiac bypass surgery* [also: trometamol]

Tronolane anorectal cream, suppositories OTC *topical local anesthetic; astringent* [pramoxine HCl; zinc oxide]

Tronothane HCl cream OTC *topical local anesthetic* [pramoxine HCl]

tropabazate INN

Tropamine + capsules (discontinued 1993) OTC *dietary supplement* [multiple amino acids, vitamins & minerals]

tropanserin INN, BAN *migraine-specific serotonin receptor antagonist* [also: tropanserin HCl]

tropanserin HCl USAN *migraine-specific serotonin receptor antagonist* [also: tropanserin]

tropapride INN

tropatepine INN

tropenziline bromide INN

TrophAmine 6%; TrophAmine 10% IV infusion ℞ *total parenteral nutrition; peripheral parenteral nutrition* [multiple essential & nonessential amino acids]

Troph-Iron liquid OTC *hematinic* [ferric pyrophosphate; vitamins B_1 & B_{12}]

Trophite liquid OTC *vitamin supplement* [vitamins B_1 & B_{12}]

trophosphamide [see: trofosfamide]

Tropicacyl eye drops ℞ *cycloplegic; mydriatic* [tropicamide]

tropicamide USAN, USP, INN *ophthalmic anticholinergic; cycloplegic; short-acting mydriatic*

tropigline INN, BAN

tropirine INN

tropodifene INN

troquidazole INN

trospectomycin INN, BAN *antibacterial* [also: trospectomycin sulfate]

trospectomycin sulfate USAN *antibacterial* [also: trospectomycin]

trospium chloride INN

troxerutin INN, BAN *vitamin P_4*

troxidone BAN *anticonvulsant* [also: trimethadione]

troxipide INN

troxolamide INN

troxonium tosilate INN [also: troxonium tosylate]

troxonium tosylate BAN [also: troxonium tosilate]

troxypyrrolium tosilate INN [also: troxypyrrolium tosylate]

troxypyrrolium tosylate BAN [also: troxypyrrolium tosilate]

True Test patch ℞ *investigational diagnostic aid for contact dermatitis*

Truphylline suppositories ℞ *bronchodilator* [aminophylline]

Trutol oral liquid ℞ *glucose tolerance test beverage* [glucose]
truxicurium iodide INN
truxipicurium iodide INN
trypaflavine [see: acriflavine HCl]
tryparsamide USP, INN
trypsin, crystallized USP *topical proteolytic enzyme; necrotic tissue debridement*
Tryptacin tablets OTC *dietary amino acid supplement* [L-tryptophan]
tryptizol [see: amitriptyline]
tryptizol HCl [see: amitriptyline HCl]
tryptophan (L-tryptophan) USAN, USP, INN *essential amino acid; serotonin precursor (The FDA has recalled all OTC tryptophan supplements.)*
Trysul vaginal cream ℞ *bacteriostatic* [sulfathiazole; sulfacetamide; sulfabenzamide; urea]
TSC (technetium sulfur colloid) [see: technetium Tc 99m sulfur colloid]
TSH (thyroid stimulating hormone) [see: thyrotropin]
TSPA (triethylenethiophosphoramide) [see: thiotepa]
T-Stat 2% topical solution ℞ *topical antibiotic for acne vulgaris* [erythromycin]
T-Tabs (trademarked form) *"T"-imprinted tablets*
T-Tussin CF liquid OTC *expectorant; decongestant; antitussive* [guaifenesin; phenylpropanolamine HCl; dextromethorphan hydrobromide; alcohol]
T-Tussin DM liquid OTC *expectorant; antitussive* [guaifenesin; dextromethorphan hydrobromide; alcohol]
T-Tussin Expectorant liquid OTC *expectorant* [guaifenesin]
T-Tussin PE liquid OTC *expectorant; decongestant* [guaifenesin; pseudoephedrine HCl; alcohol]
tuaminoheptane USP, INN *adrenergic; vasoconstrictor*
tuaminoheptane sulfate USP
tuberculin USP *dermal tuberculosis test*

tuberculin, crude [see: tuberculin]
tuberculin, old (OT) [see: tuberculin]
Tuberculin Mono-Vacc Test (O.T.) single-use intradermal puncture test device ℞ *tuberculosis skin test* [old tuberculin]
tuberculin purified protein derivative (PPD) [see: tuberculin]
Tuberculin Tine Test, Old single-use intradermal puncture test device ℞ *tuberculosis skin test* [old tuberculin]
tuberculosis vaccine [see: BCG vaccine]
Tubersol intradermal injection ℞ *tuberculosis skin test* [tuberculin purified protein derivative]
Tubex (trademarked delivery system) *cartridge-needle unit*
tubocurarine chloride USP, INN, BAN *neuromuscular blocker; muscle relaxant*
tubocurarine chloride HCl pentahydrate [see: tubocurarine chloride]
tubulozole INN *antineoplastic; microtubule inhibitor* [also: tubulozole HCl]
tubulozole HCl USAN, INN *antineoplastic; microtubule inhibitor* [also: tubulozole]
Tucks Hemorrhoidal cream OTC *astringent* [hamamelis water]
Tucks ointment (discontinued 1991) OTC *astringent* [hamamelis water]
Tucks; Tucks Take-Alongs anorectal pads OTC *astringent; antiseptic; antifungal* [witch hazel; glycerin; benzalkonium chloride; citric acid; methylparaben]
tuclazepam INN
Tuinal Pulvules (capsules) ℞ *sedative; hypnotic* [amobarbital sodium; secobarbital sodium]
tulobuterol INN, BAN
tumor necrosis factor (TNF) *investigational immunomodulator for AIDS*
Tums Plus; Tums with Simethicone liquid OTC *antacid; antiflatu-*

lent [calcium carbonate; simethicone]

Tums; Tums E-X chewable tablets, liquid OTC *antacid* [calcium carbonate]

tungsten *element* (W)

Turbinaire (trademarked form) *intranasal aerosol*

Tusal IM injection ℞ *analgesic; antipyretic; anti-inflammatory; antirheumatic* [sodium thiosalicylate]

Tusquelin syrup ℞ *decongestant; antihistamine; antitussive* [phenylpropanolamine HCl; phenylephrine HCl; chlorpheniramine maleate; dextromethorphan hydrobromide]

Tuss-Ade extended-release capsules ℞ *decongestant* [phenylpropanolamine HCl; caramiphen edisylate]

Tussafed syrup, pediatric drops ℞ *antitussive; antihistamine; decongestant* [carbinoxamine maleate; pseudoephedrine HCl; dextromethorphan hydrobromide; alcohol]

Tussafin Expectorant liquid ℞ *decongestant; antitussive; expectorant* [pseudoephedrine HCl; hydrocodone bitartrate; guaifenesin; alcohol]

Tuss-Allergine Modified T.D. capsules ℞ *decongestant; antitussive* [phenylpropanolamine HCl; caramiphen edisylate]

Tussanil DH liquid ℞ *decongestant; antihistamine; antitussive* [phenylephrine HCl; chlorpheniramine maleate; hydrocodone bitartrate; alcohol]

Tussanil DH tablets ℞ *decongestant; antitussive; expectorant; analgesic* [phenylpropanolamine HCl; hydrocodone bitartrate; guaifenesin; salicylamide]

Tussanil Plain syrup ℞ *decongestant; antihistamine* [phenylephrine HCl; chlorpheniramine maleate; alcohol]

Tussar DM Cough syrup ℞ *antitussive; antihistamine; decongestant* [dextromethorphan hydrobromide; chlorpheniramine maleate; pseudoephedrine HCl]

Tussar SF; Tussar-2 liquid ℞ *antitussive; antihistamine; expectorant* [codeine phosphate; pseudoephedrine HCl; guaifenesin; alcohol]

Tuss-DA liquid ℞ *decongestant; antitussive* [dextromethorphan; pseudoephedrine HCl]

Tuss-DM tablets OTC *antitussive; expectorant* [dextromethorphan hydrobromide; guaifenesin]

Tussex Cough syrup OTC *decongestant; antitussive; expectorant* [dextromethorphan hydrobromide; phenylephrine HCl; guaifenesin]

Tussgen liquid ℞ *decongestant; antitussive* [pseudoephedrine HCl; hydrodocone bitartrate; alcohol]

Tuss-Genade Modified sustained-release capsules ℞ *decongestant; antitussive* [phenylpropanolamine HCl; caramiphen edisylate]

Tusside liquid (discontinued 1992) ℞ *antitussive; expectorant* [dextromethorphan hydrobromide; iodinated glycerol]

Tussigon tablets ℞ *antitussive* [hydrocodone bitartrate; homatropine methylbromide]

Tussionex extended-release suspension ℞ *antihistamine; antitussive* [chlorpheniramine polistirex; hydrocodone polistirex]

Tussi-Organidin DM liquid ℞ *antitussive; expectorant* [dextromethorphan hydrobromide; iodinated glycerol]

Tussi-Organidin liquid ℞ *antitussive; expectorant* [codeine phosphate; iodinated glycerol]

Tussirex syrup, sugar-free liquid ℞ *antitussive; antihistamine; decongestant; analgesic* [codeine phosphate; pheniramine maleate; phenylephrine HCl; sodium citrate; sodium salicylate]

Tussi-R-Gen DM liquid ℞ *antitussive; expectorant* [dextromethorphan hydrobromide; iodinated glycerol]

Tussi-R-Gen liquid ℞ *antitussive; expectorant* [codeine phosphate; iodinated glycerol]

Tuss-LA sustained-release tablets ℞ *decongestant; expectorant* [pseudoephedrine HCl; guaifenesin]

Tusso-DM liquid ℞ *antitussive; expectorant* [iodinated glycerol; dextromethorphan hydrobromide]

Tussogest extended-release capsules ℞ *decongestant; antitussive* [phenylpropanolamine HCl; caramiphen edisylate]

Tuss-Ornade Spansules (sustained-release capsules), liquid ℞ *antitussive; decongestant* [caramiphen edisylate; phenylpropanolamine HCl]

Tusstat syrup ℞ *antihistamine; antitussive* [diphenhydramine HCl]

tuvatidine INN

T-Vites tablets OTC *vitamin/mineral supplement* [multiple vitamins & minerals; biotin]

TVP-101 *investigational antiparkinsonism agent*

12 Hour Antihistamine Nasal Decongestant Tablets OTC *decongestant; antihistamine* [pseudoephedrine sulfate; dexbrompheniramine maleate]

12 Hour Cold Capsules OTC *decongestant; antihistamine* [phenylpropanolamine HCl; chlorpheniramine maleate]

12 Hour nasal spray OTC *nasal decongestant* [oxymetazoline HCl]

Twice-A-Day nasal spray OTC *nasal decongestant* [oxymetazoline HCl]

Twilite caplets OTC *antihistaminic sleep aid* [diphenhydramine HCl]

Twin-K liquid ℞ *potassium supplement* [potassium gluconate; potassium citrate]

Twin-K-Cl liquid (discontinued 1991) ℞ *potassium supplement* [potassium gluconate; potassium citrate; ammonium chloride]

256U87 ℞ *investigational suppressant for HIV-related herpes simplex and zoster*

TwoCal HN liquid OTC *oral nutritional supplement*

Two-Dyne capsules ℞ *analgesic; antipyretic; sedative* [acetaminophen; caffeine; butalbital]

tybamate USAN, NF, INN *minor tranquilizer*

Ty-Cold tablets OTC *decongestant; antihistamine; antitussive; analgesic* [pseudoephedrine HCl; chlorpheniramine maleate; dextromethorphan hydrobromide; acetaminophen]

tyformin BAN [also: tiformin]

tylcalsin [see: calcium acetylsalicylate]

tylemalum [see: carbubarb]

Tylenol, Children's chewable tablets, elixir, oral suspension OTC *analgesic; antipyretic* [acetaminophen]

Tylenol Allergy Sinus caplets, gelcaps OTC *decongestant; antihistamine; analgesic* [pseudoephedrine HCl; chlorpheniramine maleate; acetaminophen]

Tylenol Cold, Children's liquid, chewable tablets OTC *pediatric decongestant, antihistamine and analgesic* [pseudoephedrine HCl; chlorpheniramine maleate; acetaminophen]

Tylenol Cold caplets, tablets OTC *decongestant; antihistamine; antitussive; analgesic* [pseudoephedrine HCl; chlorpheniramine maleate; dextromethorphan hydrobromide; acetaminophen]

Tylenol Cold & Flu Medication powder OTC *decongestant; antihistamine; antitussive; analgesic* [pseudoephedrine HCl; chlorpheniramine maleate; dextromethorphan hydrobromide; acetaminophen]

Tylenol Cold & Flu No Drowsiness Formula powder OTC *decongestant; antitussive; analgesic* [pseudoephedrine HCl; dextromethorphan hydrobromide; acetaminophen]

Tylenol Cold Medication effervescent tablets OTC *decongestant; antihistamine; analgesic* [phenylpropanolamine HCl; chlorpheniramine maleate; acetaminophen]

Tylenol Cold Multi Symptom Plus Cough, Children's liquid OTC *decongestant; antihistamine; antitussive; analgesic* [pseudoephedrine HCl; chlorpheniramine maleate; dextromethorphan hydrobromide; acetaminophen]

Tylenol Cold Night Time liquid OTC *decongestant; antihistamine; antitussive; analgesic* [pseudoephedrine HCl; diphenhydramine HCl; dextromethorphan hydrobromide; acetaminophen; alcohol]

Tylenol Cough liquid OTC *antitussive; analgesic* [dextromethorphan hydrobromide; acetaminophen]

Tylenol Cough with Decongestant liquid OTC *decongestant; antitussive; analgesic* [pseudoephedrine HCl; dextromethorphan hydrobromide; acetaminophen; alcohol]

Tylenol Headache Plus caplets OTC *analgesic; antipyretic; antacid* [acetaminophen; calcium carbonate]

Tylenol Infant's Drops solution, suspension OTC *analgesic; antipyretic* [acetaminophen]

Tylenol Multisymptom tablets, caplets (name changed to Tylenol Cold in 1992) (discontinued 1991)

Tylenol Multisymptom liquid (discontinued 1992) OTC *decongestant; antihistamine; antitussive; analgesic* [pseudoephedrine HCl; chlorpheniramine maleate; dextromethorphan hydrobromide; acetaminophen]

Tylenol No. 1, No. 2, No. 3 & No. 4 [see: Tylenol with Codeine]

Tylenol No Drowsiness Cold caplets, gelcaps OTC *decongestant; antitussive; analgesic* [pseudoephedrine HCl; dextromethorphan hydrobromide; acetaminophen]

Tylenol PM caplets, tablets OTC *antihistamine; analgesic* [diphenhydramine HCl; acetaminophen]

Tylenol Sinus Medication tablets, caplets, gelcaps OTC *decongestant; analgesic* [pseudoephedrine HCl; acetaminophen]

Tylenol tablets, caplets, liquid, gelcaps OTC *analgesic; antipyretic* [acetaminophen]

Tylenol with Codeine elixir ℞ *analgesic* [acetaminophen; codeine phosphate]

Tylenol with Codeine No. 1, No. 2, No. 3 & No. 4 tablets ℞ *analgesic* [acetaminophen; codeine phosphate]

tylosin INN, BAN

Tylox capsules ℞ *narcotic analgesic* [oxycodone HCl; acetaminophen]

tyloxapol USAN, USP, INN *detergent; wetting agent*

Tymatro troches (discontinued 1991) OTC *topical anesthetic; oral antiseptic* [benzocaine; cetylpyridinium chloride]

Tympagesic ear drops ℞ *topical local anesthetic; analgesic; decongestant* [phenylephrine HCl; antipyrine; benzocaine]

typhoid vaccine USP *active bacterin for typhoid fever (Salmonella typhi)*

typhus vaccine USP

Tyrobenz lozenges (discontinued 1992) OTC *topical anesthetic* [benzocaine]

tyromedan INN *thyromimetic* [also: thyromedan HCl]

tyromedan HCl [see: thyromedan HCl]

tyropanoate sodium USAN, USP *cholecystographic radiopaque medium* [also: sodium tyropanoate]

tyrosine (L-tyrosine) USAN, USP, INN *nonessential amino acid;* symbols: Tyr, Y

Tyrosum Cleanser liquid, packets OTC *topical acne cleanser* [isopropanol; acetone]

tyrothricin USP, INN *antibacterial*

Tyzine nasal spray, nose drops, pediatric drops ℞ *nasal decongestant* [tetrahydrozoline HCl]

U

U-87201E ℞ *investigational antiviral for AIDS*

UAA tablets ℞ *urinary anti-infective; analgesic; antispasmodic; acidifier* [methenamine; phenyl salicylate; atropine sulfate; methylene blue; hyoscyamine; benzoic acid]

UAD cream, lotion ℞ *topical anti-infective; corticosteroid* [clioquinol; hydrocortisone]

UAD Otic ear drop suspension ℞ *topical corticosteroidal anti-inflammatory; antibiotic* [hydrocortisone; neomycin sulfate; polymyxin B sulfate]

ubenimex INN

ubidecarenone INN

ubisindine INN

Ucephan oral solution ℞ *(orphan: hyperammonemia prevention in urea cycle enzymopathy)* [sodium benzoate; sodium phenylacetate]

UCG-Slide Test kit ℞ *in vitro diagnostic aid for urine pregnancy test*

U-Cort cream ℞ *topical corticosteroid* [hydrocortisone acetate]

Uendex ℞ *investigational antiviral for AIDS; (orphan: cystic fibrosis)* [dextran sulfate]

U-Eze tablets (discontinued 1991) ℞ *urinary anti-infective; antiseptic; analgesic; antispasmodic* [methenamine; sodium biphosphate; phenyl salicylate; methylene blue; hyoscyamine sulfate]

ufenamate INN

ufiprazole INN

uldazepam USAN, INN *sedative*

ulinastatin INN

ulobetasol INN *topical corticosteroidal anti-inflammatory* [also: halobetasol propionate]

ULR-LA long-acting tablets ℞ *decongestant; expectorant* [phenylpropanolamine HCl; guaifenesin]

Ultra B-50 tablets (discontinued 1992) OTC *vitamin supplement* [multiple B vitamins; folic acid; biotin; inositol; choline; lecithin]

Ultra Derm lotion, bath oil OTC *moisturizer; emollient*

Ultra KLB6 tablets OTC *dietary supplement* [vitamin B_6; multiple food supplements]

Ultra Mide 25 lotion OTC *moisturizer; emollient; keratolytic* [urea]

Ultra Tears eye drops OTC *ocular moisturizer/lubricant*

Ultra Vent (trademarked delivery system) *jet nebulizer*

Ultra Vita Time tablets OTC *dietary supplement* [multiple vitamins, minerals & food products; iron; folic acid; biotin]

Ultra Vitamin A & D tablets (discontinued 1992) OTC *vitamin supplement* [vitamins A & D]

UltraBrom PD timed-release capsules OTC *decongestant; antihistamine* [pseudoephedrine HCl; brompheniramine maleate]

Ultracal liquid OTC *total enteral nutrition*

UltraCare Disinfectant/Neutralizer System kit OTC *two-step contact lens disinfectant* [hydrogen peroxide]

Ultracef capsules, tablets, oral suspension ℞ *cephalosporin-type antibiotic* [cefadroxil monohydrate]

Ultra-Freeda; Ultra Freeda Iron Free tablets OTC *geriatric vitamin/mineral supplement* [multiple vitamins & minerals; folic acid; biotin]

Ultraject prefilled syringe ℞ *investigational contrast agent*

Ultralan liquid OTC *oral nutritional supplement*

Ultralente Iletin I subcu injection OTC *antidiabetic* [insulin zinc (beef-pork)]

Ultralente Insulin suspension for injection OTC *antidiabetic* [extended insulin zinc (beef)]

Ultram ℞ *investigational analgesic*

Ultramicrosize Griseofulvin tablets ℞ *systemic antifungal* [griseofulvin (ultramicrosize)]

Ultraprin tablets OTC *analgesic; nonsteroidal anti-inflammatory drug (NSAID); antipyretic* [ibuprofen]

Ultrase MT 12; Ultrase MT 20; Ultrase MT 24 capsules ℞ *digestive enzymes* [pancrelipase]

Ultravate ointment, cream ℞ *topical corticosteroidal anti-inflammatory* [halobetasol propionate]

Ultrazyme Enzymatic Cleaner tablets OTC *contact lens enzymatic cleaner*

umespirone INN

Unasyn powder for IV or IM injection, ADD-vantage vials ℞ *penicillin-type antibiotic* [ampicillin sodium; sulbactam sodium]

Unavit Therapeutic tablets OTC *vitamin/mineral supplement* [multiple vitamins & minerals]

Unavit-M tablets OTC *vitamin/mineral supplement* [multiple vitamins & minerals]

10-undecenoic acid [see: undecylenic acid]

undecoylium chloride-iodine

undecylenic acid USP *antifungal*

Undoguent ointment (discontinued 1991) ℞ *topical antifungal* [undecylenic acid; zinc undecylenate]

Unguentine aerosol spray OTC *topical local anesthetic* [benzocaine]

Unguentine ointment OTC *minor burn treatment* [phenol; zinc oxide; eucalyptus oil]

Unguentine Plus cream OTC *topical local anesthetic; antiseptic; antifungal* [lidocaine HCl; chloroxylenol; phenol]

Uni-Ace infant drops OTC *analgesic; antipyretic* [acetaminophen]

Unibase OTC *ointment base*

Uni-Bent Cough syrup OTC *antihistamine; antitussive* [diphenhydramine HCl]

Unicap capsules, tablets OTC *vitamin supplement* [multiple vitamins; folic acid]

Unicap Jr. chewable tablets OTC *vitamin supplement* [multiple vitamins; folic acid]

Unicap M; Unicap T tablets OTC *vitamin/mineral/iron supplement* [multiple vitamins & minerals; iron; folic acid]

Unicap Plus Iron tablets OTC *vitamin/iron supplement* [multiple vitamins; iron; folic acid]

Unicap Sr. tablets OTC *vitamin/mineral/iron supplement* [multiple vitamins & minerals; iron; folic acid]

Unicard ℞ *investigational antihypertensive; vasodilator* [dilevalol]

Unicomplex T & M tablets OTC *vitamin/mineral/iron supplement* [multiple vitamins & minerals; iron; folic acid]

Uni-Decon sustained-release tablets ℞ *decongestant; antihistamine* [phenylpropanolamine HCl; phenylephrine HCl; chlorpheniramine maleate; phenyltoloxamine citrate]

Uni-Dur ℞ *investigational antiasthmatic* [theophylline]

Unifiber powder OTC *bulk laxative* [powdered cellulose]

unifocon A USAN *hydrophobic contact lens material*

Unilax softgel, capsules OTC *laxative; stool softener* [docusate sodium; phenolphthalein]

Unimatic (delivery system) [prefilled syringe]

Unipak (packaging form) *dispensing pack*

Unipen film-coated tablets, capsules, powder for IV or IM injection ℞ *bactericidal antibiotic (penicillinase-resistant penicillin)* [nafcillin sodium monohydrate]

Uniphyl timed-release tablets ℞ *bronchodilator* [theophylline]

Unipres tablets ℞ *antihypertensive* [hydrochlorothiazide; reserpine; hydralazine HCl]

Uniquin (foreign name for U.S. product Maxaquin)

Uniserts (trademarked form) *suppositories*

Unisol; Unisol 4 solution OTC *contact lens rinsing and storage solution* [saline solution]

Unisom Nighttime Sleep-Aid tablets OTC *antihistaminic sleep aid* [doxylamine succinate]

Unitrol timed-release capsules OTC *diet aid* [phenylpropanolamine HCl]

Uni-Tussin DM syrup OTC *antitussive; expectorant* [dextromethorphan hydrobromide; guaifenesin; alcohol]

Uni-Tussin syrup OTC *expectorant* [guaifenesin; alcohol]

universal antidote (activated charcoal, magnesium hydroxide, tannic acid) *general-purpose gastric adsorbent/detoxicant*

Univial (trademarked form) *single-dose vials*

Unna's boot [see: Dome-Paste bandage]

Urabeth tablets ℞ *postsurgical cholinergic bladder muscle stimulant* [bethanechol chloride]

Uracel 5 enteric-coated tablets OTC *analgesic; antipyretic; anti-inflammatory* [sodium salicylate]

Uracid capsules ℞ *urinary acidifier to control ammonia production* [racemethionine]

uracil mustard USAN, USP *antineoplastic* [also: uramustine]

uradal [see: carbromal]

uralenic acid [see: enoxolone]

uramustine INN *antineoplastic* [also: uracil mustard]

Uranap; Uranap 500 capsules OTC *urinary acidifier to control ammonia production; oral amino acid supplement* [racemethionine]

uranin [see: fluorescein sodium]

uranium *element (U)*

urapidil INN, BAN

urea USP *osmotic diuretic; keratolytic; emollient*

urea peroxide [see: carbamide peroxide]

Ureacin-10 lotion OTC *moisturizer; emollient; keratolytic* [urea]

Ureacin-20 cream OTC *moisturizer; emollient; keratolytic* [urea]

Ureacin-40 cream ℞ *for removal of dystrophic nails* [urea]

Ureaphil IV infusion ℞ *osmotic diuretic* [urea]

Urecholine tablets, subcu injection ℞ *postsurgical cholinergic bladder muscle stimulant* [bethanechol chloride]

uredepa USAN, INN *antineoplastic*

uredofos USAN, INN *veterinary anthelmintic*

urefibrate INN

***p*-ureidobenzenearsonic acid** [see: carbarsone]

urethan NF [also: urethane]

urethane INN, BAN [also: urethan]

urethane polymers [see: polyurethane foam]

Urethrin injection ℞ *investigational treatment of urinary incontinence*

Urex tablets ℞ *urinary antibacterial* [methenamine hippurate]

Uricult OTC *in vitro diagnostic aid for bacteriuria and uropathogens*

Uridon Modified tablets ℞ *urinary anti-infective; analgesic; antispasmodic; acidifier* [methenamine; phenyl salicylate; atropine sulfate; methylene blue; hyoscyamine; benzoic acid]

Urimar-T tablets ℞ *urinary anti-infective; antiseptic; analgesic; antispasmodic* [methenamine; sodium biphosphate; phenyl salicylate; methylene blue; hyoscyamine sulfate]

Urimed Modified Formula tablets ℞ *urinary anti-infective; analgesic; antispasmodic; acidifier* [atropine sulfate; hyoscyamine sulfate; methenamine; methylene blue; phenyl salicylate; benzoic acid]

Urinary Antiseptic No. 2 tablets ℞ *urinary anti-infective; analgesic; antispasmodic; acidifier* [methenamine; phenyl salicylate; atropine sulfate; methylene blue; hyoscyamine; benzoic acid]

Urised tablets ℞ *urinary anti-infective; analgesic; antispasmodic; acidifier* [methenamine; phenyl salicylate; atropine sulfate; methylene blue; hyoscyamine; benzoic acid]

Urisedamine tablets ℞ *urinary anti-infective; antispasmodic* [methenamine mandelate; hyoscyamine]

Urispas film-coated tablets ℞ *urinary antispasmodic* [flavoxate HCl]

Uristix; Uristix 4 reagent strips OTC *in vitro diagnostic aid for multiple urine products*

Uritab tablets ℞ *urinary anti-infective; analgesic; antispasmodic; acidifier* [methenamine; phenyl salicylate; atropine sulfate; methylene blue; hyoscyamine; benzoic acid]

Uri-Tet capsules ℞ *antibacterial* [oxytetracycline HCl]

Uritin tablets ℞ *urinary anti-infective; analgesic; antispasmodic; acidifier* [methenamine; phenyl salicylate; atropine sulfate; methylene blue; hyoscyamine; benzoic acid]

Urobak tablets ℞ *broad-spectrum bacteriostatic* [sulfamethoxazole]

Urobiotic-250 capsules ℞ *urinary anti-infective* [oxytetracycline HCl; sulfamethizole; phenazopyridine HCl]

Urocit-K tablets ℞ *urinary alkalizer; (orphan: calcium kidney stone prophylaxis)* [potassium citrate]

Urodine tablets ℞ *urinary analgesic* [phenazopyridine HCl]

urofollitrophin BAN *follicle-stimulating hormone (FSH)* [also: urofollitropin]

urofollitropin USAN, INN *follicle-stimulating hormone (FSH); (orphan: anovulation)* [also: urofollitrophin]

urogastrone *(orphan: corneal transplant surgery)*

Urogesic Blue tablets ℞ *urinary anti-infective; antiseptic; analgesic; antispasmodic* [methenamine; sodium biphosphate; phenyl salicylate; methylene blue; hyoscyamine sulfate]

Urogesic tablets ℞ *urinary analgesic* [phenazopyridine HCl]

urokinase USAN, INN, BAN *plasminogen activator; thrombolytic enzyme*

Uro-KP-Neutral film-coated tablets ℞ *phosphorus supplement* [disodium phosphate; dipotassium phosphate; monobasic sodium phosphate]

Urolene Blue tablets ℞ *urinary anti-infective/antiseptic; antidote to cyanide poisoning* [methylene blue]

Uro-Mag capsules OTC *antacid; magnesium supplement* [magnesium oxide]

uronal [see: barbital]

Uro-Phosphate tablets ℞ *urinary anti-infective; acidifier* [methenamine; sodium biphosphate]
Uroplus SS; Uroplus DS tablets ℞ *anti-infective; antibacterial* [trimethoprim; sulfamethoxazole]
Uroqid-Acid; Uroqid-Acid No. 2 tablets ℞ *urinary anti-infective; acidifier* [methenamine mandelate; sodium acid phosphate]
Uro-Ves tablets ℞ *urinary anti-infective; analgesic; antispasmodic; acidifier* [methenamine; phenyl salicylate; atropine sulfate; methylene blue; hyoscyamine; benzoic acid]
Urovist Cysto intracavitary instillation ℞ *urologic radiopaque agent* [diatrizoate meglumine]
Urovist Meglumine DIU/CT injection ℞ *parenteral renal radiopaque agent* [diatrizoate meglumine]
Urovist Sodium 300 injection ℞ *parenteral radiopaque agent* [diatrizoate sodium]
Ursinus Inlay-Tabs (tablets) OTC *decongestant; analgesic* [pseudoephedrine HCl; aspirin]
ursodeoxycholic acid INN, BAN *anticholelithogenic; (orphan: primary biliary cirrhosis)* [also: ursodiol]
ursodiol USAN *anticholelithogenic; (orphan: primary biliary cirrhosis)* [also: ursodeoxycholic acid]
Ursofalk ℞ *(orphan: primary biliary cirrhosis)* [ursodiol]
ursulcholic acid INN
Uticort cream, lotion, gel ℞ *topical corticosteroid* [betamethasone benzoate]

V

VAAP (vincristine, asparaginase, Adriamycin, prednisone) *chemotherapy protocol*
VAB; VAB-I (vinblastine, actinomycin D, bleomycin) *chemotherapy protocol*
VAB-II (vinblastine, actinomycin D, bleomycin, cisplatin) *chemotherapy protocol*
VAB-III (vinblastine, actinomycin D, bleomycin, cisplatin, chlorambucil, cyclophosphamide) *chemotherapy protocol*
VAB-V (vinblastine, actinomycin D, bleomycin, cyclophosphamide, cisplatin) *chemotherapy protocol*
VAB-6 (vinblastine, actinomycin D, bleomycin, [cyclophosphamide, cisplatin]) *chemotherapy protocol*
VABCD (vinblastine, Adriamycin, bleomycin, CCNU, DTIC) *chemotherapy protocol*
VAC; VAC pulse; VAC standard (vincristine, actinomycin D, cyclophosphamide) *chemotherapy protocol*
VAC; VAC pulse; VAC standard (vincristine, Adriamycin, cyclophosphamide) *chemotherapy protocol*
VACA (vincristine, Adriamycin, cyclophosphamide, actinomycin D) *chemotherapy protocol*
VACAD (vincristine, Adriamycin, cyclophosphamide, actinomycin D, dacarbazine) *chemotherapy protocol*
vaccinia immune globulin (VIG) USP *passive immunizing agent*
vaccinia immune human globulin [now: vaccinia immune globulin]

VACP (VePesid, Adriamycin, cyclophosphamide, Platinol) *chemotherapy protocol*
VAD (vincristine, Adriamycin, dexamethasone) *chemotherapy protocol*
Vademin-Z capsules OTC *vitamin/mineral supplement* [multiple vitamins & minerals]
vadocaine INN
VAD/V (vincristine, Adriamycin, dexamethasone, verapamil) *chemotherapy protocol*
VAFAC (vincristine, amethopterin, fluorouracil, Adriamycin, cyclophosphamide) *chemotherapy protocol*
Vag vaginal cream (discontinued 1991) ℞ *bacteriostatic; antiseptic; vulnerary* [sulfanilamide; aminacrine HCl; allantoin]
Vagilia vaginal cream (discontinued 1992) ℞ *bacteriostatic; antiseptic; vulnerary* [sulfisoxazole; aminacrine HCl; allantoin]
Vaginex vaginal cream OTC *counterirritant* [tripelennamine HCl]
Vagisec Douche solution ℞ *vaginal cleansing and deodorizing*
Vagisec Plus vaginal suppositories ℞ *antiseptic* [aminacrine HCl]
Vagisil cream OTC *topical local anesthetic; antipruritic; antifungal* [benzocaine; resorcinol]
Vagistat vaginal ointment in prefilled applicator ℞ *antifungal* [tioconazole]
Vagitrol vaginal cream (discontinued 1992) ℞ *bacteriostatic* [sulfanilamide]
VAI (vincristine, actinomycin D, ifosfamide) *chemotherapy protocol*
Valadol tablets (discontinued 1991) OTC *analgesic; antipyretic* [acetaminophen]
valconazole INN
Valdeine tablets (discontinued 1991) ℞ *narcotic analgesic* [codeine phosphate; aspirin; caffeine]
valdetamide INN

valdipromide INN
Valdrene syrup (discontinued 1991) ℞ *antitussive* [diphenhydramine HCl]
valepotriate [see: valtrate]
Valergen 10; Valergen 20; Valergen 40 IM injection ℞ *estrogen replacement therapy; antineoplastic for prostatic cancer* [estradiol valerate in oil]
Valertest No. 1 IM injection ℞ *estrogen/androgen for menopausal vasomotor symptoms* [estradiol valerate; testosterone enanthate]
Valesin tablets (discontinued 1991) OTC *analgesic; antipyretic; anti-inflammatory* [acetaminophen; aspirin; salicylamide]
valethamate bromide NF
Valihist tablets OTC *antihistamine; decongestant; analgesic; antipyretic* [chlorpheniramine maleate; phenylephrine HCl; acetaminophen; caffeine]
valine (L-valine) USAN, USP, INN *essential amino acid; symbols:* Val, V
Valisone ointment, cream, lotion ℞ *topical corticosteroid* [betamethasone valerate]
Valisone Reduced Strength cream ℞ *topical corticosteroid* [betamethasone valerate]
Valium tablets, Tel-E-Dose packs, IV or IM injection, Tel-E-Ject syringes ℞ *sedative; anxiolytic; skeletal muscle relaxant; anticonvulsant adjunct* [diazepam]
Valmid Pulvules (capsules) (discontinued 1991) ℞ *hypnotic* [ethinamate]
valnoctamide USAN, INN *tranquilizer*
valofane INN
Valorin Super tablets OTC *analgesic; antipyretic* [acetaminophen; caffeine]
Valorin; Valorin Extra tablets OTC *analgesic; antipyretic* [acetaminophen]
valperinol INN

Valpin 50 tablets (discontinued 1992) ℞ *anticholinergic; treatment of peptic ulcer; antisecretory* [anisotropine methylbromide]

Valprin tablets OTC *analgesic; nonsteroidal anti-inflammatory drug (NSAID); antipyretic* [ibuprofen]

valproate pivoxil INN

valproate semisodium INN *anticonvulsant* [also: divalproex sodium; semisodium valproate]

valproate sodium USAN *anticonvulsant*

valproic acid USAN, USP, INN, BAN *anticonvulsant*

valpromide INN

Valrelease sustained-release capsules ℞ *sedative; anxiolytic; skeletal muscle relaxant; anticonvulsant adjunct* [diazepam]

valtrate INN

VAM (VP-16-213, Adriamycin, methotrexate) *chemotherapy protocol*

VAMP (vincristine, actinomycin, methotrexate, prednisone) *chemotherapy protocol*

VAMP (vincristine, amethopterin, mercaptopurine, prednisone) *chemotherapy protocol*

vanadium *element (V)*

Vancenase AQ nasal spray ℞ *intranasal steroidal anti-inflammatory* [beclomethasone dipropionate]

Vancenase nasal inhalation aerosol ℞ *intranasal steroidal anti-inflammatory* [beclomethasone dipropionate]

Vanceril oral inhalation aerosol ℞ *corticosteroid for bronchial asthma* [beclomethasone dipropionate]

Vancocin Pulvules (capsules), powder for oral solution, powder for IV or IM injection ℞ *glycopeptide-type antibiotic* [vancomycin HCl]

Vancoled powder for IV or IM injection ℞ *glycopeptide-type antibiotic* [vancomycin HCl]

vancomycin INN, BAN *tricyclic glycopeptide bactericidal antibiotic* [also: vancomycin HCl]

vancomycin HCl USP *tricyclic glycopeptide bactericidal antibiotic* [also: vancomycin]

Vancor Intravenous powder for IV injection (discontinued 1992) ℞ *antibiotic* [vancomycin HCl]

vaneprim INN

Vanex Expectorant liquid ℞ *antitussive; decongestant; expectorant* [hydrocodone bitartrate; pseudoephedrine HCl; guaifenesin; alcohol]

Vanex Forte film-coated caplets ℞ *decongestant; antihistamine* [phenylpropanolamine HCl; phenylephrine HCl; chlorpheniramine maleate; pyrilamine maleate]

Vanex-HD liquid ℞ *antitussive; decongestant; antihistamine* [hydrocodone bitartrate; phenylephrine HCl; chlorpheniramine maleate]

Vanex-LA long-acting tablets ℞ *decongestant; expectorant* [phenylpropanolamine HCl; guaifenesin]

Vanicream OTC *cream base*

vanilla NF *flavoring agent*

vanillin NF *flavoring agent*

***N*-vanillylnonamide** [see: nonivamide]

***N*-vanillyloleamide** [see: olvanil]

vanitiolide INN

Vanoxide lotion OTC *keratolytic for acne* [benzoyl peroxide]

Vanoxide-HC lotion ℞ *keratolytic for acne; topical corticosteroid* [benzoyl peroxide; hydrocortisone]

Vanquish caplets OTC *analgesic; antipyretic; anti-inflammatory* [acetaminophen; aspirin; caffeine; magnesium hydroxide; aluminum hydroxide]

Vanseb shampoo, cream, lotion OTC *antiseborrheic; keratolytic* [sulfur; salicylic acid]

Vanseb-T cream shampoo, lotion shampoo OTC *antiseborrheic; anti-*

psoriatic; keratolytic [coal tar; salicylic acid; sulfur]
Vansil capsules ℞ *anthelmintic* [oxamniquine]
Vantin film-coated tablets, granules for suspension ℞ *cephalosporin-type antibiotic* [cefpodoxime proxetil]
vanyldisulfamide INN
VAP (vinblastine, actinomycin D, Platinol) *chemotherapy protocol*
VAP (vincristine, Adriamycin, prednisone) *chemotherapy protocol*
VAP (vincristine, Adriamycin, procarbazine) *chemotherapy protocol*
vapiprost INN, BAN *antagonist to thromboxane A_2* [also: vapiprost HCl]
vapiprost HCl USAN *antagonist to thromboxane A_2* [also: vapiprost]
Vapo-Iso solution for nebulization (discontinued 1991) ℞ *bronchodilator for bronchial asthma and bronchospasm* [isoproterenol]
Vaponefrin solution for inhalation OTC *bronchodilator for bronchial asthma* [racepinephrine]
Vaporole (dosage form) *inhalant*
vapreotide USAN *antineoplastic*
Vaqta ℞ *investigational hepatitis vaccine*
varicella-zoster immune globulin (VZIG) USP *passive immunizing agent*
Varivax ℞ *investigational chickenpox vaccine*
Vascor film-coated tablets ℞ *antianginal* [bepridil HCl]
Vascoray injection ℞ *parenteral radiopaque agent* [iothalamate meglumine; iothalamate sodium]
Vaseretic 10-25 tablets ℞ *antihypertensive* [enalapril maleate; hydrochlorothiazide]
Vasocidin eye drops ℞ *topical ophthalmic corticosteroidal anti-inflammatory; bacteriostatic* [prednisolone sodium phosphate; sodium sulfacetamide]
Vasocidin ophthalmic ointment ℞ *topical ophthalmic corticosteroidal anti-inflammatory; bacteriostatic* [prednisolone acetate; sodium sulfacetamide]
VasoClear A eye drops OTC *topical ocular decongestant; astringent; antiseptic* [naphazoline HCl; zinc sulfate]
VasoClear eye drops OTC *topical ocular vasoconstrictor* [naphazoline HCl]
Vasocon Regular eye drops ℞ *topical ocular vasoconstrictor* [naphazoline HCl]
Vasocon-A eye drops ℞ *topical ocular decongestant/antihistamine* [naphazoline HCl; antazoline phosphate]
Vasoderm; Vasoderm-E cream ℞ *topical corticosteroid* [fluocinonide]
Vasodilan tablets ℞ *peripheral vasodilator* [isoxsuprine HCl]
vasopressin (VP) USP, INN *posterior pituitary hormone; antidiuretic*
vasopressin tannate USP *posterior pituitary hormone; antidiuretic*
Vasoprost ℞ *investigational prostaglandin drug*
Vasosulf eye drops ℞ *ophthalmic decongestant/bacteriostatic* [sodium sulfacetamide; phenylephrine HCl]
Vasotec IV injection ℞ *antihypertensive; angiotensin-converting enzyme inhibitor* [enalaprilat]
Vasotec tablets ℞ *antihypertensive; angiotensin-converting enzyme inhibitor* [enalapril maleate]
Vasoxyl IV or IM injection ℞ *vasopressor used in shock* [methoxamine HCl]
VAT (vinblastine, Adriamycin, thiotepa) *chemotherapy protocol*
VATD; VAT-D (vincristine, ara-C, thioguanine, daunorubicin) *chemotherapy protocol*
VATH (vinblastine, Adriamycin, thiotepa, Halotestin) *chemotherapy protocol*
Vatronol [see: Vicks Vatronol]
VAV (VP-16-213, Adriamycin, vincristine) *chemotherapy protocol*
Vaxsyn HIV-1 ℞ *investigational antiviral for AIDS (orphan)* [human T-

lymphotropic virus type III gp160 antigens]

Vazepam tablets, IV or IM injection ℞ *anticonvulsant; anxiolytic; skeletal muscle relaxant* [diazepam]

VB (vinblastine, bleomycin) *chemotherapy protocol*

VBA (vincristine, BCNU, Adriamycin) *chemotherapy protocol*

VBAP (vincristine, BCNU, Adriamycin, prednisone) *chemotherapy protocol*

VBC (VePesid, BCNU, cyclophosphamide) *chemotherapy protocol*

VBD (vinblastine, bleomycin, DDP) *chemotherapy protocol*

VBM (vinblastine, bleomycin, methotrexate) *chemotherapy protocol*

VBMCP (vincristine, BCNU, melphalan, cyclophosphamide, prednisone) *chemotherapy protocol*

VBMF (vincristine, bleomycin, methotrexate, fluorouracil) *chemotherapy protocol*

VBP (vinblastine, bleomycin, Platinol) *chemotherapy protocol*

VC (vincristine) [q.v.]

VCAP (vincristine, cyclophosphamide, Adriamycin, prednisone) *chemotherapy protocol*

V-CAP III (VP-16-213, cyclophosphamide, Adriamycin, Platinol) *chemotherapy protocol*

VCF (vaginal contraceptive film) OTC *spermicidal contraceptive* [nonoxynol 9]

VCF (vincristine, cyclophosphamide, fluorouracil) *chemotherapy protocol*

V-Cillin K tablets, powder for oral solution ℞ *bactericidal antibiotic* [penicillin V potassium]

VCMP (vincristine, cyclophosphamide, melphalan, prednisone) *chemotherapy protocol*

VCP (vincristine, cyclophosphamide, prednisone) *chemotherapy protocol*

VCR (vincristine) [q.v.]

V-Dec-M sustained-release tablets ℞ *decongestant; expectorant* [pseudoephedrine HCl; guaifenesin]

VDP (vincristine, daunorubicin, prednisone) *chemotherapy protocol*

vecuronium bromide USAN, INN, BAN *neuromuscular blocker; muscle relaxant*

Veetids '125'; Veetids '250' powder for oral solution ℞ *bactericidal antibiotic* [penicillin V potassium]

Veetids '250'; Veetids '500' film-coated tablets ℞ *bactericidal antibiotic* [penicillin V potassium]

vegetable oil, hydrogenated NF *tablet and capsule lubricant*

Vehicle/N; Vehicle/N Mild OTC *lotion base*

VeIP (Velban, ifosfamide, Platinol) *chemotherapy protocol*

Velban powder for IV injection ℞ *antineoplastic* [vinblastine sulfate]

velnacrine INN *cholinesterase inhibitor* [also: velnacrine maleate]

velnacrine maleate USAN *cholinesterase inhibitor* [also: velnacrine]

Velosef capsules, oral suspension, powder for IV or IM injection ℞ *cephalosporin-type antibiotic* [cephradine]

Velosulin Human suspension for injection OTC *antidiabetic* [insulin (human)]

Velosulin suspension for injection OTC *antidiabetic* [insulin (pork)]

Velsar powder for IV injection (discontinued 1992) ℞ *antineoplastic* [vinblastine sulfate]

Veltane tablets ℞ *antihistamine* [brompheniramine maleate]

Veltap Lanatabs (sustained-release tablets), elixir ℞ *decongestant; antihistamine* [phenylpropanolamine

HCl; phenylephrine HCl; brompheniramine maleate]
Velvachol OTC *cream base*
venlafaxine INN, BAN *antidepressant* [also: venlafaxine HCl]
venlafaxine HCl USAN *antidepressant* [also: venlafaxine]
Venoglobulin-I; Venoglobulin-S powder for IV infusion ℞ *passive immunizing agent* [immune globulin]
Venomil subcu or IM injection ℞ *venom sensitivity testing; allergenic hyposensitization therapy* [extracts of honeybee, yellow jacket, yellow hornet, white-faced hornet, mixed vespid & wasp venom]
Ventolin inhalation aerosol ℞ *bronchodilator* [albuterol]
Ventolin Rotacaps (capsules for inhalation), Nebules (solution for inhalation), syrup, tablets ℞ *bronchodilator* [albuterol sulfate]
VePesid IV injection, capsules ℞ *antineoplastic for testicular and small cell lung cancers* [etoposide]
veradoline INN *analgesic* [also: veradoline HCl]
veradoline HCl USAN *analgesic* [also: veradoline]
veralipride INN
verapamil USAN, INN, BAN *coronary vasodilator; calcium channel blocker*
verapamil HCl USAN, USP *antianginal; antiarrhythmic; calcium channel blocker*
veratrylidene-isoniazid [see: verazide]
verazide INN, BAN
Verazinc capsules OTC *zinc supplement* [zinc sulfate]
Vercyte tablets ℞ *antineoplastic* [pipobroman]
Verelan sustained-release capsules ℞ *antianginal; antiarrhythmic; antihypertensive* [verapamil HCl]
Vergo cream (discontinued 1992) OTC *topical keratolytic* [calcium pantothenate; ascorbic acid; starch]

Vergogel gel OTC *topical keratolytic* [salicylic acid]
Vergon capsules OTC *anticholinergic; antihistamine; antivertigo agent; motion sickness preventative* [meclizine]
verilopam INN *analgesic* [also: verilopam HCl]
verilopam HCl USAN *analgesic* [also: verilopam]
Verin timed-release tablets (discontinued 1992) OTC *analgesic; antipyretic; anti-inflammatory* [aspirin]
verlukast USAN, INN *bronchodilator; antiasthmatic*
Vermox chewable tablets ℞ *anthelmintic* [mebendazole]
verofylline USAN, INN *bronchodilator; antiasthmatic*
veronal [see: barbital]
veronal sodium [see: barbital sodium]
Verr-Canth liquid ℞ *topical keratolytic* [cantharidin]
Verrex liquid ℞ *topical keratolytic* [salicylic acid; podophyllum]
Verrusol liquid ℞ *topical keratolytic* [salicylic acid; podophyllum; cantharidin]
Versacaps prolonged-action capsules ℞ *decongestant; expectorant* [pseudoephedrine HCl; guaifenesin]
Versed IV or IM injection, Tel-E-Ject syringes ℞ *general anesthetic adjunct; preoperative sedative* [midazolam HCl]
Vertab capsules OTC *antinauseant; antiemetic; antivertigo; motion sickness preventative* [dimenhydrinate]
Verukan solution ℞ *topical keratolytic* [salicylic acid; lactic acid]
Verukan-20 (discontinued 1992) ℞ *topical keratolytic* [salicylic acid; lactic acid]
Verukan-HP solution ℞ *topical keratolytic* [salicylic acid]
vesnarinone USAN, INN *cardiotonic*
vesperal [see: barbital]
Vesprin IV or IM injection ℞ *antipsychotic; antiemetic* [triflupromazine HCl]

vetrabutine INN, BAN
V-Gan 25; V-Gan 50 injection ℞ *antihistamine; motion sickness; sleep aid; antiemetic; sedative* [promethazine HCl]
Viaflex (trademarked form) *ready-to-use IV*
Vianain *(orphan: enzymatic debridement of severe burns)* [ananain/comosain]
Vi-Aquamin Forte capsules (discontinued 1991) OTC *antianemic* [dried ferrous sulfate; multiple vitamins]
vibesate
Vibramycin capsules, powder for IV injection ℞ *tetracycline-type antibiotic* [doxycycline hyclate]
Vibramycin powder for oral suspension ℞ *tetracycline-type antibiotic* [doxycycline monohydrate]
Vibramycin syrup ℞ *tetracycline-type antibiotic* [doxycycline calcium]
Vibra-Tabs tablets ℞ *tetracycline-type antibiotic* [doxycycline hyclate]
VIC (vinblastine, ifosfamide, CCNU) *chemotherapy protocol*
Vicam injection ℞ *parenteral vitamin therapy* [multiple B vitamins; vitamin C]
Vicef capsules OTC *vitamin/iron supplement* [multiple vitamins; iron; folic acid]
Vicks Children's Cough syrup OTC *antitussive; expectorant* [dextromethorphan hydrobromide; guaifenesin]
Vicks Cough Drops; Vicks Ice Blue Throat Lozenges OTC *topical antipruritic/counterirritant; mild local anesthetic* [menthol]
Vicks Cough Silencers lozenges OTC *antitussive* [dextromethorphan hydrobromide; benzocaine]
Vicks Formula 44 products [see: Formula 44]
Vicks Inhaler OTC *nasal decongestant* [*l*-desoxyephedrine]

Vicks Throat Lozenges OTC *topical anesthetic; oral antiseptic; antipruritic/counterirritant* [benzocaine; cetylpyridinium chloride; menthol; camphor oil; eucalyptus oil]
Vicks VapoRub vaporizing ointment OTC *counterirritant* [camphor; menthol; eucalyptus oil; oil of turpentine]
Vicks Vatronol nose drops OTC *nasal decongestant* [ephedrine sulfate]
Vicks Vitamin C Drops (lozenges) OTC *vitamin supplement* [sodium ascorbate; ascorbic acid]
Vicodin; Vicodin ES tablets ℞ *narcotic analgesic* [hydrocodone bitartrate; acetaminophen]
Vicon Forte capsules ℞ *vitamin/mineral supplement* [multiple vitamins & minerals; folic acid]
Vicon Plus capsules OTC *vitamin/mineral supplement* [multiple vitamins & minerals]
Vicon-C capsules OTC *vitamin/mineral supplement* [multiple vitamins & minerals]
vicotrope [see: cosyntropin]
Victors Dual Action Cough Drops; Victors Vapor Cough Lozenges OTC *antipruritic/counterirritant; mild local anesthetic; antiseptic* [menthol; eucalyptus oil]
vidarabine USAN, USP, INN, BAN *antiviral*
vidarabine monohydrate *antiviral*
vidarabine phosphate USAN *antiviral*
vidarabine sodium phosphate USAN *antiviral*
Vi-Daylin ADC drops OTC *vitamin supplement* [vitamins A, D & C]
Vi-Daylin ADC Vitamins + Iron drops OTC *vitamin/iron supplement* [vitamins A, D & C; ferrous gluconate]
Vi-Daylin chewable tablets OTC *vitamin supplement* [multiple vitamins]

Vi-Daylin Multivitamin + Iron drops, chewable tablets OTC *vitamin/iron supplement* [multiple vitamins; iron]

Vi-Daylin Multivitamin liquid, drops OTC *vitamin supplement* [multiple vitamins]

Vi-Daylin Plus Iron chewable tablets, liquid OTC *vitamin/iron supplement* [multiple vitamins; ferrous gluconate]

Vi-Daylin/F ADC drops ℞ *pediatric vitamin supplement and dental caries preventative* [vitamins A, D & C; sodium fluoride]

Vi-Daylin/F ADC + Iron drops ℞ *pediatric vitamin/iron supplement and dental caries preventative* [vitamins A, D & C; sodium fluoride; ferrous sulfate]

Vi-Daylin/F chewable tablets, drops ℞ *pediatric vitamin supplement and dental caries preventative* [multiple vitamins; sodium fluoride; folic acid]

Vi-Daylin/F + Iron chewable tablets, drops ℞ *pediatric vitamin/iron supplement and dental caries preventative* [multiple vitamins; sodium fluoride; ferrous sulfate; folic acid]

Videx chewable/dispersible tablets, powder for oral solution ℞ *antiviral for advanced HIV infection and AIDS* [didanosine]

VIE (vincristine, ifosfamide, etoposide) *chemotherapy protocol*

Vifex IM injection (discontinued 1991) ℞ *antianemic; vitamin supplement* [vitamin B_{12}; folic acid]

vifilcon A USAN *hydrophilic contact lens material*

vifilcon B USAN *hydrophilic contact lens material*

Vi-Flor [see: Poly-Vi-Flor; Tri-Vi-Flor]

VIG (vaccinia immune globulin) [q.v.]

vigabatrin USAN, INN, BAN *anticonvulsant for tardive dyskinesia*

Vigomar Forte tablets OTC *vitamin/mineral/iron supplement* [multiple vitamins & minerals; iron]

Vigortol liquid OTC *geriatric vitamin/mineral supplement* [multiple B vitamins & minerals; alcohol]

Vigran film-coated tablets (discontinued 1991) OTC *vitamin supplement* [multiple vitamins; folic acid]

Vigran plus Iron tablets (discontinued 1991) OTC *antianemic* [ferrous fumarate; multiple vitamins]

viloxazine INN, BAN *antidepressant* [also: viloxazine HCl]

viloxazine HCl USAN *antidepressant; (orphan: cataplexy; narcolepsy)* [also: viloxazine]

Viminate liquid OTC *geriatric vitamin/mineral supplement* [multiple B vitamins & minerals]

viminol INN

VIMRxyn ℞ *investigational antiviral for AIDS* [hypericin]

vinafocon A USAN *hydrophobic contact lens material*

vinbarbital NF, INN [also: vinbarbitone]

vinbarbital sodium NF

vinbarbitone BAN [also: vinbarbital]

vinblastine INN *antineoplastic* [also: vinblastine sulfate]

vinblastine sulfate USAN, USP *antineoplastic* [also: vinblastine]

vinburnine INN

vincaleukoblastine sulfate [see: vinblastine sulfate]

vincamine INN, BAN

vincanol INN

vincantenate [see: vinconate]

vincantril INN

Vincasar PFS IV injection ℞ *antineoplastic* [vincristine sulfate]

vincofos USAN, INN *anthelmintic*

vinconate INN

vincristine (VC; VCR) INN *antineoplastic* [also: vincristine sulfate]

vincristine sulfate USAN, USP *antineoplastic* [also: vincristine]

vindeburnol INN
vindesine USAN, INN, BAN *antineoplastic*
vindesine sulfate USAN *antineoplastic*
vinegar [see: acetic acid]
vinepidine INN *antineoplastic* [also: vinepidine sulfate]
vinepidine sulfate USAN *antineoplastic* [also: vinepidine]
vinformide INN
vinglycinate INN *antineoplastic* [also: vinglycinate sulfate]
vinglycinate sulfate USAN *antineoplastic* [also: vinglycinate]
vinleurosine INN *antineoplastic* [also: vinleurosine sulfate]
vinleurosine sulfate USAN *antineoplastic* [also: vinleurosine]
vinmegallate INN
vinorelbine INN
vinpocetine USAN, INN
vinpoline INN
vinrosidine INN *antineoplastic* [also: vinrosidine sulfate]
vinrosidine sulfate USAN *antineoplastic* [also: vinrosidine]
vintiamol INN
vintoperol INN
vintriptol INN
vinyl alcohol polymer [see: polyvinyl alcohol]
vinyl ether USP
vinyl gamma-aminobutyric acid [see: vigabatrin]
vinylbital INN [also: vinylbitone]
vinylbitone BAN [also: vinylbital]
vinylestrenolone [see: norgesterone]
vinymal [see: vinylbital]
vinyzene [see: bromchlorenone]
vinzolidine INN *antineoplastic* [also: vinzolidine sulfate]
vinzolidine sulfate USAN *antineoplastic* [also: vinzolidine]
Vio-Bec capsules (discontinued 1992) OTC *vitamin supplement* [multiple B vitamins; vitamin C]

Vio-Bec Forte film-coated tablets (discontinued 1993) ℞ *vitamin/mineral therapy* [multiple B vitamins; vitamins C & E; folic acid; multiple minerals]
Vioform cream, ointment OTC *topical antifungal; antibacterial* [clioquinol]
Vioform-Hydrocortisone; Vioform-Hydrocortisone Mild cream, ointment ℞ *topical corticosteroid; antifungal; antibacterial* [hydrocortisone; clioquinol]
Viogen-C capsules OTC *vitamin/mineral supplement* [multiple vitamins & minerals]
Viokase tablets, powder ℞ *digestive enzymes* [pancrelipase]
viomycin INN [also: viomycin sulfate]
viomycin sulfate USP [also: viomycin]
Viopan-T film-coated tablets OTC *geriatric vitamin/mineral supplement* [multiple vitamins & minerals; folic acid; biotin]
viosterol in oil [see: ergocalciferol]
VIP (VePesid, ifosfamide, Platinol) *chemotherapy protocol*
VIP-B (VP-16, ifosfamide, Platinol, bleomycin) *chemotherapy protocol*
viprostol USAN, INN, BAN *hypotensive; vasodilator*
viprynium embonate BAN *anthelmintic* [also: pyrvinium pamoate]
viqualine INN
viquidil INN
Vira-A IV infusion ℞ *antiviral for herpes simplex and herpes zoster* [vidarabine monohydrate]
Vira-A ophthalmic ointment ℞ *ophthalmic antiviral* [vidarabine monohydrate]
Viranol gel ℞ *topical keratolytic* [salicylic acid; lactic acid]
Viranol Gel Ultra ℞ *topical keratolytic* [salicylic acid]

Virazole powder for inhalation aerosol ℞ *antiviral; (orphan: hemorrhagic fever with renal syndrome)* [ribavirin]
virginiamycin USAN, INN *antibacterial; veterinary food additive*
virginiamycin factor M₁ [see: virginiamycin]
virginiamycin factor S [see: virginiamycin]
viridofulvin USAN, INN *antifungal*
Virilon capsules ℞ *androgen for male hypogonadism, impotence and breast cancer* [methyltestosterone]
Virogen Herpes slide test OTC *in vitro diagnostic aid for herpes simplex virus antigen*
Virogen HSV Antibody slide test (discontinued 1993) OTC *in vitro diagnostic aid for herpes simplex virus antibody*
Virogen Rotatest OTC *in vitro diagnostic aid for fecal rotavirus*
Virogen Rubella Microlatex Test OTC *in vitro diagnostic aid for rubella virus antibody*
Virogen Rubella slide test OTC *in vitro diagnostic aid for rubella virus antibody*
Viro-Med tablets OTC *decongestant; antihistamine; antitussive; analgesic* [pseudoephedrine HCl; chlorpheniramine maleate; dextromethorphan hydrobromide; acetaminophen]
Viroptic Drop-Dose (eye drops) ℞ *ophthalmic antiviral* [trifluridine]
viroxime USAN, INN *antiviral*
viroxime component A [see: zinviroxime]
viroxime component B [see: enviroxime]
Visalens Soaking/Cleaning solution (discontinued 1992) OTC *contact lens cleaning and soaking solution*
Visalens Wetting solution (discontinued 1992) OTC *contact lens wetting solution*

Viscoat solution ℞ *viscoelastic agent for ophthalmic surgery* [sodium chondroitin; sodium hyaluronate]
Visidex II reagent strips (discontinued 1991) OTC *in vitro diagnostic aid for blood glucose*
Visine A.C. eye drops OTC *topical ocular decongestant; astringent; antiseptic* [tetrahydrozoline HCl; zinc sulfate]
Visine L.R. eye drops OTC *topical ocular decongestant* [oxymetazoline HCl]
Visine; Visine Extra eye drops OTC *topical ocular decongestant* [tetrahydrozoline HCl]
Visken tablets ℞ *antihypertensive; β-blocker* [pindolol]
visnadine INN, BAN
visnafylline INN
Vi-Sol [see: Ce-Vi-Sol; Poly-Vi-Sol; Tri-Vi-Sol]
Vistacon IM injection ℞ *anxiolytic* [hydroxyzine HCl]
Vistaject-25; Vistaject-50 IM injection ℞ *anxiolytic* [hydroxyzine HCl]
Vistaquel 50 IM injection ℞ *anxiolytic* [hydroxyzine HCl]
Vistaril capsules, oral suspension ℞ *anxiolytic* [hydroxyzine pamoate]
Vistaril IM injection ℞ *anxiolytic* [hydroxyzine HCl]
vistatolon INN *antiviral* [also: statolon]
Vistazine 50 IM injection ℞ *anxiolytic* [hydroxyzine HCl]
Vita Bee C-800 tablets OTC *vitamin supplement* [multiple B vitamins; vitamins C & E; folic acid]
Vita-bee with C Captabs (capsule-shaped tablets) OTC *vitamin supplement* [multiple B vitamins; vitamin C]
Vita-Bob softgel capsules OTC *vitamin supplement* [multiple vitamins; folic acid]
Vita-C crystals OTC *vitamin supplement* [ascorbic acid]

VitaCarn oral solution ℞ *carnitine replenisher for deficiency of genetic origin or end-stage renal disease (orphan)* [levocarnitine]

Vit-A-Drops eye drops OTC *ocular moisturizer/lubricant* [vitamin A]

Vita-Feron tablets OTC *hematinic* [iron; folic acid; vitamin B$_{12}$]

Vitafōl film-coated caplets ℞ *vitamin/iron/calcium supplement* [multiple vitamins; ferrous fumarate; calcium carbonate; folic acid]

Vitafōl syrup ℞ *hematinic* [ferric pyrophosphate; multiple B vitamins; folic acid]

Vita-Kaps Filmtabs (film-coated tablets) (discontinued 1993) ℞ *vitamin supplement* [multiple vitamins]

VitaKaps-M Filmtabs (film-coated tablets) (discontinued 1993) OTC *vitamin/mineral/iron supplement* [multiple vitamins & minerals; iron]

Vita-Kid chewable wafers OTC *vitamin supplement* [multiple vitamins; folic acid]

Vital B-50 protein-coated timed-release tablets OTC *vitamin supplement* [multiple B vitamins; folic acid; biotin; bromelain]

Vital High Nitrogen powder OTC *oral nutritional supplement*

Vitalets chewable tablets OTC *vitamin/mineral/iron supplement* [multiple vitamins & minerals; iron; biotin]

Vitalize SF liquid OTC *hematinic* [ferric pyrophosphate; multiple B vitamins; folic acid]

vitamin A USP *vitamin; antixerophthalmic; topical emollient*

vitamin A acid [see: tretinoin]

vitamin A palmitate

vitamin A$_1$ [see: retinol]

vitamin B$_1$ [see: thiamine HCl]

vitamin B$_1$ mononitrate [see: thiamine mononitrate]

vitamin B$_2$ [see: riboflavin]

vitamin B$_3$ [see: niacin; niacinamide]

vitamin B$_5$ [see: calcium pantothenate]

vitamin B$_6$ [see: pyridoxine HCl]

vitamin B$_8$ [see: adenosine phosphate]

vitamin B$_{12}$ [now: cyanocobalamin]

vitamin B$_c$ [see: folic acid]

vitamin B$_t$ [see: carnitine]

vitamin C [see: ascorbic acid]

vitamin D (vitamins D$_2$ and/or D$_3$) [see: ergocalciferol (D$_2$); cholecalciferol (D$_3$)]

vitamin D$_1$ [see: dihydrotachysterol]

vitamin D$_2$ [see: ergocalciferol]

vitamin D$_3$ [see: cholecalciferol]

vitamin E USP *vitamin E supplement; topical emollient*

vitamin E-TPGS (tocopheryl polyethylene glycol succinate) [see: tocophersolan]

vitamin G [see: riboflavin]

vitamin H [see: biotin]

vitamin K$_1$ [see: phytonadione]

vitamin K$_2$ [see: menaquinone]

vitamin K$_3$ [see: menadione]

vitamin K$_4$ [see: menadiol sodium diphosphate]

vitamin M [see: folic acid]

vitamin P [see: bioflavonoids]

vitamin P$_4$ [see: troxerutin]

vitamins A & D (topical) *emollient*

Vitaneed liquid OTC *oral nutritional supplement*

Vita-Plus B-12 injection ℞ *vitamin B$_{12}$ therapy* [cyanocobalamin]

Vita-Plus E softgels OTC *vitamin supplement* [vitamin E]

Vita-Plus G softgel capsules OTC *geriatric vitamin/mineral supplement* [multiple vitamins & minerals]

Vita-Plus H softgel capsules OTC *vitamin/mineral/iron supplement* [multiple vitamins & minerals; iron]

Vitarex tablets OTC *vitamin/mineral/iron supplement* [multiple vitamins & minerals; iron]

Vitazin capsules (discontinued 1992) OTC *vitamin/mineral supplement* [multiple vitamins & minerals]

Vite E cream OTC *emollient* [vitamin E]

Vitec cream OTC *emollient* [vitamin E]

Vitrax injection (discontinued 1991) ℞ *ophthalmic surgery aid* [sodium hyaluronate in balanced salt solution]

Vitron-C chewable tablets OTC *hematinic* [ferrous fumarate; ascorbic acid]

Vitron-C-Plus tablets OTC *hematinic* [ferrous fumarate; ascorbic acid]

Vivactil film-coated tablets ℞ *tricyclic antidepressant* [protriptyline HCl]

Vivalan *(orphan: cataplexy; narcolepsy)* [viloxazine HCl]

Vivarin tablets OTC *CNS stimulant; analeptic* [caffeine]

Vivonex T.E.N. single-serving packets OTC *total enteral nutrition* [multiple vitamins & minerals; essential & nonessential amino acids]

Vivotif Berna enteric-coated capsules ℞ *typhoid vaccine* [typhoid vaccine]

Vi-Zac capsules OTC *vitamin/zinc supplement* [vitamins A, C & E; zinc]

V-Lax powder OTC *bulk laxative* [psyllium hydrophilic mucilloid]

Vlemasque paste, cream (discontinued 1991) OTC *keratolytic for acne* [sulfurated lime topical solution]

Vlem-Dome liquid concentrate (discontinued 1991) OTC *wet dressing* [lime sulfur solution]

Vleminckx' solution (discontinued 1991) OTC *wet dressing* [calcium pentasulfide; calcium thiosulfate]

VLP (vincristine, L-asparaginase, prednisone) *chemotherapy protocol*

VM-26PP (VM-26, procarbazine, prednisone) *chemotherapy protocol*

VMAD (vincristine, methotrexate, Adriamycin, actinomycin D) *chemotherapy protocol*

VMCP (vincristine, melphalan, cyclophosphamide, prednisone) *chemotherapy protocol*

VMP (VePesid, mitoxantrone, prednimustine) *chemotherapy protocol*

VOCAP (VP-16-213, Oncovin, cyclophosphamide, Adriamycin, Platinol) *chemotherapy protocol*

volazocine USAN, INN *analgesic*

Volmax tablets ℞ *investigational antiasthmatic* [albuterol]

Voltaren enteric-coated tablets ℞ *nonsteroidal anti-inflammatory drug (NSAID); antiarthritic; analgesic* [diclofenac sodium]

Voltaren eye drops ℞ *ocular nonsteroidal anti-inflammatory* [diclofenac sodium]

Voltaren Retard ℞ *investigational sustained-release antiarthritic* [diclofenac sodium]

von Willebrand's factor [see: antihemophilic factor]

Vontrol tablets ℞ *antiemetic; antivertigo agent* [diphenidol HCl]

vortel [see: clorprenaline HCl]

VōSol HC Otic ear drops ℞ *topical corticosteroidal anti-inflammatory; antibacterial/antifungal* [hydrocortisone; acetic acid]

VōSol Otic ear drops ℞ *antibacterial/antifungal* [acetic acid]

voxergolide INN

Voxsuprine tablets ℞ *peripheral vasodilator* [isoxsuprine HCl]

VP (vasopressin) [q.v.]

VP (vincristine, prednisone) *chemotherapy protocol*

VP-L-asparaginase (vincristine, prednisone, L-asparaginase) *chemotherapy protocol*

VPB (vinblastine, Platinol, bleomycin) *chemotherapy protocol*

VPBCPr (vincristine, prednisone, vinblastine, chlorambucil, procarbazine) *chemotherapy protocol*

VPCA (vincristine, prednisone, cyclophosphamide, ara-C) *chemotherapy protocol*

VPCMF (vincristine, prednisone, cyclophosphamide, methotrexate, fluorouracil) *chemotherapy protocol*
VPP (VePesid, Platinol) *chemotherapy protocol*
Vumon IV infusion ℞ *antineoplastic for acute lymphoblastic leukemia (orphan)* [teniposide]

V.V.S. vaginal cream ℞ *bacteriostatic* [sulfathiazole; sulfacetamide; sulfabenzamide; urea]
Vytone cream ℞ *topical corticosteroid; antifungal; antibacterial* [hydrocortisone; iodoquinol]
VZIG (varicella-zoster immune globulin) [q.v.]

W

Wampole One-Step hCG test kit ℞ *in vitro diagnostic aid for urine/serum pregnancy test*
warfarin INN, BAN *anticoagulant* [also: warfarin potassium]
warfarin potassium USP *anticoagulant* [also: warfarin]
warfarin sodium USP *anticoagulant*
Wart Remover liquid OTC *topical keratolytic* [salicylic acid]
wart-aid cream (discontinued 1992) OTC *topical keratolytic* [calcium pantothenate; ascorbic acid; starch]
Wart-Off liquid OTC *topical keratolytic* [salicylic acid]
water, purified USP *solvent*
water, tritiated [see: tritiated water]
water moccasin snake antivenin [see: antivenin (Crotalidae) polyvalent]
water-d₂ [see: deuterium oxide]
wax, carnauba NF *tablet-coating agent*
wax, emulsifying NF *emulsifying and stiffening agent*
wax, microcrystalline NF *stiffening and tablet-coating agent*
wax, white NF *stiffening agent*
wax, yellow NF *stiffening agent*
Wehamine IV or IM injection (discontinued 1991) ℞ *antinauseant; antiemetic; antivertigo; motion sickness preventative* [dimenhydrinate]

Wehdryl injection ℞ *antihistamine; motion sickness preventative; sleep aid; antiparkinsonian* [diphenhydramine HCl]
Wehgen IM injection ℞ *estrogen replacement therapy; antineoplasic for prostatic and breast cancer* [estrone]
Wehless-105 capsules, Timecelles (sustained-release capsules) ℞ *anorexiant* [phendimetrazine tartrate]
Weightrol tablets ℞ *anorexiant* [phendimetrazine tartrate]
Wellbutrin tablets ℞ *antidepressant* [bupropion HCl]
Wellcovorin powder for IV infusion ℞ *leucovorin "rescue" after methotrexate therapy; (orphan: adjunct to colorectal cancer therapy)* [leucovorin calcium]
Wellcovorin tablets ℞ *leucovorin "rescue" after methotrexate therapy; antidote to folic acid antagonist overdose* [leucovorin calcium]
Wellferon *(orphan: Kaposi sarcoma; human papillomavirus)* [interferon alfa-n1]
Wesprin tablets OTC *analgesic; antipyretic; anti-inflammatory; antirheumatic* [aspirin, buffered with aluminum hydroxide and magnesium hydroxide]
Westcort ointment, cream ℞ *topical corticosteroid* [hydrocortisone valerate]

western equine encephalitis (WEE) immune globulin *investigational immunizing agent*

Wet-N-Soak PLUS solution OTC *contact lens wetting/soaking solution*

Wet-N-Soak solution (discontinued 1992) OTC *contact lens wetting/soaking solution*

Wetting & Soaking solution OTC *contact lens wetting/soaking solution*

Wetting solution OTC *contact lens wetting solution*

wheat germ oil [see: vitamin E]

White Cloverine Salve ointment OTC *skin protectant* [white petrolatum]

White Cod Liver Oil Concentrate capsules, chewable tablets OTC *vitamin supplement* [cod liver oil (source of vitamins A & D); vitamin E]

White Cod Liver Oil Concentrate with Vitamin C chewable tablets OTC *vitamin supplement* [cod liver oil (source of vitamins A & D); vitamin C]

white lotion USP *astringent; topical protectant*

white mineral oil [see: petrolatum, white]

white ointment [see: ointment, white]

white petrolatum [see: petrolatum, white]

white phenolphthalein [see: phenolphthalein]

white wax [see: wax, white]

Whitfield's ointment [see: benzoic & salicylic acids]

Whitfield's ointment OTC *topical antifungal; keratolytic* [benzoic acid; salicylic acid]

Whitsphill Full Strength ointment (discontinued 1991) OTC *topical antifungal; keratolytic* [benzoic acid; salicylic acid]

whole blood [see: blood, whole]

whole root rauwolfia [see: rauwolfia serpentina]

Wibi lotion OTC *moisturizer; emollient*

widow spider species antivenin [now: antivenin (Latrodectus mactans)]

Wigraine suppositories ℞ *migraine-specific vasoconstrictor* [ergotamine tartrate; caffeine; tartaric acid]

Wigraine tablets ℞ *migraine-specific vasoconstrictor* [ergotamine tartrate; caffeine]

Wigrettes sublingual tablets (discontinued 1991) ℞ *agent for migraine* [ergotamine tartrate]

wild cherry syrup USP

WinGel chewable tablets, liquid OTC *antacid* [aluminum hydroxide; magnesium hydroxide]

WinRho SD ℞ *investigational treatment for idiopathic thrombocytopenic purpura* [anti-Rh immune globulin]

Winstrol tablets ℞ *anabolic steroid for hereditary angioedema* [stanozolol]

wintergreen oil [see: methyl salicylate]

Wintersteiner's compound F [see: hydrocortisone]

witch hazel [see: hamamelis water]

Wolfina tablets (discontinued 1992) ℞ *antihypertensive; antipsychotic* [rauwolfia serpentina (whole root)]

Women's Daily Formula capsules OTC *vitamin/calcium/iron supplement* [multiple vitamins; calcium; iron; folic acid]

Wonder Ice gel OTC *counterirritant* [menthol]

Wondra lotion OTC *moisturizer; emollient* [lanolin]

wood creosote [see: creosote carbonate]

Woolley's antiserotonin [see: benanserin HCl]

Wyamine Sulfate IV or IM injection ℞ *vasopressor used in shock* [mephentermine sulfate]

Wyamycin S film-coated tablets ℞ *macrolide antibiotic* [erythromycin stearate]

Wyanoids rectal suppositories OTC *vasoconstrictor; astringent* [ephedrine sulfate; belladonna extract; boric acid; zinc oxide; bismuth salts]

Wycillin and Probenecid two prefilled disposable syringes for IM injection + two tablets (discontinued 1992) ℞ *antibiotic for Neisseria gonorrhoeae* [penicillin G procaine (syringes); probenecid (tablets)]

Wycillin IM injection, Tubex (cartridge-needle units) ℞ *bactericidal antibiotic* [penicillin G procaine]

Wydase IV or subcu injection ℞ *adjuvant to increase absorption and dispersion of injected drugs* [hyaluronidase]

Wygesic tablets ℞ *narcotic analgesic* [propoxyphene HCl; acetaminophen]

Wymox capsules, powder for oral suspension ℞ *penicillin-type antibiotic* [amoxicillin trihydrate]

Wytensin tablets ℞ *antihypertensive* [guanabenz acetate]

X

xamoterol USAN, INN, BAN *cardiac stimulant*
Xanax SR ℞ *investigational sustained-release anxiolytic* [alprazolam]
Xanax tablets ℞ *anxiolytic* [alprazolam]
xanoxate sodium USAN *bronchodilator*
xanoxic acid INN
xanthan gum NF *suspending agent*
xanthinol niacinate USAN *peripheral vasodilator* [also: xantinol nicotinate]
xanthiol INN
xanthiol HCl [see: xanthiol]
xanthocillin BAN [also: xantocillin]
xanthotoxin [see: methoxsalen]
xantifibrate INN
xantinol nicotinate INN *peripheral vasodilator* [also: xanthinol niacinate]
xantocillin INN [also: xanthocillin]
xantofyl palmitate INN
127Xe [see: xenon Xe 127]
133Xe [see: xenon Xe 133]
xenalamine [see: xenazoic acid]
xenaldial [see: xenygloxal]
xenalipin USAN, INN *hypolipidemic*
xenazoic acid INN
xenbucin USAN, INN *antihypercholesterolemic*

xenbuficin [see: xenbucin]
xenipentone INN
xenon *element* (Xe)
xenon (^{133}Xe) INN *radioactive agent* [also: xenon Xe 133]
xenon Xe 127 USP *diagnostic aid; medicinal gas; radioactive agent*
xenon Xe 133 USAN, USP *radioactive agent* [also: xenon (^{133}Xe)]
xenthiorate INN
xenygloxal INN
xenyhexenic acid INN
xenysalate INN, BAN *topical anesthetic; antibacterial; antifungal* [also: biphenamine HCl]
xenysalate HCl [see: biphenamine HCl]
xenytropium bromide INN
Xerac AC liquid ℞ *topical acne cleanser* [aluminum chloride hexahydrate; anhydrous ethyl alcohol]
Xerac BP5; Xerac BP10 gel OTC *topical keratolytic for acne* [benzoyl peroxide]
Xerac gel OTC *antibacterial; exfoliant* [microcrystalline sulfur; isopropyl alcohol]
Xero-Lube oral spray OTC *saliva substitute*

xibenolol INN
xibornol INN, BAN
xilobam USAN, INN *muscle relaxant*
ximoprofen INN
xinidamine INN
xinomiline INN
xipamide USAN, INN *antihypertensive; diuretic*
xipranolol INN
Xomazyme-791 *(orphan: metastatic colorectal adenocarcinoma)* [anti-TAP-72 immunotoxin]
Xomazyme-H65 *(orphan: graft vs. host disease; graft rejection)* [CD5-T lymphocyte immunotoxin]
xorphanol INN *analgesic* [also: xorphanol mesylate]
xorphanol mesylate USAN *analgesic* [also: xorphanol]
X-Prep Bowel Evacuant Kit-1 liquid, tablet & suppository in a kit OTC *pre-procedure bowel evacuant* [X-Prep liquid (q.v.); Senokot-S tablets (q.v.); Rectolax suppository (q.v.)]
X-Prep Bowel Evacuant Kit-2 liquid, granules & suppository in a kit OTC *pre-procedure bowel evacuant* [X-Prep liquid (q.v.); Citralax granules (q.v.); Rectolax suppository (q.v.)]
X-Prep liquid OTC *pre-procedure bowel evacuant* [senna extract; alcohol]
X-Seb Plus shampoo OTC *antiseborrheic; keratolytic; antibacterial; antifungal* [salicylic acid; pyrithione zinc]
X-Seb shampoo OTC *antiseborrheic; keratolytic* [salicylic acid]
X-seb T Plus shampoo OTC *antiseborrheic; antipsoriatic; keratolytic* [coal tar; salicylic acid; menthol]

X-seb T shampoo OTC *antiseborrheic; antipsoriatic; keratolytic* [coal tar; salicylic acid]
xylamidine tosilate INN *serotonin inhibitor* [also: xylamidine tosylate]
xylamidine tosylate USAN *serotonin inhibitor* [also: xylamidine tosilate]
xylazine INN *analgesic; veterinary muscle relaxant* [also: xylazine HCl]
xylazine HCl USAN *analgesic; veterinary muscle relaxant* [also: xylazine]
xylitol NF *sweetened vehicle*
Xylocaine 10% Oral spray ℞ *mucous membrane anesthetic* [lidocaine HCl]
Xylocaine HCl injection ℞ *injectable local anesthetic* [lidocaine HCl]
Xylocaine HCl IV for Cardiac Arrhythmias IV injection, IV admixture ℞ *antiarrhythmic* [lidocaine HCl]
Xylocaine IV, IM or subcu injection ℞ *anesthetic; antiarrhythmic* [lidocaine HCl]
Xylocaine ointment, jelly ℞ *mucous membrane anesthetic* [lidocaine HCl]
Xylocaine ointment OTC *topical local anesthetic* [lidocaine]
Xylocaine; Xylocaine Viscous solution ℞ *mucous membrane anesthetic* [lidocaine HCl]
xylocoumarol INN
xylofilcon A USAN *hydrophilic contact lens material*
xylometazoline INN, BAN *vasoconstrictor; nasal decongestant* [also: xylometazoline HCl]
xylometazoline HCl USP *vasoconstrictor; nasal decongestant* [also: xylometazoline]
Xylo-Pfan tablets OTC *intestinal function test* [xylose]
xylose (D-xylose) USP *intestinal function test*
xyloxemine INN

Y

yatren [see: chiniofon]
169Yb [see: pentetate calcium trisodium Yb 169]
169Yb [see: ytterbium Yb 169 pentetate]
yeast, dried NF
yeast cell derivative *claimed to promote wound healine*
Yelets tablets OTC *vitamin/mineral/iron supplement* [multiple vitamins & minerals; ferrous fumarate; folic acid]
yellow ferric oxide [see: ferric oxide, yellow]
yellow fever vaccine USP *active immunizing agent for yellow fever*
yellow mercuric oxide [see: mercuric oxide, yellow]
yellow ointment [see: ointment, yellow]
yellow phenolphthalein [see: phenolphthalein, yellow]
yellow precipitate [see: mercuric oxide, yellow]
yellow wax [see: wax, yellow]
yerba santa [see: eriodictyon]
YF-Vax subcu injection R *yellow fever vaccine* [yellow fever vaccine]
Y-Itch cream (discontinued 1991) OTC *topical local anesthetic; antiseptic* [benzocaine; dibucaine; tetracaine; benzalkonium chloride]
Yocon tablets R *no approved uses; sympatholytic; mydriatic; aphrodisiac* [yohimbine HCl]
Yodoxin tablets, powder R *amebicide* [iodoquinol]
yohimbic acid INN
yohimbine HCl *claimed to be an aphrodisiac; no FDA-sanctioned uses*
Yohimex tablets R *no approved uses; sympatholytic; mydriatic; aphrodisiac* [yohimbine HCl]
ytterbium *element (Yb)*
ytterbium Yb 169 pentetate USP *radioactive agent*
yttrium *element (Y)*
Yutopar IV infusion, tablets R *arrest preterm labor* [ritodrine HCl]

Z

zabicipril INN
zacopride INN *antiemetic; peristaltic stimulant* [also: zacopride HCl]
zacopride HCl USAN, INN *antiemetic; peristaltic stimulant* [also: zacopride]
Zadaxin R *investigational hepatitis B treatment*
Zaditen R *investigational antiasthmatic* [ketotifen]
zafuleptine INN
zalcitabine USAN *antiviral; (orphan: AIDS)*
zalospirone INN *anxiolytic* [also: zalospirone HCl]
zalospirone HCl USAN *anxiolytic* [also: zalospirone]
zaltidine INN, BAN *antagonist to histamine H_2 receptors* [also: zaltidine HCl]
zaltidine HCl USAN *antagonist to histamine H_2 receptors* [also: zaltidine]
Zanosar powder for IV injection R *antineoplastic for metastatic islet cell carcinoma of pancreas* [streptozocin]
zanoterone USAN *antiandrogen*
Zantac film-coated tablets, syrup, IV or IM injection R *gastric and duodenal ulcer treatment; histamine H_2 antagonist* [ranitidine HCl]

Zantryl capsules ℞ *appetite suppressant* [phentermine HCl]
zapizolam INN
zaprinast INN, BAN
zardaverine INN
Zarontin capsules, syrup ℞ *anticonvulsant* [ethosuximide]
Zaroxolyn tablets ℞ *diuretic; antihypertensive* [metolazone]
Zartan capsules ℞ *cephalosporin-type antibiotic* [cephalexin monohydrate]
zatosetron INN *antimigraine* [also: zatosetron maleate]
zatosetron maleate USAN *antimigraine* [also: zatosetron]
Z-Bec tablets OTC *vitamin/zinc supplement* [multiple vitamins; zinc sulfate]
ZBT Baby powder OTC *topical diaper rash treatment* [talc]
ZE Caps soft capsules OTC *dietary supplement* [vitamin E; zinc gluconate]
Zeasorb powder OTC *absorbent* [microporous cellulose; talc]
Zeasorb-AF powder OTC *topical antifungal* [tolnaftate]
Zebeta film-coated tablets ℞ *antihypertensive; β-blocker* [bisoprolol fumarate]
Zebrax capsules (discontinued 1991) ℞ *anticholinergic; anxiolytic* [clidinium bromide; chlordiazepoxide HCl]
Zefazone powder for IV injection ℞ *cephalosporin-type antibiotic* [cefmetazole sodium]
zein NF *coating agent*
Zeisin Autohaler (metered-dose inhaler) ℞ *investigational antiasthmatic*
Zemo lotion (discontinued 1991) OTC *antipruritic; mild anesthetic; counterirritant* [alcohol; phenol; methyl salicylate]
Zemo ointment (discontinued 1991) OTC *antipruritic; counterirritant* [bismuth subnitrate; methyl salicylate; menthol; triclosan]

Zenate Prenatal film-coated tablets ℞ *vitamin/calcium/iron supplement* [multiple vitamins; calcium; iron; folic acid]
zenazocine mesylate USAN *analgesic*
Zentinic capsules (discontinued 1991) OTC *antianemic* [ferrous fumarate; multiple B vitamins; vitamin C; folic acid]
Zentron chewable tablets (discontinued 1991) OTC *antianemic* [ferrous fumarate; multiple B vitamins; vitamin C]
Zentron liquid (discontinued 1991) OTC *antianemic* [ferrous sulfate; multiple B vitamins; vitamin C]
zepastine INN
Zephiran Chloride tincture, tincture spray, aqueous solution, disinfectant concentrate, towelettes OTC *topical antiseptic* [benzalkonium chloride]
zephirol [see: benzalkonium chloride]
Zephrex film-coated tablets ℞ *decongestant; expectorant* [pseudoephedrine HCl; guaifenesin]
Zephrex LA timed-release tablets ℞ *decongestant; expectorant* [pseudoephedrine HCl; guaifenesin]
zeranol USAN, INN *anabolic*
Zeroxin-5; Zeroxin-10 gel ℞ *topical keratolytic for acne* [benzoyl peroxide]
Zestoretic tablets ℞ *antihypertensive; angiotensin-converting enzyme inhibitor; diuretic* [hydrochlorothiazide; lisinopril]
Zestril tablets ℞ *antihypertensive; angiotensin-converting enzyme inhibitor* [lisinopril]
Zetar Emulsion bath oil ℞ *antipsoriatic; antiseborrheic; antipruritic; emollient* [coal tar]
Zetar shampoo OTC *antiseborrheic; antipsoriatic; antipruritic; antibacterial* [coal tar]
zetidoline INN, BAN
Zetran IV or IM injection ℞ *skeletal muscle relaxant; anxiolytic* [diazepam]

Z-gen tablets OTC *vitamin/zinc supplement* [multiple vitamins; zinc]
zidapamide INN
zidometacin USAN, INN *anti-inflammatory*
zidovudine USAN, INN, BAN *antiviral for AIDS and AIDS-related complex (orphan)*
ZilaBrace gel (discontinued 1991) OTC *oral topical anesthetic for braces* [benzocaine]
Zilactin Medicated gel OTC *astringent for oral canker and herpes lesions* [tannic acid]
Zilactol Medicated liquid OTC *astringent for pre-emergent oral herpes lesions* [tannic acid]
ZilaDent gel OTC *oral topical anesthetic* [benzocaine]
zilantel USAN, INN *anthelmintic*
Zileuton ℞ *investigational anti-inflammatory for asthma, ulcerative colitis and rheumatoid arthritis*
zileuton USAN, INN *5-lipoxygenase inhibitor*
zilpaterol INN
zimeldine INN, BAN *antidepressant* [also: zimeldine HCl]
zimeldine HCl USAN *antidepressant* [also: zimeldine]
zimelidine HCl [now: zimeldine HCl]
zimidoben INN
Zinacef powder for IV or IM injection ℞ *cephalosporin-type antibiotic* [cefuroxime sodium]
zinc *element (Zn)*
Zinc 15 tablets OTC *zinc supplement* [zinc sulfate]
Zinc 220 capsules OTC *zinc supplement* [zinc sulfate]
zinc acetate USP *(orphan: Wilson's disease)*
zinc acetate, basic INN
zinc acetate dihydrate [see: zinc acetate]
zinc bacitracin [see: bacitracin zinc]
zinc caprylate *antifungal*
zinc carbonate USAN *zinc supplement*
zinc chloride USP *astringent; dentin desensitizer; dietary zinc supplement*
zinc chloride Zn 65 USAN *radioactive agent*
zinc complex bacitracins [see: bacitracin zinc]
zinc gelatin USP
zinc gluconate USP *dietary zinc supplement*
zinc oleate NF
zinc oxide USP *astringent; topical protectant; emollient; antiseptic*
zinc peroxide, medicinal USP
zinc phenolsulfonate NF *not generally regarded as safe and effective as an antidiarrheal*
zinc propionate *antifungal*
zinc pyrithione [see: pyrithione zinc]
zinc stearate USP *dusting powder; tablet and capsule lubricant; antifungal*
zinc sulfate USP *astringent; dietary zinc supplement*
zinc sulfate heptahydrate [see: zinc sulfate]
zinc sulfate monohydrate [see: zinc sulfate]
Zinc Sulfide Compound Lotion, Improved (discontinued 1992) OTC *topical acne treatment* [zinc sulfide; sulfur]
zinc sulfocarbolate [see: zinc phenolsulfonate]
Zinc Trace Metal Additive IV injection (discontinued 1992) ℞ *intravenous nutritional therapy* [sinc sulfate]
zinc undecylenate USP *antifungal*
zinc valerate USP
Zinc-220 capsules OTC *zinc supplement* [zinc sulfate]
Zinca-Pak IV injection ℞ *intravenous nutritional therapy* [zinc sulfate]
Zincate capsules ℞ *zinc supplement* [zinc sulfate]
zinc-eugenol USP

Zincfrin eye drops OTC *topical ocular decongestant; astringent; antiseptic* [phenylephrine HCl; zinc sulfate]

Zincon shampoo OTC *antiseborrheic; antibacterial; antifungal* [pyrithione zinc]

zindotrine USAN, INN *bronchodilator*

zindoxifene INN

Zinecard ℞ *(orphan: doxorubicin-induced cardiomyopathy)* [dexrazoxane]

Zinkaps-220 capsules OTC *zinc supplement* [zinc sulfate]

zinoconazole INN *antifungal* [also: zinoconazole HCl]

zinoconazole HCl USAN *antifungal* [also: zinoconazole]

zinostatin USAN, INN *antineoplastic*

zinterol INN *bronchodilator* [also: zinterol HCl]

zinterol HCl USAN *bronchodilator* [also: zinterol]

zinviroxime USAN, INN *antiviral*

zipeprol INN

Ziradryl lotion OTC *topical antihistamine; astringent; antiseptic* [diphenhydramine HCl; zinc oxide; alcohol]

zirconium *element (Zr)*

zirconium oxide *astringent*

Zithromax capsules ℞ *macrolide antibiotic* [azithromycin dihydrate]

Zixoryn *(orphan: neonatal hyperbilirubinemia)* [flumecinol]

⁶⁵Zn [see: zinc chloride Zn 65]

ZNP cleansing bar OTC *antiseborrheic; antibacterial; antifungal* [pyrithione zinc]

zocainone INN

Zocor tablets ℞ *antihyperlipidemic* [simvastatin]

Zodeac-100 tablets ℞ *vitamin/mineral/iron supplement* [multiple vitamins & minerals; ferrous fumarate; folic acid; biotin]

zofenopril INN, BAN *angiotensin-converting enzyme (ACE) inhibitor* [also: zofenopril calcium]

zofenopril calcium USAN *angiotensin-converting enzyme (ACE) inhibitor* [also: zofenopril]

zofenoprilat INN *antihypertensive* [also: zofenoprilat arginine]

zofenoprilat arginine USAN *antihypertensive* [also: zofenoprilat]

zoficonazole INN

Zofran tablets, IV infusion ℞ *antiemetic for cancer chemotherapy* [ondansetron HCl]

Zoladex subcu implant ℞ *palliative hormonal therapy for prostatic carcinoma* [goserelin acetate]

zolamine INN *antihistamine; topical anesthetic* [also: zolamine HCl]

zolamine HCl USAN *antihistamine; topical anesthetic* [also: zolamine]

zolazepam INN, BAN *sedative* [also: zolazepam HCl]

zolazepam HCl USAN *sedative* [also: zolazepam]

zolenzepine INN

zolertine INN *antiadrenergic; vasodilator* [also: zolertine HCl]

zolertine HCl USAN *antiadrenergic; vasodilator* [also: zolertine]

Zolicef powder for IV or IM injection ℞ *cephalosporin-type antibiotic* [cefazolin sodium]

zolimidine INN

zoliprofen INN

zoliridine [see: zolimidine]

Zoloft film-coated tablets ℞ *antidepressant* [sertraline]

zoloperone INN

zolpidem INN, BAN *imidazopyridine-type sedative/hypnotic* [also: zolpidem tartrate]

zolpidem tartrate USAN *imidazopyridine-type sedative/hypnotic* [also: zolpidem]

Zolyse ophthalmic solution ℞ *enzymatic zonulolytic for intracapsular lens extraction* [chymotrypsin]

zomebazam INN

zomepirac INN, BAN *analgesic; anti-inflammatory* [also: zomepirac sodium]

zomepirac sodium USAN, USP *analgesic; anti-inflammatory* [also: zomepirac]

zometapine USAN *antidepressant*

Zonalon ℞ *investigational topical antipruritic*

Zone-A Forte lotion ℞ *topical corticosteroid; local anesthetic* [hydrocortisone acetate; pramoxine]

Zone-A lotion, cream (discontinued 1993) ℞ *topical corticosteroid; anesthetic* [hydrocortisone acetate; pramoxine]

zonisamide USAN, INN, BAN *anticonvulsant*

Zonite Douche solution concentrate OTC *antiseptic; antipruritic/counterirritant; vaginal cleansing and deodorizing* [benzalkonium chloride; menthol; thymol]

Zophren (European name for U.S. product Zofran)

zopiclone INN, BAN

zopolrestat USAN *antidiabetic; aldose reductase inhibitor*

zorbamycin USAN *antibacterial*

ZORprin Zero Order Release tablets ℞ *analgesic; antipyretic; anti-inflammatory; antirheumatic* [aspirin]

zorubicin INN *antineoplastic* [also: zorubicin HCl]

zorubicin HCl USAN *antineoplastic* [also: zorubicin]

Zostrix; Zostrix-HP cream OTC *topical analgesic* [capsaicin]

zotepine INN

Zovirax capsules, tablets, oral suspension, ointment, IV infusion ℞ *antiviral for herpes simplex, herpes zoster, and adult-onset chickenpox* [acyclovir]

Zovirax powder for IV infusion ℞ *antiviral* [acyclovir sodium]

zoxazolamine NF, INN

Z-Pro-C tablets (discontinued 1991) ℞ *dietary supplement* [zinc gluconate; ascorbic acid]

zuclomifene INN

zuclomiphene USAN

zuclopenthixol INN, BAN

Zurinol tablets ℞ *uricosuric for gout* [allopurinol]

Zydone capsules ℞ *narcotic analgesic* [hydrocodone bitartrate; acetaminophen]

zylofuramine INN

Zyloprim tablets ℞ *xanthine oxidase inhibitor for gout; (orphan: ex vivo preservation of kidneys for transplantation)* [allopurinol]

Zymacap capsules OTC *vitamin supplement* [multiple vitamins; folic acid]

Zymase capsules containing enteric-coated spheres ℞ *digestive enzymes* [pancrelipase]

APPENDIX A
Sound Alikes

Listed below are 924 pairs of drugs that sound alike or sufficiently alike that they may be confused in transcription. The list is not all-inclusive, and we would appreciate hearing of any additions the reader might suggest. You may wish to refer to this list when it has been difficult to hear the whole word. You should also periodically review the list to be certain that you are not confusing similar-sounding drugs.

A-Caine	Anocaine
Accurbron	Accutane
Accutane	Accurbron
Achromycin	actinomycin
Achromycin	Aureomycin
Actidil	Actifed
Actifed	Actidil
actinomycin	Achromycin
actinomycin	Aureomycin
Adapin	Atabrine
Adapin	Ativan
Adapin	Betapen
Advil	Avail
Aerolone	Aralen
Aerolone	Arlidin
Afrin	Afrinol
Afrin	aspirin
Afrinol	Afrin
Agoral	Argyrol
Ak-Mycin	Akne-Mycin
Akne-Mycin	Ak-Mycin
Alamag	Alma-Mag
Aldactazide	Aldactone
Aldactone	Aldactazide
Aldomet	Aldoril
Aldoril	Aldomet
Aldoril	Elavil
Allergan	allergen
Allergan	Auralgan
allergen	Allergan
allergen	Auralgan
Alma-Mag	Alamag

505

Appendix A

Ambenyl	Aventyl
Amicar	Amikin
Amikin	Amicar
amitriptyline	nortriptyline
amoxapine	amoxicillin
amoxapine	Amoxil
amoxicillin	amoxapine
Amoxil	amoxapine
Anafranil	enalapril
Analbalm	Analpram
Analpram	Analbalm
Ancobon	Oncovin
Anocaine	A-Caine
Anturane	Artane
Anusol	Aplisol
APAC	APAP
APAP	APAC
Aplisol	Anusol
Aplisol	Apresoline
Appedrine	aprindine
Appedrine	ephedrine
Apresoline	Aplisol
Apresoline	Priscoline
aprindine	Appedrine
aprindine	ephedrine
ara-C	ERYC
Aralen	Aerolone
Aralen	Arlidin
Argyrol	Agoral
Arlidin	Aerolone
Arlidin	Aralen
Artane	Anturane
aspirin	Afrin
Atabrine	Adapin
Atarax	Marax
atenolol	timolol
Ativan	Adapin
Ativan	Avitene
Auralgan	Allergan
Auralgan	allergen
Aureomycin	Achromycin
Aureomycin	actinomycin
Avail	Advil
Aventyl	Ambenyl
Aventyl	Bentyl
Avitene	Ativan
Azlin	Mezlin
azolimine	Azulfidine

Azulfidine	azolimine
Bacid	Banacid
bacitracin	Bacitrin
bacitracin	Bactrim
Bacitrin	bacitracin
Bactocill	Pathocil
Bactrim	bacitracin
Banacid	Bacid
Banophen	Barophen
Banthine	Brethine
Barophen	Banophen
Belladenal	belladonna
Belladenal	Benadryl
belladonna	Belladenal
Beminal	Benemid
Benadryl	Belladenal
Benadryl	Bentyl
Benadryl	Benylin
Benadryl	Caladryl
Benemid	Beminal
Benoxyl	PanOxyl
Bentyl	Aventyl
Bentyl	Benadryl
Bentyl	Bontril
Benylin	Benadryl
Benylin	Betalin
Betalin	Benylin
Betapen	Adapin
Betapen	Phenaphen
Bichloracetic acid	dichloroacetic acid
Bicillin	V-Cillin
Bicillin	Wycillin
bleomycin	Cleocin
boil	Boyol
Bontril	Bentyl
Bontril	Vontrol
Boyol	boil
Brethine	Banthine
Bretylol	Brevital
Brevital	Bretylol
Bromfed	Bromphen
Bromophen	Bromphen
Bromphen	Bromfed
Bromphen	Bromophen
Broncholate	Brondelate
Brondecon	Bronitin
Brondelate	Broncholate
Bronitin	Brondecon

butabarbital	butalbital
butalbital	butabarbital
butalbital	Butibel
Butazolidin	Butisol
Butibel	butalbital
Butisol	Butazolidin
Byclomine	Hycomine
Bydramine	Hydramine
Caladryl	Benadryl
calcitonin	calcitriol
calcitriol	calcitonin
Capastat	Cepastat
Capitrol	captopril
captopril	Capitrol
Catapres	Catarase
Catapres	Combipres
Catapres	Ser-Ap-Es
Catarase	Catapres
cefazolin	cephalexin
cefazolin	cephalothin
cefotaxime	cefoxitin
cefoxitin	cefotaxime
ceftizoxime	cefuroxime
cefuroxime	ceftizoxime
Cepastat	Capastat
cephalexin	cefazolin
cephalexin	cephalothin
cephalothin	cefazolin
cephalothin	cephalexin
cephapirin	cephradine
cephradine	cephapirin
chlorpheniramine	chlorphentermine
chlorphentermine	chlorpheniramine
cimetidine	dimethicone
clarithromycin	erythromycin
Cleocin	bleomycin
Cleocin	Lincocin
Clinoxide	clioxanide
Clinoxide	Clipoxide
clioxanide	Clinoxide
Clipoxide	Clinoxide
clomiphene	clonidine
clonidine	clomiphene
clonidine	Klonopin
clonidine	Loniten
clonidine	quinidine
clotrimazole	co-trimoxazole
co-trimoxazole	clotrimazole

Appendix A 509

Codafed	Codaphen
Codaphen	Codafed
Codegest	Codehist
Codehist	Codegest
Colestid	colistin
colestipol	colistin
colistin	Colestid
colistin	colestipol
Combipres	Catapres
Cort-Dome	Cortone
Cortenema	quart enema
Cortin	Cotrim
cortisone	Cortizone
Cortizone	cortisone
Cortone	Cort-Dome
Cotrim	Cortin
Coumadin	Kemadrin
cytarabine	vidarabine
dacarbazine	Dicarbosil
dacarbazine	procarbazine
dactinomycin	daunorubicin
Dalmane	Dialume
danthron	Dantrium
Dantrium	danthron
Daranide	Daraprim
Daraprim	Daranide
Daricon	Darvon
Darvocet-N	Darvon-N
Darvon	Daricon
Darvon-N	Darvocet-N
daunorubicin	dactinomycin
daunorubicin	doxorubicin
Decaderm	Decadron
Decadron	Decaderm
Decadron	Percodan
Deconal	Deconsal
Deconsal	Deconal
Delacort	Delcort
Delcort	Delacort
Demerol	Demulen
Demerol	dicumarol
Demerol	Dymelor
Demerol	Temaril
Demolin	Demulen
Demulen	Demerol
Demulen	Demolin
Dermacort	DermiCort
DermiCort	Dermacort

deserpidine	desipramine
Desferal	Disophrol
desipramine	deserpidine
desoximethasone	dexamethasone
Desoxyn	digitoxin
Desoxyn	digoxin
dexamethasone	desoximethasone
Dexedrine	dextran
dextran	Dexedrine
dextran	dextrin
dextrin	dextran
Dialume	Dalmane
Dicarbosil	dacarbazine
dichloroacetic acid	Bichloracetic acid
dicumarol	Demerol
digitoxin	Desoxyn
digitoxin	digoxin
digoxin	Desoxyn
digoxin	digitoxin
Dilantin	Dilaudid
Dilaudid	Dilantin
Dimacol	dimercaprol
dimenhydrinate	diphenhydramine
dimercaprol	Dimacol
Dimetabs	Dimetane
Dimetabs	Dimetapp
Dimetane	Dimetabs
Dimetapp	Dimetabs
dimethicone	cimetidine
diphenhydramine	dimenhydrinate
Diphenylin	Dyphenylan
Disophrol	Desferal
Disophrol	disoprofol
Disophrol	Stilphostrol
disoprofol	Disophrol
Ditropan	Intropin
Diutensen	Salutensin
dobutamine	dopamine
Dommanate	Dramanate
Donnagel	Donnatal
Donnatal	Donnagel
Donnazyme	Entozyme
dopamine	dobutamine
dopamine	Dopram
Dopar	Dopram
Dopram	dopamine
Dopram	Dopar
doxorubicin	daunorubicin

Dramanate	Dommanate
Dyazide	Thiacide
Dyazide	thiazides
Dymelor	Demerol
Dymelor	Pamelor
Dyphenylan	Diphenylin
Dyrenium	Pyridium
Ecotrin	Edecrin
Edecrin	Ecotrin
Edecrin	Ethaquin
Elavil	Aldoril
Elavil	Enovil
Elavil	Equanil
Elavil	Mellaril
emetine	Emetrol
Emetrol	emetine
enalapril	Anafranil
Endal	Intal
Enduron	Imuran
Enduron	Inderal
Enduronyl	Inderal
Enovil	Elavil
Entozyme	Donnazyme
ephedrine	Appedrine
ephedrine	aprindine
Epifrin	epinephrine
Epifrin	EpiPen
Epinal	Epitol
epinephrine	Epifrin
EpiPen	Epifrin
Epitol	Epinal
Equanil	Elavil
erythromycin	clarithromycin
ERYC	ara-C
Esidrix	Lasix
Esimil	Estinyl
Esimil	Isomil
Estinyl	Esimil
Estratab	Ethatab
ethacridine	ethacrynic
ethacrynic	ethacridine
Ethaquin	Edecrin
Ethatab	Estratab
ethinamate	ethionamide
ethionamide	ethinamate
Eurax	Serax
Eurax	Urex
Euthroid	Synthroid

Euthroid	thyroid
Eutonyl	Eutron
Eutron	Eutonyl
Evac-Q-Kit	Evac-Q-Kwik
Evac-Q-Kwik	Evac-Q-Kit
Feosol	Feostat
Feosol	Fer-in-Sol
Feosol	Festal
Feostat	Feosol
Fer-in-Sol	Feosol
Festal	Feosol
Festal	Festalan
Festalan	Festal
Feverall	Fiberall
Fiberall	Feverall
Fioricet	Lorcet
Fiorinal	Florinef
Flaxedil	Flexeril
Flexeril	Flaxedil
Florinef	Fiorinal
fluocinolone	fluocinonide
fluocinonide	fluocinolone
folacin	Fulvicin
Fostex	pHisoHex
Fulvicin	folacin
Fulvicin	Furacin
Furacin	Fulvicin
Gamastan	Garamycin
Gantanol	Gantrisin
Gantrisin	Gantanol
Garamycin	Gamastan
Garamycin	kanamycin
Garamycin	Terramycin
Gelfoam	Ger-O-Foam
Genapap	Genatap
Genatap	Genapap
gentamicin	Jenamicin
gentamicin	kanamycin
Ger-O-Foam	Gelfoam
glucose	Glutose
Glutose	glucose
Glycotuss	Glytuss
Glytuss	Glycotuss
Gonak	Gonic
Gonic	Gonak
guaifenesin	guanfacine
guanethidine	guanidine
guanfacine	guaifenesin

guanidine	guanethidine
Guiatuss	Guiatussin
Guiatussin	Guiatuss
Haldol	Halenol
Haldol	Halog
Halenol	Haldol
Halog	Haldol
Halotestin	Halotex
Halotestin	Halotussin
Halotex	Halotestin
Halotussin	Halotestin
Hespan	Histastan
Hexadrol	Hexalol
Hexalen	Hexalol
Hexalol	Hexadrol
Hexalol	Hexalen
Hiprex	Hispril
Hispril	Hiprex
Histastan	Hespan
Histastan	Histatime
Histatime	Histastan
Hycodan	Hycomine
Hycodan	Vicodin
Hycomine	Byclomine
Hycomine	Hycodan
Hycomine	Vicodin
Hydergine	Hydramine
Hydramine	Bydramine
Hydramine	Hydergine
Hydramine	Hydramyn
Hydramine	Hytramyn
Hydramyn	Hydramine
Hydropane	Hydropine
Hydrophen	Hydropine
Hydropine	Hydropane
Hydropine	Hydrophen
Hygroton	Regroton
Hyper-Tet	HyperHep
Hyper-Tet	Hyperstat
HyperHep	Hyper-Tet
HyperHep	Hyperstat
Hyperstat	Hyper-Tet
Hyperstat	HyperHep
Hyperstat	Nitrostat
Hytone	Vytone
Hytramyn	Hydramine
Ilosone	inosine
Imferon	imipramine

Imferon	Imuran
imipramine	Imferon
imipramine	Norpramin
imipramine	trimipramine
Imuran	Enduron
Imuran	Imferon
Inderal	Enduron
Inderal	Enduronyl
Inderal	Inderide
Inderide	Inderal
Indocin	Lincocin
Indocin	Minocin
inosine	Ilosone
insulin	inulin
Intal	Endal
Intropin	Ditropan
Intropin	Isoptin
inulin	insulin
Ismelin	Ritalin
Isomil	Esimil
Isoptin	Intropin
Isopto Carpine	Isopto Eserine
Isopto Eserine	Isopto Carpine
Isordil	Isuprel
Isuprel	Isordil
Jenamicin	gentamicin
K-LOR	Kaochlor
K-LOR	Klor
kanamycin	Garamycin
kanamycin	gentamicin
Kaochlor	K-LOR
kaolin	Kaon
Kaon	kaolin
Kaopectate	Kapectalin
Kapectalin	Kaopectate
Kay Ciel	KCl
KCl	Kay Ciel
Keflet	Keflex
Keflet	Keflin
Keflex	Keflet
Keflex	Keflin
Keflin	Keflet
Keflin	Keflex
Kemadrin	Coumadin
Kenalog	Ketalar
Ketalar	Kenalog
Klonopin	clonidine
Klor	K-LOR

Klotrix	Liotrix
Komex	Koromex
Koromex	Komex
lanolin	Lanoline
Lanoline	lanolin
Lanoxin	Levoxine
Lasix	Esidrix
Lasix	Lidex
levallorphan	levorphanol
levodopa	methyldopa
levorphanol	levallorphan
levothyroxine	liothyronine
Levoxine	Lanoxin
Lidex	Lasix
Lidex	Lidox
Lidex	Wydase
Lidox	Lidex
Lincocin	Cleocin
Lincocin	Indocin
liothyronine	levothyroxine
Liotrix	Klotrix
Loniten	clonidine
Lorcet	Fioricet
Lotrimin	Otrivin
Luminal	Tuinal
Maalox	Marax
Mandol	nadolol
Marax	Atarax
Marax	Maalox
Marcaine	Narcan
mazindol	mebendazole
Mebaral	Medrol
Mebaral	Mellaril
Mebaral	Tegretol
mebendazole	mazindol
Meclan	Meclomen
Meclan	Mezlin
Meclomen	Meclan
Medrol	Mebaral
Mellaril	Elavil
Mellaril	Mebaral
Mellaril	Moderil
meperidine	meprobamate
mephenytoin	Mephyton
mephenytoin	Mesantoin
Mephyton	mephenytoin
Mephyton	methadone
meprobamate	meperidine

516 Appendix A

Meprospan	Naprosyn
Mesantoin	mephenytoin
Mesantoin	Mestinon
Mesantoin	Metatensin
Mestinon	Mesantoin
Mestinon	Metatensin
Metahydrin	Metandren
Metandren	Metahydrin
metaproterenol	metoprolol
Metatensin	Mesantoin
Metatensin	Mestinon
metaxalone	metolazone
methadone	Mephyton
methenamine	methionine
methionine	methenamine
methixene	methoxsalen
methoxsalen	methixene
methyldopa	levodopa
metolazone	metaxalone
Metopirone	metyrapone
metoprolol	metaproterenol
metyrapone	Metopirone
metyrapone	metyrosine
metyrosine	metyrapone
Mezlin	Azlin
Mezlin	Meclan
MICRhoGAM	microgram
microgram	MICRhoGAM
Midrin	Mydfrin
Milontin	Miltown
Milontin	Mylanta
Miltown	Milontin
Minocin	Indocin
Minocin	Mithracin
Minocin	niacin
Mithracin	Minocin
mithramycin	mitomycin
mitomycin	mithramycin
mitomycin	Mity-Mycin
mitomycin	Mutamycin
Mity-Mycin	mitomycin
Moban	Mobidin
Moban	Modane
Mobidin	Moban
Modane	Moban
Modane	Mudrane
Moderil	Mellaril
Modicon	Mylicon

Moi-Stir	moisture
moisture	Moi-Stir
Mudrane	Modane
Mutamycin	mitomycin
Myambutol	Nembutal
Mydfrin	Midrin
Mydfrin	Myfedrine
Myfedrine	Mydfrin
Mylanta	Milontin
Myleran	Mylicon
Mylicon	Modicon
Mylicon	Myleran
nadolol	Mandol
Naldecon	Nalfon
Nalfon	Naldecon
Naprosyn	Meprospan
Naprosyn	naproxen
Naprosyn	Natacyn
naproxen	Naprosyn
Narcan	Marcaine
Nardil	Norinyl
Natacyn	Naprosyn
Nembutal	Myambutol
Neomixin	neomycin
neomycin	Neomixin
niacin	Minocin
Nicobid	Nitro-Bid
Nilstat	Nitrostat
Nilstat	nystatin
Nitro-Bid	Nicobid
nitroglycerin	Nitroglyn
Nitroglyn	nitroglycerin
Nitrostat	Hyperstat
Nitrostat	Nilstat
Nitrostat	nystatin
Norinyl	Nardil
Norlutate	Norlutin
Norlutin	Norlutate
Norpramin	imipramine
nortriptyline	amitriptyline
nystatin	Nilstat
nystatin	Nitrostat
Omnipen	Unipen
Oncovin	Ancobon
Ophthochlor	Ophthocort
Ophthocort	Ophthochlor
Orabase	Orinase
Oracin	orarsan

Oracin	Orasone
orarsan	Oracin
orarsan	Orasone
Orasone	Oracin
Orasone	orarsan
Oretic	Oreton
Oreton	Oretic
Orex	Ornex
Orinase	Orabase
Orinase	Ornade
Orinase	Ornex
Orinase	Tolinase
Ornade	Orinase
Ornade	Ornex
Ornex	Orex
Ornex	Orinase
Ornex	Ornade
Ortho-Creme	Orthoclone
Orthoclone	Ortho-Creme
Otobiotic	Urobiotic
Otrivin	Lotrimin
oxymetazoline	oxymetholone
oxymetholone	oxymetazoline
oxymetholone	oxymorphone
oxymorphone	oxymetholone
Pamelor	Dymelor
Panarex	Panorex
Panasol	Panscol
Panorex	Panarex
PanOxyl	Benoxyl
Panscol	Panasol
Pantopon	Parafon
Parafon	Pantopon
paramethadione	paramethasone
paramethasone	paramethadione
Pathilon	Pathocil
Pathocil	Bactocill
Pathocil	Pathilon
Pathocil	Placidyl
Pavabid	Pavased
Pavased	Pavabid
Pavatine	Pavatym
Pavatym	Pavatine
Paverolan	Pavulon
Pavulon	Paverolan
penicillamine	penicillin
penicillin	penicillamine
penicillin	Polycillin

Pentazine	Phenazine
pentobarbital	phenobarbital
Pentothal	pentrinitrol
pentrinitrol	Pentothal
Percodan	Decadron
Perdiem	Pyridium
Periactin	Taractan
Persantine	Pertofrane
Pertofrane	Persantine
Phazyme	Pherazine
phenacetin	phenazocine
Phenaphen	Betapen
Phenaphen	Phenergan
Phenazine	Pentazine
Phenazine	phenelzine
Phenazine	Phenoxine
Phenazine	Pherazine
phenazocine	phenacetin
phenelzine	Phenazine
phenelzine	Phenylzin
Phenergan	Phenaphen
Phenergan	Theragran
phenobarbital	pentobarbital
Phenoxine	Phenazine
phentermine	phentolamine
phentolamine	phentermine
phentolamine	Ventolin
Phenylzin	phenelzine
Pherazine	Phazyme
Pherazine	Phenazine
pHisoHex	Fostex
physostigmine	pyridostigmine
physostigmine	Prostigmin
piperacetazine	piperazine
piperazine	piperacetazine
Pitocin	Pitressin
Pitressin	Pitocin
Placidyl	Pathocil
Pod-Ben	Podoben
Podoben	Pod-Ben
Podoben	Podofin
Podofin	Podoben
Podofin	podophyllin
podophyllin	Podofin
Polycillin	penicillin
Ponstel	Pronestyl
pralidoxime	pramoxine
pralidoxime	pyridoxine

Pramosone	pramoxine
pramoxine	pralidoxime
pramoxine	Pramosone
prazepam	prazepine
prazepam	Prazosin
prazepine	prazepam
Prazosin	prazepam
prednisolone	prednisone
prednisone	prednisolone
Priscoline	Apresoline
procaine	Procan
Procan	procaine
procarbazine	dacarbazine
Prolene	proline
proline	Prolene
promazine	Promethazine
Promethazine	promazine
Pronestyl	Ponstel
Prostigmin	physostigmine
Protamine	Protopam
Protopam	Protamine
Psorex	Serax
Pyridium	Dyrenium
Pyridium	Perdiem
Pyridium	pyridoxine
Pyridium	pyrithione
Pyridium	pyritidium
pyridostigmine	physostigmine
pyridoxine	pralidoxime
pyridoxine	Pyridium
pyrithione	Pyridium
pyritidium	Pyridium
quart enema	Cortenema
Quarzan	Questran
Questran	Quarzan
quinacrine	quinidine
Quinatime	quinidine
quinidine	clonidine
quinidine	quinacrine
quinidine	Quinatime
quinidine	quinine
quinine	quinidine
recombinant	Recombinate
Recombinate	recombinant
Reglan	Regonol
Regonol	Reglan
Regroton	Hygroton
Repan	Riopan

Restoril	Vistaril
Rifadin	rifampin
Rifadin	Ritalin
rifampin	Rifadin
Riopan	Repan
Ritalin	Ismelin
Ritalin	Rifadin
Salutensin	Diutensen
Sepo	Septa
Septa	Sepo
Septa	Septra
Septra	Septa
Ser-Ap-Es	Catapres
Serax	Eurax
Serax	Psorex
Serax	Urex
Serax	Xerac
Serentil	Surital
Simplet	Singlet
Singlet	Simplet
Soprodol	Sopronol
Sopronol	Soprodol
stilbestrol	Stilphostrol
Stilphostrol	Disophrol
Stilphostrol	stilbestrol
Streptase	Streptonase
Streptonase	Streptase
Sulf-10	Sulten-10
Sulfa-Trip	Sulfatrim
sulfamethizole	sulfamethoxazole
sulfamethoxazole	sulfamethizole
sulfathiazole	sulfisoxazole
Sulfatrim	Sulfa-Trip
sulfisoxazole	sulfathiazole
Sulten-10	Sulf-10
Surital	Serentil
Synthroid	Euthroid
Tagamet	Tegopen
Taractan	Periactin
Taractan	Tinactin
Tedral	Teldrin
Tegopen	Tagamet
Tegopen	Tegrin
Tegretol	Tegrin
Tegrin	Tegopen
Tegrin	Tegretol
Teldrin	Tedral
Temaril	Demerol

522   Appendix A

Temaril	Tepanil
Tepanil	Temaril
Tepanil	Tofranil
Terramycin	Garamycin
testolactone	testosterone
testosterone	testolactone
thallium	Valium
Theoclear	Theolair
Theocolate	Theolate
Theolair	Theoclear
Theolair	Thyrolar
Theolate	Theocolate
Thera-Flur	TheraFlu
TheraFlu	Thera-Flur
Theragran	Phenergan
Theravite	Therevac
Therevac	Theravite
Thiacide	Dyazide
Thiacide	thiazides
thiazides	Dyazide
thiazides	Thiacide
Threostat	Triostat
Thyrar	Thyrolar
thyroid	Euthroid
Thyrolar	Theolair
Thyrolar	Thyrar
Ticar	Tigan
Tigan	Ticar
timolol	atenolol
Tinactin	Taractan
TobraDex	Tobrex
tobramycin	Trobicin
Tobrex	TobraDex
Tofranil	Tepanil
Tolinase	Orinase
Topic	Topicort
Topicort	Topic
Triafed	Trifed
triamcinolone	Triaminicin
Triaminic	Triaminicin
Triaminic	TriHemic
Triaminicin	triamcinolone
Triaminicin	Triaminic
triamterene	trimipramine
Trifed	Triafed
TriHemic	Triaminic
trimeprazine	trimipramine

trimethaphan	trimethoprim
trimethoprim	trimethaphan
trimipramine	imipramine
trimipramine	triamterene
trimipramine	trimeprazine
Triostat	Threostat
Trobicin	tobramycin
Tronolane	Tronothane
Tronothane	Tronolane
Tuinal	Luminal
Tuinal	Tylenol
Tussafed	Tussafin
Tussafin	Tussafed
Tussex	Tussionex
Tussex	Tussirex
Tussi-Organidin	Tussi-R-Gen
Tussi-R-Gen	Tussi-Organidin
Tussionex	Tussex
Tussionex	Tussirex
Tussirex	Tussex
Tussirex	Tussionex
Tylenol	Tuinal
Unipen	Omnipen
Uracel	uracil
Uracel	Urised
Uracid	uracil
Uracid	Urised
Uracid	Urocit
uracil	Uracel
uracil	Uracid
Urex	Eurax
Urex	Serax
Urised	Uracel
Urised	Uracid
Urised	Urispas
Urispas	Urised
Urobiotic	Otobiotic
Urocit	Uracid
V-Cillin	Bicillin
V-Cillin	Wycillin
Valium	thallium
Valium	Valpin
Valmid	Valpin
Valpin	Valium
Valpin	Valmid
Valpin	Valprin
Valpin	Velban
Valprin	Valpin

Vasocidin	Vasodilan
Vasodilan	Vasocidin
Vasosulf	Velosef
Velban	Valpin
Velosef	Vasosulf
Ventolin	phentolamine
Vicodin	Hycodan
Vicodin	Hycomine
vidarabine	cytarabine
Vigran	Wigraine
Vistaril	Restoril
Vitron	Vytone
Vontrol	Bontril
Vytone	Hytone
Vytone	Vitron
Wigraine	Vigran
Wycillin	Bicillin
Wycillin	V-Cillin
Wydase	Lidex
Xanax	Zantac
Xerac	Serax
Zantac	Xanax
Zarontin	Zaroxolyn
Zarontin	Zentron
Zaroxolyn	Zarontin
Zaroxolyn	Zeroxin
Zentron	Zarontin
Zeroxin	Zaroxolyn

APPENDIX B
Investigational Code Names

A code name is a temporary identification assigned to a product by the manufacturer. The number or letter-number combination is used while the substance in undergoing testing, before a generic name is given. Below are 3017 code names and their subsequently assigned generic names.

10275-S	epitiostanol
106223	cefamandole nafate
110264	cefaparole
125 I NM-113	iomethin I 125
1314 TH	ethionamide
131 I NM-113	iomethin I 131
1380U	baquiloprim
1589 RB	pefloxacin
16726	symetine HCl
16842	bitoscanate
1709 CERM	niaprazine
177 J.D.	aminocaproic acid
1875 CERM	fepromide
18894	nifungin
194-B	zolamine HCl
20025	clorprenaline HCl
205 E	calcium dobesilate
21401-Ba	tribenoside
21679-CH	malethamer
22-708	endralazine mesylate
24281	mitocarcin
249-16	deditonium bromide
2-5410-3A	iodixanol
256U87	generic not yet assigned—see main list
26383	thiphencillin potassium
26P	aliflurane
27165	temefos
27,267 R.P.	zopiclone
27-400	cyclosporine
28002	epipropidine
29060-LE	vinblastine sulfate
2936	proscillaridin
29866	levopropoxyphene napsylate
2-PAM chloride	pralidoxime chloride

30038CB	minaprine HCl
3-01003	guanoxan sulfate
3-01029	guanoclor sulfate
30109	noracymethadol HCl
30639	polyethadene
3123L	puromycin
31518	pyrroliphene HCl
31595C	mitosper
31814	heteronium bromide
32-046	edetate dipotassium
32379	dromostanolone propionate
32645	vinleurosine sulfate
33006	acetohexamide
33355	mestranol
33379	flurandrenolide
33876	anthelmycin
34977	capreomycin sulfate
349 C59	moxipraquine
35483	cyclothiazide
360 medical fluid	dimethicone
36781	vinrosidine sulfate
36-801	etifoxine
37 162 R.P.	suproclone
37231	vincristine sulfate
38000	clometherone
38253	cephalothin sodium
38389	levopropylcillin potassium
38489	nortriptyline HCl
38851	bolmantalate
39435	cephaloglycin
3 MS	hydroxytoluic acid
3TC	generic not yet assigned—see main list
40 045	articaine
40045	trimetazidine
40602	cephaloridine
4091 C.B.	benfurodil hemisuccinate
41071	cefalonium
41-123	clazolam
41 982 RP	pefloxacin mesylate
42-348	lifibrate
42406	metoquizine
42-548	mazindol
4306 CB	clorazepate dipotassium
4311 CB	clorazepate monopotassium
43-663	guanoxabenz
43-715	proquazone
43853	clobenoside
44089	valproic acid

44106	toquizine
44328	dexproxibutene
46083	cefazolin sodium
46236	dobutamine HCl
46-790	fluproquazone
46 R.P.	benzylsulfamide
47-210 (as sodium)	tetriprofen
47599	pyrazofurin
47657	apramycin
47663	tobramycin
48-674	furacrinic acid
49040	vinglycinate sulfate
4909 RP	chlorproethazine HCl
49825	nylestriol
4A65	imidocarb HCl
4-C-32	ticlopidine HCl
4-MP	fomepizole
5048	dimethisterone
5052	acetylcysteine
5054	prodilidine HCl
5058	oxybutynin chloride
5071	megestrol acetate
5107	chloral betaine
516 MD	cinnarizine
5190	amidephrine mesylate
52230	pyrrolnitrin
53183	aranotin
53-32C	ticlopidine HCl
5373	melengestrol acetate
53858	fenoprofen
57C65	cloguanamil
59156	enpromate
5IUDR	idoxuridine
60284	cyclophenazine HCl
611 C 65	thenium closylate
640/1	cefuracetime
640/359	cefuroxime
64716	cinoxacin
65-318	bidimazium iodide
66-269	pretamazium iodide
66873	cephalexin
673-082	nexeridine HCl
67314	monensin
68618	mycophenolic acid
69323	fenoprofen calcium
711 SE	pipratecol
7162 RP	trimipramine
7432-S	ceftibuten

786-723	anilopam HCl
79907	lergotrile
79 T61	lucanthone HCl
80066	bufilcon A
8088 C.B.	benfotiamine
8102 CB	bamifylline HCl
83636	lergotrile mesylate
8599 R.P. mesylate	fonazine mesylate
882	generic not yet assigned—see main list
A-118	sultroponium
A-12253A	nebramycin
A-16612	teroxalene HCl
A-17624	ditolamide
A-19120	paragyline HCl
A-19757	encyprate
A-1981-12	prodilidine HCl
A-20968	piposulfan
A-2205	profadol HCl
A-2371	plicamycin
A-2655	dioxamate
A-27053	chromonar HCl
A-272	rutamycin
A-3217	ocfentanil HCl
A-32686	proscillaridin
A-3331	brifentanil HCl
A-33547	remoxipride
A-35957	altrenogest
A-4020 Linz	midodrine HCl
A 40664 (as tartrate)	raclopride
A-41-304	desoximetasone
A-4180	isometamidium chloride
A-4492	pentamorphone
A 46 745	gestrinone
A-4696	actaplanin
A-4828	trofosfamide
A-53986	fostedil
A-5610	azelastine HCl
A 5MP	adenosine phosphate
A-60386X	beractant
A-61589	docebenone
A-65006	lansoprazole
A-7283	guanoctine HCl
A-8103	pipobroman
A-82	nitroxoline
A-8999	aspartocin
AA-861	docebenone
AAFC	flurocitabine
AB08	doxycycline fosfatex

AB-100	uredepa
AB-103	benzodepa
AB-132	meturedepa
AB-A 663	cimaterol
Abbott-16900	teflurane
Abbott-19957	lorbamate
Abbott-22370	trimetozine
Abbott-24091	berythromycin
Abbott-34842	butamben picrate
Abbott-35616	clorazepate dipotassium
Abbott-36581	butamirate citrate
Abbott-38579	protirelin
Abbott-38642	fosfonet sodium
Abbott-39083	clorazepate monopotassium
Abbott-40728	cetocycline HCl
Abbott-41070	gonadorelin acetate
Abbott-43326	carteolol HCl
Abbott-43818	leuprolide acetate
Abbott 44090	valproate sodium
Abbott-44747	astromicin sulfate
Abbott-45975	terazosin HCl
Abbott-46811	cefsulodin sodium
Abbott-47631	estazolam
Abbott-48999	cefotiam HCl
Abbott-50192 (HCl)	cefmenoxime HCl
Abbott-50711	divalproex sodium
Abbott-56268	clarithromycin
Abbott-56619	difloxacin HCl
Abbott-61827	tosufloxacin
Abbott-62254	temafloxacin HCl
Abbott-64662	enalkiren
ABOB	moroxydine
AC 1198	dimethadione
AC 1370	cefpimizole
AC 263,780	cimaterol
AC 3810	bamifylline HCl
AC4464	torsemide
AC-528	dioxation
AC-601	buramate
ACC-9089	flestolol sulfate
AD 106	cicrotoic acid
AD-810	zonisamide
ADD-3878	ciglitazone
ADR-033	tripamide
AE-705W	neutramycin
AE-9	feclobuzone
AF-1161	trazodone HCl
AF-2139	dapiprazole HCl

AF-438 (as citrate)	oxolamine
AF-634	proxazole citrate
AF-864	benzydamine HCl
AG-1749	lansoprazole
AG-3	chromonar HCl
AG-337	generic not yet assigned—see main list
AG 58107	ioxitalamic acid
Agent M-01	sucrosofate potassium
AGN 20	metamfazone
AGN 511 (as HCl)	prazitone
AGN 616	fantridone HCl
AGR-1240	minaprine
AH 19065	ranitidine HCl
AH 22216	lamtidine
AH 23844 (lavoltidine)	lavoltidine succinate
AH 23844A	lavoltidine succinate
AH 25352X	sufotidine
AH 3923	salmefamol
AH 5158A	labetalol HCl
AH 8165D	fazadinium bromide
AHR-10282B	bromfenac sodium
AHR-10718	suricainide maleate
AHR-1118	pridefine HCl
AHR-11190-B	zacopride HCl
AHR-11325-D	rocastine HCl
AHR-1680	fenpipalone
AHR-224	pyroxamine maleate
AHR-2277 (as HCl)	lenperone
AHR-2438B	polignate sodium
AHR-3000	butaperazine
AHR-3002	fenfluramine HCl
AHR-3015	cintazone
AHR-3018	apazone
AHR-3053	carbocysteine
AHR-3070-C	metoclopramide HCl
AHR-438	metaxalone
AHR-4698	isosorbide mononitrate
AHR-504	glycopyrrolate
AHR-5531C	dazopride fumarate
AHR-5850D	amfenac sodium
AHR-6134	cloroperone HCl
AHR-619	doxapram HCl
AHR 6646	duoperone fumarate
AHR-8559	fluzinamide
AHR-857	sulfameter
AHR-9377	tampramine fumarate
AI-27,303	cetamolol HCl
AICA	orazamide

A IX	demecycline
AL02145	apraclonidine HCl
AL02725	pyrithione sodium
Al-0361	hydroxyphenamate
AL 0559	fenamole
AL-1021	carperone
AL1577A	levobetaxolol HCl
AL 20 (as HCl)	clemizole
AL-721	generic not yet assigned—see main list
AL 842	deterenol HCl
ALCA	alcloxa
ALDA	aldioxa
Allergan 211	idoxuridine
ALO 1401-02	betaxolol HCl
AL-T150	oxyfilcon A
AL-T30	vinafocon A
AM-684-Beta	relomycin
AMA 1080(2Na)	carumonam sodium
AMR-69	pirfenidone
AN 1317	perimetazine
AN 1324	glybuzole
anesthetic compound no. 347	enflurane
ANP 246	clofexamide
ANP 3260	clofezone
antibiotic 241a	biniramycin
antibiotic A-5283	natamycin
antifoam A	simethicone
antifoam AF	simethicone
AO-407	hydrofilcon A
AOMA	surfomer
AO-PLUTO	mesifilcon A
AP 67	chlorthenoxazine
APM	aspartame
APSAC	anistreplase
AQ-110	tretoquinol
AR 12008	trapidil
AR-121	generic not yet assigned—see main list
ARC I-K-1	methopholine
ARDF 26	gliquidone
AS 101	arsanilic acid
AS-17665	nifurthiazole
ASA 158/5 (as phosphate)	benproperine
ASL-279	dopamine HCl
ASL-601	acecainide HCl
ASL-603	bretylium tosylate
ASL-607	pentastarch
ASL-8052	esmolol HCl
Asta 3746	ciclonium bromide

Astra 1512	prilocaine HCl
Astra 1572	iron sorbitex
AT-101	isosorbide
AT-125	acivicin
AT-2266	enoxacin
AT 327	tipepidine
AW 10	sitogluside
AW 105-843	naftifine HCl
AW 14'2333	perlapine
AW-14'2446	clodazon HCl
AY-11,440	clogestone acetate
AY-11,483	estrofurate
AY-15,613	citenamide
AY-20,385	nequinate
AY-20,694	dexpropranolol HCl
AY-21,011	practolol
AY-21,367	furobufen
AY-21,554	talopram HCl
AY-22,124	intriptyline HCl
AY-22,214	taclamine HCl
AY-22,241	actodigin
AY-22,284A	alrestatin sodium
AY-22,469	deprostil
AY-23,028	butaclamol HCl
AY-23,289	prodolic acid
AY-23,713	pirandamine HCl
AY-23,946	tandamine HCl
AY-24,031	gonadorelin HCl
AY-24,169	dexclamol HCl
AY-24,236	etodolac
AY-24,269	proroxan HCl
AY-24,559	doxaprost
AY-24,856	pareptide sulfate
AY-25,329	azaclorzine HCl
AY-25,712	acifran
AY-27,110	ciladopa HCl
AY-27,255	vinpocetine
AY-27,773	tolrestat
AY-28,228	atiprosin maleate
AY-28,768	pelrinone HCl
AY-30,715	pemedolac
AY-5312	chlorhexidine HCl
AY-5710	magaldrate
AY-6108	ampicillin
AY-61122	methallibure
AY-61123	clofibrate
AY-62014	butriptyline HCl
AY-62021	clopenthixol

AY-62022	medrogestone
AY 6204 (as HCl)	pronetalol
AY-64043	propranolol HCl
AY-6608	pentagastrin
AY-8682	cyheptamide
AZQ	diaziquone
AZT-P-ddI	generic not yet assigned—see main list
B 10610	iodoxamic acid
B 11420	iopronic acid
B 1312 (as HCl)	bupranolol
B 1464	guanacline sulfate
B1Q 16	hedaquinium chloride
B-2311	morinamide
B-35251	mitocromin
B-360	paroxypropione
B-4130	iodamide
B-436	prenylamine
Ba 13155 (as tartrate)	meladrazine
Ba-20684	etonitazene
Ba-29038	boldenone undecylenate
Ba-29837	deferoxamine HCl
Ba-30803	benzoctamine HCl
BA 32644	niridazole
Ba-32968	delfantrine
Ba-33112	deferoxamine mesylate
Ba-34,276 (as HCl salt)	maprotiline
Ba-34,647	baclofen
BA 36278A	cephacetrile sodium
Ba-39,089	oxprenolol HCl
Ba-40088	proxibutene
Ba 41166/E	rifampin
BA 4164-8	diflumidone sodium
Ba-41795	codactide
BA 4197	flucrylate
BA 4223	triflumidate
BA 7602-06	talniflumate
BA 7604-02	talosalate
BA 7605-06	talmetacin
BAQD 10	dequalinium chloride
BASF 43915	pelretin
BASF 47011	doretinel
BAX 1400Z	dimethadione
BAX 1515	sutilains
BAX 1526	chymopapain
BAX 2739Z	bamifylline HCl
BAX 422Z	albutoin
BAY 1500	mefruside
BAY 1521	noxiptiline

BAY 2353	niclosamide
BAY 4059 Va	brotianide
BAY 4503	propiram fumarate
BAY 5097	clotrimazole
BAY 9002	naftalofos
Bay a 1040	nifedipine
BAY B 4231	glisoxepide
Bay d 1107	etofenamate
BAY d 8815 (HCl)	amidantel
Bay e 5009	nitrendipine
BAY e 9736	nimodipine
Bayer 1362	butaperazine
Bayer 1420	propanidid
Bayer 205	suramin sodium
Bayer 21199	coumaphos
Bayer 2502	nifurtimox
Bayer 3231	triaziquone
Bayer 5360	metronidazole
Bayer 9015	niclofolan
Bayer 9037	quintiofos
Bayer 9053	phoxim
Bayer A 128	aprotinin
Bayer L 1359	metrifonate
BAY g 2821	muzolimine
Bay g 5421	acarbose
Bay g 6575	nafazatrom
BAY h 2049	daniquidone
Bay h 4502	bifonazole
Bay h 5757	febantel
BAY i 7433	copovithane
Bay k 5552	nisoldipine
BAY m 1099	miglitol
BAYNAC	fenfluthrin
BAY o 1248	emiglitate
Bay o 9867 monohydrate	ciprofloxacin HCl
Bay q 3939	ciprofloxacin
Bay q 4218	butaprost
BAY q 7821	ipsapirone HCl
BAY V1 4718	etisomicin
BAY V1 6045	flumethrin
BAY Va 1470	xylazine HCl
Bay VA 9387	etisazole
BAY Va 9391	olaquindox
BAY Vh 5757	febantel
Bay Vi 9142	toltrazuril
BAY Vk 4999	fuzlocillin
Bay Vl 1704	cyfluthrin
Bay Vn 6528	fenfluthrin

Bay Vp 2674	enrofloxacin
BB-K8	amikacin sulfate
BC-105	pizotyline
BCM	mannomustine
BCX 2600	stiripentol
BCX-34	generic not yet assigned—see main list
BDH 1298	megestrol acetate
BDH 1921	melengestrol acetate
Be-100	ibuprofen piconol
Be-1293	xipamide
BE 419	ioglycamic acid
BG 8301	teceleukin
BL 191	pentoxifylline
BL-3912A	dimoxamine HCl
BL-4162a	anagrelide HCl
BL-5111	tiodazosin
BL-5572M	proxorphan tartrate
BL-5641A	etintidine HCl
BL-P 1322	cephapirin sodium
BL-P 1462	suncillin sodium
BL-P 1761	sarpicillin
BL-P 1780	sarmoxicillin
BL-P 804	hetacillin
BL-R 743	intrazole
BL-S578	cefadroxil
BL-S640	cefatrizine
BL-S786	ceforanide
BM02.015	torsemide
BM 13.177	sulotroban
BM 13.505	daltroban
BM 14.190	carvedilol
BM 15.075	bezafibrate
BM 22.145	isosorbide mononitrate
BM 41.332	ciamexon
BM 51052	carazolol
BMY 13805-1	gepirone HCl
BMY 13859-1	tiospirone HCl
BMY-21891	belfosdil
BMY-25182	cefbuperazone
BMY-26517	pemirolast potassium
BMY-28142	cefepime
BMY-30120	chlorhexidine phosphanilate
BMY-41606	vapreotide
BMY-45622	generic not yet assigned—see main list
BN-1270	cicletanine
BP-1184	guanoctine HCl
BP 400	pimethixene
BRL-1241	methicillin sodium

BRL 12594	ticarcillin cresyl sodium
BRL-1288	benapryzine HCl
BRL-1341	ampicillin
BRL 13856	clopirac
BRL 14151	clavulanic acid
BRL 14151K	clavulanate potassium
BRL 14777	nabumetone
BRL-1621	cloxacillin sodium
BRL-1702	dicloxacillin
BRL 17421 (as sodium)	temocillin
BRL-2039	floxacillin
BRL-2064	carbenicillin disodium
BRL 2288	ticarcillin disodium
BRL 2333	amoxicillin
BRL 2534	azidocillin
BRL 26921	anistreplase
BRL-284	levopropylcillin potassium
BRL 29060	paroxetine
BRL 30892	denbufylline
BRL-3475	carbenicillin phenyl sodium
BRL 34915	cromakalim
BRL 38705	epsiprantel
BRL 40015	diproteverine
BRL 4664	nonabine
BRL 4910A	mupirocin
BRL-804	hetacillin
BRL 8988 HCl	talampicillin HCl
BS 100-141	guanfacine HCl
B.S. 6534	bufenadrine
BS 6748	xyloxemine
BS 6987	deptropine citrate
BS 7161D (as HCl)	pytamine
B.S. 7173-D	xylocoumarol
BS 749	metacetamol
B.S. 7561 (as HCl)	tixadil
B.S. 7573-a	acridorex
BS 7723 (as maleate)	tropirine
BS 7977 D (as dihydrochloride)	xipranolol
BSH	borocaptate sodium B 10
BSSG	sitogluside
BT 621 (as HCl)	todralazine
BTPABA, PFT	bentiromide
BTS 13622	hexaprofen
BTS 17345	fluprofen
BTS 18,322	flurbiprofen
BTS 24332	esflurbiprofen
BTS 49 465	flosequinan
BU-2231A	talisomycin

BW 12C generic not yet assigned—see main list
BW 207U xenalipin
BW 234U dihydrochloride rimcazole HCl
BW 248U sodium acyclovir sodium
BW 301U isethionate piritrexim isethionate
BW 325U trifenagrel
BW 33A atracurium besylate
BW 33-T-57 methisazone
BW 356-C-61 gloxazone
BW 430C lamotrigine
BW-467-C-60 bethanidine sulfate
BW 49-210 diaveridine
BW 532U cinflumide
BW 56-158 allopurinol
BW 56-72 trimethoprim
BW-57-322 azathioprine
BW 57-323 thiamiprine
BW 58-271 rolodine
BW-61-32 stilbazium iodide
BW 63-90 butacetin
BW 647U HCl bipenamol HCl
BW 64-9 butoxamine HCl
BW 72U trimethoprim sulfate
BW 759U ganciclovir
BW 825C acrivastine
BW A256C palatrigine
BW A509U zidovudine
BW A515U desciclovir
BW A770U mesylate crisnatol mesylate
BW A938U dichloride doxacurium chloride
BW B1090U mivacurium chloride
Bx 311 cinoxolone
BX 341 bifluranol
BX 363A (as disodium salt) cicloxolone
BX 591 acefluranol
BX 650A ipsalazide
BX 661A balsalazide
BZ 55 carbutamide
C-11925 phanquone
C-12669 demecolcine
C-1428 cyclarbamate
C 1656 clometacin
C-238 pridinol
C-3 capobenate sodium
C-3 capobenic acid
C-434 trimedoxime bromide
C-49802B-Ba oxaprotiline HCl
Ca 1022 carbutamide

CA-7	brinolase
CAM-807	bialamicol HCl
CAS 276	molsidomine
CB 1048	chlornaphazine
CB 10615	nifurmazole
CB 11 (as HCl)	phenadoxone
CB 11380	nifurizone
CB 12592	subendazole
CB-154	bromocriptine
CB-154 mesylate	bromocriptine mesylate
CB 1664	aceprometazine
CB 1678	propiomazine
CB 2201	amfepentorex
CB-30038	minaprine
CB 302	ferric fructose
CB 3025	melphalan
CB 304	azaribine
CB 309	fenabutene
CB-311	somatropin
CB 313	mitotane
CB-337	meglutol
CB 3697	racefemine
CB 4260	nortetrazepam
CB 4261	tetrazepam
CB 4857	menitrazepam
CB 4985	acequinoline
CB 804	bucloxic acid
CCA	lobenzarit sodium
C.C.I. 12923	minaxolone
CCI 15641	cefuroxime axetil
CCI 18773	cloticasone propionate
CCI 18781	fluticasone propionate
CCI 23628	cefuroxime pivoxetil
CCI 4725	clobetasol propionate
CCI 5537	clobetasone butyrate
CDDD 1815	alprenoxime HCl
CDDD 2803	adaprolol maleate
CEPH (as HCl)	todralazine
CERM 1978	bepridil HCl
CERM 730	amoproxan
CG 201	bevonium metilsulfate
CG-315E	tramadol HCl
CGA-23654	nitroscanate
CGA 72662	cyromazine
CGP-14221/E	cefotiam HCl
CGP 21690E	oxiracetam
CGP 2175C	metoprolol fumarate
CGP-2175E	metoprolol tartrate

CGP 23339AE	pamidronate disodium
CGP-7174/E	cefsulodin sodium
CGP 7760B	prenalterol HCl
CGP 9000	cefroxadine
CGS 10078B	bendacalol mesylate
CGS 10746B	pentiapine maleate
CGS 10787D	prinomide tromethamine
CGS 13080	pirmagrel
CGS 13945	pentopril
CGS 14824A HCl	benazepril HCl
CGS 14831	benazeprilat
CGS 15040A	serazapine HCl
CGS 16617	libenzapril
CGS 5391B (anhydrous)	enolicam sodium
CGS 7135A	azaloxan fumarate
CGS 7525A	aptazapine maleate
CH 3565	triclosan
CHX-100	masoprocol
CI-100	acetosulfone sodium
CI-107	argipressin tannate
CI-301	bialamicol HCl
CI-336	carbocloral
CI-366	ethosuximide
CI-379	benzilonium bromide
CI-395	phencyclidine HCl
CI 403A	pararosaniline pamoate
CI-406	oxymetholone
CI-416	triclofenol piperazine
CI-419	fenimide
CI 427	prodilidine HCl
CI-433	clamoxyquin HCl
CI 440	flufenamic acid
CI-456	diapamide
CI-473	mefenamic acid
CI-501	cycloguanil pamoate
CI-515	guanoxyfen sulfate
CI-546	alipamide
CI 556	acedapsone
CI-572	profadol HCl
CI-581	ketamine HCl
CI-583	meclofenamic acid
CI-633	clioxanide
CI-634	tiletamine HCl
CI-636	sulfacytine
CI-642	butirosin sulfate
CI 673	vidarabine
CI-686 HCl	trebenzomine HCl
CI-705	methaqualone

540 Appendix B

CI-716	zolazepam HCl
CI-718	bentazepam
CI-719	gemfibrozil
CI-720	gemcadiol
CI-781	zometapine
CI 787	tioperidone HCl
CI-825	pentostatin
CI-874	indeloxazine HCl
CI-879	pramiracetam HCl
CI-879 (sulfate)	pramiracetam sulfate
CI-880	amsacrine
CI-881	ametantrone acetate
CI-882	sparfosate sodium
CI-888	procaterol HCl
CI-897	tebuquine
CI-898	trimetrexate
CI-904	diaziquone
CI-906	quinapril HCl
CI-907	indolapril HCl
CI-908	dezaguanine
CI-908 mesylate	dezaguanine mesylate
CI-909	tiazofurin
CI-911	rolziracetam
CI-912	zonisamide
CI-914	imazodan HCl
CI-919	enoxacin
CI-920	fostriecin sodium
CI-928	quinaprilat
CI-942	piroxantrone HCl
CI-945	gabapentin
CI-970	tacrine HCl
CIBA 1906	thiambutosine
CJ 91B	olsalazine sodium
CK-0383	verofylline
CK-0569 (as the base)	ipexidine mesylate
CK-1752A	sematilide HCl
CL 10304	aminocaproic acid
CL 106359	triamcinolone acetonide sodium phosphate
CL 112,302	buprenorphine HCl
CL 115,347	viprostol
CL 118,532	triptorelin
CL 12,625	natamycin
CL-1388R	guanadrel sulfate
CL 13,900	puromycin
CL 14377	methotrexate
CL 16,536	puromycin HCl
CL-1848C	etoxadrol HCl

CL 203,821	cetaben sodium
CL 205925	iprocinodine HCl
CL 206,214	butamisole HCl
CL 206,576	sulbenox
CL 206,797	cypothrin
CL 216,942	bisantrene HCl
CL 217,658	imcarbofos
CL 220,075	bicifadine HCl
CL 22415	demecycline
CL 227,193	piperacillin sodium
CL 232,315	mitoxantrone HCl
CL 2422	guancydine
CL 25477	azetepa
CL 26193	simtrazene
CL 27,071	descinolone acetonide
CL 273,703	maduramicin
CL 274,471	colestolone
CL 284,635	cefixime
CL 287,088	nemadectin
CL 287,389	nilvadipine
CL 297,939	bisoprolol; bisoprolol fumarate
CL 298,741	tazobactam
CL 301,423	moxidectin
CL 307,579	tazobactam sodium
Cl 337	azaserine
CL 34433	triamcinolone hexacetonide
CL 34699	amcinonide
CL 36467	methotrimeprazine
CL 369	ketamine HCl
CL 39743	methotrimeprazine
CL 39808	thozalinone
CL 399	tiletamine HCl
CL 40881	ethambutol HCl
CL 48156	imidoline HCl
CL 5,279	nithiamide
CL 53415	cyproximide
CL 54131	piperamide maleate
CL 54998	brocresine
Cl-583 Na salt	meclofenamate sodium
CL 59112	roletamide
CL 61965	triamcinolone acetonide sodium phosphate
CL 62,362	loxapine
CL-639C	dioxadrol HCl
Cl-64,976	zilantel
CL 65205	boxidine
CL 65336	tranexamic acid
CL 65,562	triflocin

Cl-661	oxiramide
CL 67,772	amoxapine
Cl-683	ripazepam
CL 71563	loxapine succinate
Cl-775	bevantolol HCl
Cl-808	vidarabine phosphate
Cl-808 sodium	vidarabine sodium phosphate
CL 82204	fenbufen
CL 83,544	felbinac
Cl-845	pirmenol HCl
CL 84,633	nimidane
CL-867	piridicillin sodium
Cl-871	piracetam
CL 88,893	clazolimine
CL 90,748	azolimine
CL-911C	dexoxadrol HCl
CL-912C	levoxadrol HCl
CL 98984	cinodine HCl
CLY-503	simfibrate
CM 31-916	ceftiofur sodium
CN-10,395	ethosuximide
CN-14,329-23A	cycloguanil pamoate
CN-15,573-23A	pararosaniline pamoate
CN-15,757	azaserine
CN-16146	carbocloral
CN-17,900-2B	clamoxyquin HCl
CN-1883	acedapsone
CN-20,172-3	benzilonium bromide
CN-25,253-2	phencyclidine HCl
CN-27,554	flufenamic acid
CN-34,799-5A	guanoxyfen sulfate
CN-35355	mefenamic acid
CN-36,337	diapamide
CN-38,474	alipamide
CN 38703	methaqualone
CN-52,372-2	ketamine HCl
CN-54521-2	tiletamine HCl
CN-5834-5931B	triclofenol piperazine
CN 59,567	clioxanide
CO 405	butidrine
compound 109168	nifluridide
compound 112531	vindesine
compound 113878	ciprefadol succinate
compound 113935	pentomone
compound 122587	drobuline
compound 133314	trioxifene mesylate
compound 24266	pentetate calcium trisodium Yb 169
compound 42339	acronine

compound 469	isoflurane
compound 497	dieldrin
compound 53616	frentizole
compound 56063	melizame
compound 57926	sinefungin
compound 68-198	diamfenetide
compound 79891	narasin
compound 81929	dobutamine
compound 83405	cefamandole
compound 83846	aprindine HCl
compound 85287	nibroxane
compound 89218	nisoxetine
compound 904	alexidine
compound 90459	benoxaprofen
compound 90606	isamoxole
compound 93819	fluretofen
compound 99170	aprindine
compound 99638	cefaclor
compound LY 131126	butopamine
compound S	zidovudine
CP-10,188	fenclonine
CP-10,303-8	quinterenol sulfate
CP-10,423-16	pyrantel pamoate
CP-10,423-18	pyrantel tartrate
CP 1044 J3	bufexamac
CP-11,332-1	quinazosin HCl
CP-12,009-18	morantel tartrate
CP-12,252-1	thiothixene HCl
CP-12,299-1	prazosin HCl
CP-12,521-1	piquizil HCl
CP-12,574	tinidazole
CP-13,608	tesicam
CP-14,185-1	hoquizil HCl
CP-14,368-1	lometraline HCl
CP-14,445-16	oxantel pamoate
CP-15,464-2	carbenicillin indanyl sodium
CP-15,467-61	lithium carbonate
CP 1552 S	milacemide HCl
CP-15-639-2	carbenicillin disodium
CP-15,973	sudoxicam
CP-16,171	piroxicam
CP-16,171-85	piroxicam olamine
CP-16,533-1	verapamil
CP 172 AP	clopirac
CP-18,524	tibric acid
CP-19,106-1	trimazosin HCl
CP-20,961	avridine
CP-22,341	temodox

CP-22,665	flumizole
CP-24,314-1	pirbuterol HCl
CP-24,314-14	pirbuterol acetate
CP-24,441-1	tametraline HCl
CP-24,877	drinidene
CP-25,673	tiazuril
CP-26,154	tolimidone
CP-27,634	gliamilide
CP-28,720	glipizide
CP-31,081	polydextrose
CP-32,387	pirolate
CP-33,994-2	pirbenicillin sodium
CP-34,089	sulprostone
CP-36,584	flutroline
CP-38,754	plauracin
CP-44,001-1	nantradol HCl
CP-45,634	sorbinil
CP-45,899-2	sulbactam sodium
CP-45,899-99	sulbactam benzathine
CP-47,904	sulbactam pivoxil
CP-48,810-27	fanetizole mesylate
CP-48,867-9	ristianol phosphate
CP-49,952	sultamicillin
CP-50,556-1	levonantradol HCl
Cp-51,974-1	sertraline HCl
CP-52,640-2	cefoperazone sodium
CP-54,802	alitame
CP-556S	suloctidil
CP-57,361-01	zaltidine HCl
CP-62,993	azithromycin
CP-65703	ampiroxicam
CP-66,248-2	tenidap sodium
CP-73,049	binfloxacin
CP-76,136-27	danofloxacin mesylate
Cpd 109514	nabilone
Cpd. 5411	iopentol
CR/662	tipepidine
CS-151	crofilcon A
CS-514	pravastatin sodium
CS-807	cefpodoxime proxetil
CSAG-144	mebeverine HCl
CTR 6110	nitrodan
CV 57533	xenyhexenic acid
CV 58903	xenazoic acid
CY-116	aminocaproic acid
CY 153	acexamic acid
CY 39	psilocybine
D 00079	anoxomer

D-1262	cloxypendyl
D-1593	diapamide
D-1721	alipamide
D-1959 HCl	reproterol HCl
D2083	desonide
D 237	cloforex
D-254	pipazethate
D-365	verapamil
D 4028	enprofylline
D 47	sulbentine
d4T	stavudine
D 7093	mesna
D-775	homofenazine
D-9998	flupirtine maleate
DA 1773	sodium picosulfate
DA 2370	feprazone
DA-398	epirizole
DA 688	gefarnate
DA-708	teflurane
DA-808	nafcaproic acid
DA-893	roflurane
DA-914	nafiverine
DA-992	naftypramide
DAC	decitabine
D.A.T.	acetiamine
DATC	tiocarlide
DBV	buformin
DCH 21 (as sodium salt)	exiproben
DETF	metrifonate
DF 118	dihydrocodeine bitartrate
DH-524	fenmetozole HCl
DH-581	probucol
DIM-SA	succimer
DL 152	bietaserpine
DL-164	tiodonium chloride
DL-588	napactadine HCl
DL-8280	ofloxacin
dl HM-PAO	exametazime
dl HM-PAO	hexametazime
DMI	desipramine HCl
DMSC	doxycycline fosfatex
DT-3	detrothyronine
DT-327	clopamide
D-Trp LHRH-PEA	deslorelin
DU-21220	ritodrine
DU-21445	tiprenolol HCl
DU 22550 (as sulfate)	caproxamine
DU 23000 (maleate)	fluvoxamine

DU-23187	quincarbate
Dup 785	brequinar sodium
DV-1006	cetraxate HCl
DW-61	flavoxate HCl
DW-62	dimefline HCl
DW 75	norleusactide
E-0659	azelastine HCl
E-106-E (as cyclamate)	furfenorex
E 141	ethamsylate
E-2663	bentiromide
E 39	inproquone
E-52	pentafilcon A
E-614	tripamide
E 9002	naftalofos
EA-166	guanoxyfen sulfate
EDU	edoxudine
EE$_3$ME	mestranol
EGTA	egtazic acid
EGYT 201	bencyclane fumarate
EHB 776	foscarnet sodium
EL10	dehydroepiandrosterone
EL349	somidobove
EL737	ractopamine HCl
EL-857	apramycin
EL870	tilmicosin
EL-974	ticarbodine
ELD 950	eledoisin
EMBAY 8440	praziquantel
EMD 15 700	nitrefazole
EMD 19698 (as hydrogen maleate)	peratizole
EMD 33 512	bisoprolol
EMD 9806	pramiverine
EN-1010	pyrrocaine
EN-141	josamycin
EN-15304	naloxone HCl
EN-1620A	nalmexone HCl
EN-1639A (as HCl)	naltrexone
EN-1661L	bisobrin lactate
EN-1733A	molindone HCl
EN-2234A	nalbuphine HCl
EN-313	moricizine
EN-970	fluquazone
ENT-20852	butonate
ENT-23969	carbaril
ENT-25567	naftalofos
ENT 29,106	nimidane
EPO	epoetin alfa
EPOCH	epoetin beta

ES 304	nicofuranose
ET-394	tribromsalan
ET-495	piribedil
ETTN	propatyl nitrate
EU-1063	proquinolate
EU-1085	leniquinsin
EU-1093	buquinolate
EU-1806	nafronyl oxalate
EU-2826	benurestat
EU-2972	nolinium bromide
EU-3120	acodazole HCl
EU-3325	triafungin
EU-3421	oxifungin HCl
EU-4093	azumolene sodium
EU-4200	piribedil
EU-4534	flurofamide
EU-4584	tolfamide
EU-4891	diacetolol HCl
EU-4906	sitogluside
EU-5306	pefloxacin
EUDR	edoxudine
EX 10-029-C	elantrine
EX 10-781	metizoline HCl
EX 12-095	eterobarb
EX 4355	desipramine HCl
EX 4810	ambuside
Ex 4883	rolicyprine
EXP-105-1	amantadine HCl
EXP 126	rimantadine HCl
EXP 338	midaflur
EXP 999	metopimazine
F 1500	succisulfone
F 1983	pyrovalerone HCl
F28249α	nemadectin
F-368	dantrolene
F-413	clodanolene
F-440	dantrolene sodium
F-605 (as the sodium)	clodanolene
F 6066	cyclofenil
F-691	furodazole
F-776	orpanoxin
F-853	nitrafudam HCl
Fa 402	fentonium bromide
FBA 1420	propanidid
FBA 4059	brotianide
FBB 4231	glisoxepide
FBB 6896	clenpirin
FC-1157a	toremifene citrate

FER-1443	ticlatone
FG 5111	melperone
FI 5852	oxabolone cipionate
F.I. 6146	buzepide metiodide
FI 6337	metergoline
FI 6339 (as the base)	daunorubicin HCl
F.I. 6426	stallimycin HCl
F.I. 6654	caroxazone
F.I. 6820	brofoxine
FK 027	cefixime
FK 235	nilvadipine
FK-565	generic not yet assigned—see main list
FK 749	ceftizoxime sodium
FLA 731	remoxipride
FPL 12924AA	remacemide HCl
FPL 58668KC	probicromil calcium
FPL 59002	nedocromil
FPL 59002KC	nedocromil calcium
FPL 59002KP	nedocromil sodium
FPL 59360	minocromil
FPL 60278	dopexamine
FPL 60278AR	dopexamine HCl
FPL.670	cromolyn sodium
FR 13749	ceftizoxime sodium
FR 17027	cefixime
FU-02	fumoxicillin
FWH 399	troxonium tosilate
G-201	generic not yet assigned—see main list
G-203	fluocinonide
G-24480	dimpylate
G-25178	prodeconium bromide
G-25766	clorindione
G 26,872	phenbutazone sodium glycerate
G 30320	clofazimine
G-32883	carbamazepine
G-33040	opipramol HCl
G-33182	chlorthalidone
G 34586	clomipramine HCl
G-35020	desipramine HCl
G 35259	ketipramine fumarate
G-4	dichlorophen
G-704,650	alendronate sodium
GEA 654	alaproclate
GM 6001	generic not yet assigned—see main list
Go 1213	atolide
Go 1733	suloxifen oxalate
Go 2782	iproxamine HCl
Go 3026A	ciclafrine HCl

Go-560	febarbamate
Go 919	piprozolin
GOE 3450	gabapentin
Goedecke 3282	ozolinone
Gp120	generic not yet assigned—see main list
GP-121	phencyclidine HCl
GP 31406	depramine
GP 45840	diclofenac sodium
GP 51084	glibutimine
GPA-878	metazamide
GR 20263	ceftazidime
GR 2/1214	clobetasone butyrate
GR 2/1574	alfadolone
GR 2/234	alfaxalone
GR 2/443 (as propionate)	doxibetasol
GR 2/925	clobetasol propionate
Gr 30921	mitoquidone
GR 32191 (vapiprost)	vapiprost HCl
GR 32191B	vapiprost HCl
GR 33207	ovandrotone albumin
GR 33343 X	salmeterol
GR 38032F	ondansetron HCl
GR 412	dodeclonium bromide
GR 43175C	sumatriptan succinate
GR 43659X	lacidipine
GR50360A	fluparoxan HCl
GR 50692	cefempidone
GR 53992B (GX 1296B)	teludipine HCl
GR 63178K	fosquidone
GS-1339	dymanthine HCl
GS 2147	sancycline
GS-2876	methacycline
GS-2989	meclocycline
GS-3065	doxycycline
GS-3159	carbenicillin potassium
GS 393	generic not yet assigned—see main list
GS-6244	carbadox
GS-6742	sulfomyxin
GS-7443	mequidox
GS-95	thiethylperazine maleate
H 102/09 HCl	zimeldine HCl
H 104/08	pamatolol sulfate
H 133/22	prenalterol HCl
H 154/82	felodipine
H 168/68	omeprazole
H 365	paroxypropione
H 3774	alibendol
H 4132	dotefonium bromide

H 4170	tolpiprazole
H 4723	clobazam
H 56/28	alprenolol HCl
HB 115	nifurprazine
HB 419	glyburide
H.B.F. 386	cactinomycin
HC 1528	decoquinate
HC 20,511 fumarate	ketotifen fumarate
HF 1854	clozapine
HF 1927	dibenzepin HCl
HF-2159	clothiapine
HF 241	bufeniode
HGP-2	adaprolol maleate
HGP-5	alprenoxime HCl
HH105	butetamate
HH 197	butamirate citrate
HL 267	dipenine bromide
HL 362	colforsin
HL 523 (as HCl)	tiformin
HMD	oxymetholone
Hoe 045	articaine
HOE 062 (roxatidine)	roxatidine acetate HCl
Hoe 105	citenazone
HOE 118	piretanide
HOE 216V	luxabendazole
HOE 280	ofloxacin
HOE 296	ciclopirox olamine
Hoe 296V	resorantel
HOE 304	desoximetasone
HOE 36801	etifoxine
HOE 39-893d	penbutolol sulfate
HOE 42-440	tiamenidine HCl
HOE440	tiamenidine
Hoe 473	aclantate
HOE 498	ramipril
HOE 760	roxatidine acetate HCl
HOE 766	buserelin acetate
HOE 777	prednicarbate
Hoe 881V	fenbendazole
HOE 893d	penbutolol sulfate
HOE 984	nomifensine maleate
Hoechst 10495	norpipanone
Hoechst 10582	normethadone
HP 029	velnacrine maleate
HP 128	suronacrine maleate
HP 1598	guanoxyfen sulfate
HP 3522	brocrinat
HP 494	fluradoline HCl

HP 522	brocrinat
HP 549	isoxepac
HPA-23	generic not yet assigned—see main list
HPEK-1	tetroquinone
hPTH 1-34 (acetate salt)	teriparatide acetate
HR 376	clobazam
HR 756	cefotaxime sodium
HR 810 sulfate	cefpirome sulfate
HR 930	fosazepam
HRP 543	dazepinil HCl
HRP 913	neflumozide HCl
HS-592	clemastine
HSP 2986	pramiverine
HT-11	cloperastine
HTO	tritiated water
HUF-2446	clodazon HCl
HY-185	carbocloral
[123]I labeled IMP	iofetamine HCl I 123
[123]I-M123	iofetamine HCl I 123
I-653	desflurane
IA-307	acetosulfone sodium
ICI 118,587	xamoterol
ICI 118,630	goserelin
ICI 125,211	tiotidine
ICI 128,436	ponalrestat
ICI 136,753	tracazolate
ICI 141,292	epanolol
ICI 156,834	cefotetan
ICI 194660	meropenem
ICI 28257	clofibrate
ICI 29661	pyrimitate
ICI 32865	etoglucid
ICI-33,828	methallibure
ICI 35,868	propofol
ICI 38174 (as HCl)	pronetalol
ICI 45520	propranolol HCl
ICI 45763 (as HCl)	toliprolol
ICI 46,474	tamoxifen citrate
ICI 46683	oxyclozanide
I.C.I. 47,319	dexpropranolol HCl
ICI 48213	cyclofenil
ICI 50,123	pentagastrin
I.C.I. 50,172	practolol
I.C.I. 54,450	fenclozic acid
ICI 54,594 (as sodium salt)	brofezil
ICI 55,052	nequinate
ICI 55,897	clobuzarit
ICI 58,834	viloxazine HCl

ICI 59118	razoxane
ICI 66,082	atenolol
ICI 80,008 (as sodium salt)	fluprostenol sodium
ICI 80,996	cloprostenol sodium
ICI 81,008	fluprostenol sodium
ICI 8173	quindoxin
ICI-U.S. 457	octazamide
ICN-542	ribaminol
ICRF 159	razoxane
IL-17803A (as HCl)	acebutolol
IL-19552	pipotiazine palmitate
IL 22811 HCl	meptazinol HCl
IL 5902	spiramycin
IL 6001	trimipramine
IL-6302 mesylate	fonazine mesylate
IMI-28	epirubicin HCl
IMI 30	idarubicin HCl
IMI 58	esorubicin HCl
IN 1060	cyprolidol HCl
IN 29-5931B	triclofenol piperazine
IN 379	pimetine HCl
IN 461	benzindopyrine HCl
IN 511	phenyramidol HCl
IN 836	fenyripol HCl
INF-1837	flufenamic acid
INF-3355	mefenamic acid
INF 4668	meclofenamic acid
IPA	riboprine
IS 2596	domoxin
I.S. 499	poldine methylsulfate
ISIS 2105	generic not yet assigned—see main list
isomer A	zuclomiphene
isomer B	enclomiphene
Janssen R 4929	benzetimide HCl
JAV 852	benfosformin
JB-8181	desipramine HCl
JD-96	vinylbital
JF-1	nalmefene
JL-1078	dihexyverine HCl
JL 512	fenadiazole
JM-8	carboplatin
JM-9	iproplatin
K 11941	alfaprostol
K-17	thalidomide
K-1900	nimorazole
K-38	glycyclamide
K-386	glycyclamide
K 4024	glipizide

K 4277	indoprofen
K 9147	tolciclate
KABI 925	emylcamate
KAT 256 (as HCl)	clobutinol
KB-944	fostedil
KB 95	benzpiperylon
K-F 224	naftoxate
KL-255 (as HCl)	bupranolol
Ko 1173 Cl	mexiletine HCl
KO 1366	bunitrolol
Ko 592 (as HCl)	toliprolol
KS 33	oxyridazine
KW-110	aceglutamide aluminum
KWD 2019	terbutaline sulfate
L-1573	cysteamine
L-1633	sodium dibunate
L-1718	osalmid
L-1777	medazomide
L 2197	benzarone
L-2214	benzbromarone
L 2329	benziodarone
L 2642	etabenzarone
L-3428	amiodarone
L-364,718	devazepide
L-4269	pyridarone
L-5103 Lepetit	rifampin
L-5418	diftalone
L 542	mercurobutol
L-554	tritoqualine
L 566	dibemethine
L 5818 (as HCl)	coumazoline
L-6257	oxetorone fumarate
L-637,510	nelezaprine maleate
L-6400	fluazacort
L-647,339	naxagolide HCl
L-669,455	dexibuprofen lysine
L-67	prilocaine HCl
L-696,229	generic not yet assigned—see main list
L-697,661	generic not yet assigned—see main list
L-749	salacetamide
L 75 1362B	colforsin
L-8	lypressin
L 8027	nictindole
L-9394	butoprozine HCl
LA-012 (as HCl)	quatacaine
LA 1221 (as HCl)	butalamine
LA III	diazepam
LA 391	sodium picosulfate

La 6023	metformin
LAC-43	bupivacaine HCl
LAS 3876	almagate
LAS 9273	clebopride
LAS W-090	ebastine
LB 125	cyprodenate
LB-46	pindolol
LB-502	furosemide
LC 44	flupentixol
LD 2351 (as hydrobromide)	butopiprine
LD 2480	piprocurarium iodide
LD 2630	difencloxazine HCl
LD 2988	folescutol
LD 3055	oxypyrronium bromide
LD 335	propyromazine bromide
LD 3394	fenozolone
LD 3612	paraflutizide
LD 4644	pipebuzone
LD 935	dipiproverine HCl
Leo 114	polyestradiol phosphate
levo-BC-2605	oxilorphan
levo-BC-2627	butorphanol
levo-BC-2627 tartrate	butorphanol tartrate
levo-BL-4566	moxazocine
LJ 206	carbocysteine
LJC 10,141	felbinac
LL 1530	nadoxolol
LL-705W	neutramycin
LM-1404	lortalamine
LM 176	cobamamide
LM 192	viquidil
LM 2717	clobazam
LM-427	rifabutin
LM-94	hymecromone
L.N. 107	broparestrol
LS-121	nafronyl oxalate
LS 519 C12	pirenzepine HCl
LU3-010	talopram HCl
LVD	dextran 40
LY 048 740	avilamycin
LY061188	cephalexin HCl
LY097964	cefetamet
LY099094	vindesine sulfate
LY104208	vinzolidine sulfate
LY 108380	doxpicomine HCl
LY110140	fluoxetine HCl
LY 119863	vinepidine sulfate
LY120363	flumezapine

LY121019	cilofungin
LY 122512	anitrazafen
LY 12271-72	viroxime
LY 122772	enviroxime
LY 123508	lorzafone
LY 127123	enviradene
LY 127623	metkephamid acetate
LY 127809	pergolide mesylate
LY 127935	moxalactam disodium
LY 135837	indecainide HCl
LY137998	somatropin
LY 139037	nizatidine
LY 139381	ceftazidime
LY 139603	tomoxetine HCl
LY 141894	amflutizole
LY 146032	daptomycin
LY 150378	clofilium phosphate
LY 150720	picenadol HCl
LY156758	raloxifene HCl
LY163502	quinelorane HCl
LY163892	loracarbef
LY167005	proinsulin human
LY171555	quinpirole HCl
LY171883	tomelukast
LY 174008	dobutamine tartrate
LY 175326	isomazole HCl
LY177370	tilmicosin
LY177837	somidobove
LY 186655	tibenelast sodium
LY188011	gemcitabine
LY188011 HCl	gemcitabine HCl
LY 195115	indolidan
LY 237216	dirithromycin
LY281067	sergolexole maleate
LYO31537	ractopamine HCl
M-1028 (Meiji)	haloprogin
M-14	rifamycin
M-141	spectinomycin HCl
M 285	cyprenorphine HCl
M. 5050	diprenorphine
M-811	salverine
M. 99 (as HCl)	etorphine
MA 1277	zolertine HCl
MA 1291	quipazine maleate
MA 1337	cloperidone HCl
MA-1443	letimide HCl
MA-540	quinuclium bromide
MA-593	salethamide maleate

MAS-1	polyglyconate
Material A	pentetate calcium trisodium Yb 169
M&B 15497	decoquinate
M&B 16942A	diacetolol HCl
M&B 17803A (as HCl)	acebutolol
M&B 22948	zaprinast
M&B 33153	oxoprostol
M&B 39831	temozolomide
M&B 5062 A	amicarbalide
M&B 782 (as isethionate)	propamidine
MB 800 (as isethionate)	pentamidine
M&B 9302	clorgiline
MBR-4164-8	diflumidone sodium
MBR-4197	flucrylate
MBR 4223	triflumidate
MCE	metergoline
McN-1075	fenmetramide
McN-1107	clominorex
McN-1210	pyrinoline
McN-1231	fluminorex
McN-1546	flumetramide
McN-1589	mixidine
McN-2378	mefenidil
McN-2378-46	mefenidil fumarate
McN-2453	azepindole
McN-2559	tolmetin
McN-2559-21-98	tolmetin sodium
McN-2783-21-98	zomepirac sodium
McN-3113	xilobam
McN-3377-98	fenobam
McN-3495	pirogliride tartrate
McN-3716	methyl palmoxirate
McN-3802 (anhydrous free acid)	palmoxirate sodium
McN-3802-21-98	palmoxirate sodium
McN 3935	linogliride
McN-3935	linogliride fumarate
McN-4097-12-98	fenoctimine sulfate
McN-4853	topiramate
McN-742	aminorex
McN-A-2673-11	etoperidone HCl
McN-A-2833	perindopril
McN-A-2833-109	perindopril erbumine
McN-JR-13,558-11	fetoxylate HCl
McN-JR-15,403-11	difenoxin
McN-JR-1625	haloperidol
McN-JR-16,341	penfluridol
McN-JR-2498	trifluperidol
McN-JR-4263-49	fentanyl citrate

McN-JR-4584	benperidol
McN-JR-4749	droperidol
McN-JR-4929-11	benzetimide HCl
McN-JR-6218	fluspirilene
McN-JR-6238	pimozide
McN-JR-7242-11	difluanine HCl
McN-JR-7904	lidoflazine
McN-JR-8299-11	tetramisole HCl
McN-R-1162-22	potassium glucaldrate
McN-R-1967	fenretinide
McN-R-726-47	poldine methylsulfate
McN-R-73-Z	rotoxamine
McN-X-181	valnoctamide
McN-X-94	capuride
MD 141	ethamsylate
MD 2028	fluanisone
MD 67350 (as maleate)	cinepazide
MDL 14,042	lofexidine HCl
MDL 17,043	enoximone
MDL 19,205	piroximone
MDL 19,744	tipentosin HCl
MDL 257	zindotrine
MDL 458	deflazacort
MDL 473	rifapentine
MDL 507	teicoplanin
MDL 71,754	vigabatrin
MDL 71,782 A	eflornithine HCl
MDL 72,422	tropanserin HCl
MER-29	triparanol
MER-41	clomiphene citrate
M.G. 13054	fenquizone
M.G. 13608	domiodol
M.G. 143	sulmarin
M.G. 1559	xenbucin
Mg 4833	fencibutirol
M.G. 5454	guaiapate
MG 559	metamfepramone
M.G. 5771	butixirate
M.G. 624	stilonium iodide
M.G. 652	oxamarin HCl
M.G. 8823	exaprolol HCl
M.G. 8926 (as HCl)	droprenilamine
MH-532	phenprobamate
MI-216	iothalamic acid
Mi-85	apazone
MJ 10061	benzbromarone
MJ 12,175-170	tiprinast meglumine
MJ 12,880-1	tipropidil HCl

MJ 13,105-1	bucindolol HCl
MJ 13401-1-3	fenprinast HCl
MJ 13,754-1	nefazodone HCl
MJ 1986	indriline HCl
MJ 1987	mesuprine HCl
MJ 1988	quazodine
MJ 1992	soterenol HCl
MJ 1998	metalol HCl
MJ 1999	sotalol HCl
MJ 4309-1	oxybutynin chloride
MJ 505	phenyramidol HCl
MJ 9022-1	buspirone HCl
MJ 9067-1	encainide HCl
MJ 9184-1	zinterol HCl
MJF 10,938	xipamide
MJF 11567-3	cefadroxil
MJF-12264	tegafur
MJF 12637	suloctidil
MJF 9325	ifosfamide
MK-0681	trientine HCl
MK-0787	imipenem
MK-0936	abamectin
MK-130 (as the base)	cyclobenzaprine HCl
MK-188	zeranol
MK-196	indacrinone
MK-208	famotidine
MK-217	alendronate sodium
MK-240	protriptyline HCl
MK-250	emylcamate
MK-329	devazepide
MK-341	tranilast
MK-351	methyldopa
MK-360	thiabendazole
MK-366	norfloxacin
MK-401	clorsulon
MK-417	sezolamide HCl
MK-422	enalaprilat
MK-458	naxagolide HCl
MK-521	lisinopril
MK 57	methyldesorphine
MK-595	ethacrynic acid
MK-621	efrotomycin
MK-678	seglitide acetate
MK-733	simvastatin
MK-791	cilastatin sodium
MK-801	dizocilpine maleate
MK-803	lovastatin
MK-906	finasteride

ML-1024	theofibrate
ML 1034	celucloral
MO-1255	encyprate
MO-911	pargyline HCl
MP-10013	iogulamide
MP-1051	silodrate
MP 2032	iocarmic acid
MP 2032-meglumine	iocarmate meglumine
MP-271	iosefamic acid
MP 302 (with ioxaglate sodium)	ioxaglate meglumine
MP 328	ioversol
MP 4006	albumin, aggregated
MP 4018	stannous pyrophosphate
MP-537	iomethin I 125; iomethin I 131
MP-600	betiatide
MP-6026	ioglucol
MP-620	iocetamic acid
MP 7010	stannous sulfur colloid
MP-8000	ioglucomide
MPV-1248	atipamezole
MPV-1440	dexmedetomidine
MPV-253 AII	detomidine HCl
MPV-785	medetomidine HCl
MRL 38	hexadiline
MRL-41	clomiphene citrate
MRP-10	pentetate calcium trisodium Yb 169
MSL-109	generic not yet assigned—see main list
MTS 263	tropenziline bromide
MY-25 (as bitartrate)	metergotamine
MY-33-7 (as HCl)	lotucaine
MYC 8003	mocimycin
MZ-144	rimazolium metilsulfate
N-0252	laurocapram
N-137	carbetimer
N-3	methetoin
N-399	xenytropium bromide
N-553 (as HCl)	tolperisone
N-7009	flupentixol
N-7020	meprotixol
N-714	chlorprothixene
N-746	clopenthixol
NA-119	bromamid
NA 274	bromhexine HCl
NA-66	pimeclone
NAB 365	clenbuterol
NASH	borocaptate sodium B 10
NAT-327	trimoxamine HCl
NAT-333	fenspiride HCl

NB 68	dacuronium bromide
NC-123	mesoridazine
NC 1264	thonzonium bromide
NC 150	phenazopyridine HCl
NC-1968	fungimycin
NC-7197	esproquin HCl
NCNU	pentamustine
ND 50	octopamine
NDC 0082-4155	daunorubicin HCl
NDR 263	propenzolate HCl
NDR 304	ethyl dibunate
NDR-5061A	aletamine HCl
NDR-5523A	trimoxamine HCl
NDR-5998A	fenspiride HCl
NE-19550	olvanil
NE 97221	piridronate sodium
NF-1010	nifurdazil
NF-1088	nifurquinazol
NF-1120	nifurimide
NF-1425	furazolium tartrate
NF-161	nifursemizone
NF-246	nifuradene
NF-602	levofuraltadone
NF-71	nifurmerone
NF-84	nifuraldezone
NF-902 (as HCl)	levofuraltadone
NF-963	furazolium chloride
NG-29	generic not yet assigned—see main list
NIB	nabitan HCl
NIH 2933	dimepheptanol
NIH 7574	benzethidine
NIH 7607	etonitazene
NIH 7667	noracymethadol HCl
NIH 7672	methopholine
NIH 8805	buprenorphine HCl
NK 1006	bekanamycin
NK-631	peplomycin sulfate
NKK-105	malotilate
NPAP	prajmalium bitartrate
NPT 15392	nosantine
NSD 1055	brocresine
Nu-1779	betaprodine
Nu-1932	betameprodine
NU-2121	nicotinyl alcohol
NU-445	sulfisoxazole diolamine
NY-198	lomefloxacin HCl
ODA 914	demoxytocin
OM 401	generic not yet assigned—see main list

OM-977	etaminile
OMDS	dipyrithione
OPC-1085	carteolol HCl
OPC-8212	vesnarinone
ORF 10131	norgestimate
ORF 11676	nalmefene
ORF 15244	thymopentin
ORF 15817	edoxudine
ORF 15927	rioprostil
ORF 16600	bemarinone HCl
ORF 17070	histrelin
ORF 18704	pelretin
ORF 20257	doretinel
ORF 20485	tepoxalin
ORF 22164	atosiban
ORF 22867	bemoradan
ORF-8063	triflubazam
ORF 9326	nisterime acetate
ORG 10172	danaparoid sodium
ORG 3770	mirtazapine
Org 817	epimestrol
Org GB 94	mianserin HCl
Org NA 97	pancuronium bromide
ORG NC 45	vecuronium bromide
Org OD 14	tibolone
P 071	cetirizine HCl
P-1011	dicloxacillin sodium
P-113	saralasin acetate
P-12	oxacillin sodium
P-1306	glyparamide
P-1496	zeranol
P-1560	taleranol
P-165	azaserine
P-1742	fluperolone acetate
P-1779	althiazide
P-1888	isosulfan blue
P-2105	epithiazide
P-248	levopropylcillin potassium
P-25	cloxacillin sodium
P-2525	polythiazide
P-2530	methalthiazide
P-2647	benzquinamide
P-286	ioxaglic acid
P-301	hydroxyphenamate
P-3693A	doxepin HCl
P-3896	guanisoquin sulfate
P-4125	isosulfan blue
P-4385B	clothixamide maleate

P-4599	cidoxepin HCl
P-463	fenamole
P-4657 B	thiothixene
P-50	ampicillin
P-5227	pinoxepin HCl
P-638	puromycin
P 7	lauroguadine
P-71	lycetamine
P 71-0129	fendosal
P-7138	nifurpirinol
P 720549	isoxepac
P 76 2494A	fluradoline HCl
P 76 2543	dazepinil HCl
P 78 3522	brocrinat
P79 3913	neflumozide HCl
PA-144	plicamycin
PAA-3854	clamoxyquin HCl
PAA-701	bialamicol HCl
2-PAM chloride	pralidoxime chloride
PAM-MR-1165	acedapsone
PAM-MR-807-23a	cycloguanil pamoate
PAMN (as methonitrate)	prampine
PASIT	glyprothiazol
PAT	fenamole
PB 89 (as HCl)	fominoben
p-BIDA	butilfenin
PC-1421	piperacetazine
PC-603	iproclozide
PD 107779	enoxacin
PD-110843	zonisamide
PD 90,695-73	dezaguanine mesylate
PD-93	piromidic acid
PDB	prifinium bromide
pentapeptide DSDPR	pentigetide
PF-26	mepramidil
PFA-186	salicylate meglumine
PG 430	febuverine
PG-501	mazaticol
PH 218	edogestrone
pierrel-TQ 86	azipramine HCl
PIXY321	generic not yet assigned—see main list
PK 10169	enoxaparin
PM 1807	fenimide
PM-185184	secnidazole
PM-1952	fenacetinol
PM-3944	flucetorex
PM-671	ethosuximide
PN 200-110	isradipine

POLI 67	tetrydamine
POR 8	ornipressin
PP 563	cyhalothrin
PPI-002	generic not yet assigned—see main list
PR-0818-156A	verilopam HCl
PR-122	generic not yet assigned—see main list
PR-225	generic not yet assigned—see main list
PR-239	generic not yet assigned—see main list
PR-320	molecusol & carbamazepine
PR-3847	teroxalene HCl
PR-741-976A	somantadine HCl
PR-870-714A	veradoline HCl
PR-877-530L	flavodilol maleate
PR 879-317A	oxamisole HCl
PR 934-423A	remacemide HCl
PR-G 138-CL (as HCl)	ciclosidomine
protease 1	brinolase
PS-1286	pararosaniline pamoate
PS 2383	trimetozine
PT-9	betahistine HCl
PU-239	benzilonium bromide
PY 108-068	darodipine
PZ 1511	carpipramine dihydrochloride
PZ68	pentosan polysulfate sodium
QB-1	cloquinozine
QZ-2	methaqualone
R 10.100	ethonam nitrate
R 10,948	diamocaine cyclamate
R 11,333	bromperidol
R 12,563 (as HCl)	dexamisole
R 12,564	levamisole HCl
R 1303	carbofenotion
R-13423	dicloxacillin
R 13,558	fetoxylate HCl
R-13,672	haloperidol decanoate
R 1406	phenoperidine
R-148	methaqualone
R 14,827	econazole nitrate
R 14,889	miconazole nitrate
R 14,950	flunarizine HCl
R 15,403 (as HCl)	difenoxin
R-15,454 (as nitrate salt)	isoconazole
R 15,556	orconazole nitrate
R 1575	cinnarizine
R 15,889	lorcainide HCl
R-1625	haloperidol
R 16,341	penfluridol
R 16,470 (as HCl)	dexetimide

R 1658	moperone
R 1707	glafenine
R 17,147	cyclobendazole
R 17,635	mebendazole
R 17,889	flubendazole
R 17,934	nocodazole
R 18,553	loperamide HCl
R 1881	metribolone
R 18,910	fluperamide
R 1929	azaperone
R 19,317	rodocaine
R 2028	fluanisone
R 2113	desoximetasone
R 2159	anisopirol
R 2167	fluanisone
R 22,700 (as HCl)	rodocaine
R 23,050	salantel
R 2323	gestrinone
R 23,633	fludazonium chloride
R 23,979	enilconazole
R 2453	demegestone
R-2498	trifluperidol
R-25,061	suprofen
R-25,160	cliprofen
R 25,540	imafen HCl
R 25,831 (as the free base)	carnidazole
R 26,412	sulnidazole
R 27,500	sepazonium chloride
R 28,096 (as HCl)	carnidazole
R 2858	moxestrol
R-28,644	azaconazole
R 28,930	fluspiperone
R 2962	amiperone
R 29,764	clopimozide
R 29,860	nitramisole HCl
R 30,730	sufentanil
R 31,520	closantel
R 3248	aceperone
R 33,204	declenperone
R 3345	pipamperone
R 3365	piritramide
R 33,799	carfentanil citrate
R 33800	sufentanil citrate
R 33,812	domperidone
R 34,000	doconazole
R 34,009	milenperone
R 34,301	halopemide
R-34,803	etibendazole

R 34,995	lofentanil oxalate
R 35,443	oxatomide
R 38,198	buterizine
R 39,209	alfentanil HCl
R 39,500	parconazole HCl
R 3959	clometacin
R 4082	propyperone
R 41,400	ketoconazole
R-41,468	ketanserin
R-42,470	terconazole
R-4263	fentanyl citrate
R 4318	floctafenine
R 43,512	astemizole
R 4444	duometacin
R-45,486	flumeridone
R-4584	benperidol
R-46,541	bromperidol decanoate
R 46,846	tubulozole HCl
R 4714	oxiperomide
R-47,465	pirenperone
R-4749	droperidol
R 48	chlornaphazine
R 4845	bezitramide
R 5046	cinperene
R 50,547	levocabastine HCl
R 50 970	metrenperone
R 51 163	tameridone
R 51,211	itraconazole
R-51,469	mioflazinc HCl
R 5147	spiperone
R 516	cinnarizine
R-51,619	cisapride
R 5188	spiroxatrine
R-52	mannosulfan
R 52,245	setoperone
R-53,200	altanserin tartrate
R 5385	acoxatrine
R 54,718	transcainide
R-548	tricetamide
R 55,667	ritanserin
R 5808	spiramide
R58425	loperamide oxide
R 58735	sabeluzole
R 610	racemoramide
R 6109	spirilene
R 6218	fluspirilene
R 6238	pimozide
R62,690	clazuril

R 62 818	lorcinadol
R 6438	antazonite
R64,433	diclazuril
R 64 766	risperidone
R65,824	nebivolol
R 661	buzepide metiodide
R 67408	fenclofenac
R 7242	difluanine HCl
R 7464	propoxate
R 7904	lidoflazine
R 798	rimiterol hydrobromide
R 8025	antienite
R-803	furaprofen
R 805	nimesulide
R 8141	antienite
R-8193	antafenite
R 8284	proclonol
R 8299	tetramisole HCl
R-830	prifelone
R-830T	prifelone
R-835	ibafloxacin
R 9298	seperidol HCl
RA-8	dipyridamole
RA-C-384	iodocetylic acid I 123
RC-160	vapreotide
RC-167	niceverine
RC-172	aldioxa
RC-173	alcloxa
RC-27109	nifuroxazide
RC 61-91	ifenprodil
RCH 314	benhepazone
RCM 258	fepentolic acid
RD 11654	ibufenac
RD 17345	fluprofen
RD 2801	pyritidium bromide
Rd 292	fenpentadiol
RD 328	pasiniazid
RD 406	cyprodenate
RD 9338 (as HCl)	norbudrine
Rec 15 0122	nifurpipone
Rec 15/1476	fenticonazole nitrate
Rec 7/0267	dimefline HCl
REV 3659-(S)	pivopril
REV 6000A	delapril HCl
RG 12986	generic not yet assigned—see main list
RG 270	iomeglamic acid
RG 83894	generic not yet assigned—see main list
RGH 1106	pipecuronium bromide

RH-32,565	uredofos
RH-565	uredofos
RHC 2871	eclazolast
RHC 2906	flordipine
RHC 3659-(S)	pivopril
RHC 3988	quazolast
RI-64	pifexole
Riker 52G	aprotinin
Riker 594	sulthiame
Riker 595	butaperazine
Riker 601	triaziquone
RIT 1140	apicycline
RMI 10,482A	metizoline HCl
RMI 16,238	eterobarb
RMI 16,289	enclomiphene
RMI 16,312	zuclomiphene
RMI 80,029	elantrine
RMI 8090DJ	quindecamine acetate
RMI 81,182EF	cilobamine mesylate
RMI 81,968	medroxalol
RMI 81,968 A	medroxalol HCl
RMI 83,027	rolicyprine
RMI 83,047	ambuside
RMI 9,384A	desipramine HCl
RMI 9918	terfenadine
RMP-7	generic not yet assigned—see main list
Ro 03-8799	pimonidazole
Ro 10-1670/000	acitretin
Ro 10-6338	bumetanide
Ro 10-9070	amdinocillin
Ro 10-9071	amdinocillin pivoxil
Ro 10-9359	etretinate
Ro 11-1163/000	moclobemide
Ro 11-1430	motretinide
Ro 11-1781/023	tiapamil HCl
Ro 12-0068/000	tenoxicam
Ro 13-5057	aniracetam
Ro 13-6438/006	quazinone
RO 13-8996	oxiconazole nitrate
Ro-13-9297	lornoxicam
Ro 13-9904	ceftriaxone sodium
Ro 14-4767/000	amorolfine
RO 1-5155	nicotinyl alcohol
Ro 15-1788/000	flumazenil
Ro 1-6794	dextrorphan
Ro 17-2301/006	carumonam sodium
Ro 1-9334/19	dehydroemetine
Ro 1-9569	tetrabenazine

Ro 20-5720/000	carprofen
Ro 21-0702	flurocitabine
Ro 21-3981/001	midazolam maleate
Ro 21-3981/003	midazolam HCl
Ro 21-5535	calcitriol
Ro 21-5998	mefloquine
Ro 21-5998/001	mefloquine HCl
Ro 21-6937/000	trimoprostil
Ro 21-8837/001	estramustine phosphate sodium
Ro 22-1319/003	piquindone HCl
Ro 22-2296/000	estramustine
Ro 22-3747/000	tiacrilast
Ro 22-3747/007	tiacrilast sodium
Ro 22-7796	cifenline
Ro 22-7796/001	cifenline succinate
Ro 22-8181	interferon alfa-2a
Ro 22-9000	alfaprostol
Ro 2-2985	lasalocid
Ro 23-0731/000	sedecamycin
Ro 23-3544/000	ablukast
Ro 23-3544/001	ablukast sodium
Ro 23-6019	teceleukin
Ro 23-6240/000	fleroxacin
Ro 2-3773	clidinium bromide
Ro 2-9757	fluorouracil
Ro 2-9915	flucytosine
Ro-31-2848/006	cilazapril
Ro 31-3113	cilazaprilat
Ro-31-3948/000	romazarit
Ro 4-0403	chlorprothixene
Ro 4-1544-6	sodium stibocaptate
Ro 4-1778/1	methopholine
Ro 4-2130	sulfamethoxazole
Ro 4-3780	isotretinoin
RO 4-3816	alcuronium chloride
Ro 4-4393	sulfadoxine
Ro 4-4602	benserazide
Ro 4-5282	mefenorex HCl
Ro 4-5360	nitrazepam
Ro 4-6467/1	procarbazine HCl
Ro 48347	trengestone
Ro 5-0690	chlordiazepoxide HCl
Ro 5-2092	demoxepam
Ro 5-2807	diazepam
Ro 5-3059	nitrazepam
RO 5-3307/1	debrisoquin sulfate
Ro 5-3350	bromazepam
Ro 5-4023	clonazepam

Ro 5-4200	flunitrazepam
Ro 5-4556	medazepam HCl
Ro 5-4645/010	coumermycin sodium
Ro 5-6901	flurazepam HCl
Ro 5-9110/1	dorastine HCl
Ro 5-9754	ormetoprim
Ro 6-4563	glibornuride
Ro 7-0207	ornidazole
Ro 7-0582	misonidazole
Ro 7-1554	ipronidazole
Ro 7-4488/1	cuprimyxin
RP 12222	penmesterol
RP 13057 (as the base)	daunorubicin HCl
RP 13607	clotioxone
RP 14539	secnidazole
RP 16091	metiazinic acid
RP 19552	pipotiazine palmitate
R.P. 19,583	ketoprofen
R.P. 20 578	bamnidazole
RP 22,050 HCl	zorubicin HCl
RP 22410	glisoxepide
RP 2254	glyprothiazol
RP 2259	glybuthiazol
RP 2512 (as isethionate)	pentamidine
RP 2921	aminothiazole
RP 2987	diethazine HCl
RP 3854	melarsoprol
RP 4763 (as sodium salt)	difetarsone
RP 5171	proadifen HCl
RP 6484	etymemazine HCl
RP 6847	oxomemazine
RP 6870	inproquone
RP 7044	methotrimeprazine
RP 7204	cyamemazine
RP 7293	pristinamycin
RP 7891	glybuzole
RP 8595	dimetridazole
RP 8823	metronidazole
RP 8909	periciazine
RP 9159	perimetazine
RP 9671	nosiheptide
RP 9778	protionamide
RP 9921	aprotinin
RP 9955	melarsonyl potassium
RR No. 32705	rutamycin
RS-11988	laidlomycin propionate potassium
RS-1301	delmadinone acetate
RS-1320	flunisolide acetate

RS-21361	imiloxan HCl
RS-21592	ganciclovir
RS-21592 sodium	ganciclovir sodium
R&S 218-M	alletorphine
RS-2208	amadinone acetate
RS-2252	flucloronide
RS-2362	procinonide
RS-2386	ciprocinonide
RS-3268R	nandrolone cyclotate
RS-3540	naproxen
RS-35887	butoconazole nitrate
RS-35887-00-10-3	butoconazole nitrate
RS-35909-00-00-0	ticabesone propionate
RS-3650	naproxen sodium
RS-3694R	cormethasone acetate
RS-37326	anirolac
RS-37449	temurtide
RS-3999	flunisolide
RS-4034	naproxol
RS-40584	flumoxonide
RS-40974-00-00-0	tiopinac
RS-43179	lonapalene
RS-43285	ranolazine HCl
RS-4464	triclonide
RS-44872	sulconazole nitrate
RS-44872-00-10-3	sulconazole nitrate
RS-4691	cloprednol
RS-49014	tazifylline HCl
R&S 5205-M	homprenorphine
RS-6245	tazolol HCl
RS-6818	xanoxate sodium
RS-68439	detirelix acetate
RS-69216	nicardipine HCl
RS-69216-XX-07-0	nicardipine HCl
RS-7337	tixanox
RS-82856	lixazinone sulfate
RS-82917-030	tifurac sodium
RS-84043	fenprostalene
RS-84135	enprostil
RS-85446-007	timobesone acetate
RS-8858	oxfendazole
RS-9390	prostalene
RS-94991-298	nafarelin acetate
RU 15060	tiaprofenic acid
Ru 15750	floctafenine
RU-1697	trenbolon acetate
RU-19110	halofuginone hydrobromide
RU-2267	altrenogest

RU 2323	gestrinone
RU 24756	cefotaxime sodium
RU 28965	roxithromycin
RU 38882	inocoterone acetate
RU 486	mifepristone
RU 882	inocoterone acetate
RU 965	roxithromycin
RWJ 10131	norgestimate
RWJ 15817	edoxudine
RWJ 15927	rioprostil
RWJ 16600	bemarinone HCl
RWJ 17070	histrelin
RWJ 18704	pelretin
RWJ 20257	doretinel
RWJ 20485	tepoxalin
RWJ 22164	atosiban
RX 6029-M HCl	buprenorphine HCl
Rx 67408	fenclofenac
RX77989	pentamorphone
S 10036	fotemustine
S-1210	bietaserpine
S-1320	budesonide
S 1530	nimetazepam
S-16820	prifelone
S-210	morsuximide
S-222	ditazole
S-2395	tertatolol
S-2539F	phenothrin
S-25930	ibafloxacin
S 314	fusafungine
S 4105	medibazine
S 5614	dexfenfluramine
S-62	chlorphentermine HCl
S 7	fenticlor
S 73 4118	piretanide
S 77 0777	prednicarbate
S-940	naftalofos
S-9490	perindopril
S-9490-3	perindopril erbumine
S-9780	perindoprilat
SA-267	dipenine bromide
SB 7505	ibopamine
SBW-22	ketorfanol
SC 10363	megestrol acetate
SC 11585	oxandrolone
SC 11800	ethynodiol diacetate
SC-12350	nitralamine HCl
SC-12937	azacosterol HCl

SC-13504	ropizine
SC-13957	disopyramide phosphate
SC-14207	metogest
SC-14266	canrenoate potassium
SC-16148	silandrone
SC 1749 (as sodium salt)	menbutone
SC-18862	aspartame
SC-19198	methynodiol diacetate
SC-21009	norgestomet
SC-23992	prorenoate potassium
SC-25469	pinadoline
SC-26100	difenoximide HCl
SC-26304	dicirenone
SC-26438	pirolazamide
SC-26714	mexrenoate potassium
SC-27123	octriptyline phosphate
SC-27166	nufenoxole
SC-27761	pranolium chloride
SC-29333	misoprostol
SC-31828	disobutamide
SC-32642	metronidazole HCl
SC-32840	oxagrelate
SC-33643	bemitradine
SC-33963	reclazepam
SC-34301	enisoprost
SC-35135	edifolone acetate
SC-36602	actisomide
SC-37681	gemeprost
SC-38390	zinoconazole HCl
SC-39026	lodelaben
SC-4642	norethynodrel
SC-47111	lomefloxacin HCl
SC-47111A	lomefloxacin
SC-47111B	lomefloxacin mesylate
SC-7031	disopyramide
SC-7294	propetandrol
SC-7525	bolandiol dipropionate
SC-9376	canrenone
SC-9880	flurogestone acetate
SCE-1365 (Takeda) (base)	cefmenoxime HCl
Sch 1000-Br-monohydrate	ipratropium bromide
Sch 10144	tolnaftate
Sch 10159	triclofos sodium
Sch 10304	clonixin
Sch 10595	bupicomide
Sch 10649	azatadine maleate
Sch 11460	betamethasone dipropionate
Sch 11572	meclorisone dibutyrate

Sch 11973	tosifen
Sch 12041	halazepam
Sch 12149	pazoxide
Sch 12169	closiramine aceturate
Sch 12650	dazadrol maleate
Sch 12679	trepipam maleate
Sch 12707	clonixeril
Sch 13166 D fumarate	domazoline fumarate
Sch 13430.2KH$_2$PO$_4$	megalomicin potassium phosphate
Sch 13475 sulfate	sisomicin sulfate
Sch 13521	flutamide
Sch 13949W Sulfate	albuterol sulfate
Sch 14342	betamicin sulfate
Sch 14714	flunixin
Sch 14714 meglumine	flunixin meglumine
Sch 14947	rosaramicin
Sch 14947.NaH$_2$PO$_4$	rosaramicin sodium phosphate
Sch 14947 stearate	rosaramicin stearate
Sch 15280	azanator maleate
Sch 15427	carmantadine
Sch 15507	dopamantine
Sch 15698	fletazepam
Sch 15719W	labetalol HCl
Sch 16134	quazepam
Sch 16524	repromicin
Sch 17894	rosaramicin propionate
Sch 18020W	beclomethasone dipropionate
Sch 18667	rosaramicin butyrate
Sch 19741	picotrin diolamine
Sch 19927	dilevalol HCl
Sch 20569	netilmicin sulfate
Sch 21420	isepamicin
Sch 21480	tioxidazole
Sch 22219	alclometasone dipropionate
Sch 22591	pentisomicin
Sch 25298	florfenicol
Sch 2544	cycliramine maleate
Sch 28316Z	indenolol
Sch 29851	loratadine
Sch 30500	interferon alfa-2b
Sch 31353	dexamethasone acefurate
Sch 32088	mometasone furoate
Sch 32481	netobimin
Sch 33844	spirapril HCl
Sch 33861	spiraprilat
Sch 3444	parapenzolate bromide
Sch 35852	cisconazole
Sch 39720	ceftibuten

Sch 4358	meprednisone
Sch 4831	betamethasone
Sch 4855	pseudoephedrine sulfate
Sch 6620	prednazate
Sch 6673	acetophenazine maleate
Sch 6783	diazoxide
Sch 7056	acrisorcin
Sch 9384	oxymetazoline HCl
Sch 9724	gentamicin sulfate
Scha-306	cintazone
SCL-70	alofilcon A
SCT 1	salcatonin
SCTZ (as edisylate)	clomethiazole
SD 1223-01	trazitiline
SD 1248-17 (as HCl)	tropatepine
SD 14112	sulclamide
SD 149-01	feneritrol
SD 15803	vincofos
SD 17102	meticrane
SD 1750	dichlorvos
SD 2102-18	acrocinonide
SD 2124-01	procinolol
SD 25	dicarfen
SD 270-07 (as succinate)	oxaprazine
SD 270-31 (as disuccinate)	oxaflumazine
SD 271-12	clobenzorex
SD 27115 (as cyclamate)	furfenorex
SD 286-03	cimemoxin
SD 7859	clofenvinfos
SDZ MSL-109	sevirumab
SE 1702	gliclazide
SeHCAT	tauroselcholic acid
SF 86-327	terbinafine
SG-75	nicorandil
SGD 301-76	oxiconazole nitrate
SH 100	oxapium iodide
SH 1040	gestaclone
SH 1051	glicetanile sodium
SH 2.1139/H 248 AB	ioxotrizoic acid
SH 213 AB	iotroxic acid
SH 240	moxnidazole
SH 263	droxacin sodium
SH 3.1168	gliflumide
SH 567	methenolone acetate
SH 582	gestonorone caproate
SH 601	methenolone enanthate
SH 714	cyproterone acetate
SH 717	glymidine sodium

SH 723	mesterolone
SH 741	clomegestone acetate
SH 742	fluocortolone
SH 770	fluocortolone caproate
SH 818	clocortolone acetate
SH 863	clocortolone pivalate
SH 926	iodamide
SH 968	diflucortolone pivalate
SH B 331	gestodene
SH E 199	etoformin HCl
SH G 318 AB	sermetacin
SH H 200 AB	ioglicic acid
SH H 239 AB	ioseric acid
SH K 203	fluocortin butyl
SH L 451 A	gadopentetate dimeglumine
SJ 1977	methixene HCl
SK&F 102,362	nilvadipine
SKF 105657	epristeride
SK&F 110679	generic not yet assigned—see main list
SK&F 12866	clorethate
SKF 13338	ampyrimine
SK&F 13364-A	thyromedan HCl
SK&F 1340	dimefadane
SK&F 14287	idoxuridine
SK&F 14336	clomacran phosphate
SK&F 15601A	toliodium chloride
SKF 16046	anisacril
SK&F 18,667	poloxalene
SK&F 1995	dicloralurea
SKF 20716	periciazine
SK&F 2208	hetaflur
SK&F 24529	lobendazole
SKF 2599	doxenitoin
SK&F 28175	fluotracen HCl
SK&F 29044	parbendazole
SK&F 30310	oxibendazole
SK&F 3050	cortodoxone
SKF 33134-A	amiodarone
SK&F 38094	dectaflur
SK&F 38095	olaflur
SK&F 39162	auranofin
SK&F 39186	amicloral
SK&F 40383	carbuterol HCl
SK&F 41558	cefazolin sodium
SK&F 478	diphenidol
SK&F 478-A	diphenidol HCl
SK&F 478-J	diphenidol pamoate
SK&F 51	octodrine

SK&F 5116	methotrimeprazine
SK&F 525-A	proadifen HCl
SK&F 53705-A	sulfonterol HCl
SK&F 59962	cefazaflur sodium
SK&F 61636	bromoxanide
SK&F 62698	ticrynafen
SK&F 62979	albendazole
SK&F 63797	dribendazole
SK&F 6539	flurothyl
SK&F 69634	clopipazan mesylate
SK&F 70230-A	pipazethate
SK&F 72517	elfazepam
SK&F 7690	benorterone
SK&F 7988	virginiamycin
SK&F 82526-J	fenoldopam mesylate
SKF-8318	xenazoic acid
SK&F 8542	triamterene
SK&F 88373-Z	ceftizoxime sodium
SKF 8898-A	moroxydine
SK&F 92058	metiamide
SK&F 92657-A$_2$	prizidilol HCl
SK&F 92676-A$_3$	impromidine HCl
SK&F 92994-A$_2$	oxmetidine HCl
SK&F 92994-J$_2$	oxmetidine mesylate
SK&F 93319	icotidine
SK&F 93479	lupitidine HCl
SK&F 93574	donetidine
SK&F 93944	temelastine
SK&F 94836	siguazodan
SK&F 95587	sulotroban
SK&F 96148	daltroban
SKF 9976 (as citrate)	oxolamine
SK&F D-39304	cephradine
SK&F D-75073-Z	cefonicid monosodium
SK&F D-75073-Z$_2$	cefonicid sodium
SL 501	chlophedianol HCl
SL 75 177-10	cicloprolol HCl
SL 75.212-10	betaxolol HCl
SL 76 002	progabide
SL 77 499-10	alfuzosin HCl
SL 79.229-00	fengabine
SL 80.0342-00	alpidem
SL 80.0750-23N	zolpidem tartrate
SL 81.0142-00	tolgabide
SM-1213 (free base)	amiprilose HCl
SM-3997	tandospirone citrate
SMP 68-40	pyrabrom
SMP-78 Acid S	ambruticin

SMS-201-995	octreotide
SMS-201-995 ac	octreotide acetate
SN-166 (as the sodium salt)	glucosulfone
SN-263	sodium amylosulfate
S.N. 44	insulin, dalanated
SN 654	mepartricin
SNR 1804	clamidoxic acid
SP-106	nabitan HCl
SP-119	tinabinol
SP-175	nabazenil
SP-204	menabitan HCl
SP-304	pirnabine
SP-325	naboctate HCl
SP54	pentosan polysulfate sodium
SP63	otilonium bromide
SPA-S-132	partricin
SPA-S-160	mepartricin
SPA-S-510	piroxicam cinnamate
SPA-S-565	rifametane
SPC 297 D	azidocillin
SPI-77	mitopodozide
SQ 10,269	carbiphene HCl
SQ 10,496	thiazesim HCl
SQ 10,643	cinanserin HCl
SQ 1089	hydroxyurea
SQ 11,302	epicillin
SQ 11436	cephradine
SQ 11725	nadolol
SQ 13050	econazole nitrate
SQ 13,396	iopamidol
SQ 13847	pirquinozol
SQ 14055	tiamulin
SQ 14,225	captopril
SQ 1489	thiram
SQ 15,101	algestone acetophenide
SQ 15,102	amcinafal
SQ 15,112	amcinafide
SQ 15,659	rolitetracycline
SQ 15,860	glyhexamide
SQ 15,874	pipazethate
SQ 16,123	methicillin sodium
SQ 16,150	estradiol enanthate
SQ 16360	fusidate sodium
SQ 16374	methenolone enanthate
SQ 16,401	halquinols
SQ 16,423	oxacillin sodium
SQ 16496	methenolone acetate
SQ 16,603	fusidic acid

SQ 18566	halcinonide
SQ 19844	sincalide
SQ 20009	etazolate HCl
SQ 20824	cicloprofen
SQ 20881	teprotide
SQ 2128	ethoxazene HCl
SQ 21982	iodoxamic acid
SQ 21983	iopronic acid
SQ 22022 (dihydrate)	cephradine
SQ 22947	tiamulin fumarate
SQ 26490	naflocort
SQ 26776	aztreonam
SQ 26962	mebrofenin
SQ 26991	zofenopril calcium
SQ 27,239	tipredane
SQ 28555	fosinopril sodium
SQ 30217	technetium Tc 99m teboroxime
SQ 30836	tigemonam dicholine
SQ-31,000	pravastatin sodium
SQ 65396	cartazolate
SQ 82291	oximonam
SQ 82531	gloximonam
SQ 82629	oximonam sodium
SQ 83360	pirazmonam sodium
SQ 9343	phytate sodium
SQ 9453	dimethyl sulfoxide
SQ 9538	testolactone
SQ 9993	estradiol undecylate
[85]Sr	strontium nitrate Sr 85
SR-202	mifobate
SR 2508	etanidazole
SR-7037	belfosdil
SR 720-22	metolazone
SRG 95213	diazoxide
St 1085 (as the base)	midodrine HCl
ST12	dexamethasone dipropionate
St 1411	dimepregnen
ST-155	clonidine HCl
ST-155-BS	clonidine
ST 375	tolonidine
St 567-BR (as hydrobromide)	alinidine
ST 600	flutonidine
ST-813	oxiconazole nitrate
ST 9067	azintamide
STA-307	tiomesterone
St. Peter 224	midodrine HCl
Su-10568	clortermine HCl
Su-13437	nafenopin

Su-18137	cyproquinate
Su 21524	pirprofen
Su-4885	metyrapone tartrate
Su-5864	guanethidine sulfate
Su-6518	dimethindene maleate
Su-8341	cyclopenthiazide
Su-9064	metoserpate HCl
SUM 3170	loxapine
SUR 2647	sumacetamol
SYD-230	clioxanide
synthetic TRH	protirelin
T-1220	piperacillin sodium
T-1551	cefoperazone sodium
T-1982	cefbuperazone
T-2636	sedecamycin
T-2636A	sedecamycin
T-88	generic not yet assigned—see main list
TA-3090	clentiazem maleate
TA 5901	cefempidone
TAP031 (as the base)	fertirelin acetate
TAP-144	leuprolide acetate
TAT-3	picoperine
TATBA	triamcinolone hexacetonide
Tc924 (DPD)	butedronate tetrasodium
Tc99m-MP 4006	technetium Tc 99m albumin aggregated
Tc99m RP-30A	technetium Tc 99m sestamibi
Tc-MAG$_3$	technetium Tc 99m mertiatide
TE-031	clarithromycin
TE 114	tiemonium iodide
tenite butyrate formula 264 H4	cabufocon B
TH 1165a (as hydrobromide salt)	fenoterol
TH-1321	protionamide
Th-152	metaproterenol sulfate
TH-2151	hydracarbazine
TH-2180	propanidid
Th 322	metrifudil
THFES (HM)	zeranol
TLC ABLC	generic not yet assigned—see main list
TLC C-53	generic not yet assigned—see main list
TMB-4	trimedoxime bromide
TNO-6	spiroplatin
TP-21	thioridazine
TP-5	thymopentin
TPN-12	sulforidazine
TPS-23	mesoridazine
TR-2378	broperamole
TR-2515	pelanserin HCl

TR-2855	cromitrile sodium
TR-2985	ropitoin HCl
TR-3369	indorenate HCl
TR-4698	rioprostil
TR-495	methaqualone
TR-4979	butaprost
TR-5109	conorphone HCl
TR-5379M	xorphanol mesylate
trans AMCHA	tranexamic acid
TS 408	hydrocortisone buteprate
TSAA-291	oxendolone
TTFD	fursultiamine
TVP-101	generic not yet assigned—see main list
TVX485	etofenamate
TWSB; TWSb	sodium stibocaptate
U-10,136	alprostadil
U-10,149	lincomycin
U-10,858	minoxidil
U-10,974	flumethasone
U-10,997	mibolerone
U-11100A	nafoxidine HCl
U-12,019E	methylprednisolone sodium phosphate
U-12,062	dinoprostone
U-12,241	cirolemycin
U-12898	bluensomycin
U-13,933	asperlin
U-14,583	dinoprost
U-14,583E	dinoprost tromethamine
U-14,743	porfiromycin
U-15167	nogalamycin
U-15,614	trestolone acetate
U-15,965	lydimycin
U-17312E	etryptamine acetate
U-17,323	fluorometholone acetate
U-17835	tolazamide
U-18,409AE	spectinomycin HCl
U-18,496	azacitidine
U-18,573	ibuprofen
U-18,573G	ibuprofen aluminum
U-19183	sparsomycin
U-19,646	chlorphenesin carbamate
U-19,718	kalafungin
U-19763	bolasterone
U-19,920	cytarabine
U-19920A	cytarabine HCl
U-2032	kethoxal
U-20,661	steffimycin
U-21,251	clindamycin

U-22020	indoxole
U-22,550	calusterone
U-22,559A	dexoxadrol HCl
U-24,729A	mirincamycin HCl
U-24,792	lomofungin
U-24,973A	melitracen HCl
U-25,179 E	clindamycin palmitate HCl
U-25,873	ranimycin
U-26,225A	tramadol HCl
U-26,452	glyburide
U-27,182	flurbiprofen
U-28,009	denofungin
U-28,288D	guanadrel sulfate
U-28,508	clindamycin phosphate
U-28,774	ketazolam
U-29,479	scopafungin
U-30,604	zorbamycin
U-31,889	alprazolam
U-31,920	uldazepam
U-32,070E	calcifediol
U-32,921	carboprost
U-32,921E	carboprost tromethamine
U-33,030	triazolam
U-34,865	diflorasone diacetate
U-36,059	amitraz
U-36,384	carboprost methyl
U-41,123	adinazolam
U-41,123F	adinazolam mesylate
U-42,126	acivicin
U-42,585E	lodoxamide tromethamine
U-42,718	lodoxamide ethyl
U-42,842	arbaprostil
U-43,120	paulomycin
U-4527	cycloheximide
U-46,785	meteneprost
U-47,931E	bromadoline maleate
U-48,753E	eclanamine maleate
U-52,047	menogaril
U-53,059	itazigrel
U-53,217	epoprostenol
U-53,217A	epoprostenol sodium
U-53,996H	tazadolene succinate
U-54,461	bropirimine
U-54,555	metronidazole phosphate
U-54,669F	losulazine HCl
U-56,321	timefurone
U-57,930E	pirlimycin HCl
U-5956	filipin

U-6013	isoflupredone acetate
U-60,257	piriprost
U-60,257B	piriprost potassium
U-61,431F	ciprostene calcium
U-62066E	spiradoline mesylate
U-63,196	cefpimizole
U-63,196E	cefpimizole sodium
U-63287	ciglitazone
U-63,366F	trospectomycin sulfate
U-63,557A	furegrelate sodium
U-64279A	ceftiofur HCl
U-64279E	ceftiofur sodium
U-66858	bunaprolast
U-67,590A	methylprednisolone suleptanate
U-69689E	fertirelin acetate
U-6987	carbutamide
U-70138	paldimycin
U-71038	ditekiren
U-72107A	pioglitazone HCl
U-72791A	cefmetazole sodium
U-74006F	tirilazad mesylate
U-75630	ibuprofen piconol
U-76252	cefpodoxime proxetil
U-77,233	ormaplatin
U-7743	mercufenol chloride
U-7750	streptovarycin
U-7800	fluprednisolone
U-8344	uracil mustard
U-8471	medrysone
U-87201E	atevirdine mesylate
U-935	amiquinsin HCl
U-9889	streptozocin
UCB 1402	decloxizine
UCB 1474	chlorbenzoxamine HCl
UCB 1549	minepentate
UCB 1967	dropropizine
UCB 2073	etoxeridine
UCB 3928	fedrilate
UCB 4445	buclizine HCl
UK-11,443	primidolol
UK-18,892	butikacin
UK-20,349	tioconazole
UK-2054	famotine HCl
UK-2371	memotine HCl
UK-25,842	oxfenicine
UK-31,214	propikacin
UK-31,557	carbazeran
UK-33,274-27	doxazosin mesylate

UK-3540-1	amedalin HCl
UK-3557-15	daledalin tosylate
UK-37,248-01	dazoxiben HCl
UK-38,485	dazmegrel
UK-4271	oxamniquine
UK-48,340-11	amlodipine maleate
UK-48,340-26	amlodipine besylate
UK-49,858	fluconazole
UK-61260-27	nanterinone
UK-61,689	semduramicin
UK-61,689-2	semduramicin sodium
UK-73,300	candoxatril
UK-738	ethybenztropine
UK-73,967	candoxatrilat
UM 952	buprenorphine HCl
UP 106	propizepine
UP 107	bepiastine
UP 164	morniflumate
UP 74	nixylic acid
UP 83	niflumic acid
USV 3659-(S)	pivopril
V-C 13	dichlofenthion
VK-57	glyprothiazol
VM-26	teniposide
VP-16-213	etoposide
W-1015	nisobamate
W 10168	vifilcon A
W-1372	beloxamide
W 1655	phenazopyridine HCl
W 1760A	namoxyrate
W-19053 (as HCl)	etidocaine
W 1929	colistimethate sodium
W 2180	suxemerid sulfate
W 2197	pentrinitrol
W 2291A	mimbane HCl
W-2354	seclazone
W 2394A	pemerid nitrate
W-2395	meseclazone
W 2426	chlorphentermine HCl
W 2900A	etozolin
W-2946M	reproterol HCl
W-2964M	flupirtine maleate
W 2965 A	acetryptine
W-2979M	azelastine HCl
W 3207B	modaline sulfate
W 3366A	quindonium bromide
W3395	algestone acetonide
W 3399	quingestrone

W 3566	quinestrol
W 3580B	ampyzine sulfate
W-36095	tocainide
W 3623	cyprazepam
W 3676	sulazepam
W 3699	piprozolin
W 37	buformin
W 3746	cetophenicol
W 3976B	triampyzine sulfate
W 4020	prazepam
W 42782	iproxamine HCl
W 43026A	ciclafrine HCl
W 4425	almadrate sulfate
W 4454A	estrazinol hydrobromide
W 4540	quingestanol acetate
W 4565	oxolinic acid
W 4600	algeldrate
W 4701	hexedine
W 4744	mecloqualone
W 4869	prednival
W-5219	proglumide
W 5494A	naranol HCl
W 5733	atolide
W 5759A	tilidine HCl
W-583	mebutamate
W 5975	betamethasone benzoate
W 6309	difluprednate
W 6412A	bunolol HCl
W 6439A	suloxifen oxalate
W 6495	oxisuran
W 7000A	levobunolol HCl
W 713	tybamate
W 7320	alclofenac
W7783	ambruticin
W 8495	isoxicam
WA 184	sitogluside
W-A 335	danitracen
WE352	triflubazam
We941	brotizolam
We 973-BS	ciclotizolam
WG-253	rimiterol hydrobromide
WG 537 (as acetate)	flumedroxone
WH 5668	propanidid
WHR-1051B	biclodil HCl
WHR-1142A	lidamidine HCl
WHR-2908A	lofepramine HCl
WHR-5020	etofenamate
WHR-539	fenclorac

Win 11,318	bupivacaine HCl
Win 11450	benorilate
Win 11,464	fludorex
Win 11,530	menoctone
Win 11831	lorajmine HCl
Win 13,146	teclozan
Win 1344	gamfexine
Win 13820	becanthone HCl
Win 14833	stanozolol
Win 17625	azastene
Win 17665	topterone
Win 17,757	danazol
Win 1783	isomethadone
Win 18,320	nalidixic acid
Win 18,320-3	nalidixate sodium
Win 18,413-2	solypertine tartrate
Win 18,501-2	oxypertine
Win 18,935	milipertine
Win 19356	clorindanic acid
Win 20,228	pentazocine
Win 20,740	cyclazocine
Win 21,904	alexidine
Win 23,200	volazocine
Win 24,540	trilostane
Win 24,933	hycanthone
Win 25,347	nimazone
Win 25,978	amfonelic acid
Win 27147-2	cyclindole
Win 27,914	nivazol
Win 29194-6	carbantel lauryl sulfate
Win 31,665	alpertine
Win 32,729	epostane
Win 32,784	bitolterol mesylate
Win 3406	isoetharine
Win 34,276	ketazocine
Win 34284	oxarbazole
Win 34886	nisbuterol mesylate
Win 35150	flucindole
Win 35,213	rosoxacin
Win 35833	ciprofibrate
Win 38020	arildone
Win 38770	azarole
Win 39103	metrizamide
Win 39424	iohexol
Win 40014	quinfamide
Win 40350	durapatite
Win 40680	amrinone
Win 40808-7	sulfinalol HCl

Win 41464-2	octenidine HCl
Win 41,464-6	octenidine saccharin
Win 41528-2	fezolamine fumarate
Win 42156-2	tonazocine mesylate
Win 42,202	fosarilate
Win 42964-4	zenazocine mesylate
Win 44,441-3	quadazocine mesylate
Win 47,203-2	milrinone
Win 48,049	ofornine
Win 48,098-6	pravadoline maleate
Win 49,016	medorinone
Win 49,375	amifloxacin
Win 49,375-3	amifloxacin mesylate
Win 5063	racephenicol
Win 5063-2	thiamphenicol
Win 51,181-2	napamezole HCl
Win 51,711	disoxaril
Win 54,177-4	ipazilide fumarate
Win 5563-3	colterol mesylate
Win 771	hydroxypethidine
Win 8851-2	tyropanoate sodium
Win 90,000	cicletanine
Win 9154	inositol niacinate
Win 9317	propatyl nitrate
Wl 140	calcium polycarbophil
Wl 287	euprocin HCl
Wl 291	zolamine HCl
WP-973	chlorhexidine phosphanilate
WR 142,490	mefloquine
WR-171669	halofantrine HCl
WR 180,409	enpiroline phosphate
WR-228,258	tebuquine
WR-2721	ethiofos
WV 569 (as HCl)	norfenefrine
WX 14812	alofilcon A
WX 14822	hydrofilcon A
WX 2412	fungimycin
Wy-1359	propiomazine
WY-15,705	ciramadol
WY-15,705 HCl	ciramadol HCl
WY-16,225	dezocine
WY-18,251	tilomisole
Wy-2039	etoxeridine
WY-20,788	penamecillin
WY-21,743	oxaprozin
WY-21,894	fentiazac
Wy 21901	indoramin
WY-21,901 HCl	indoramin HCl

WY-22811 HCl	meptazinol HCl
WY-23,409	ciclazindol
WY-24,081 HCl	tiquinamide HCl
WY-24,377	isotiquimide
Wy-2445	carphenazine maleate
WY-25,021	rolgamidine
Wy-2837	potassium aspartate & magnesium aspartate
Wy-2838	potassium aspartate & magnesium aspartate
Wy-3263	iprindole
Wy-3277	nafcillin sodium
Wy-3467	diazepam
Wy-3475	norbolethone
Wy-3478	sodium oxybate
Wy-3498	oxazepam
Wy-3707	norgestrel
Wy-3917	temazepam
Wy-4036	lorazepam
WY-4082	lormetazepam
WY-40,972	lutrelin acetate
WY-42,362 HCl	recainam HCl
WY-42,362 tosylate	recainam tosylate
WY-44,417 sodium	apalcillin sodium
WY-44,635	cefpiramide
WY-45,030	venlafaxine HCl
Wy-4508	cyclacillin
WY-460E	thiazinamium chloride
WY-47384	gevotroline HCl
WY-47,663 acetate	anaritide acetate
WY-48624	enciprazine HCl
WY-48986	risotilide HCl
WY-5104	levonorgestrel
Wy-806	oxethazaine
Wy-8138	bisoxatin acetate
Wy-8678	guanabenz
WY-8678 acetate	guanabenz acetate
X-1497	methicillin sodium
XLG	polyglactin 910
XM-72	polybutester
XU 62-320	fluvastatin sodium
XZ-450	azithromycin
Y 3642	tinoridine
Y 4153 (as HCl)	clocapramine
Y 6124 (as HCl)	bufetolol
YC-93	nicardipine HCl
YM-09330	cefotetan disodium
YTR-830H	tazobactam

Z 326	fentonium bromide
Z 424	viminol
Z-4828	trofosfamide
Z4942	ifosfamide
Z 6000	troxerutin
ZK 10 720	ioprocemic acid
ZK 39 482	iotrolan
ZK 57 671	sulprostone
ZK 62 711	rolipram
ZK 71 630	iotetric acid
ZK 76 604	pirazolac
ZK 79 112	iotasul

APPENDIX C
Abbreviations Used with Medications and Dosages

Abbreviation	Literally	Meaning
a.c.	ante cibum	before meals or food
ad	ad	to, up to
A.D.	auris dextra	right ear
ad lib.	ad libitum	at pleasure
A.L.	auris laeva	left ear
a.m., A.M.	ante meridiem	morning
Aq.	aqua	water
A.S.	auris sinistra	left ear
A.U.	aures unitas	both ears
	auris uterque	each ear
b.i.d.	bis in die	twice daily
b.m.	bowel movement	bowel movement
cc	cubic centimeter	cubic centimeter
d.	die	day
et	et	and
g	gram	gram
gt., gtt.	gutta	a drop
h.	hora	hour
h.s.	hora somni	at bedtime
IM*	intramuscular	intramuscular
IV*	intravenous	intravenous
mcg	microgram	microgram
mg	milligram	milligram
ml	milliliter	milliliter
O.D.	oculus dexter	right eye
O.L.	oculus laevus	left eye
O.S.	oculus sinister	left eye
O.U.	oculus uterque	each eye
p.c.	post cibum	after meals
p.m., P.M.	post meridiem	afternoon or evening
p.o.	per os	by mouth
p.r.n.	pro re nata	as needed

*Some references suggest that IM and IV be typed with periods to distinguish from Roman numerals, but we believe context is sufficient to make this distinction.

Abbreviation	Literally	Meaning
q.a.d.	quaque alternis die	every other day
q.d.	quaque die	every day
q.h.	quaque hora	every hour
q.i.d.	quater in die	four times a day
q.o.d.		every other day
q.s.	quantum satis	sufficient quantity
q.s. ad	quantum satis ad	a sufficient quantity to make
℞, Rx	recipe	take, a recipe
Sig.	signetur	label
s.o.s.	si opus sit	if there is need
stat	statim	at once, immediately
t.i.d.	ter in die	three times a day
tsp.	teaspoonful	teaspoonful